Pharmacology

Edited by
Robert A. Meyers

Related Titles

Meyers, R. A. (ed.)

Encyclopedia of Molecular Cell Biology and Molecular Medicine

16 Volume Set

2005

ISBN: 978-3-527-30542-1

Kayser, O., Müller, R. H. (eds.)

Pharmaceutical Biotechnology

Drug Discovery and Clinical Applications

2004

ISBN: 978-3-527-30554-4

Knäblein, J. (ed.)

Modern Biopharmaceuticals

Design, Development and Optimization

2005

ISBN: 978-3-527-31184-2

Pharmacology

From Drug Development to Gene Therapy

Edited by

Robert A. Meyers

Volume 2

WILEY-
VCH

WILEY-VCH Verlag GmbH & Co. KGaA

The Editor

Dr. Robert A. Meyers
RAMTECH LIMITED
122, Escalle Lane
Larkspur, CA 94939
USA

■ All books published by Wiley-VCH are carefully produced. Nevertheless, authors, editors, and publisher do not warrant the information contained in these books, including this book, to be free of errors. Readers are advised to keep in mind that statements, data, illustrations, procedural details or other items may inadvertently be inaccurate.

Library of Congress Card No.: applied for

British Library Cataloguing-in-Publication Data: A catalogue record for this book is available from the British Library.

Bibliographic information published by the Deutsche Nationalbibliothek
Die Deutsche Nationalbibliothek lists this publication in the Deutsche Nationalbibliografie; detailed bibliographic data are available on the Internet at http://dnb.d-nb.de.

© 2008 WILEY-VCH Verlag GmbH & Co. KGaA, Weinheim

Composition: Laserwords Private Ltd., Chennai, India
Printing: Betz-Druck GmbH, Darmstadt
Bookbinding: Litges & Dopf GmbH, Heppenheim

Printed in the Federal Republic of Germany
Printed on acid-free paper

ISBN 978-3-527-32343-2

Contents

Preface   ix

Color Plates   xvii

Volume 1

Part I   Drug Development   1

1   Medicinal Chemistry   3
   David J. Triggle

2   Biotransformations of Drugs and Chemicals   39
   Paul R. Ortiz de Montellano

3   Disposition and Clearance Prediction of Drug Bioavailability   63
   William Bains

4   Pharmacokinetics and Pharmacodynamics of Biotech Drugs   107
   Bernd Meibohm and Hartmut Derendorf

5   Targeting and Intracellular Delivery of Drugs   137
   Ruth Duncan

6   Pharmacogenomics and Drug Design   179
   Philip Dean, Paul Gane, and Edward Zanders

7   Chemistry, Biology, and Drug Design of Synthetic Peptides   193
   Tomi K. Sawyer

8   Structure-based Drug Design and NMR-based Screening   225
   David J. Craik and Richard J. Clark

9   Receptor Targets in Drug Discovery   315
   Michael Williams, Christopher Mehlin, Rita Raddatz, and David J. Triggle

10   Therapeutic Compounds in Nature as Leads for New Pharmaceuticals   359
   Antony D. Buss, Brian Cox, and Roger D. Waigh

Pharmacology. From Drug Development to Gene Therapy. Edited by Robert A. Meyers.
Copyright © 2008 Wiley-VCH Verlag GmbH & Co. KGaA, Weinheim
ISBN: 978-3-527-32343-2

11 Cancer Stem Cells   419
    Michael F. Clarke and Andrew T. Hass

12 Plant-based Expression of Biopharmaceuticals   441
    Jörg Knäblein

Part II   Innovative Therapeutic Approaches   467

13 Genetic Engineering of Antibody Molecules   469
    Manuel L. Penichet and Sherie L. Morrison

14 Exploiting Model Organisms for Disease Intervention   493
    Caretha L. Creasy, George P. Livi, and Christine Debouck

15 Pharmacology and Emerging Clinical Application of RNA   519
    Sailen Barik and Vira Bitko

16 Biochemistry of HIV Therapeutics   555
    Raveendra Dayam and Nouri Neamati

17 Xenotransplantation in Pharmaceutical Biotechnology   579
    Gregory J. Brunn and Jeffrey L. Platt

18 RNA Interference   599
    John G. Doench and Carl Novina

19 Genomic Approaches in Targeted Therapy   627
    Anna C. Maroney and Sergey E. Ilyin

20 Therapeutic Angiogenesis   639
    Mary E. Gerritsen

21 Oligonucleotides   679
    Olaf Heidenreich and Georg Sczakiel

Volume 2

Part III   Cancer Therapeutics   701

22 Molecular Oncology   703
    Miguel H. Bronchud

23 Theoretical Foundations of Cancer Chemotherapy   755
    Nicholas B. La Thangue

24 Antitumor Steroids   775
    Guy Leclercq

25 Immunotoxins and Recombinant Immunotoxins in Cancer Therapy   795
    Yoram Reiter and Avital Lev

Part IV   Gene Therapy   827

26 Liposome Gene Transfection   829
    Nancy Smyth Templeton
27 Genetic Vaccination   855
    Joerg Reimann, Martin Schleef, and Reinhold Schirmbeck

28 Vectors and Gene Therapy   879
    Edward A. Burton, David J. Fink, and Joseph C. Glorioso

29 Somatic Gene Therapy   933
    M. Schweizer, E. Flory, C. Münk, Uwe Gottschalk, and K. Cichutek

30 Virus-free Gene Transfer Systems in Somatic Gene Therapy   951
    Oliver Kayser and Albrecht F. Kiderlen

31 Gene Therapy and Cardiovascular Diseases   969
    Michael E. Rosenfeld and Alan D. Attie

32 Vector System: Plasmid DNA   1001
    Rajkumar Banerjee and Leaf Huang

33 Vector Targeting in Gene Therapy   1045
    Yosuke Kawakami and David T. Curiel

    Index   1081

Preface

This treatise on pharmacology was compiled from a selection of key articles from the recently published 16 volume *Encyclopedia of Molecular Cell Biology and Molecular Medicine* (ISBN 978-3-527-30542-1, http://www.meyers-emcbmm.de/). This two volume publication is composed of 33 detailed articles arranged in four sections covering Drug Development; Innovative Therapeutic Approaches; Cancer Therapeutics; and Gene Therapy. The articles were prepared by eminent researchers from many of the major molecular biology and pharmacology research institutions spanning the globe.

Leading participating academic institutions include: the University of California, San Francisco; the University of Michigan, Ann Arbor; the University of California, Los Angeles; the University of Southern California; the Mayo Clinic; the Massachusetts Institute of Technology; the Dana-Farber Cancer Institute; Harvard Medical School; the Baylor College of Medicine; the University of Florida, Gainesville; the Welsh School of Pharmacy, Cardiff University; the University of Queensland, Brisbane, Australia; the University of Strathclyde, Glasgow, Scotland; the Paul-Ehrlich-Institut, Langen, Germany; the Robert Koch-Institut, Berlin; Germany; the University of Tübingen, Tübingen, Germany; University of Ulm, Ulm, Germany; the University of Lübeck, Lübeck, Germany; University of Glasgow, Glasgow, UK; Université Libre de Bruxelles, Brussels, Belgium; Pharmaceutical Biology, Rijksuniversiteit Groningen, Groningen, The Netherlands; the Technion-Israel Institute of Technology, Haifa, Israel; the Indian Institute of Chemical Technology, Hyderabad, India; and the Hospital General of Granollers, Barcelona, Spain.

The research groups of major pharmaceutical firms also participated including: Novartis Pharma Research Centre, Horsham, UK; Schering AG, Berlin, Germany; GlaxoSmithKline Pharmaceutical Research & Development, Collegeville, PA; Johnson & Johnson Pharmaceutical Research & Development, Spring House, PA; as well as ARIAD Pharmaceuticals, Cambridge, MA and Exelixis, South San Francisco.

Each article begins with a concise definition of the subject and its importance, followed by the body of the article and extensive references for further reading. The references are divided into secondary references (books and review articles) and primary research papers. Each subject is presented on a first-principle basis, including detailed figures,

Pharmacology. From Drug Development to Gene Therapy. Edited by Robert A. Meyers.
Copyright © 2008 Wiley-VCH Verlag GmbH & Co. KGaA, Weinheim
ISBN: 978-3-527-32343-2

tables and drawings. Because of the self-contained nature of each article, some overlap among articles on related topics occurs. Extensive cross-referencing is provided to help the reader expand his or her range of inquiry.

The master publication, which is the basis of the Pharmacology set, is the *Encyclopedia of Molecular Cell Biology and Molecular Medicine*, which is the successor and second edition of the VCH *Encyclopedia of Molecular Biology and Molecular Medicine*, and covers the molecular and cellular basis of life at a university and professional researcher level. The first edition, published in 1996–1997 was utilized in libraries around the world. This second edition is double the first edition in length and comprises the most detailed treatment of both molecular and cell biology available today. The Board with twelve Nobel laureates and I believe that there is a serious need for this publication, even in view of the vast amount of information available on the World Wide Web and in text books and monographs. We feel that there is no substitute for our tightly organized and integrated approach to selection of articles and authors and implementation of peer review standards for providing an authoritative single-source reference for undergraduate and graduate students, faculty, librarians and researchers in industry and government.

Our purpose is to provide a comprehensive foundation for the expanding number of molecular biologists, cell biologists, pharmacologists, biophysicists, biotechnologists, biochemists and physicians as well as for those entering the field of molecular cell biology and molecular medicine from majors or careers in physics, chemistry, mathematics, computer science and engineering. For example, there is an unprecedented demand for physicists, chemists and computer scientists who will work with biologists to define the genome, proteome and interactome through experimental and computational biology.

The Board and I first divided all of molecular cell biology and molecular medicine into primary topical categories and each of these was further defined into subtopics. The following is a summary of the topics and subtopics:

- Nucleic Acids: amplification, disease genetics overview, DNA structure, evolution, general genetics, nucleic acid processes, oligonucleotides, RNA structure, RNA replication and transcription.
- Structure Determination Technologies Applicable to Biomolecules: chromatography, labeling, large structures, mapping, mass spectrometry, microscopy, magnetic resonance, sequencing, spectroscopy, x-ray diffraction.
- Proteins, Peptides and Amino Acids: analysis, enzymes, folding, mechanisms, modeling, peptides, structural genomics (proteomics), structure, types.
- Biomolecular Interactions: cell properties, charge transfer, immunology, recognition, senses.
- Molecular Cell Biology of Specific Organisms: algae, amoeba, birds, fish, insects, mammals, microbes, nematodes, parasites, plants, viruses, yeasts.
- Molecular Cell Biology of Specific Organs or Systems: excretory, lymphatic, muscular, neurobiology, reproductive, skin.
- Molecular Cell Biology of Specific Diseases: cancer, circulatory, endocrine, environmental stress, immune, infectious diseases, neurological, radiation.
- Biotechnology: applications, diagnostics, gene altered animals, bacteria and fungi, laboratory techniques, legal, materials, process engineering, nanotechnology, production of classes or specific molecules, sensors, vaccine production.

- Biochemistry: carbohydrates, chirality, energetics, enzymes, biochemical genetics, inorganics, lipids, mechanisms, metabolism, neurology, vitamins.
- Pharmacology: chemistry, disease therapy, gene therapy, general molecular medicine, synthesis, toxicology.
- Cellular Biology: developmental cell biology, diseases, dynamics, fertilization, immunology, organelles and structures, senses, structural biology, techniques.

We then selected some 340 article titles and author or author teams to cover the above topics. Each article is designed as a self-contained treatment. Each article begins with a key word section, including definitions, to assist the scientist or student who is unfamiliar with the specific subject area. The encyclopedia includes more than 3000 key words, each defined within the context of the particular scientific field covered by the article. In addition to these definitions, the glossary of basic terms found at the back of each volume, defines the most commonly used terms in molecular and cell biology. These definitions should allow most readers to understand articles in the encyclopedia without referring to a dictionary, textbook or other reference work.

Larkspur, March 2008

Robert A. Meyers
Editor-in-Chief

List of Contributors

Alan D. Attie
Department of Biochemistry, University of Wisconsin-Madison, Madison, WI, USA

William Bains
Choracle Ltd., 37 The Moor, Melbourn, Royston, UK

Rajkumar Banerjee
Indian Institute of Chemical Technology, Hyderabad, India

Sailen Barik
University of South Alabama, Mobile, AL, USA

Vira Bitko
University of South Alabama, Mobile, AL, USA

Miguel H. Bronchud
Hospital General of Granollers, Barcelona, Spain

Gregory J. Brunn
Transplantation Biology Program, Mayo Clinic, Rochester, MN and Department of Pharmacology and Experimental Therapeutics, Mayo Clinic, Rochester, MN, USA

Edward A. Burton
University of Pittsburgh, Pittsburgh, PA, USA

Antony D. Buss
MerLion Pharmaceuticals Pte. Ltd, Science Park II, Singapore

K. Cichutek
Paul-Ehrlich-Institut, Langen, Germany

Michael F. Clarke
Department of Hematology and Oncology, The University of Michigan, Ann Arbor, MI, USA

Richard J. Clark
University of Queensland, Brisbane, Australia

Brian Cox
Novartis Pharma Research Centre, Horsham, UK

David J. Craik
University of Queensland, Brisbane, Australia

Caretha L. Creasy
Division of Genomic & Proteomic Sciences, GlaxoSmithKline Pharmaceutical Research & Development, Collegeville, PA, USA

David T. Curiel
University of Alabama at Birmingham, Birmingham, UK

Pharmacology. From Drug Development to Gene Therapy. Edited by Robert A. Meyers.
Copyright © 2008 Wiley-VCH Verlag GmbH & Co. KGaA, Weinheim
ISBN: 978-3-527-32343-2

Raveendra Dayam
University of Southern California, Los Angeles, CA, USA

Philip Dean
DeNovo Pharmaceuticals Limited, Cambridge, UK

Christine Debouck
Division of Genomic & Proteomic Sciences, GlaxoSmithKline Pharmaceutical Research & Development, Collegeville, PA, USA

Hartmut Derendorf
University of Florida, Gainesville, FL, USA

John G. Doench
Massachusetts Institute of Technology, Cambridge, MA, USA

Ruth Duncan
Welsh School of Pharmacy, Cardiff University, Cardiff, UK

David J. Fink
University of Michigan, Ann Arbor, MI, USA

E. Flory
Paul-Ehrlich-Institut, Langen, Germany

Paul Gane
DeNovo Pharmaceuticals Limited, Cambridge, UK

Mary E. Gerritsen
Exelixis, South San Francisco, CA, USA

Joseph C. Glorioso
University of Michigan, Ann Arbor, MI, USA

Uwe Gottschalk
Paul-Ehrlich-Institut, Langen, Germany

Andrew T. Hass
Cellular and Molecular Biology Program, The University of Michigan, Ann Arbor, MI, USA

Olaf Heidenreich
Department of Molecular Biology, Institute for Cell Biology, University of Tübingen, Tübingen, Germany

Leaf Huang
University of Pittsburgh, Pittsburgh, PA, USA

Sergey E. Ilyin
Johnson & Johnson Pharmaceutical Research & Development, Spring House, PA, USA

Yosuke Kawakami
University of Alabama at Birmingham, Birmingham, UK

Oliver Kayser
Pharmaceutical Biology, Rijksuniversiteit Groningen, Groningen, The Netherlands

Albrecht F. Kiderlen
Robert Koch-Institut, Berlin, Germany

Jörg Knäblein
Schering AG, Berlin, Germany

Nicholas B. La Thangue
Division of Biochemistry and Molecular Biology, Davidson Building, University of Glasgow, Glasgow, UK

Guy Leclercq
Institut J. Bordet, Université Libre de Bruxelles, Brussels, Belgium

Avital Lev
Technion-Israel Institute of Technology, Haifa, Israel

George P. Livi
Division of Genomic & Proteomic Sciences, GlaxoSmithKline Pharmaceutical Research & Development, Collegeville, PA, USA

Anna C. Maroney
Johnson & Johnson Pharmaceutical
Research & Development, Spring House,
PA, USA

Christopher Mehlin
University of Washington, Seattle, WA, USA

Bernd Meibohm
The University of Tennessee Health Science
Center, Memphis, TN, USA

Sherie L. Morrison
Department of Microbiology, Immunology,
and Molecular Genetics, University of
California, Los Angeles, CA, USA

C. Münk
Paul-Ehrlich-Institut, Langen, Germany

Nouri Neamati
University of Southern California, Los
Angeles, CA, USA

Carl Novina
Cancer Immunology and AIDS, Dana-
Farber Cancer Institute, and Department
of Pathology, Harvard Medical School,
Boston, MA, USA

Paul R. Ortiz de Montellano
Department of Pharmaceutical Chemistry,
University of California, San Francisco, CA,
USA

Manuel L. Penichet
Department of Microbiology, Immunology,
and Molecular Genetics, University of
California, Los Angeles, CA, USA

Jeffrey L. Platt
Transplantation Biology Program, Mayo
Clinic, Rochester, MN and Departments of
Surgery, Immunology and Pediatrics, Mayo
Clinic, Rochester, MN, USA

Rita Raddatz
Cephalon Incorporated, West Chester, PA,
USA

Joerg Reimann
University of Ulm, Ulm, Germany

Yoram Reiter
Technion-Israel Institute of Technology,
Haifa, Israel

Michael E. Rosenfeld
Department of Pathobiology, University of
Washington, Seattle, WA, USA

Tomi K. Sawyer
ARIAD Pharmaceuticals, Cambridge, MA,
USA

Reinhold Schirmbeck
University of Ulm, Ulm, Germany

Martin Schleef
Plasmid Factory, Bielefeld, Germany

M. Schweizer
Paul-Ehrlich-Institut, Langen, Germany

Georg Sczakiel
Institute for Molecular Medicine, University
of Lübeck, Lübeck, Germany

Nancy Smyth Templeton
Department of Molecular and Cellular Biol-
ogy, Baylor College of Medicine, Houston,
TX, USA

David J. Triggle
State University of New York, Buffalo, NY,
USA

Roger D. Waigh
University of Strathclyde, Glasgow,
Scotland, UK

Michael Williams
Cephalon Incorporated, West Chester, PA,
USA

Edward Zanders
DeNovo Pharmaceuticals Limited,
Cambridge, UK

Color Plates

Phytomedics (tobacco):

- Root secretion, easy recovery
- Greenhouse contained tanks
- High density tissue
- Salts and water only
- Tobacco is well characterized
- Stable genetic system

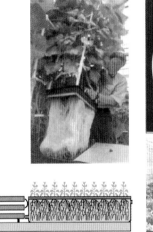
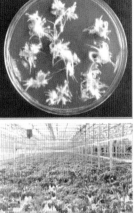

Fig. 6 (p. 455) Secretion of the biopharmaceuticals via tobacco roots. The tobacco plants are genetically modified in such a way that the protein is secreted via the roots into the medium ("rhizosecretion"). In this example, the tobacco plant takes up nutrients and water from the medium and releases GFP (Green Fluorescent Protein). Examination of root cultivation medium by its exposure to near ultraviolet-illumination reveals the bright green-blue fluorescence characteristics of GFP in the hydroponic medium (left flask in panel lower left edge). The picture also shows a schematic drawing of the hydroponic tank, as well as tobacco plants at different growth stages, for example, callus, fully grown, and greenhouse plantation. Source: Knäblein J. (2003) *Biotech: A New Era in the New Millennium – Biopharmaceutic Drugs Manufactured in Novel Expression Systems*, DECHEMA-Jahrestagung der Biotechnologen, Munich, Germany, 21.

Pharmacology. From Drug Development to Gene Therapy. Edited by Robert A. Meyers.
Copyright © 2008 Wiley-VCH Verlag GmbH & Co. KGaA, Weinheim
ISBN: 978-3-527-32343-2

ICON Genetics (tobacco):
- Viral transfection
- Fast development
- High protein yields
- Coexpression of genes

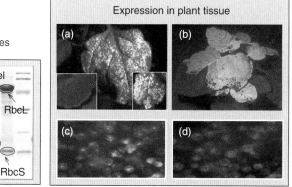

Fig. 7 (p. 456)   Viral transfection of tobacco plants. This new generation platform for fast (1 to 2 weeks), high-yield (up to 5 g kg^{-1} fresh leaf weight) production of biopharmaceuticals is based on proviral gene amplification in a nonfood host. Antibodies, antigens, interferons, hormones, and enzymes could successfully be expressed with this system. The picture shows development of initial symptoms on a tobacco following the Agrobacterium-mediated infection with viral vector components that contain a GFP gene (a); this development eventually leads to a systemic spread of the virus, literally converting the plant into a sack full of protein of interest within two weeks (b). The system allows to coexpress two proteins in the same cell, a feature that allows expression of complex proteins such as full-length monoclonal antibodies. Panels (c) and (d) show the same microscope section with the same cells, expressing Green Fluorescent Protein (c) and Red Fluorescent Protein (d) at the same time. The yield and total protein concentration achievable are illustrated by a Coomassie gel with proteins in the system: GFP (protein of interest), CP (coat protein from wild-type virus), RbcS and RbcL (small and large subunit of ribulose-1,5-bisphosphate carboxylase). Source: Knäblein J. (2003) *Biotech: A New Era in the New Millennium – Biopharmaceutic Drugs Manufactured in Novel Expression Systems*, DECHEMA-Jahrestagung der Biotechnologen, Munich, Germany, 21.

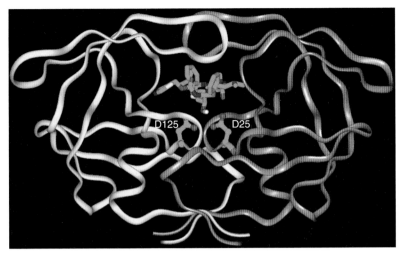

Fig. 5 (p. 564) Crystal structure of HIV-1 protease (PR) complexed with ritonavir (PDB1HXW). The two monomers of the PR are represented as ribbon models (yellow and magenta). The two catalytic aspartate residues (D25 and D125) are rendered as ball and stick models while the ritonavir is represented by a stick model. The hydroxyl group of the ritonavir occupies the space between two aspartate residues.

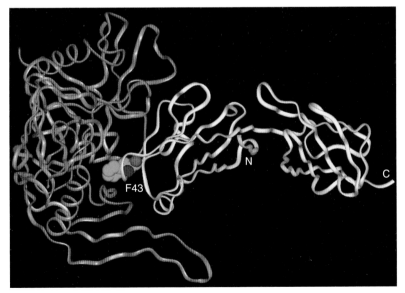

Fig. 8 (p. 569) The ribbon diagram of crystal structure shows binding of gp120 (magenta) to CD4 receptor (yellow). The F43 (shown as CPK model) of CD4 protrudes into a hydrophobic cavity on gp120. In this orientation, the CD4 binding cavity on gp120 is clearly visible.

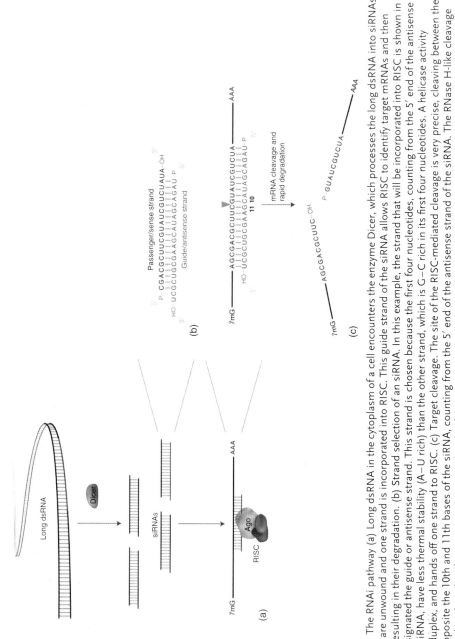

Fig. 1 (p. 603) The RNAi pathway (a) Long dsRNA in the cytoplasm of a cell encounters the enzyme Dicer, which processes the long dsRNA into siRNAs. These siRNAs are unwound and one strand is incorporated into RISC. This guide strand of the siRNA allows RISC to identify target mRNAs and then cleave them, resulting in their degradation. (b) Strand selection of an siRNA. In this example, the strand that will be incorporated into RISC is shown in red, and is designated the guide or antisense strand. This strand is chosen because the first four nucleotides, counting from the 5′ end of the antisense strand of the siRNA, have less thermal stability (A–U rich) than the other strand, which is G–C rich in its first four nucleotides. A helicase activity unwinds this duplex, and hands off one strand to RISC. (c) Target cleavage. The site of the RISC-mediated cleavage is very precise, cleaving between the nucleotides opposite the 10th and 11th bases of the siRNA, counting from the 5′ end of the antisense strand of the siRNA. The RNase H-like cleavage leaves a free hydroxyl on the 5′ region (i.e. the capped end) of the mRNA, and a phosphate on the 3′ half (i.e. the polyadenylated end).

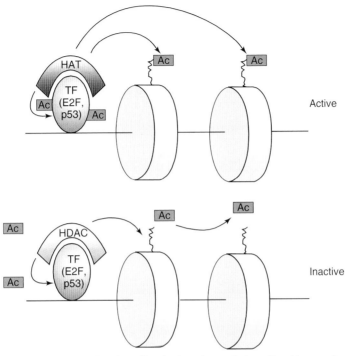

Fig. 4 (p. 764) Acetylation control in the cell cycle. Acetylation (Ac) mediated by acetyltransferases (HATS) can target histone tails in the form of nucleosomes (yellow) or transcription factors (TF) involved in cell cycle control, like E2F and p53. In most cases so far studied, acetylation appears to activate transcription. In contrast, deacetylation mediated by histone deacetylases (HDAC) causes transcriptional inactivity by targeting histones in nucleosomes, leading to a more transcriptionally inert state, together with dampening the activity of transcription factors.

Part III
Cancer Therapeutics

Pharmacology. From Drug Development to Gene Therapy. Edited by Robert A. Meyers.
Copyright © 2008 Wiley-VCH Verlag GmbH & Co. KGaA, Weinheim
ISBN: 978-3-527-32343-2

22
Molecular Oncology

Miguel H. Bronchud
Hospital General of Granollers, Barcelona, Spain

1	The Molecular and Clonal Evolution of a Cancer	707
2	Cancer as a Disease Process of Key Regulatory Pathways	713
3	Main Types of Molecular Markers of Cancer Cells: Genetic and Epigenetic Changes	721
4	The Era of 'Targeted Therapies'	726
4.1	Threats and Opportunities	726
4.1.1	Threats	726
4.1.2	Opportunities	732
	Bibliography	750
	Books and Reviews	750
	Primary Literature	751

Keywords

Angiogenesis
This is the biological process that leads to the formation of new blood vessels, and involves the proliferation of endothelial cells and their morphological association into functional capillaries.

Apoptosis
This is the Biological process that describes the complex mechanisms of "programed cell death," eventually leading to endonuclease driven fragmentation of DNA and

Pharmacology. From Drug Development to Gene Therapy. Edited by Robert A. Meyers.
Copyright © 2008 Wiley-VCH Verlag GmbH & Co. KGaA, Weinheim
ISBN: 978-3-527-32343-2

chromatin by a number of Caspase-dependent or Caspase-independent biochemical events.

Binary State (of Regulatory Molecules)
Most, if not all, biochemical regulatory proteins can be present at any one time in an "on" or an "off" molecular form, with regard to one or more of their functions.

Carcinogenesis
This is now recognized to be a progressive, usually rather slow, multistep process involving sequential mutations, failure of adequate DNA repair, activation of oncogenes, loss of tumor suppressor function, epigenetic changes, and a gradual (or less frequently, rapid) transition from benign to malignant phenotypes.

Cellular Adhesion
Downregulation of 'adherens junctions' (AJ) assembly by mutations, hypermethylation, or transcriptional repression of the adhesion molecule E-Cadherin, has been described in several malignancies, and particularly in human diffuse gastric carcinomas, lobular breast cancers and familial gastric cancers. In many ways, E-cadherin behaves as a tumor suppressor gene, while beta-catenin behaves as a potentially potent oncogene.

Cell Cycle Checkpoints
Mammalian cells can remain quiescent (in Go phase of their cell cycle) for long periods of time, but the right combination of growth factors can induce them to enter G1 and then, if no impediment occurs, progress through S-phase (DNA replication), G2, and mitosis, and complete their cell division.

Chemoprevention
The treatment of carcinogenesis, its prevention, inhibition or reversal.

Drug Resistance
Surprisingly, conventional chemotherapy and radiotherapy work not because cancer cells are especially more "sensitive" to their cytotoxic effects than normal cells, but because normal cells can usually recover faster and more efficiently than cancer cells. Normal tissues virtually never develop resistance to chemotherapy, but human cancers are frequently chemo- or radio-resistant when they are diagnosed, or can become resistant following cytotoxic treatments, because of multiple pharmacological, cell kinetic or molecular mechanisms.

Growth Factors
They were defined in the 1970s, long before their molecular characterization and purification, as *substances other than nutrients required by cells in vitro for their survival, proliferation, and differentiation.*

Intraepithelial Neoplasia
Intraepithelial neoplasia (IEN) is a moderate to severe dysplasia that occurs on the carcinogenic pathway from normal tissue to malignant cancer.

Oncogenes

These are growth control genes present in the human genome (as "proto-oncogenes"), as well as in the genomes of most, if not all, multicellular organisms. Incorrect expression or mutation of an oncogene usually results in "Gain of Function" and unregulated cell growth, as seen in malignant cells.

Mutations

The molecular changes in DNA associated with carcinogenesis are not very different from those associated with genetic variation and molecular evolution of organisms and species. These changes include local changes in DNA sequences, rearrangement of DNA segments within the genome, and (in the case of viral carcinogenesis) horizontal transfer of a DNA (or RNA) segment originating in another kind of organism.

Proteasomes

The average human cell contains about 30 000 proteasomes, each of which contains several protein-digesting proteases. Among other functions, they control the intracellular half-life of important regulatory proteins.

Stromal cells and Cancer

Stromal cells are all cells in a tumor that are not the cancer cells.

Tumor Antigens

These are molecules that contain the epitope determinants recognized by T cells that specifically target tumor cells.

Tumor Suppressor Genes

Unlike oncogenes, tumor suppressor genes (formerly "antioncogenes") display the function of suppressing cellular proliferation, and/or maintaining cellular differentiation, facilitating normal cellular adhesion mechanisms, stopping entry into the cell cycle (G1, S-phase, mitosis or G2) to allow DNA-repair mechanisms, maintaining normal cellular shape and cell contact inhibition mechanisms, and promoting normal differentiation and senescence.

Molecular Oncology can be defined as *that branch of medical science that looks at the cancer problem from a molecular point of view*. For several reasons, "molecular oncology" represents "the heart of the matter" of cancer.

As it would be quite an ambitious, and virtually impossible, task to pretend to cover the whole subject of "Molecular Oncology" in a single unipersonal review, what follows is a short personal view of what the author regards as the basic molecular understanding of cancer in the year 2004, and the more likely therapeutic implications of this new molecular knowledge.

We should not forget the huge prevalence of malignant diseases in the developed world. Cancers are probably responsible for one-third of deaths in men in industrialized countries and for almost one-fourth in women. At the beginning of the twenty-first century, these diseases still cause a lot of human suffering, despite very significant progress in their early detection, improvements in radical treatments (local or systemic), and better medical control of iatrogenic side effects of chemotherapies.

In the same way as the invention and later refinement of the microscope eventually led to the discovery and classification of pathological microorganisms, the discovery of DNA, RNA, proteins, proteoglycans and other regulatory molecules (including lipids, arachidonic acid derivatives, steroids, and sex hormones) is rapidly leading to a better and deeper understanding of cancer, and remains the best promise to lead to better and more effective methods for cancer prevention, early detection, prognostic classifications, and cure.

This is because it is currently believed that cancer can be truly understood in terms of those molecular changes, genetic and epigenetic, that gradually lead a given cell clone, within a given tissue field, to develop a certain "competitive advantage" over neighboring cell clones, enabling the transformed cell clone to gradually displace its neighbors and grow into a neoplastic tissue. Finally, this "new tissue" can go on to transform itself into a malignant neoplasia, leading to invasion of local organs, or distant spread (generally through the bloodstream, the lymphatic system, or both). The growth of cancer cells at distant sites is called *metastasis*.

"Cancer" is a state, whereas "carcinogenesis" is a process. Key to the multistep genetic nature of cancer is that carcinogenesis is "progressive." In most epithelial tissues, progression means the sequential accumulation of somatic mutations, or even epigenetic changes (like abnormal DNA methylation patterns). In some cases of familial predisposition to cancer, some of these mutations are inherited.

Gradually, a given target tissue experiences a transition from normal histology, to proliferative and/or dysplastic changes, to so-called *intraepithelial neoplasia (IEN)*, which can be early or severe, to superficial cancers *(in situ)*, and finally to invasive disease. In some instances, this process of malignant transformation may be aggressive and relatively rapid (e.g. in the presence of a DNA repair-deficient genotype, or an aggressive oncogenic virus, or a lethal combination of "oncogenic hits"), but in general these changes occur over a long period of time, like 3 to 30 years.

The problem is that in the past two and a half decades there has been an "explosion" of information, rather than true knowledge, about the molecular aspects of cancer. More than 300 different genes and their respective protein products have been described as being directly or indirectly linked to cancer. The number of such 'cancer-related genes' is constantly increasing and the final figure could well be more than 1000. Although it seems reasonable to believe that some, or many, of these 'cancer-related' genes may represent the *consequence* rather than the *cause* of the cellular development of the cancer cell phenotype, the 'trees' are so many that there is a real risk of missing the "wood."

Indeed, some believe that, in the not too distant future, relevant information will pass from the Molecular Pathology Laboratory to the busy Cancer Clinical Units only with the help of clever computer programs. Before clinicians can make up their minds about the curability or incurability of any given cancer, and in order to decide which sequence and combination of drugs to use to treat a particular patient, they will have to consult a computer program and the Molecular Pathology Laboratory. Although there is still no treatment for any of the major lethal cancers that is as effective as, say, antibiotics are against infections, there is vast accumulated knowledge of the fine regulatory mechanisms that are deranged in cancer cells, and this undoubtedly promises new therapeutic insights. For example, selective oral tyrosine-kinase inhibitors (Gleevec), for chronic myeloid leukemia, and specific monoclonal antibodies (Herceptin) for breast cancer or some lymphomas (Mabthera), have been introduced into routine clinical use.

In contrast to the situation twenty years ago, not only do we now know of many molecular targets to design new drugs for the chemoprevention or treatment of cancer but, paradoxically, we have an apparent excess of targets for our current resources of drug development worldwide. The Human Genome Project has completed its first basic human genome map well ahead of schedule, and it is likely to give us further insights and more potential targets. It is now estimated that the human genome contains some 35 000 genes, which is less than had originally been estimated by most researchers. Many of these genes are well characterized and their functions in various pathways are known. But the real function of the majority of these human genes remains inconclusive. In other words, the rate-limiting step in true progress against cancer is the amount of resources we can spend, and the optimization and coordination of this huge research process, rather than a shortage or lack of therapeutic targets.

Selecting the right targets for cancer therapy can make a big difference. If, for example, we were clever or lucky enough to correctly guess the right targets for the main human cancers, and if large multinational pharmaceutical companies agreed to focus their efforts and enormous resources on these right targets, then revolutionary new cancer treatments might become available for clinical testing within 5 to 10 years. But, if we got it wrong, or not enough importance was given to this war against cancer by politicians or business people, then it might take another 20 or 30 years, or even more.

1
The Molecular and Clonal Evolution of a Cancer

In view of the fact that the incidence of most of the common epithelial cancers is age related, the British epidemiologists Armitage and Doll had already calculated, in 1958, that for some of the common solid tumors the logarithm of cancer incidence should be linearly related to the logarithm of a person's age. If such an interpretation holds good, then we could deduce, from the slope of the death rate from cancer of the large intestine in relation to age (plotted logarithmically), that about 6 mutations are needed to produce a cancer of the large intestine.

This guess is extraordinary if one thinks that more or less the same conclusion was reached, based on molecular genetic knowledge, by the American scientists Fearon and Vogelstein in their classic work on colorectal tumorigenesis. The 'multistep mutations' theory of cancer was also supported by epidemiological evidence, and by the 'initiation and promotion' models of carcinogenesis. A characteristic feature of most forms of carcinogenesis is the long period that elapses between initial application of the carcinogen and the time the first cancers appear. It is necessary to apply coal tar repeatedly to the skin of a mouse for several months before any tumors are detectable. Similarly, most common human cancers can take 3 to 30 years or more to develop.

The chemical carcinogenesis experimental models also helped to identify at least two classes of carcinogenic compounds: the initiators and the promoters. For example, if a group of mice are fed a small amount of the carcinogen dimethylbenzanthracene (DMBA), this produces widespread irreversible alterations (presumably mutations) in the cells of each mouse. Subsequent irritation of the skin by painting it twice a week with croton oil (the "promoter") eventually results in the local appearance of tumors. These tumors will appear even if croton oil is not started until 16 weeks after the DMBA feeding, but no tumors arise if either DMBA or croton oil is given alone or if the order of the treatments is reversed. In several aspects, estrogens (in the case of breast cancer) and testosterone (in the case of prostate cancer) have also been regarded as potential tumor promoters.

Other insights into the "genetic" nature of tumorigenesis came from studies on viral carcinogenesis, and from seminal observations in the uncommon retinal cancers in children.

The discovery of tumor oncogenes and tumor suppressor genes almost twenty years ago opened the way to the study of the molecular epidemiology of cancer. It soon became apparent that in general more than one somatic mutational event is needed for malignant transformation, the possible exception being the uncommon hereditary retinoblastomas, already described by the "two-hits model" proposed by Knudson.

Later, it was found that certain carcinogens are linked to selective (though not entirely "specific") mutational events. For example, researchers have described molecular linkages between exposure to carcinogens and cancer types, in p53 mutational spectra of hepatocellular carcinoma, skin cancers, and lung cancer. In 1990, Fearon and Vogelstein proposed a molecular model for colorectal carcinogenesis, based on the sequential accumulation of genetic events in key regulatory genes along the sequence from adenoma to carcinoma.

More recently, in 1997, Kinzler and Vogelstein proposed the concept of two different types of carcinogenic genetic events: those involving "gatekeeper" genes, characterized by their control of net cellular proliferation, and those involving "caretaker" genes, associated with maintenance of genomic integrity. Examples of gatekeeper genes include APC and beta-catenin in colon epithelium, Rb in retinal epithelial cells, NF1 in Schwann cells, and VHL in kidney cells. Thus, it is proposed that an alteration in APC leads to a derangement of the cellular proliferation pathway that is important for maintaining a constant cell population, at least in colonic cells. The identification of other gatekeeper genes is anticipated, and some may be genes crucial to morphogenetic events of specific tissues. Unlike gatekeeper genes, caretaker genes generally maintain genomic stability and are not involved directly in the initiation of the neoplastic process, but their mutations enhance the probability of mutations in other genes, including those in the gate-keeper class. Because multiple mutations are found in cancer cells, the existence of a "mutator phenotype" was suggested by Loeb in 1991 as being an important step in tumor development. Candidate mutator genes are involved in multiple cellular functions needed for maintaining genetic stability, such as DNA repair, DNA replication, chromosomal segregation, cell cycle control, and apoptosis.

Some individuals may be predisposed to cancer because of inherited mutations of some key genes. This has attracted considerable attention in recent times, particularly in relationship to genes having susceptibility for breast cancer and colon cancer.

The genetic alterations in oncogenes generally lead to an increased function of the protein, whereas, in general, tumor suppressor genes are inactivated during carcinogenesis with apparent loss-of-function of the protein. However, the mechanisms of activation or inactivation are multiple, and their precise effects on gain- or loss-of-function are incompletely understood. *K-ras* and *H-ras* genes are examples of oncogenes that are preferentially altered by point mutation (codons 12, 13 and 61), generating a protein with constant GTPase activity. The *c-myc* gene can be activated by chromosomal translocation (in some leukemias) or by gene amplification (in some solid tumors). The *p53* and *Rb* tumor suppressor genes are often knocked out by point mutation in one allele and by deletion (loss of heterozygosity) at the other. Others, like *p16*, have high rates of homozygous deletions or promoter hypermethylation. Some genetic defects are fairly characteristic for a given tissue type (most colorectal cancers have APC or beta-catenin mutations). But the "same players" are frequently involved in different tumors. Each human cancer can be regarded as a different molecular entity, with a different matrix of molecular targets, and it evolves with time (even as a result of systemic or local therapies).

However, it would be a mistake to believe that all common epithelial human cancers follow these clear-cut histological sequential patterns from adenoma to carcinoma. In fact, only a minority of the commonest type of breast cancers (infiltrating ductal carcinomas, or IDC) arise from ductal carcinoma *in situ*. Thus, the molecular changes leading to IDC, accounting for almost 70% of all breast cancers, can happen before the histological features associated with DCIS become evident. DCIS is characterized by a proliferation of malignant epithelial cells confined to the mammary ducts without light microscopic evidence of invasion through the basement membrane into the surrounding stroma; but IDC, by definition, show signs of invasion of stromal tissue, often with vascular and/or lymphatic vessel involvement. In other words, conventional histological and radiological techniques (e.g. bilateral mammograms) cannot detect with adequate precision the ongoing carcinogenic events in many cases of women at risk.

Patients with head and neck squamous cell carcinoma (HNSCC) often develop multiple (pre)malignant lesions, ranging from leucoplakia to other cancers. This led Slaughter et al, way back in 1953, to postulate the concept of "field cancerization." The incidence rate of second primary tumors following a first diagnosis of HNSCC is 10 to 35%, depending both on the location of the first primary tumor and the age of the patient. The carcinogens associated with HNSCC (alcohol and tobacco smoking) are thought to induce mucosal changes in the entire upper aerodigestive tract (UADT), causing multiple genetic abnormalities in the whole tissue region. Similar arguments apply also to other tobacco-related cancers, like transitional cell carcinomas of the urogenital tract or bronchogenic carcinomas. An alternative theory for these observations is based on the premise that any transforming event is rare and that the multiple lesions arise because of the widespread migration of transformed cells through the whole UADT. However, most field changes appear to be induced by smoking, supporting the theory of carcinogen-induced field cancerization rather than field cancerization due to migrated transformed cells.

Other possible causes of "field carcinogenic events" can involve hormonal factors (e.g. changes in the ovaries, breasts or prostate), inflammation and hyperemia (increased proliferative and angiogenic activity in chronic cystitis, gastritis, esophagitis or colitis), chronic viral infections (e.g. Hepatitis B virus for hepatocarcinomas, Epstein-Barr virus for nasopharyngeal carcinomas or some lymphomas), aberrant methylation linked to aging, free-radical induced DNA damage (e.g. for cancers of the gastrointestinal tract), skin exposed to ultraviolet irradiation (e.g. actinic keratosis and squamous cell carcinomas), ionizing radiation-induced damage, or aberrant morphogenetic pathways. It is also possible that different carcinogenic pathways operate in different tissue fields belonging to the same organ. For example, adenocarcinomas of the right side of the colon are often associated with clinical and molecular characteristics different from those of adenocarcinomas of the colorectal region.

Even in breast cancer, the reported incidence of multicentric or multifocal lesions in areas away from the primary tumor in mastectomy specimens ranges from 9 to 75%, depending on the definition of multicentricity, the extent of tissue sampling and differences in the histological techniques of examination. Therefore, multifocality or multicentricity of breast cancers may in fact be a lot more common than is currently acknowledged.

In this context, the old "Field Cancerization" theory by Slaughter, and the more recent "Multi-step Carcinogenesis" model by Fearon and Vogelstein can now come together in a single model: Sequential Field Cancerization.

If it does require some seven sequential carcinogenic "genetic hits" in a single cellular clone for a malignant tumor to develop, it is mathematically more likely to occur in a tissue with a high background of genetic alterations in neighboring cellular clones, than in a tissue with a low background of such alterations, or with no detectable carcinogenic mutations at all (Figs. 1 and 2).

The probability of a single clone accumulating 7 independent but sequential genetic alterations leading to a malignant phenotype, without any similar events occurring in neighboring cells, would seem to be rather low. This simple conclusion, and our ability to measure "background carcinogenesis" in different parts of the body, might lead to several unexpected implications. Technology is just beginning to be sufficiently sensitive to start testing the hypothesis. One potential technical problem is that in premalignant tissue, the "signal" (e.g. relevant oncogenetic lesions) might be muted by the "noise" (normal genome of most of the cells in the tissue), until the premalignant clones have expanded enough to become more numerous locally than normal cells. However, it is only a matter of time before this goal is technically achievable.

A possible future objective is the development of a combined histological

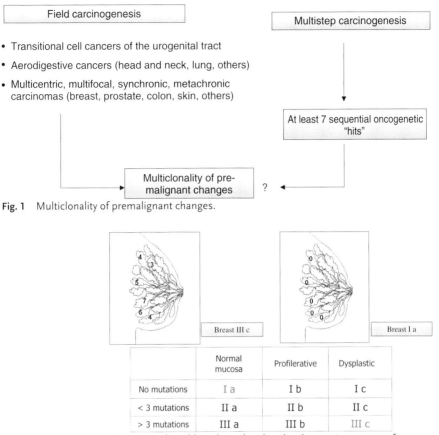

Fig. 1 Multiclonality of premalignant changes.

Fig. 2 Combined histological and molecular staging system of premalignant changes. Numbers inside the drawings refer to numbers of relevant gene mutations/deletions/amplifications identified in various regions of the breasts. Carcinogenic pathways may differ depending on the specific combination of genetic (and epigenetic) changes. (Reproduced from Bronchud, M. H. (2002) Is cancer really a "local" cellular clonal disease?, *Medical Hypothesis* **59**, 560–565. With Permission of Elsevier Science.)

and molecular staging system (Fig. 2). For example, after a follow-up of 5 to 10 years, one would expect more new cancers to develop in group IIIc of Fig. 2 (dysplastic changes and three or more significant mutations identified), than in group Ia (normal histology and no mutations identified).

There is a growing number of experimental findings in support of this complex concept. Among the first was the observation by Azadeh Stark and colleagues from various American institutions, that women with benign breast biopsies, demonstrating both HER-2/neu amplification and a proliferative histopathological diagnosis (either typical or atypical hyperplasia), may be at a substantially increased risk for subsequent breast cancer (up to more than sevenfold) compared to normal.

The clinical application of this concept and technology should help to classify patients into various relative risk groups early in the development of a malignant disease, allowing a tailor-made program for follow-up and screening, as well as more appropriate chemopreventive and therapeutic interventions. For example, a suitable combination of relevant biomarkers might help clinicians to identify smokers at high risk of developing lung cancers (approximately 10 to 15% of frequent smokers). Being confronted with a personal risk of cancer, rather than a general statistical risk, is a potent motivation to quit smoking and to undergo more frequent health checks (like high-resolution CT scans to detect isolated pulmonary nodules).

Some smokers may be protected because of genetic polymorphisms of enzymes involved in the molecular activation of pre-carcinogens present in tobacco, whereas others may be more vulnerable to the carcinogenic effects because of genetic defects in DNA-repair enzymes. Some molecular changes associated with aging and carcinogenesis might be epigenetic (e.g. promoter hypermethylation) rather than genetic. Even some pediatric malignancies might be secondary to abnormal morphogenetic events *in utero*.

It has been estimated that in the USA alone some 30% of people above the age of 60 can be found, by colonoscopy, to have adenomas of the colon, 70% or more of men above the age of 80 will have IEN of the prostate, 30% of people aged 60 or more have actinic keratosis on their skins, 20% of sexually active women above the age of 40 may have some degree of cervical IEN, at least 40% of heavy smokers can show metaplastic or dysplastic changes in their bronchial mucosa, and some 20% of women with dense mammograms and aged more than 50 may show atypical cells on ductal washings from the nipple or ultrasound-guided fine-needle aspirates.

The use of a battery of genetic or protein biomarkers relevant to each of the main cancer types may soon help us to better define individual cancer risks, and to measure background carcinogenesis in individual tissue samples. Perhaps, not too long from now, oncology units will be devoted to the treatment of carcinogenesis just as much as to the treatment of cancer.

One crucial difference between normal cells and transformed cells *in vivo*, which is difficult to prove experimentally but can be deduced, is that during cancer development, the effects of mutations are likely to be persistent, whereas most regulatory intercellular signals (particularly of "paracrine" nature) in normal cells are likely to be terminated by changes in cell position, production of signals, or modulatory effects on membrane receptor state. In normal tissues, the quantitative levels of signaling have been shown to be very important; signaling episodes, moreover, can have very different frequencies, and a specific cell can be influenced by a long-term signal while responding to a different signal of shorter duration. This does require that normal cells can sometimes remember a decision indefinitely, and can terminate their response to a specific signal, so that exposure to a new signal, or even the same signal, can subsequently produce a different molecular response.

The fact that cancer cells have lost, at least in part, this "position-dependent" obedience to signals, to the extent that they can even grow into distant metastases, makes them life threatening to their host organisms. Some sort of position dependence, however, is likely to remain even for most cancer cells, because their site of seeding and metastatic growth is not random, but depends on a number of cell adhesions and microenvironmental predisposing factors.

2
Cancer as a Disease Process of Key Regulatory Pathways

The basic mechanisms controlling classical metabolic regulatory pathways have been known for many years. For example, the "citric acid cycle" (postulated by Krebs in 1937), the central role of ATP in energy-transfer cycles (postulated mainly by Lipmann in 1939–41), and Mitchell's intriguing hypothesis (1961) to explain the mechanism of oxidative and photosynthetic phosphorylation, to name but a few, have been part of biochemistry textbooks for decades. Some twenty years ago, the structure of DNA had already been known for over twenty years before that, and yet eminent scientists were pessimistic about real therapeutic progress in oncology.

In contrast, regulatory pathways involved in the complex regulation of cell growth, differentiation, senescence, and cell death are only recently being gradually understood. Although we are still largely unable to draw schematically precise cell-type-specific regulatory pathways, research efforts are intensifying, and our knowledge is rapidly expanding.

Growth and differentiation must be tightly controlled in any organism. Curious though it may seem, recent research suggests that fractal networks for transporting the materials essential for life, for example, nutrients, water, and oxygen, may be prime movers in determining shape and form (morphology) in Nature. A series of key papers by Geoffrey B. West, a theoretical physicist at Los Alamos National Laboratory, James H. Brown, a biology professor at the University of New Mexico,

and Brian J. Enquist, a postdoctoral biologist at the nonprofit Santa Fe Institute, have reduced to just three general principles the allometric scaling laws, that are major determinants of most anatomical and physiological variables of organisms as they increase in body size.

In the year 2001, which was the hundredth anniversary of the institution of the Nobel Prizes, three of the leading investigators in the field of Cell Cycle Control were awarded the Nobel Prize for Physiology and Medicine. The American scientist Leland H. Hartwell of the Fred Hutchinson Cancer Research Center, and the British scientists R. Timothy Hunt and Sir Paul M. Nurse, both at the Imperial Cancer Research Fund in London, received this prestigious award for 'the confluence of two different approaches to learning about the molecular machinery regulating the cell cycle'.

While Hartwell was screening for temperature-sensitive mutants in the yeast *Saccharomyces cerevisiae* in the 1960s and 1970s, he identified a large series of genes that, in mutant form, arrested mitosis. This led him, and former postdoctoral researcher Ted Weinert, to hypothesize that 'checkpoints' regulate the sequence of events in mitosis (3). Even as Hartwell was uncovering these genes, Paul Nurse was identifying, in a different yeast (*Schizosaccharomyces pombe*), a protein kinase (CDC2) that is a key component of the maturation factors that drive cell division. Nurse then took a human cDNA library and eventually cloned a human CDC2, having observed the striking structural homology of these key regulatory molecules, that indicated a high degree of evolutionary conservation in different species.

Working at the Marine Biological Laboratory in Woods Hole, Mass., in the early-1980s, Hunt solved a crucial piece of the cell cycle puzzle. In sea urchin oocytes, and later in frogs, Hunt identified proteins whose levels rose and fell throughout the cell cycle. He called them *cyclins*, and they were later found to be necessary in activating the ever-present kinases, like CDC2. Together a cyclin and a cyclin-dependent kinase (CDK) push the cells along the cell cycle regulatory checkpoints.

Previous work by others had already opened the path to these important findings. For instance, back in the early-1970s two scientists, Yoshio Masui and L. Dennis Smith, transferred the cytoplasm from activated frog oocytes to naïve oocytes arrested in meiosis, and identified a substance they called *MPF* (*maturation promotion factor*). Almost twenty years later, that substance proved to be none other than the CDK/Cyclin heterodimer.

In the year 2002 the Nobel Prize was awarded for seminal discoveries in another key area of biological relevance: the genetic regulation of organ development and programed cell death, or apoptosis. The winners of the Prize were the British scientists Sydney Brenner and John Sulston, and the American scientist Robert Horvitz. They discovered that specific genes control the cellular death program in the nematode worm *Caenorhabditis elegans*. This worm, approximately 1-mm long, has a short generation time and is transparent, which makes it possible to follow cell division directly under the microscope. The fertilized egg cell undergoes a series of cell divisions leading to cell differentiation and cell specialization, eventually producing the adult worm. In this organism, all cell divisions and differentiations are invariant that is, identical from individual to individual. This made it possible to gradually construct a precise cell lineage for all cell divisions. During the development of the organism, 1090 cells are generated, but precisely 131 of these cells are eliminated by programed cell death. This results in an adult nematode (the hermaphrodite), composed of 959 somatic cells. Again, most of the multiple genes controlling programed cell death have human equivalents (Apoptosis Pathways).

Thanks to the Human Genome Project, we now know that there are between 30 000 and 35 000 genes in the Human Genome, and 18 000 in the nematode worm. Both the Cell Cycle Control genes and the Programed Cell Death genes are crucial for carcinogenesis, and obvious targets for cancer therapy. In fact, optimal curative cancer therapies should include combinations of drugs that not only cause cell cycle arrest in tumor cells, but also lead to their apoptosis.

Recognizing that much of the cell's work is done not by individual proteins but by large macromolecular complexes, researchers are increasingly trying to map protein–protein interactions throughout the cell. The new term *Interactome* has been proposed to define this new type of "cartography" describing the main functional interactions of single proteins and protein macrocomplexes. For example, the map of the *C. elegans* interaction network, or interactome, links 2898 proteins (nodes) *via* 5460 interactions (edges).

It seems likely that, with time, different family patterns of "malignant interactomes" will be gradually identified, each with its unique "key pathogenetic changes" caused by the specific abnormal regulatory pathways implicated in its carcinogenesis process.

Over the past few years, researchers engaged in the nascent field of "interactomics" have been busy deconstructing these molecular machines, mapping protein–protein interactions in bacteria, yeast, fruit flies, nematodes, mice, and humans.

The resulting charts have exposed the functions of previously mysterious proteins, have helped drug companies *hone* their development efforts, and are laying the foundations for systems biology. Some proteins appear to be rather "promiscuous" in their interactions. Drugs targeting these so-called *sticky proteins* have the potential to produce troubling side effects. Pharmaceutical companies, therefore, would be better served by focusing on those molecules that appear more selective, and by limiting themselves only to the particular process they are targeting.

It must be said, however, that doubts about the validity of interactome information remain. Although "data rich," these studies produce lower-quality results than would a scientist who devotes years to a single protein. High throughput means that you do things fast, but the information can be "data-rich and analysis-poor." Again, as is true for most of Molecular Oncology today, "the trees may not allow us to see the woods."

Y2H data especially are open to question, because the technique essentially amounts to a genetic trick. It relies on artificial fusion constructs: often, mere fragments of the full-length protein are introduced into cells, forced into the nucleus, and overexpressed. False-positive results are inevitable.

The vast majority, 93%, of yeast proteins makes five or fewer connections, yet only one in five such proteins is essential.

Deletion of highly connected proteins (those joining 15 or more proteins) is three times more likely to be lethal.

Recently, Marc Vidal's team at the Dana-Farber Cancer Institute in Boston expanded this study by examining coexpression of genes linked by hubs. Their conclusion: all hubs are not created equal. Some, called *party hubs,* contain proteins that interact simultaneously, whereas *date hubs* contain proteins that interact at different times and locations.

The Dana–Farber group infers a modular architecture for the proteome, in which date and party hubs operate at different organizational levels. Party hubs function to assemble individual molecular complexes, or modules. These modules, in turn, are linked at a higher level, using date hubs. Thus, the date hub calmodulin links modules for cation homeostasis; budding, cell polarity, and filament formation; protein folding and stabilization; and the endoplasmic reticulum.

There can be little doubt that if this new branch of biological research (Interactomes), develops to the point of not only mapping the functional protein–protein interactions in any given key regulatory pathways like the TGF-beta pathway but also predicting, on the basis of genomic and/ or proteomic data for any given cancer tissue, the dynamic functional consequences of the intrinsic molecular changes observed in tumor specimens, and the manner of their response to external manipulation by drugs or ionizing radiation, then we can end up with truly useful tools for both drug development and clinical follow-up.

With so much disparate data available, the challenge for researchers is to integrate that information into a single "interaction network," and then to take decisions relating to research and development of new anticancer drugs. These could, for example, be based on new visualization tools such as "Cytoscape," jointly developed by the Institute for Systems Biology at the University of California at San Diego, and the Memorial Sloan-Kettering Cancer Center in New York. Cytoscape, a technology still undergoing development, incorporates interaction data with other large-scale genomic information to build networks of cellular processes and pathways. Through the Systems Biology Markup Language (SBML), it can also communicate with other SBML-enabled programs to test mathematical simulations of cellular events.

Unraveling the twisted skeins of the relative contributions of altered regulatory pathways to the cancer phenotype of each individual cancer can be certainly annoying. Simplicity is elegant, but it can also be deceiving. In spite of the unquestionable success of many reductionistic approaches in science, we should never underestimate complexity, as often going against nonsense sensible arguments is just so much blowing against the wind.

However, at this stage of knowledge, it does seem likely, and it remains highly desirable, that most of these key regulatory cascades will converge into a number of key regulatory events: the DNA replication at multiple different sites in the genome, the coordinated expression or suppression of a battery of genes, the culmination of the developmental history and cell fate of any given clone, the progressive modification of the biological "clock-like mechanisms" that drive differentiation and aging, and the three-dimensional structure–function relationships of chromatin.

A very simplistic, and classic Cartesian, way to look at what happens in cancer cells is to describe the main functional implications of genetic events (point mutations, deletions, translocations, etc.) in binary terms (GF: gain-of-function; LF: loss-of-function *versus* N: normal function) in a table such as the one that I have called '*Matrix of Targets*'.

Each cancer may have, because of its own genetic and epigenetic backup and clonal history, a different Matrix of Targets. This adds to the complexity of potential curative therapies, but can eventually translate into therapeutic combinatorial models of several drugs or biological agents capable of stopping the growth and proliferation of cancer cells, reducing their invasive or metastatic properties, or even restoring their differentiation or apoptotic pathways.

Another way to look at things is to take the view that certain key genetic changes are the true and main pathogenetic mechanisms for any single cancer, because these key genetic changes (e.g. the abl-bcr fusion gene, associated with the Philadelphia chromosome in Chronic Myeloid Leukemia) lead to a much wider pattern of changes in gene expression, up or down, thereby consolidating the malignant phenotype: increased and unrestrained cellular proliferation, loss of contact inhibition, lack of normal differentiation or presence of abnormal differentiation, genomic instability, ectopic expression of genes, angiogenic activity, acquisition of the invasive phenotype, the ability of cells to spread and seed at distant sites, and so on.

These key "pathogenic genetic events" would drive the clonal evolution of cancer cells in a way similar to the "evolution genes" postulated by Werner Arber, elegantly described in the chapter on "Genetic Variation and Molecular Evolution" in this encyclopedia."

There is therefore a need, in Molecular Oncology, to follow very closely the rapidly accumulating knowledge on the molecular mechanisms that regulate gene expression.

Identifying genome-wide regulatory motifs is problematic because of their typically low consensus sequences. Grasping which transcription factors bind to such motifs is even more difficult, as numerous factors can bind to any one motif.

In two recent publications, Pugh and colleagues found that only 20% of yeast genes contained their TATA boxes, but they were all highly regulated in response to stresses such as heat and osmotic shock. Such genes generally use a multicomponent protein complex called *SAGA*, which is one of several complexes thought to bring the TBP to promoters. In contrast, genes without a recognizable TATA box appeared to use mainly another complex, TFIID, and were less involved in responding to stress. This could be an example of bipolar type of regulation.

Predicting gene expression from DNA sequence, and understanding the relative role of individual transcription factors in the development of normal tissues and in the oncodevelopment of cancers, are the clear goals of these technologies. However, these goals are still not within immediate reach.

Although probably no two cancers are 100% identical, in the same way as no two cancer patients are ever identical, the rational understanding of how altered regulatory pathways can lead to the development and consolidation of cancer cell clones, may provide us with some basic patterns of regulatory circuits associated with malignancy. To some extent these "biochemical maps" or "carcinogenic patterns" may be tissue dependent.

Most of these key regulatory processes, if not all, will have:

1. Upstream regulatory elements; for example, membrane-bound or membrane-associated.
2. Intermediate elements; cytosolic or bound to organelles, like mitochondria.
3. Downstream elements, transcription factors, DNA- or RNA-specific sequences.
4. Bottlenecks, Cross talk points and "Achilles heels" (Oncogene Addiction Hypothesis) of cancers.

New cancer therapies will not be directed merely towards hitting the DNA synthesizing machinery but also towards selective targets at or downstream from abnormally activated catalytic functions (thereby abrogating the abnormal stimulatory signals), or at or upstream from inactivated or missing catalytic functions (switching on parallel or alternative regulatory pathways).

In simplistic terms, the new therapeutic drugs should, for example, lock or inhibit activated proto-oncogenes in their inactive state, or somehow lock tumor suppressor proteins in their active state, which is the one normally responsible for inhibiting entry into S-phase or mitosis, or maintaining the normal differentiation and apoptotic pathways (Fig. 3). In other words, as regulatory proteins are usually present in normal cells in either an active form or an inactive form, and the chemical equilibrium between the two forms depends on the regulatory microenvironment of the cell, new targeted therapies should be able to correct, or at least limit, the malignant phenotype by restoring the normal balance between stimulatory and inhibitory signals within the cell.

This concept of regulatory pathways involved in cell behavior is the basis of a new biochemistry. Crucial alterations in this new biochemistry, perhaps as few as five distinct key molecular changes, may be enough to transform a normal human cell into a tumor cell. It appears that because of their higher complexity, human cells are more difficult to transform than rodent cells. Perhaps surprisingly, more simple organisms, such as *Drosophila*

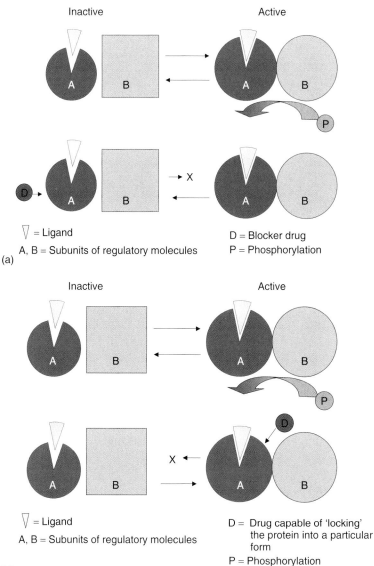

Fig. 3 Hypothetical new target-oriented therapies. (a) Oncogenes as targets. The new anticancer agents should lock the oncogenic protein in its *inactive form*, either by binding to the active site, or by binding to an allosteric regulatory site; (b) Tumor suppressors as targets. The new anticancer agents should do the opposite of what is described above. They should lock the tumor suppressor protein into its *active form*, that is, the one capable of inhibiting the cancer phenotype, by either binding to the relevant active site or to allosteric regulatory sites. (From M. H. Bronchud. (2004) *Principles of Molecular Oncology*, reprinted by permission of Humana Press.)

melanogaster flies, very rarely develop malignant cells, in spite of their ability to develop mutations in experimental systems. There has been no clear explanation for this apparent paradox.

Phosphate atoms are again involved in this "new biochemistry," because protein phosphorylation is the common end-result of many signal pathways. It was back in 1937 (the same year Krebs postulated the citric acid cycle) that C. Cori and G. Cori began their outstanding studies on glycogen phosphorylation (the main store of sugars in the liver of mammals). However, it was not until 1988 that Tonks obtained the first partial sequence of a tyrosine phosphatase. Today, it has been suggested that the human genome might contain as many as 2000 kinase genes and up to 1000 phosphatase genes.

A "normal" cell, under "normal" circumstances, probably decides nothing by itself (there is no cellular "free-will"), but merely obeys orders. Normal cells can signal each other in many different ways: through pores in the membranes (gap junctions or plasmodesmata), or because of specific membrane receptors that recognize soluble or bound ligands (endocrine, paracrine or autocrine mechanisms), or in some special cases (e.g. neurones) by synaptic transmission. However, a cancer cell (because of mutations, amplifications, translocations or deletions) makes mistakes (misinterpreting the normal orders or even making them up for the wrong reasons). And it cannot help doing so because its software has gone badly and progressively wrong. Cancer cells do not have exactly the same underlying chemistry as the normal cells of the body.

This makes them "strong," but also, paradoxically, makes them vulnerable to more specific and selective combinations of drugs.

Most of these, second, third, fourth, and so on, intracellular messengers are binary: they are either switched on or off (by phosphorylation-dephosphorylation, for example). At any one time a number of + and − signals travel from the cell membrane to the nucleus (and, perhaps, also backwards). These signals are irreversibly altered in cancer cells. The normal balance between the "on" and "off" signals is altered in cancer cells.

To reestablish the normal circuits, or to kill the cell by misleading it into apoptosis, we must learn to be clever, understand these key pathways, and develop drugs to block them or to activate alternative complementary pathways. Thus, cancer is a disease of regulatory pathways. There may not be "magic bullets" to kill all cancer cells. The signal transduction pathways involved in the proliferative response to various growth factors and mitogens are extremely complex and interactive. They do not act as simple linear cascades. The so-called *'cross talk'* is an invariable feature. The new biochemistry is essentially the network of sensing and signaling in cell homeostasis.

Several key questions remain:

1. How much selectivity can we expect to achieve with new drugs that will manipulate these complex signaling pathways?
2. Will these new drugs be cytostatic, or cytotoxic, or both?
3. How will these new drugs be obtained: serendipity; rational drug design; high-throughput screening; combinatorial chemistry; antisense technologies; gene vectors; antigrowth factors; monoclonal antibodies?
4. Will they imply chronic therapies or acute therapies?
5. Will they have new, and at times unexpected, toxicities?

6. Will some malignant clones still develop resistance to signal transduction therapy?

Some of these questions can already be answered by the available examples of targeted therapies in cancer. For example, it seems that most of the new drug entities acting on cell surface growth factor receptors, or cytosolic downstream regulatory elements, for example inhibitors of the EGFR (Epidermal Growth Factor Receptor) or associated tyrosine-kinase activities, are mainly "cytostatic" *in vivo* rather than "cytotoxic"; they are fairly nontoxic (though, at times, with new unpredicted toxicities, like acneiform skin rashes), and are best administered on a continuous long-term protocol.

A very competitive area at present is in fact represented by the pharmacology of epidermal growth factor receptor (EGFR) targeting. EGFR signaling pathways play a key role in the regulation of cell proliferation, survival, and differentiation. Monoclonal antibodies, mAbs, among which C225 (Cetuximab), and "specific" tyrosine- kinase inhibitors, TKIs, like ZD1839 (Iressa) have been developed, clearly differ in their mode of action at target level. The primary action mechanism of C225 (a chimeric mAb) is a competitive antagonism of EGFR. Independent of the phosphorylation status of the receptor, the EGFR-C225 complex is subsequently internalized. On the other hand, TKIs act on the cytosolic ATP binding domain of EGFR by inhibiting EGFR autophosphorylation. Depending on the nature of the TKI, EGFR inhibition can either be reversible, as with drugs like ZD1839 and OSI-774, or irreversible, as with PD 183 805.

There are still rather few published studies dedicated to examining in detail the various possible mechanisms of resistance to EGFR targeting, irrespective of the anti-EGFR drug considered. There is also some confusion as to the precise cytosolic and nuclear downstream effects following EGFR targeting, particularly when combined with conventional cytotoxic drugs. Moreover, although some consensual findings tend to suggest a link between the level of the EGFR protein target (as detected by IHC) and the intrinsic efficacy of the targeting drug, more pharmacodynamic studies *in vivo* are needed to establish convincing conclusions regarding EGFR levels and targeting efficacy on which clinical strategies can be based with confidence.

Some new, but not unexpected toxicities have already been described for many of these new targeted therapies. For example, the anti-VEGF monoclonal antibody Bevacizumab (Avastin), indicated in combination with intravenous (iv) 5-FU based chemotherapy as first line or second line treatment for patients with metastatic carcinoma of the colon or rectum, can result in the development of gastrointestinal perforation (2% of cases) and wound dehiscence, in some cases resulting in fatality. The appropriate interval between termination of Avastin and subsequent elective surgery required to avoid the risks of impaired wound healing/wound dehiscence has not yet been precisely determined. Moreover, this exciting new therapeutic molecule can also cause unexpected hemoptysis, and in early studies with squamous lung cancers, the incidence of serious or fatal hemoptysis reached up to 31%.

These considerations can lead to some methodological problems in the design of clinical trials. The primary endpoints in phase III randomized clinical studies should remain those reflecting survival of patients, but secondary end points should include measurable quality of life, disease-related symptoms, performance status, and time to disease progression.

On the other hand, primary endpoints in phase I and II studies should include, besides toxicity and classical pharmacokinetics, data on relative efficacy and sophisticated *in vivo* pharmacodynamics, ranging from changes in genomics (gene expression profiling) and proteomics (protein expression, intracellular localization, and posttranslational modifications) of key targets and downstream effector molecules in tumors in response to the new drug. Additional surrogate endpoints to be considered in phase II studies include relevant *in vivo* dynamic changes on positive emission scanning (PET), new dynamic molecular imaging like dynamic enhanced magnetic resonance imaging (DCE-MRI), and other methods to quantify changes in the growth kinetics of tumors, and for the subset identification of cancers that respond (*versus* those that do not respond) to the new therapies.

3
Main Types of Molecular Markers of Cancer Cells: Genetic and Epigenetic Changes

There are different types of tumor markers:

1. *Genetic markers*: In both hereditary and nonhereditary tumors. These genetic changes can be detected by conventional DNA sequencing techniques, Real-Time Kinetic PCR-based techniques (RT-PCR), gene expression microarrays and DNA microarray-based sequence analysis, comparative genomic hybridization (CGH), fluorescence *in situ* hybridization (FISH), and a variety of new rapidly evolving molecular methods.

2. *Pharmacogenetic markers*: Pharmacogenetic markers are hereditary genetic polymorphisms that may influence the *in vivo* anticancer drug metabolism (activation of pro-drugs, or de-activation), or, perhaps from a more relevant clinical point of view, the likelihood of drug-related serious toxicities because of inherited metabolic polymorphisms. Thus, as an example, genetic variants in the UDP-glucuronosyltransferase 1A1 gene products can predict the risk of subsequent treatment-related severe neutropenia by irinotecan, a fairly active cytotoxic drug in colorectal cancers.

3. *Cellular and tissue markers*: Detected by conventional histopathology or immunohistochemistry, IHC, or by more sophisticated proteomics or genomics technologies; for example, Kodadek has described "protein-function arrays" and "protein-detecting-arrays", and Kononen et al. have described "tissue microarrays" that can allow the molecular study of several hundred tumor specimens in a single paraffin block.

4. *Circulating cancer markers*: The ones traditionally used in the clinic include a variety of glycoproteins, oncofetal antigens, hormones or pro-hormones, tissue-related secreted products, and so on. Some of these are (with the main cancer types associated to increased serum levels): CEA (colon cancer, lung cancer, breast cancer, etc.), CA125 (ovarian cancer), PSA (prostate cancers), Beta-2-Microglobulin (lymphoproliferative diseases), LDH (a nonspecific marker of tumor bulk and aggressive disease in Non-Hodgkin's Lymphomas and other cancers), CA19.9 (pancreatic cancers and other cancers), CA 15.3 (breast cancer and others), HCG-*beta* (nonseminomatous

germ cell cancers), AFP (hepatocarcinomas and nonseminomatous germ cell cancers), Immunoglobulin levels (multiple myelomas), and Thyroglobulin (Thyroid carcinomas). More recent markers detectable in serum or other body fluids (including urine, feces, sputum or bronchial washings) include DNA fragments of oncogenes, soluble growth factor receptors (like HER-2), cytokines (IL-6 for metastatic renal cell carcinoma), and other substances.

Some of these markers are already used routinely in clinical practice (e.g. several circulating cancer markers are useful for the diagnosis, prognosis, and follow-up of some cancer types), while others are being investigated as a source of important prognostic information or even as predictors of response to chemotherapy or radiotherapy (e.g. several cellular and tissue markers). Still others are being explored, in the context of genetic counseling, as potentially useful to screen for hereditary cancer predisposition, for example, BRCA-1 and BRCA-2 for breast and ovarian cancers; RERs and several MMR genes (hMSH2, hMLH1, hMSH6, hPMS1, hPMS2, etc.) for families with hereditary predisposition to colon cancer (HNPCC); and the APC gene in families with FAP (familial adenomatous polyposis).

One of the most peculiar types of molecular markers in human cancer cells is the increased expression of normal or abnormal "Telomerases," and significant progress is being made in understanding how it works. In contrast, despite being implicated in many important regulatory pathways including DNA repair, protein ubiquination and cell cycle control, the exact mechanisms by which inactivation of the tumor suppressor gene BRCA1 or 2 might lead to malignant transformation, particularly in families with high risk of breast and ovarian cancers, remains speculative.

5. *Epigenetic markers*: I shall describe very briefly some of the described "epigenetic" markers. Unless genetic therapies develop to the point where it will truly be possible to perform *in vivo* some form of curative "genetic surgery," for example, either replacing a missing tumor suppressor gene with a normal wild-type counterpart, or removing an activated oncogene, in every single cancer "stem cell", or cancer "progenitor cell," and without unbearable side effects or deleterious long-term consequences, it is perhaps wiser and more relevant to consider as primary targets for therapy the epigenetic and protein elements associated with carcinogenesis, rather than just the "genetic" elements.

We should not forget that, ever since Paul Ehrlich described them in 1913, the classic biochemical targets for drug action are:

1. Inhibition of the active site of an enzyme (or competition with the natural ligand of a hormone or growth factor receptor);
2. Allosteric inhibition and false feedback inhibitors of enzymes or growth factor receptors;
3. Other inhibitors acting outside the active center (exoinhibitors);
4. Double blockade (e.g. where pairs of compounds are used together to block a single biochemical pathway).

The recent progress in the physical mapping of the Human Genome is already pointing toward a "Post-Genome Era." Automated or semiautomated devices capable of reading thousands of genes are already available. Genomics and proteomics are here to stay, but their routine use in the clinic obviously requires proof of efficacy and judicious use. Apart from technical problems inherent in these techniques, which time will solve, there are some general obstacles to realizing their promise:

1. the lack of genetic markers to cover 100% of all tumors;
2. the lack of knowledge about the functional implications of most genetic defects (the precise maps of these regulatory pathways are still under investigation, and may be to some extent tissue specific);
3. the widespread location and heterogeneity of many of the gene mutations (particularly in large genes);
4. the lack of knowledge about the prevalence of these genetic defects in an apparently healthy population (people with no detectable cancer or histologically malignant lesions; for example, presence of molecular lesions in endometriosis or in apparently normal oral or bronchial mucosa);
5. the lack of knowledge about the significance (in terms of risk of developing cancer) of each of these genetic lesions individually or in different combinations. For example, which combinations of genetic lesions are more relevant to neoplastic transformation in a given tissue?

Epigenetic markers of cancer are probably secondary and later events in most of carcinogenesis, but their importance had also been suspected for several decades. The relevance of these epigenetic changes, and particularly of changes involving the three-dimensional conformational structure of chromatin, making it more or less accessible to polymerases and Transcription Factors, have enabled these markers to gain popularity, and they can have significant therapeutic potential.

Methylation of DNA serves as an epigenetic method of modulating gene expression, and it has been demonstrated that hypermethylation silences a number of tumor suppressor genes including most of the CKIs. Epigenetic mechanisms of carcinogenesis are increasingly coming into focus. Recent findings indicate that aberrant methylation can also be detected in the smoking-damaged bronchial epithelium of cancer-free heavy smokers, suggesting it as an ideal candidate biomarker for lung cancer risk assessment, and potentially useful for the monitoring of chemoprevention trials. Of 12 lung cancer cell lines lacking a deletion or critical mutation in Rb or CDKN2A, which codes for the CKI p16(INK4A) protein, all were found to be methylated at exon 1 of the CDKN2A gene.

Other studies have also shown that underexpression of this gene CDKN2A is frequently seen in early preinvasive lesions of squamous cell carcinoma of the lung and cervix.

Some recent work in Korea, at the Samsung Biomedical Research Institute, suggests that tumor-specific methylation of the p16 gene, and other lung cancer-related genes, like Ras association domain family 1A (RASSF1A), H-cadherin, and retinoic acid receptor beta (RAR-beta) genes may be suitable biomarkers, detectable by methylation-specific polymerase chain reaction (MSP), for the early detection of nonsmall cell lung cancers in bronchial lavage fluids of smokers.

While at least three functional DNA methyltransferases have been identified, the most abundant is DNMT1, which is mainly responsible for methylation during DNA replication. DNMT1 localizes at replication foci, at least in part by interacting with the proliferating cell nuclear antigen known as PCNA, which is a subunit of DNA polimerase *delta* (that can also bind to the CKI p21 protein). The enzyme DNMT1 catalyzes the covalent addition of a methyl group from a donor S-adenosyl-methionine to the 5 position of cytosine, predominantly within the CpG dinucleotides in highly repeated transposable elements.

These elements are termed *parasitic* because of their resemblance to viral DNA and their ability to move between different chromosomal sites. During embryogenesis there is an initial generalized demethylation of DNA, followed by a specific adult pattern of methylation. While roughly half of the 5' promoter proximal elements contain CpG islands, they are not usually methylated in normal tissues. But cancers display a particular pattern of methylation. Overall they are hypomethylated, but they do have specific regions of hypermethylation, often associated with regions rich in tumor suppressor genes.

Several molecular variations of deoxycytidine have been developed to inhibit DNMT1, each modified at position 5 of the pyrimidine ring, and these have been reviewed recently. Four agents have been employed clinically: 5-azacytidine (azacitidine), 5-aza-2'-deoxycytidine (decitabine), 1-*beta*-D-arabinofuranosyl-5-azacytosine (fazarabine) and dihydro-5-azacytidine (DHAC). These agents are not new. Some are almost 40 years old, but other analogs such as ara-C and gemcitabine (already in clinical use as anticancer agents) do not inhibit methylation of DNA.

Because methylation of CpG islands in promoter-proximal regions is uncommon in normal cells, normal gene expression should be largely unaffected by these agents. But, at least in some leukemic cells, decitabine has also been found to increase the expression of the multiple drug resistance MDR1 gene product, and this could be clinically counterproductive.

Some studies with these inhibitors go back to the 1980s, for example the EORTC studies with decitabine, and others have been completed more recently. In general, response rates to these agents in solid tumors have been rather low, but more promising results have been obtained in hematological malignances. Toxicities have been similar to conventional cytotoxics: granulocytopenia, thrombocytopenia, alopecia, nausea, vomiting, and diarrhea. The reason why these drugs have not yet translated into better clinical outcomes, in spite of a sound biological basis for their activity in human malignancies, is not clear.

Acetylation and deacetylation of histones can also provide new insights into how to modify the gene expression patterns of normal and cancer cells.

Methylation of DNA has been shown to induce recruitment of histone deacetylase, which inhibits transcription, and agents have been devised that inhibit this deacetylase. The combination of a DNMT inhibitor and a histone deacetylase inhibitor might be a logical way to activate tumor suppressor gene expression (e.g. CKIs), and a number of preclinical studies are in progress.

Chromatin is no longer considered to be a passive scaffolding for nuclear DNA. At the heart of chromatin's structure is the nucleosome, a complex of DNA wound around an octamer containing two molecules each of histone proteins H2A, H2B, H3, and H4. Histones contain two distinct domains. These are: the protein's amino-terminal tails, which protrude from the nucleosome core, rich in charged amino acids such as lysine and arginine residues; and the globular histone core domain that is mainly responsible for the histone:histone interactions involved in nucleosome formation.

A number of posttranslational modifications occur in the histone tail domain, including acetylation, phosphorylation, ribosylation, methylation, ubiquitinylation, and glycosylation. Of these, the most widely studied is the acetylation of histone tail domains on specific lysine residues.

The steady-state levels of histone acetylation in the cell are maintained by a delicate balance between the action of histone acetyltransferases (HATs), and histone deacetylases (HDACs).

A number of methodological breakthroughs have allowed a better understanding of this process. Tightly compacted nucleosomes forbid general transcription factors, such as TFIID and RNA polymerase II holoenzyme, from interacting with promoter sequences of specific genes. It is becoming clear that many transcriptional activators actually direct two different types of chromatin remodeling enzymes to specific promoters: an ATP-dependent remodeling enzyme and a histone acetyltransferase.

The field of chromatin research was revamped in 1996 when C.David Allis and colleagues published evidence that the yeast Gcn5p protein, already known to positively regulate gene transcription, was actually a HAT. This acetylation may induce a conformational change that weakens nucleosomal DNA:histone interactions, making the DNA more accessible to transcription factors. Many other transcriptional coactivators have also been recently found to contain HAT activity. Other studies have identified several HDACs (including the mammalian HDAC 1 to 8), as well as large multiprotein complexes, including the so-called *RbAp*-46 and *48*

(retinoblastoma and histone binding proteins), that can undo histone acetylation and modify gene expression.

Recently, Strahl and Allis have proposed the existence of a "histone code," whereby nonhistone proteins read the patterned display of various modifications on one or more histone tails, resulting in the regulation of downstream transcriptional events.

Considering all this new knowledge, it should come as no surprise that HATs and HDACs have also become potential targets for cancer therapy. They appear to act as both oncogenes and tumor suppressors, depending upon the genetic and epigenetic contexts. One interesting example is the variety of chromosome translocations, (often an undesired consequence of previous cytotoxic chemotherapy), that can affect the mixed lineage leukemia (MLL) locus. Thus, a MLL-CBP fusion protein maintains the HAC activity of CBP, and it can be highly oncogenic as a result of the specific targeting of the fusion protein to certain genes.

The field of HATs and HDACs modulating drugs is promising, but highly complex. To achieve selectivity, HATs must be highly targeted to specific genes, and this targeting depends on several structural protein motifs such as "bromo domains" and "PHD" fingers.

Allosteric inhibitors might be more selective and clinically useful than active site inhibitors. But traditionally, chemists have learnt how to develop suitable pharmacological compounds to interfere with active sites and substrate binding, rather than to interfere with the allosteric properties of a regulatory protein, or protein complex. Even modern automated or semi-automated "high-throughput" screens are usually designed for compounds affecting enzyme activity, rather than for those altering protein–protein interactions.

This is a major challenge for the whole field of new anticancer drugs development. Learning how to modify the allosteric properties of oncogenic proteins should become an important aspect of anticancer drug research.

4
The Era of 'Targeted Therapies'

4.1
Threats and Opportunities

Although the term "target-oriented therapies" has only recently been popularized in oncological literature, it must be acknowledged that hormone receptors (e.g. estrogen receptors in breast cancer, and testosterone receptors in prostate cancer) have been used as therapeutic targets by clinical oncologists for a rather long time.

In fact, even the antimetabolite 5-fluorouracil (5-FU), that is a common constituent of many conventional chemotherapy protocols (in 2002, for example, over 2 million patients with cancer were treated worldwide with this drug), was chemically synthesized back in 1957 by Heidleberger, but can also be regarded as a biochemically targeted molecule. This is because 5-FU's activity is based on the observation that uracil is preferentially used by cancer cells, and that fluorinated analogs of this base might "selectively" inhibit the functioning of DNA and RNA in cancer cells, by forming stable ternary complexes with the enzyme thymidylate synthase (TS), resulting in thymidine starvation and inhibition of DNA synthesis.

4.1.1 Threats
From the therapeutic research point of view, the real impact of Molecular Oncology is that it has provided us with many more potential targets for drug discovery than we can handle with our present ability to understand the real priorities, and our capacity to develop valid anticancer drugs in a relatively short period of time. As we move toward this new exciting era of cancer therapies ("Targeted Therapies") we face several key problems:

1. Current cytotoxics have a very limited curative potential, except in rare cancers.

2. Most current cytotoxics are relatively "old drugs" and their patents are running out. New anticancer drugs are needed in the short term.

3. There seem to be more "potential molecular targets" for therapy than true industrial capacity to develop new effective drugs in the short term. In general, once the relevant oncoprotein is identified and purified, gene cloning allows the production of sufficient quantities to allow the determination of its main molecular mechanisms (catalytic or regulatory) and its three-dimensional structure. Appropriate molecules (e.g. those developed by empirical methods like high-throughput screening or by rational drug design) can then be tested *in vitro* and in preclinical models to determine their activity and toxicity, pharmacokinetics and pharmacodynamics. More and more oncological units will be devoted to clinical testing of new drugs, and cancer research is likely to undergo a rapid growth, provided enough resources are made available. It could, perhaps, prove globally more rewarding to concentrate on normal regulatory proteins (e.g. upstream on the cell membrane, cytosolic or associated to organelles, like mitochondria or proteasomes, or at downstream "bottlenecks", or points of "cross talk") than

on mutated oncoproteins. The problem in this case, however, is that inhibition of normal downstream regulatory oncoproteins might prove more toxic than selective inhibition of mutated oncoproteins, or inhibition of upstream membrane-bound regulatory elements. Clinical oncologists, on the other hand, are well trained to cope with important toxicities, and highly effective methods to reduce nausea and vomiting, or drug-induced myelosuppression and serious infections have been developed over the past 15 years.

4. The average cost of bringing a new anticancer drug to market is still around 500 to 800 million US dollars, and the time from discovery to the market remains around 10 to 15 years. Both need to be considerably reduced.

5. New "target oriented" therapies will probably be more effective, and less toxic, but also more narrow in their indications, thereby limiting their potential markets.

6. New targeted therapies will require more sophisticated diagnostic tools than conventional cytotoxic chemotherapies, in order to correctly identify the right subset of patients most likely to benefit from such therapies. Conventional histopathology or immunohistochemistry (IHC) will not be enough to achieve this. This will add to overall costs.

High levels of c-erbB-2 expression or c-erbB2 amplification must be used (by IHCS or FISH) to identify patients for whom Herceptin may be of benefit, but even in this group of patients only some 50% will show objective responses to the combination of Herceptin plus chemotherapy (30% if chemotherapy alone is used). The reasons for this are unclear. Theoretically, Herceptin,

by interfering with signal transduction emanating from HER-2 (again, locking the oncogenic molecule into an inactive or less active form) should reduce the potential proliferative competitive advantage of cancer cells in comparison with normal cells.

However, the additive or synergistic effects of cytotoxic drugs could be caused by as-yet-unknown effects of these drugs downstream on the signaling pathway. As a matter of fact, other inhibitors of EGFR (for example, inhibitors of the EGFR associated tyrosine-kinase activity), such as gefitinib, have not so far shown any significant survival benefit when used in the treatment of nonsmall cell lung cancer patients, in combination with platinum-based cytotoxics.

Moreover, the relationship between tumor marker levels and sensitivity to new therapies may not be linear, or may depend on yet unknown circumstantial factors.

For example, HER-2 inhibitors (in the case of Trastuzumab) can induce objective response rates in breast cancer patients, but often without clear evidence of a dose–response relationship in their response or survival, or in adverse events. The main predictor of response may be the degree of expression of the target molecule, as well as the intrinsic relevance of this target molecule to the cancer phenotype. Thus, response rates for single agent Trastuzumab in 111 assessable patients with metastatic breast cancer was 35% for patients whose tumors showed a 3+ staining of HER-2 by IHC, as compared to 0% for the case of tumors with only a 2+ staining. This suggests an interesting nonlinear relationship between marker expression and clinical response. The message, as linguists have known for a long time, is that: 'the same word in a different context can give the final sentence a very different meaning'.

Thus, drug companies are well advised to present their phase II and III clinical studies with adequate and comprehensive biochemical (genomic or proteomic, or both) pharmacodynamic data to fully persuade health authorities and clinicians about the benefits of the new therapeutic agents, and the indications for their use.

7. The applications of pharmacodynamics are becoming increasingly important. We should be able to measure, in any given tumor, the direct and indirect genomic and proteomic effects of whatever changes a new drug is producing, or is meant to produce. We should also be able to put this usually complex type of information into some kind of model, so that it can be extrapolated to other tumors with different molecular compositions. Not an easy task, but one of the most exciting challenges ahead. Sound understanding of clinical and biological knowledge, as well as intuitive parallel thinking, good communication skills and an open collaboration within multidisciplinary teams can be really helpful. Paul Workman (2004) has suggested an "Audit Trail" for each new "target oriented" anticancer drug in development:

– *Is the target expressed and is the pathway active?* It is important to understand the relationship among target expression, pathway activity, and response to a therapeutic agent.

– *Are sufficient concentrations achieved in plasma, blood, and tissues?* Obviously, if for pharmacokinetic reasons adequate concentrations of the drug are not achieved in animal studies, or in patients in phase I studies, it is pointless to proceed forward with that particular drug structure.

– *Is there activity on the desired molecular target?* For example it is common, when studying the activity of a particular kinase inhibitor, to assess the phosphorylation of a downstream substrate. Lack of activity on the target can be a reason for lack of therapeutic benefit, though it must be said that some of the new target-oriented therapies can lead to clinical benefit by apparently acting on targets (e.g. with similar "active sites") not previously foreseen or identified.

– *Is there modulation on the desired molecular target?* It may be useful also to look at "off-target effects," since the *in situ* regulatory feedback circuits can lead to unexpected biochemical changes.

– *How can we achieve the desired biological effect?* For example, which regulatory pathway (cell cycle control, apoptosis, necrosis, etc.) is to be predominantly interfered with?

– *Is a clinical benefit seen (in objective tumor response, growth inhibition, time to disease progression, survival)?*

– *Finally, but very importantly, is the molecular target really key in the pathogenesis of that particular cancer?* If so, as seems to be the case, for example, for the abl-bcr fused genes in CML, or the EWS gene translocations and rearrangements observed in many human sarcomas, then hitting the target *per se* would have beneficial therapeutic consequences. Otherwise, only one target will not be enough, and multitargeting will be required for good clinical efficacy.

8. Some form of dynamic and efficient ("parallel or sequential") coordination of projects between Diagnostics and Pharmacology, and *vice versa*, is also highly desirable. Clinicians are already faced with increasing numbers of difficult therapeutic choices, and it would be naive to believe that this increasingly complex decision-making process will be based exclusively on simple classical clinical or pathological characteristics such as the age of the patient, performance status, TNM stage (which describes the degree of local or distant growth and spread of the tumor), and conventional histopathological degrees of differentiation (SBR in breast cancer, or Gleason score in prostate cancers).

Let us look, for example, at the present clinically complex situation in two very common cancers:

1. *Colon cancer*: The introduction into clinical practice of 5 new drugs – the cytotoxics Irinotecan and Oxaliplatin, the oral cytostatic Capecitabine, and the monoclonal antibodies Cetuximab (an antagonist of EGFR), and Bevacizumab (best described as an inhibitor of angiogenesis that "traps" VEGF) – , in addition to the old classic antimetabolite "5-Fluorouracil," has dramatically increased the number of possible permutations and combinations of all active drugs in metastatic colon cancer to the extraordinary figure of 720 possible choices.

2. *Breast cancer*: A special case of targeted therapies is that of endocrine therapies for cancer, which actually constitute the first historical example of targeted therapies. For example, inhibition of estrogen (in breast cancers), or testosterone (in prostate cancers) action or production can probably be regarded as the first examples of anticancer-targeted therapies. Beatson first observed tumor regression of breast cancer in some patients following oophorectomy in 1896, but it was not until some 60 years later that estradiol receptors were identified by following the localization of radioactive estradiol in the immature rat. How hormones influence growth and behavior of malignant tissues was not known in those days, and even today a lot of questions remain unanswered.

Approximately two-thirds of all breast cancer patients have estrogen-receptor positivity in their tumor, and about half of them respond to endocrine therapy, at least initially. The reasons why the other half or so of patients with estrogen-receptor-positive tumors do not respond to endocrine therapies are rather complex and not completely understood.

Somewhat similarly, at least 80% of prostate cancer sufferers initially respond to androgen withdrawal, but regretfully the mean treatment response duration in prostate cancer is only about two years. Both types of endocrine therapy have both cytostatic and cytotoxic properties for cancer cells. Perhaps surprisingly, neither estrogen receptors (ER) nor androgen receptors (AR) have been described as proto-oncogenes, even though, at least theoretically, their mutation into activated forms could lead to some competitive advantage to affected cells. The truth is that, in contrast to the large numbers of missense AR mutations that have been found in association with androgen insensitivity syndromes, there do not seem to be many AR mutations that predispose to human prostate cancer, with the exception perhaps of a missense mutation present in the germline of 0.33% of the Finnish population and 1.91% of Finnish prostate cancer patients.

For many years, Tamoxifen, a drug that binds the estrogen receptor with high affinity and that globally acts as a partial agonist/antagonist, was the only oral endocrine therapy available for most breast cancer patients, with estrogen-receptor positive tumors. Now, however, the emergence of several new antiestrogens (the so-called *Aromatase Inhibitors*, for example, of which three different molecules have already been approved for marketing), and some clinical studies suggesting that LHRH-agonists may be equally, or more, active than conventional low-intensity chemotherapy (like CMF) as adjuvant therapy in young premenopausal women, has made decision-making algorithms significantly more complex for both clinical oncologists and breast cancer patients.

For example, as recently reviewed by Hortobagyi, with regard to conventional cytotoxic chemotherapy for breast cancer we have gradually learnt, over more than three decades of work, that the use of CMF (cyclophosphamide, methotrexate, and 5-FU) as "adjuvant chemotherapy," following primary breast surgery (to treat potential microscopic residual or metastatic disease), can reduce the odds of cancer recurrence by some 23.5%, and of cancer-related death by 17%. The use of anthracycline-containing regimens, though usually more toxic and associated with iatrogenic hair loss (alopecia) and potential cardiotoxicity, improves results by another 11 and 12% for odds of recurrence and death, respectively. Finally, the introduction of taxanes (that alter microtubular assembly in dividing cells, among many other biochemical changes) in addition to anthracyclines may result in a relative reduction in odds of recurrence, compared with no adjuvant systemic therapy, of some 40 to 60%, depending on age and hormonal status of the patient.

If tamoxifen, the partial agonist/antagonist of estrogen, is used alone as adjuvant therapy in postmenopausal women with estrogen-receptor postive breast cancers, a five years duration of treatment implies a reduction in the risk of local cancer relapse of close to 47%, and an impressive 26% reduction in the risk of cancer-related risks. A more recent large study, conducted by the National Cancer Institute of Canada, has shown that if five years of Tamoxifen, in a premenopausal estrogen-receptor-positive group of breast cancer patients, are followed by five years of an oral aromatase inhibitor called "Petrozole" (that effectively acts as a peripheral "antiestrogen"), the risk of local relapse of cancer is reduced by between 43 to 53%, depending on axillary lymph node status, with a 46% reduction in the risk of contralateral breast cancers, and a fairly significant increase in disease-free interval (and perhaps overall survival), as compared with the group of patients receiving tamoxifen alone.

To make matters even more complicated on the subject of hormonal treatments of breast cancers, a recent study with a different aromatase inhibitor (exemestane) has shown that three years of tamoxifen followed by two or three years of exemestane, produces better clinical results than the conventional five years of adjuvant Tamoxifen.

Bearing in mind these results and other considerations, even nonclinicians will easily understand why explaining the various treatment options to cancer patients and relatives, together with adequate explanations on primary treatments, like the radical surgical approach (e.g. mastectomy), *versus* the conservative (e.g. "tumorectomy plus radiotherapy") approaches, or the new "sentinel node" technologies (e.g. to spare radical axillary lymph node dissection), tend to occupy increasing amounts of time during the initial clinical consultation, and are becoming one of the most difficult tasks for all clinical oncologists.

Conclusion on the threats Unless we find new and more efficient (faster and less expensive) ways to develop new anticancer drugs, and new and more rational (as well as more practical) criteria for using them in combination, the majority of health systems will simply be unable to cope with the expected "avalanche" of new medications.

Professionals will soon be in difficulty when deciding on which combination of drugs to use in any given patient, and in exactly which combination or sequence. Patients themselves (gradually better informed, and naturally keen to actively participate in the therapeutic decision process) will become more confused, and perhaps more vulnerable to biased information or misinformation; and, last but not least, many, if not most health providers may eventually be unable to pay for all new drugs and procedures, considering the ever-increasing costs.

If we also add the rapid demographic changes (that lead to an elderly population with many more cancers) in the developed world, and the increasing political pressure to control pharmacy costs, we come to the inevitable conclusion that dealing with the cancer problem is bound to get initially more complex and expensive, before it becomes rationally more manageable and less expensive.

Molecular Oncology has a lot to do with all this, both as a partial cause of the problem, and as a possible rational solution in the mid- to long-term.

More should probably also be spent on prevention/early detection, and research on "chemoprevention." Thus, health authorities may soon ask themselves whether it makes sense to increase by 20 to 40% the overall costs of treating, for example, metastatic colon cancer or advanced lung cancers, to gain only a year or less of overall survival, rather than adopting more aggressive policies to induce people to undergo more regular colonoscopies,, under sedation, from the age of 50 (say, three times in a lifetime, at 50, 60, and 70 years of age, in the absence of high risk factors) or to simply quit smoking.

The case of AIDS is a good example. Besides a better general knowledge and control of risk factors in the populations at risk, at least within the developed world, the introduction into the clinic, well over a decade ago, of "expensive" combinations of new antiretroviral oral therapies has dramatically increased the life expectancy of HIV-infected cases, from 3 to 5 years at first, to an almost normal life expectancy or, in any case, well over 15 years of life. In this case, chronic expensive therapies "make sense," and are easily justifiable, even to the most rigorous and cost-conscious public health systems. Even under these favorable circumstances, given the fact that the HIV retrovirus in most infected patients often produces several mutant molecular forms each day, the problem of drug resistance remains. This justifies the molecular sequencing of the genome of HIV mutants and, based on the genetic variations detected, changing the individual medication to other suitable antiretroviral drugs, or putting the patient into new drug testing programs.

4.1.2 **Opportunities**

1. The activity of many of the cytotoxic agents used in clinical practice today was first detected by traditional screening methods, as in the case of murine leukemias (L1210 and P388) and murine solid tumors. But these cytotoxic drugs were essentially designed to interfere with DNA or chromosomal replication, because we were ignorant of the molecular basis of cancer.

2. As explained in this chapter, we are beginning to have enough information on the precise molecular mechanisms involved in the regulation of "cell behavior" (benign or malignant), and we shall soon be prepared to classify all the "players" (regulatory proteins) into "processes" (regulatory pathways in disease).

3. It is now possible not only to tell which are the key players in each pathway, but also how each pathway is organized (from upstream to downstream), and where we should intervene therapeutically to correct the malignant behavior of tumor cells (e.g. inhibiting angiogenesis, cell growth or the metastatic process), or to eradicate malignant cell clones (by facilitating senescence and/or apoptosis, or by stimulating the destruction of tumor cells).

4. In simplistic terms (see Fig. 3 for graphic explanation) the new therapeutic drugs should either:

   – block or inhibit activated proto-oncogenes in their inactive state, like Gleevec in the case of several Tyrosine Kinases, for example; or
   – considering the fact that most regulatory molecules have binary states (active/inactive), somehow lock or stabilize tumor suppressor proteins in their active state, which is the one normally responsible for inhibiting entry into S-phase or mitosis, and for maintaining the normal differentiation and apoptotic pathways.

5. In other words, as regulatory proteins are usually present in normal cells in either an active form or inactive form, and the chemical equilibrium between the two forms depends on the regulatory microenvironment of the cell, new targeted therapies should be able to correct, or at least limit, the malignant phenotype by restoring the normal balance between stimulatory and inhibitory signals within the cell.

6. Examples of these new types of "oncogene inhibitors" drugs are either already on the market (e.g. Gleevec or Herceptin), or in development (EGFR inhibitors, VEGF inhibitors).

The case of tumor suppressor genes is more complex, because the ideal therapy in these cases, where the problem is usually a loss-of-function mutation of the promoter (e.g. a deletion or a hypermethylation), would be a genetic replacement of the wild type. However, because of mainly technical reasons (lack of suitable vector, inefficiency of the transformation systems, lack of stability of "transfected cells," danger of oncogenetic transformation by retroviruses, etc.), the truth is that the original research enthusiasm of the 1990s regarding the clinical therapeutic application of genetic therapy programs no longer exists, even if new approaches and new techniques are under active investigation. However, as I postulated in the Second Edition of "Principles of Molecular Oncology" (Humana Press, N.J., 2004) and also in this article, there is a possibility of developing low-molecular-weight drugs capable of inhibiting the "inacti-vation of tumor suppressor function," for example, inhibitors of Rb phospho-rylation or activating "cryptic" tumor suppressor functions.

Because of the presence of either wild-type or mutant p53 protein in most human tumors, the restoration of en-dogenous p53 function in cancer cells by small-molecular-weight compounds (as shown by Bykov et al, 2002), or by the *in vivo* delivery of transducible, pro-teolytically stable p53C' d-peptides such as RI-TATp53C' (as recently shown by Snyder et al, 2004) have become promising new approaches to can-cer therapy.

7. In this way, we can hope to eventually reduce the number of potential thera-peutic targets from several hundreds to perhaps only twenty or thirty major pri-mary targets. Most of these processes, if not all, will have upstream regula-tory elements (e.g. membrane-bound or membrane-associated), intermediate elements (cytosolic or bound to or-ganelles, like mitochondria) and down-stream elements (transcription factors, DNA- or RNA-specific sequences). A critical and exciting phase will be the development of models based on the abnormal circuitry of regulatory path-ways in cancer cells. This would help us to find the "Achilles heel" of the par-ticular cancer (Weinstein, 2002), or the right combination of targets to tackle.

The main targets for cancer therapy identified so far can be summarized as follows:

Angiogenesis Biological process that le-ads to the formation of new blood vessels, and that involve the proliferation of endothelial cells and their morphological association into functional capillaries. The "angiogenesis switch" refers to the set of changes in gene expression and protein function that can change the natural local tissue balance between "inducers and inhibitors of angiogenesis," for example, secretion of growth factors like FGF (Fibroblast Growth Factors) or VEGF (Vascular Endothelial Growth Factors), or changes in membrane receptors associated with the malignant invasive phenotype and growth of tumors.

Hypoxia-inducible factors (HIF), cy-tokines, cellular adhesion molecules (CAMS) like the Integrins family, or secreted proteases like the metallopro-teinases (MMPs) can also alter the an-giogenic phenotype of tissues.

A great variety of molecules produced by normal mammalian cells can inhibit an-giogenesis, such as thrombospondin, an-giostatin, endostatin, tumstatin, arresten, and vasostatin. Of the approximately 200 compounds with antiangiogenic activity described so far, several are already in clinical testing, but we are only really be-ginning to unravel the complexities of the subject, particularly in humans.

One of the most promising approaches is the use of humanized monoclonal antibodies with the capacity to inhibit binding of VEGF to its receptor, or other inhibitors of VEGFR activation. VEGF-A is a highly specific, selective mitogen for vascular endothelial cells *in vitro*, and is produced *in vivo* by many tissues.

For example, Bevacizumab, a human-ized monoclonal antibody against VEGF, has already shown reasonably good results in clinical testing up to phase II and phase III studies. It has shown modest activity in breast cancer, but significant prolonga-tion of the time to progression of disease in metastatic renal cancer and, when added to cytotoxic chemotherapy, it significantly improved survival in patients with metastatic colorectal cancers.

Antiangiogenic therapies would no doubt be ideal adjuncts, or complementary long-term therapies, to primary surgical treatments or to chemo-radiotherapy programs. They should also reduce the problems of resistant phenotypes, considering that these new endothelial cells are normal, and have genomic stability.

"Angiolytic" substances such as Adherins and Integrins, which are inhibitors of the function of several cellular adhesion molecules, are also under investigation. In principle, they are capable of disrupting preexisting tumor blood vessels *in vivo*, thereby leading to interruption of the blood supply, and necrosis of the tumors.

Apoptosis Apoptosis is a biological process that describes the complex mechanisms of "programed cell death," eventually leading to endonuclease driven fragmentation of DNA and chromatin by a number of Caspase-dependent or Caspase-independent biochemical events. Although the mitochondrial release of cytochrome-C appears essential for at least some caspase-mediated events, mitochondrial-independent activation of caspases *via* activation of the Fas-FasLigand pathways (also known as CD95, or APO-1 pathways) is also reasonably well defined. The mitochondria are currently seen as an important convergence point for a number of pro-apoptotic or antiapoptotic members of the so-called *Bcl-2* family of proteins. However, the recent enthusiasm for "apoptosis" as the main, or only, mechanism of tumor cell death can be prudently questioned on several grounds. Except in cells of lymphoid origin, apoptosis is a relatively insignificant mode of cell death for most cells in solid tissues, and experimental conclusions based on measuring the extent of cell kill by cytotoxic agents, rather than on true effects on clonogenic survival of tumor cells, can be misleading. Thus, despite the seemingly strong case that cells die from cancer treatments (chemotherapy or radiotherapy) because of apoptosis chiefly controlled by wild-type p53, much current data do not appear to fit with this simple hypothesis. On the other hand, it seems reasonable to expect that unless new drugs are capable of inducing cell death (by necrosis or apoptosis), the therapeutic effects will be mainly "cytostatic" rather than "cytotoxic."

Clinicians, and patients of course, like to see tumors "shrink" or, ideally, to "disappear," rather than just stay "more or less the same," with "stabilization", that is, no clear tumor growth but no tumor size reduction either.

Binary state (of regulatory molecules) In ancient Chinese philosophy and medicine, the Universe we live in was clearly a model of the binary nature of things. For example, "cold" was considered to be a "Yin" pathogenic factor, and its nature is to slow things down. On the other hand, "heat or fire" was considered a "Yang" pathogenic factor, causing expansion and increased activity. In a similar sort of way, all biochemical regulatory proteins can be present at any one time in an "on" or "off" molecular form, with regard to one or more of their functions.

This "Yin" or "Yang" effect will depend, for the normal wild-type forms of regulatory proteins, on the regulatory microenvironment, and the possible conformational changes (usually allosteric) produced by a number of enzyme activities including phosphorylation/dephosphorylation, acetylation/deacetylation, farnesylation/

defarnesylation, methylation/demethylation, and so on.

Cell Cycle Checkpoints: Mammalian cells can remain quiescent (in Go phase of their cell cycle) for long periods of time, but the right combination of growth factors can induce them to enter G1 and then, if no impediment occurs, progress through S-phase (DNA replication), G2, and mitosis, and complete their cell division. Tumor doubling times can show tremendous variations. For example, some 60% of human breast cancers show tritiated thymidine incorporation rates and labeling indices of less than 4%, indicating a rather slow doubling time of tumor cells, but the rest of the breast cancers can show labeling indices between 4 and 41%. No doubt this reflects the molecular heterogeneity of breast cancers. The best and more selective anticancer drugs of the future, in this cell cycle setting, would have to tag specific cyclins (e.g. cyclin D1 and cyclin E, that can act as *de facto* potent oncogenes) for degradation. Recent research points towards a key role for Cyclin E in breast cancer, and Cyclin D1 in some non-Hodgkin's lymphomas and in colon cancer, where they act as potent oncogenes. Alternatively, marked cytostatic effects should be produced by new drugs designed to stimulate the activity of selective CKIs (Cyclin-dependent kinase inhibitors), or to lock crucial downstream elements (like the retinoblastoma protein complex) that act as *de facto* tumor suppressor genes, in order to enable them to maintain their active roles as cell cycle inhibitors.

Cell shape Surprisingly little systematic research has been published to establish the molecular links between "cell shape" and "cell behavior." Yet it makes sense to assume that both are related. For example, most differentiated epithelial cells adopt a rectangular or polygonal shape, and display a marked polarity (from their attachment to the basement membrane, to the opposite membrane surface on the lumen), as well as a solid cytoskeleton, parallel anchorage to neighboring cells, abundant cytoplasm and endoplasmic reticulum, and low, if any, migration capacity. They also display a low rate of proliferation (except at special sites like the intestinal crypts, where they change shape anyway). In general, as cells take a spindle shape (epithelial-mesenchymal transition, or *vice versa*), they become more potentially mobile and proliferative. Finally, blood cells tend to be round, with a high nuclear/cytoplasm ratio, and are both more mobile and more likely to undergo cell division if stimulated.

The so-called *blast cells*, in leukemias and lymphomas, and also in undifferentiated or poorly differentiated carcinomas, show similar changes in shape, nuclear/cytoplasmic ratio, mobility, and high- proliferative activity.

Downregulation of "adherens junctions" (AJ) assembly by mutations, hypermethylation, or transcriptional repression of the adhesion molecule E-Cadherin, have been described in several malignancies, and particularly in human diffuse gastric carcinomas, lobular breast cancers and familial gastric cancers. In many ways, E-cadherin behaves as a tumor suppressor gene, while *beta*-catenin behaves as a potentially potent oncogene. Thus, when the ratio of free cytoplasmic *beta*-catenin is too high, because (for example) of loss of E-cadherin, or because of APC mutations, an excess of *beta*-catenin is free to travel to the nucleus. This leads to the overexpression of a set of transcription factors (TCF/LEF), and of potent oncogenes such as cyclin D1 or c-myc.

When the intracellular levels of another important protein regulator (named *snail*) rise above a certain threshold, there is usually active repression of the transcription of the *E-cadherin* gene, and a promotion of the so-called *epithelial-mesenchymal transition* (*EMT*), that leads polygonal/epithelioid-shaped cells to convert into spindle/round type of cells.

Chemoprevention Chemoprevention is "the treatment of carcinogenesis, its prevention, inhibition or reversal." The term "chemoprevention" is controversial. Some may confuse the term "chemo" with "chemotherapy", and "prevention" may not be the best word to define "early detection" of cancer biomarkers. The subject is bound to grow very rapidly, both in terms of the identification, validation, and clinical relevance of cancer biomarkers, and also in terms of their impact on the quantitative estimation and prediction of individual human cancer risks.

In the relatively recent past, the possibility has been raised that pharmacological agents or nutritional modification might prevent the development of human cancer, or at least slow down its progression. The concept of chemoprevention is gaining support, although there are still significant experimental and conceptual problems associated with it. For example, if the study population is composed of normal or nearly normal subjects (such as normal volunteers, smokers without obvious disease, or people with a history of one isolated gastrointestinal polyp), very few side effects may be acceptable. In contrast, if the subjects are at high risk of cancer (e.g. have a history of familial polyposis, hereditary predisposition to breast or colon cancer, or second tumors) considerable side effects may be acceptable.

It remains possible that many of the target-oriented new drugs being developed will show clinically relevant efficacy in cancer chemoprevention studies, perhaps even superior to that shown in advanced cancers. The reason is that these target-oriented new drugs usually display tolerable or little toxicity, can be administered orally for long periods of time, and delay the growth of cell clones with a proliferative or angiogenic advantage over their normal counterparts (e.g. by interfering with growth factor signal transduction, or with the angiogenic process).

There is also significant scientific interest in certain metabolic or detoxification phenotypes that may lead to a higher cancer risk, such as aryl hydrocarbon hydroxylase activity (AHH), debrisoquine hydroxylation, and glutathione-S-transferase activity. For example, AHH activity depends on one subfamily of cytochrome P-450 microsomal enzymes that convert polycyclic aromatic hydrocarbons into carcinogenic intermediates. Case-control studies have yielded contradictory results regarding the association between AHH activity in lymphocytes and lung cancer risk. Why only a minority of heavy smokers actually develop lung cancer remains largely unknown.

Beta-carotene, the retinoids, folic acid, vitamins C and E, and tamoxifen have been reported so far in published phase III clinical chemoprevention trials. The retinoids have probably been studied the longest and, although their therapeutic index is somewhat narrow because of toxicities, they have achieved successful results in oral leukoplakia, actinic keratosis, prevention of skin cancer in xeroderma pigmentosum, and prevention of second primary tumors in squamous cell carcinoma of the head and neck. More recent, but rapidly growing, is the role of other agents, such as cyclooxygenase-two (COX-2) inhibitors in chemoprevention. COX-2, a key enzyme for the production of prostaglandins from arachidonic acid, is overexpressed in colon carcinogenesis and other malignancies.

The role of tamoxifen in chemoprevention of breast cancer has recently reached the front pages of newspapers. A recent report from the American Society of Clinical Oncology (ASCO) lists several conclusions endorsed by the Health Services Research Committee and the ASCO Board of Directors. Tamoxifen, at 20 mg/d for 5 years, may be offered to reduce the risk to women who have a defined breast cancer risk of more than or equal to 1.66%. Risk/benefit models suggest that greatest clinical benefit with least side effects is derived from the use of Tamoxifen in younger premenopausal women who are less likely to suffer thromboembolic sequelae and uterine cancers. Data confirm a substantial reduction in breast cancer risk, but do not yet demonstrate, probably because of a relatively short follow-up, an overall health benefit or increased survival. Tamoxifen is not free from side effects but health-related quality of life is not adversely affected in most cases.

Drug resistance Conventional cytotoxic chemotherapy and radiotherapy were designed to hit the DNA synthetic machinery of rapidly proliferating cells, to alter the integrity of DNA in tumor cells, or to interfere with microtubule assembly and chromosomal movements during mitosis. With these rather nonspecific forms of therapy, some relatively uncommon cancers, like many pediatric tumors, some leukemias and lymphomas, germ cell cancers, and a few other malignancies can be totally cured. And in many other cases, although these therapies do not offer much hope of cure, they can nevertheless provide

effective palliation of symptoms, and even (when used as adjuncts to primary surgical resection) increased overall survival, or at least disease-free interval. Although the judicious use of these agents, together with surgical treatments, remains the mainstay of Oncology Therapeutics, their success in curing or totally eradicating the majority of the most common cancers is limited, and usually inversely proportional to the total amount of cancer cells, among other important prognostic factors.

Surprisingly, conventional chemotherapy and radiotherapy work not because cancer cells are especially more "sensitive" to their cytotoxic effects than normal cells, but because normal cells usually can recover faster and more efficiently than cancer cells. Normal tissues virtually never develop resistance to chemotherapy, probably because they maintain the mechanisms that allow normal renewing cell populations, like the highly proliferating cells in the normal bone marrow or gastrointestinal tract, and are capable of monitoring and correctly repairing DNA damage, or induce the programed cell death (suicide) of cells with irreparable DNA damage. Unfortunately, many cancer cells that have lost these normal repair mechanisms become resistant to the action of cytotoxic treatments. In 1943, Luria and Delbruck observed that the bacterium *E.coli* developed resistance to bacterial viruses (bacteriophages), not by surviving exposure, but by expanding clones of bacteria that had spontaneously mutated to a type inherently resistant to phage infection. In other words, following a process of Darwinian selection, those clones inherently resistant to the killer phage gradually outgrow the rest of clones when exposed to the killer agent. On the basis of this model, Goldie and Coldman proposed, in 1979, a model that predicted that cancer cells mutate to drug resistance at a rate intrinsic to the genetic instability of a particular tumor. A large number of potential drug-resistance mechanisms have already been described. Some refer to the existence of multidrug resistance proteins (like the so-called *P-glycoprotein*) on the cell membranes of some cancer cells, and even normal cells of certain tissue types. These proteins can actually actively pump cytotoxic agents out of cells. Others refer to specific mechanisms of resistance unique to each cytotoxic agent. But the predominating general opinion today is that the main mechanisms of resistance to current cytotoxic therapies are more general and, as already described above, more linked to the particular set or combination of genetic and epigenetic defects in DNA-repair pathways, cell cycle control pathways and apoptosis, than to the specific molecular structure of the cytotoxic drug in question.

Growth factors   These were defined in the 1970s, long before their molecular characterization and purification, as substances other than nutrients required by cells *in vitro* for their survival, proliferation, and differentiation.

In fact, it was soon discovered that normal cells are simply unable to survive and grow *in vitro* except in the presence of serum, and fetal calf serum became the 'gold standard' critical component for culture medium. Only some transformed cells, or cancer-derived cell lines, as shown by seminal work by authors like Sporn and Todaro(1980) and Sporn and Roberts (1985), were capable of growing in serum-free medium, because these transformed cells either produce their own growth factors ("autocrine" stimulation), or had become "growth factor-independent" because of the activity of Oncogenes and the lack of activity of tumor suppressor genes.

Substantial evidence, derived from the use of recombinant growth factors *in vivo* (growth factors produced by molecular cloning, and expression of the gene product by a suitable recombinant vector), or from experiments with transgenic animals or site-directed mutagenesis, supports the notion that these substances serve similar purposes *in vivo*. Therefore, it is now widely accepted that differentiation, proliferation, and survival of most normal tissue types is controlled, at least in part, by a complex network of regulatory growth factors. These are usually glycoproteins, frequently of low molecular weight, that act at very low concentrations, in the picomolar range, by binding to specific cell membrane receptors. These receptors can be present in both high-affinity and low-affinity forms, they can be absolutely specific for one growth factor or be shared by two or more factors, and they can be membrane-bound, soluble or both. Some signaling systems, like the Wnt, depend also on the combined activity or modulation of membrane-bound "coreceptors." It has been suggested that HER-2 is also a "coreceptor."

Unlike conventional hormones, which are produced by specialized glands, most growth factors appear to be made systemically; stromal cells (e.g. fibroblasts or endothelial cells), inflammatory cells (e.g. macrophages), and activated T-lymphocytes are some of their main sources. Some perhaps surprising findings regarding the production and secretion of specific growth factors, point to the kidney as being the main physiological producer of erythropoietin (that stimulates the production of red blood cells), and the liver as the main physiological producer of thrombopoietin, also called *MGDF* (*megakaryocyte growth and differentiation factor*), a key regulatory molecule in the production of platelet precursors.

Most standard conventional chemotherapy protocols were designed based on the kinetics of recovery of the bone marrow in response to cytotoxic agents, because neutropenia and thrombocytopenia can easily become doselimiting. The successful introduction into clinical practice (in the mid-1980s) of recombinant human colony-stimulating factors, such as G-CSF (Granulocyte Colony-stimulating Factor, or Filgrastim) and GM-CSF (Granulocyte-Macrophage Colony-stimulating Factor, or Sargramostim), led to a marked decreased in iatrogenic morbidity and mortality.

The use of recombinant human colony-stimulating factors has, according to Chu and DeVita Jr (2002) revolutionized chemotherapy treatments, by playing an important role in decreasing the incidence of infections and the need for hospitalization, and in enabling the maintenance of the optimal dose intensity of chemotherapy treatments for chemosensitive malignancies.

Most human growth factors are "pleiotropic." That is to say, they can modify several cell types and several key regulatory pathways at once, rather than being absolutely cell-type-specific, and display some degree of "redundancy." For example, even in the absence (in experimental animal systems like gene knockout mice) of highly cell-type-specific growth factors like the erythropoietin gene (*EPO*) or the granulocyte colony-stimulating factor genes (*G-CSF*), these gene-deficient animals can still survive with background production of endogenous red blood cells (normally driven by *EPO*), and/or white blood cells (normally driven by *G-CSF*).

It would be over-optimistic to expect growth factor inhibitors alone to prove to be highly effective anticancer agents. On the other hand, the combination of growth factor inhibitors and conventional cytotoxics, or other inhibitors of key signal transduction pathways, might prove valid as human anticancer therapies.

Intraepithelial neoplasia Intraepithelial neoplasia (IEN) is characterized as a moderate to severe dysplasia that occurs on the carcinogenic pathway from normal tissue to malignant cancers. Accumulation of genetic and epigenetic lesions results in the typical phenotypic changes associated with cancer cells, including loss of cell cycle control points, defects in DNA repair, aberrant methylation patterns, and defects in the apoptosis pathways. Because this process of carcinogenesis often requires many years, and most of the common epithelial human cancers increase in frequency, at times almost exponentially, from the age of 45 to 55 to old age, identification of IEN by histopathological or molecular means (genomics or proteomics analysis) can offer a window of opportunity for intervention in the progression of the malignancy.

Clinical studies for the early detection, and primary or secondary prevention of cancer (chemoprevention) are already ongoing for bladder cancers, breast cancers, cervical cancers, colon cancers, endometrial cancers, esophageal cancers, lung cancers, ovarian cancers, prostate cancers, skin cancers, and so on.

Oncogenes These are growth control genes that are present in the human genome (as "proto-oncogenes"), as well as in the genomes of most, if not all, multicellular organisms. Incorrect expression or mutation of an oncogene usually results in gain of function and unregulated cell growth, as seen in malignant cells. Many of them are part of the complex cell's signal transduction pathways, including cell membrane growth factor receptors, or intracytoplasmic proteins. These signal proteins may be an intracytoplasmic piece of the receptor molecule, or another molecule activated just inside the membrane. Tyrosine kinase is an example of a signal molecule. The first signal may serve only as an intermediary, affecting a change in a second messenger. The G proteins, for example (belonging to the *Ras* oncogene family) are a group of intracytoplasmic second-messenger molecules. The intracellular cascade of signals eventually reaches the nucleus, leading to changes in gene expression and cell behavior. Of the over 100 oncogenes that have been identified so far, most are key players in these signal transduction pathways.

Mutations The molecular changes in DNA associated with carcinogenesis are not very different from those associated with genetic variation and molecular evolution of organisms and species, and include local changes in DNA sequences, rearrangement of DNA segments within the genome, and (in the case of viral carcinogenesis) horizontal transfer of a DNA (or RNA) segment originating in another kind of organism.

Basic definitions of these three different natural strategies that allow for genetic variations have been explained in detail in this same Encyclopedia by the Nobel Laureate Werner Arber (Biozentrum, University of Basel).

Point mutation, for example, means the replacement of a single correct nucleotide within a gene by an incorrect one, and can occur as a result of one of several mutagenic events. Mutagenic chemicals (e.g. from cigarette smoking) enter the cell and bind to DNA, forming a structure called a *DNA adduct* which, during replication of the DNA molecule, will lead to an incorrect nucleotide substitution.

Mutagenic chemicals can damage DNA in many other ways, such as by methylation of a nucleotide. Radiation can cause single strand breaks. In general, it is thought that most, but not all, carcinogens are mutagenic. In contrast, the so-called *Tumor Promoters* are substances that by themselves do not cause mutagenic events, but amplify, directly or indirectly, preexisting cellular clones with mutations.

There are at least 16 ways to reduce or abolish the function of a gene product: delete the entire gene, ensure loss of the relevant chromosome, delete part of the gene, disrupt the gene structure (by a translocation or an inversion), insert a sequence into the gene, inhibit or prevent transcription, promoter mutation reducing mRNA levels, decrease mRNA stability, inactivate donor splice sites (causing read-through into intron), inactivate donor or acceptor splice sites (causing exon to be skipped), activate cryptic splice sites, introduce a frameshift in translation, convert a codon into a stop codon, replace an essential aminoacid, prevent posttranscriptional processing, or prevent correct cellular localization of product. Mutation of a gene is not the only way to abolish its function (e.g. long-range chromatin alterations, abnormal methylation and/or imprinting). For example, in human neoplasms *p16* is silenced in at least three ways: homozygous deletion, methylation of the promoter, and point mutation. The first two represent the majority of inactivation events in most primary cancers. *P16* is a very common early event in cancer progression and is frequently seen in premalignant lesions. The importance of *p16* is probably similar to that of *p53*. Mutations in the *p53* gene have been found in some 30% of human tumors, and wild-type *p53* has been reported to suppress tumorigenesis and promote apoptosis (236). The p53 protein is a potent transcription factor and may promote transcription of genes that are also involved in carcinogenesis and angiogenesis.

Loss-of-function mutations usually produce recessive phenotypes, so that as long as one allele remains normal there are no significant phenotypic changes. However, for a limited number of genes, a 50% reduction in the dosage of the gene can lead to phenotypic changes (dosage effect). Certain regulatory functions are inherently dosage-sensitive: for example, gene products which compete with each other to determine a developmental or metabolic switch, or that cooperate with each other in interactions with fixed stoichiometry, or those whose function depends on partial or variable occupancy of a receptor or DNA binding site.

Less frequently, mutations can lead to gain-of-function, rather than loss-of-function. For example, they can result in the ability to acquire a new substrate, overexpression of the gene product, the receptor being turned permanently 'on', the ion channel being inappropriately open, structurally abnormal multimers, chimeric gene, the ability to bind to new DNA sequences, or the ability to trap and inactivate important regulatory molecules. If a protein has several catalytic and allosteric domains (e.g. at a regulatory network bottleneck), destruction or loss-of-function of only one of these domains can allow others to be inappropriately activated.

It is, at least theoretically, possible that some carcinogenic events may include both loss of the natural function of the gene product, and gain of a function not normally associated with that particular gene product. For example, a truncated protein might be unable to perform the original function of the native protein, but could still interact functionally with other regulatory proteins by exposing the remaining protein domains.

Proteasomes The average human cell contains about 30 000 proteasomes, each of which contains several protein-digesting proteases. These complexes help regulate a variety of important cellular functions besides the cell cycle, such as the response to viral infection, the so-called *"stress responses,"* abnormal protein catabolism, neural and muscular degeneration, antigen processing, DNA repair, and even cellular differentiation. In fact, at least in principle, diseases can develop if the system is either overactive or underachieving. This research field is rapidly evolving, and a number of proteasome inhibitors are now under development. In fact, at least one of them (Bortezomib) has already been approved by the FDA for the clinical treatment of refractory multiple myelomas.

When the cell needs to destroy a protein, it usually marks it with a chain of small polypeptides called *ubiquitin*. The ubiquitin–proteasome pathway degrades 90% of all abnormal, misfolded proteins, and all of the short-lived regulatory proteins in the cell. These short-lived proteins, whose half-lives are less than three hours, account for 10 to 20% of all cellular proteins. As a result, proteasome inhibitors do not target individual cellular functions, but they usually affect a broad spectrum of functions.

The research area that has evolved fairly rapidly in recent years is that of the so-called *Ubiquitin-Proteasome Pathways*. This involves the processes of selective intracellular protein degradation. For example, the intracellular levels of cyclins, proteins required for cell cycling, are strictly controlled, and seem to be crucial for the normal functioning of several regulatory cell cycle checkpoints. Indeed, the activity of cyclins appears to be mainly regulated by cyclin levels, rather than by intrinsic molecular changes. Cyclin-dependent Kinase Inhibitor(CKI) protein levels are also strictly controlled throughout the cell cycle, and their degradation is also dependent on the ubiquitin-proteasome pathways.

At least theoretically, selective degradation of cyclins (that often act as oncogenes) but selective inhibition of degradation of CKIs (like *p16* or *p27*, that act as tumor suppressor genes) would provide cancer clinicians with new and powerful tools to fight cancer cells.

The overall regulatory process is rather complex. For example, in normal proliferating cells, the *CKI p27* is actively degraded. The ubiquitin-conjugating enzyme Cdc34, which is a ubiquitin ligase (formed of at least four subunits: the F-box protein Skp2, Skp1, Cul1 and Roc1), and Cks1 are required for the transfer of ubiquitin to phosphorylated *p27*. In a self-amplification process, CDKs phosphorylate *p27* on Thr 187, allowing *p27* recognition by the Skp2 subunit of the ubiquitin ligase.

Stromal cells and cancer Stromal cells are all those cells in a tumor that are not cancer cells. They form the tumor microenvironment and, unlike tumor cells (which are usually monoclonal), they are polyclonal, and contain a mixture of mesenchymal cells (fibroblasts, for example), inflammatory cells (macrophages), immune cells (lymphocytes), antigen-presenting cells (dendritic cells), and other circumstantial cell types. The tumor microenvironment is extremely important for cancer growth, and often it represents the end-result of

a perverse gradual mechanism of invasion and destruction by the mutated cancer cells (the "evil terrorists") of the tissues of the host (or "victim").

In other words, cancer cells often direct themselves the building of the stromal cell tissue microenvironment, in order to allow an even better growth advantage over normal cells, to evade any possible immune resistance, and to continue their invasion of normal structures.

One illustrative example of the sophisticated mechanisms that can lead to normal tissue destruction by cancer cells is the formation of osteolytic lesions in multiple myeloma. Multiple myelomas are a class of cancer cells derived from precursors of B-cell lymphocytes. They are usually diagnosed by detecting abnormally high-monoclonal serum levels of an immunoglobulin (heavy or light chains, or both, of any type), associated with an increase in plasma cells within the bone marrow, of different degrees of morphological differentiation. They can be localized to one site, but more often they are already disseminated in multiple sites at the time of clinical presentation. Although they are usually more frequent in old age, they can also affect young people. The associated symptoms are difficult to control clinically, because multiple myelomas can lead to multiple osteolytic lesions ("holes" in the bones), generalized loss of bone density, pathological bone fractures, and insufficient hemopoiesis (blood production). These conditions produce a tendency to develop infections because of immune suppression (reduced levels of protective immunoglobulins and normal white blood cells), and bleeding problems (because of the reduced levels of platelets). Myelomas are usually treatable (but seldom curable), by a combination of chemotherapy, radiotherapy, and intravenous biphosphonates, that are potent inhibitors of osteoclastic activation.

Some recent work has suggested that myeloma cancer cells modify the normal and dynamic "yin and yang," of bone formation (e.g. osteoblast function) and destruction (osteoclast function). The cancer cells achieve this by, among other mechanisms, secreting RANKL (receptor activator of nuclear factor-kB ligand), a potent stimulator of osteoclast function, and by increasing the degradation of 'Osteoprotegerin', the natural soluble antagonist of RANKL.

Furthermore, Tian and colleagues, by comparing different patterns of gene expression in 57 of approximately 10 000 genes in two subsets of myeloma patients (those with focal osteolytic lesions in bone, and those without), have recently demonstrated that some myeloma cells also secrete a soluble molecule called *DKK1*, that binds to an important class of growth factor "coreceptors" that can affect the Wnt-signaling pathway, resulting in decreased activity of osteoblasts. This might explain the loss of bone density in patients, and why normal osteoblasts in myeloma patients do not fill (with new bone) the "holes" made by myeloma cells themselves, or by their secreted pro-osteolytic substances.

A potential therapeutic approach to ameliorating the bone-specific morbidity of multiple myeloma is by the administration of a suitable antibody against DKK1. The development of new inhibitors of RANKL would also prove useful. In this way, the molecular approach would help toward the restoration of the normal microenvironment.

Tumor antigens They can be defined as molecules that contain the epitope determinants recognized by Tcells that specifically target tumor cells. For many years the underlying principle of tumor immunologists was that cells of the immune system can normally recognize tumors as distinct from the normal tissues (nonself), or as a danger to the organism, and eliminate them (concept of "immunosurveillance"). Although it has now been clearly shown that many, but probably not all, tumors (for example, melanomas) display "tumor antigens", as discrete molecular entities, various mechanisms have been implicated in the resistance of tumors to immune attack: modulation of NK (natural killer cells) receptors, secretion of inhibitory cytokines, recruitment of accessory cells that may thwart immune function, downregulation of molecules critical for antigen-presentation, costimulation of immune cells, and so on.

All these potential mechanisms, and others, can lead to 'tumor editing', so that it is no longer recognized by the normal immune system as 'foreign' and therefore dangerous.

Tumor suppressor genes Unlike oncogenes, Tumor suppressor genes (formerly "antioncogenes") display the function of suppressing cellular proliferation, and/or maintaining cellular differentiation, facilitating normal cellular adhesion mechanisms, stopping entry into the cell cycle (G1, S-phase, mitosis or G2) to allow DNA-repair mechanisms, maintaining normal cellular shape, cell contact inhibition mechanisms, and so on.

Tumor suppressor genes are either underexpressed in cancer cells, because of genetic deletions or promoter hypermethylation, or have undergone other forms of loss of function genetic or epigenetic changes. For example, abnormal *p53* function can be the result of the acquisition of point mutations, posttranslation inactivation through binding to other regulatory proteins (such as the so-called *MDM2*), enhanced degradation (e.g. by the activity of the E6 protein of carcinogenic human papilloma viruses), or other mechanisms like decreased translation of wild-type *p53* by the folate-dependent enzyme thymidylate synthase. In these cases, depending on the cellular context and microenvironment, cancer cells are unable to undergo cell cycle arrest and/or apoptosis in response to the DNA damage produced by cytotoxic chemotherapy or radiotherapy.

Reversion of the malignant phenotype was demonstrated, over three decades ago, by the classical "cell fusion" experiments by Henry Harris, at Oxford. The loss of particular chromosomes in hybrid normal-malignant cells, or the gain of normal chromosomes when fusing normal cells with particular types of malignant cells *in vitro*, led to the first experimental data to back the hypothesis of "antioncogenes," or tumor suppressor genes. Later experiments in the 1980s and 1990s, with the help of gene transfer methods including modified retroviruses and adenovirus, have given more support to the idea that in many cases the malignant phenotype of cancer cells can be reversed, *in vitro* and *in vivo*, by replacing a key tumor suppressor gene. However, because of the technical difficulties and the potential dangers of gene therapy in patients, these findings have not yet led to clinically relevant forms of gene therapy.

An alternative approach, based on the binary state of most regulatory molecules, as proposed in "Principles of Molecular Oncology" (2004), is to develop drugs that can lock *in vitro* and '*in vivo*' a particular tumor suppressor protein into its active "tumor suppressor function" (Fig. 3).

The tumor suppressor paradigm characteristically calls for loss of both functional copies of the gene and indeed many, though not all, tumor suppressor genes must undergo biallelic inactivation in order to sustain a true loss-of-function effect.

An example is the PTEN tumor suppressor pathway.

In 1997, PTEN (phosphatase and tensin homolog deleted on chromosome10), was cloned and mapped to cytoband 10q23, a region of chromosome 10 that undergoes frequent somatic deletion in some malignant human tumors, in particular, in endometrial cancers (almost 50%), some brain tumors (e.g. 30–40% of glioblastoma multiforme, and to a lesser extent anaplastic astrocytomas), metastatic prostate cancers (20–60%) and malignant melanomas.

Discordance between the rate of "loss of heterozygosity" (LOH) and the rate of mutation of the second allele of the *PTEN* gene, has led some to suggest that a second tumor suppressor gene is located in the 10q23 region, but this difference could also due to other reasons: (1) technical inability to detect second mutational events (low sensitivity); (2) a gene dosage-effect where loss of one allele of *PTEN* may have a partial tumor promoting effect; c) epigenetic alterations in the *PTEN* gene, the mRNA, or corresponding protein; d) cooperation between loss of only one allele of *PTEN* and a genetic event in another not-yet-identified gene. The PTEN protein is also regulated by phosphorylation. In particular the serine/threonine kinase CK2, upregulated in many cancers, phosphorylates the PTEN C-terminal tail and reduces PTEN activity, raising the possibility that phosphorylation of PTEN by CK2 might be a mechanism contributing to the downregulation of PTEN in certain human cancers retaining a wild-type PTEN allele. In consequence, inhibitors of CK2 might prove useful therapeutic agents in some cancers.

Whatever be the reasons, loss of PTEN tumor suppressor protein leads to constitutive activation of the PIP3 (phosphatidylinositol-3,4,5-trisphosphate) pathway, with important downstream consequences, *via* the molecular participation of Oncogenic Protein Pathways (like Akt pathways and the m-TOR protein that derives its name from "mammalian target of rapamycin"). This process results in significant changes in cell cycle progression, survival, cell spreading and motility, and even in the angiogenic properties of tumor cells.

This PTEN/PI3K molecular system provides an example of an elegant "on-off switch" that has been evolved as "nutrient and growth factor response pathways"where the switch moves to "on" position when PI3 kinase (PI3K) deposits a phosphate group on the D3 position of the inositol ring, while it is turned "off" when the PTEN removes the phosphate group from the same position.

Another important example of a TS that can prove to be a valid target for cancer therapy is *p53*. Underactivity of *p53*, caused by loss-of-function mutations, encourages the growth of cancer, whereas its overactivity can accelerate the aging process and cell death. Following some elegant pioneering work by Snyder and colleagues (recently reviewed by David Lane in the New England Journal of Medicine), a synthetic 34-amino-acid peptide, made of *d*-amino acids, rather than the conventional *l*-amino acids, and called *RI-TATp53C*, has been shown to be a potent activator of DNA-binding and tumor suppressor functions in both wildtype and mutant *p53*. In preclinical models, this synthetic peptide, that cannot be degraded by proteases and is internalized into cancer

cells by a lipid-raft-dependent pinocytosis mechanism, has been shown to achieve complete cures in a mouse model of terminal peritoneal lymphoma.

New cancer therapies will be directed not merely to hit the DNA synthetic machinery, but to hit selective targets at or downstream from abnormally activated catalytic functions (thereby abrogating the abnormal stimulatory signals), or at or upstream from inactivated or missing catalytic functions (switching on parallel or alternative regulatory pathways).

Multitargeting The "oncogene addiction hypothesis", first put forward by Weinstein, emphasizes the importance of oncogenes or tumor suppressor genes in the maintenance and initial development of any given cancer. In other words, some cancers are extremely dependent on only one or a few oncogenic changes, and may be inhibited by one or a few target-oriented drugs. The correction of a key oncogenetic lesion in a cancer that has undergone a multitude of other activating oncogenic events may nevertheless provide anticancer effects. Although the main clinical examples of such 'Achilles heels' of cancers are provided by relatively unusual tumors like chronic myeloid leukemia, and c-KIT mutants like GIST-tumor (both very sensitive to the therapeutic effects of Imatinib), the situation in most common solid tumors is probably more complex. For example, even in breast cancers that express, by IHC, huge numbers of HER-2 targets (tumors considered to be candidates for Herceptin must express positivity of HER-2 in over 80% of cells, or positivity for FISH with a chromosome amplified ratio of 17 or more), the use of Trastuzumab may lead to response rates of only around 30% when used alone, and 50% when combined with conventional cytotoxic chemotherapy. The use of new HSP90 inhibitors can tackle several carcinogenic targets at once, the so-called *hallmark traits of cancer*, because HSP90 is a molecular chaperone that stabilizes several mutated and overexpressed "client" signaling molecules such as many oncogenic kinases or even the catalytic component of telomerase. Inhibition of HSP90 leads to incorrect folding and subsequent degradation of oncogenic client proteins through the ubiquitin-proteasome pathways, but this "promiscuity" of action of HSP90 inhibitors can also lead to less specificity, lower anticancer potency and more potential iatrogenic side effects.

Other multitarget agents currently undergoing clinical development include: (1) SU11248, an oral multitargeted kinase inhibitor with direct antitumor as well as antiangiogenic activity, *via* the targeting of the VEGF, platelet-derived growth factor, KIT, and FLT3 receptor tyrosine kinases; (2) PTK87/ZK 222584, an potent orally administered inhibitor of the VEGF-mediated Flt-1 and Kinase Domain-containing Receptor(KDR) family of tyrosine kinases; (3) BAY 43–9006, again an orally given drug that inhibits Raf-1, but also other membrane receptors and molecular targets; (4) CCI-779, a novel mammalian target of rapamycin (m-TOR) kinase inhibitor, that may be useful in tumors with *PTEN* mutations, or alterations in the Akt activity pathways, regulated by PI3-kinase and *PTEN* suppressor genes.

One obvious regulatory pathway with direct relevance to cancer therapeutics is Cell Cycle Control.

From an almost 'military' point of view, the 'heart of the matter' of tumor cell growth and survival is more likely to be in the nucleus of cancer cells (downstream), than on the cell membranes (upstream).

The role of cyclin D1 in circumventing the cell-cycle checkpoints has been known to be crucial for the pathogenesis of some nonHodgkins Lymphomas and also in colon cancer, and its relationship with intracellular catenin levels have recently come to light. In most cancers, a defect in the retinoblastoma checkpoint is what allows cells to divide uncontrollably and excessively. But usually, in colon cancer, this checkpoint is surprisingly free of defect, and for a long time it was unclear how colon cancer cells achieved a proliferative advantage over their normal counterparts. Then several researchers started to link the intracellular catenin levels with the tumor suppressor protein known as *adenomatous polyposis coli* (*APC*).

The search was on for the target of *beta*-catenin. Osamu Tetsu and Frank McCormick at the University of California in San Francisco published a key paper in 1999, linking intracellular catenin directly with increased expression of cyclin D1, thereby prompting cells to enter the S-phase.

High levels of cyclin D1 override the checkpoint in colonic epithelial cells, generating a population of cells that will not be totally transformed, but might acquire further mutations, for example in *Ras* or other oncogenes, to acquire the truly malignant phenotype. The two pathways, Ras and beta catenin-APC, somehow converge into the same apparent bottleneck activating the expression of cyclin D1.

Similarly, cyclin E has a pivotal role in transducing the mitogenic stimulus of several hormones, cytokines, and extracellular growth factors. Transient expression of cyclin E induces the formation and activation of CDK2 complexes and, as explained before, pRb is again a key substrate. It seems that pRb must be phosphorylated by CDK4/cyclin D before being phosphorylated by CDK2/cyclin E.

Recent evidence suggests that levels of total cyclin E (and low-molecular-weight cyclin E) in tumor tissue, as measured by Western blot assays, correlate strongly with survival in patients with breast cancer.

In a retrospective analysis of 395 patients with breast cancer with a median follow-up of 6.4 years, high levels of truncated or total cyclin E correlate with poor disease-specific survival. Among patients with early (stage I) breast cancer, all those with low levels of cyclin E were alive at seven years, as compared with none of those with expression of high levels of cyclin E. If these findings are confirmed by others, then determination of cyclin E levels by an immunohistochemical assay might soon become routine in oncology units. Stimulation of the proliferation of breast cancer cells by estrogens and growth factors is also accompanied by increased cyclin E levels and the formation of active cyclin E−cdk2 complexes.

From the above arguments, it is obvious that selective inhibitors of cyclin E and D are good candidates for cancer therapy. Molecules designed to inhibit the binding of these cyclins to their corresponding pockets in CDKs (particularly CDK2 and CDK4) are being designed and developed, and some might soon be under preclinical development. Structural studies, for example, have focused on how RXL (cyclin-binding motif) and LXCXE (part of cyclin structure) contribute to substrate selection. The RXL motif in *p27* is thought to bind to a hydrophobic surface on cyclin A. This surface is conserved between cyclins A,B,D and E (lying opposite to the CDK2-binding site).

Cyclin-dependent Kinase Inhibitors (CKIs) can provide us with basic clues on how proliferation is normally controlled *in*

vivo, on new classes of clinically relevant prognostic factors in cancer, and on how to develop molecular mimetics with high affinity for CDKs, and similarly potent inhibitory actions. Synthetic d-peptides (as opposed to naturally occurring l-peptides) are also being investigated in this context as potential allosteric pharmacological regulators of CKIs.

Molecular dynamics simulations can provide complementary information on the nature of these interactions. Owing to the large contact surface between both proteins, it is difficult to design a single small-molecular-weight drug capable of embracing all the interactions deduced from the crystal structures and the molecular dynamic simulations. However, increasing insight into the design of small molecules with sufficient selectivity to alter the T-loop conformation and distortion of the ATP binding site is gradually been achieved. Moreover, the development of short-chain synthetic peptides capable of inhibiting normal binding of p16 to CDK4 can allow a better understanding of the key structure, activity and allosteric properties of these complex molecular interactions.

Gene transfer experiments, for example transfection into tumor cells in culture of active CKI genes, has enabled several laboratories to test the principle of the induction of tumor regression by the activation, or transfer, of CKI activity A good illustration of this is that ectopic p18 expression inhibits growth and induces apoptosis of multiple myeloma (MM) cells. In about a quarter of human MM cell lines, cyclin D1 is overexpressed because the *cyclin D1* gene is brought under the influence of immunoglobulin heavy chain (IgH) enhancer and promoter elements by chromosomal translocation t(11;14) (q13;q32). The CKI p18 predominantly binds to CDK6 and, to a lesser extent, to

CDK4 and inactivates their kinase activity. Furthermore, p18 can efficiently block CDK6 phosphorylation by CAK/cyclin H1. Cell lines transfected with an inducible p18 expression vector not only exhibited growth inhibition, but also apoptosis.

Microinjection of CKI proteins has also confirmed other biological activities of CKIs. For example, injection of the CKI p21 and p27 in *Xenopus laevis* embryos blocked centrosome duplication. The centrosome nucleates the polymerization of microtubules and duplicates once per cell cycle starting at the G1-S transition, and plays a major role in organizing the poles of the mitotic spindle. The inhibition of normal centrosome function by p21 and p27 can also arrest cell growth, and lead to abnormal segregation of chromosomes.

Another unexpected property of CKI is the reported ability of p21 (WAF1/CIP1) to restore hormone responsiveness to estrogen-receptor (ER)-negative breast cancer cells. Again, the overexpression of p21 with a tetracycline-inducible gene transfer vector can make ER-negative, p21-negative breast cancer cells sensitive to growth inhibition by anti-estrogens. A strong positive association has been found between the expression of p21 and the presence of ER in tumor samples from 60 patients with breast cancer.

Besides gene therapy approaches, *in vivo* protein and peptide transduction systems are also being investigated by several laboratories. Recombinant proteins, like recombinant human colony-stimulating factors, have been used in cancer patients for some 15 years already. However, the inability of molecules larger than 600 daltons to cross the plasma membrane has restricted the pharmacological use of proteins to those which function outside the cell, for example, by binding to specific cell membrane receptors. Most tumor suppressors, on the other hand, are intracellular, and therefore cannot be administered to patients as recombinant proteins directly.

At first sight, the retinoblastoma (Rb) protein is the true bottleneck of most of these cell cycle–controlling pathways. In 1986-87 the tumor suppressor *Rb* gene, first identified because it mutated in hereditary retinoblastomas, was cloned by three different laboratories headed by eminent molecular biologists: Robert A. Weinberg and Thaddeus Dryja, William Benedict and Yuen-Kai Fung, and Wen-Hwa Lee. It is a rather large gene, over 200-kb long, and with 27 exons. It codifies for a nuclear protein of 928 amino acids, which is constitutively expressed during the cell cycle, but with characteristic cell cycle dependent varying degrees of phosphorylation.

Phosphorylation of pRb is carried out initially by D-type cyclins (in protein complexes with CDK4 or CDK6) followed later by cyclin E/CDK2. Virtually all human tumors tested so far show mutations that directly or indirectly alter the normal function of *Rb*. Nearly all tumor-derived *pRb* mutants have lost the ability to repress E2F-responsive genes, and reintroduction by gene transfer of wild-type pRb into Rb $-/-$ tumor cells leads to restoration of E2F control and cell cycle arrest. There are at least six human *E2F* genes (*E2F*1 to *E2F*6) and their protein products bind to specific DNA sequences as heterodimers with either DP1 or DP2 proteins. It is now clear that binding to pRb converts the E2F family from transcriptional activators to potent transcriptional repressors. E2F6, unlike the other E2F family members, is an intrinsic transcriptional repressor and does not apparently interact with pRb family members.

Hyperphosphorylated pRb is unable to maintain the binding and inactivation of E2F, and free E2F molecules lead to transcription of multiple genes involved in the initiation of DNA synthesis and cellular proliferation.

Using gene expression profiling methods (Affymetrix GeneChips) it has been possible to demonstrate changes in the expression of over 200 genes, most of them involved in cell cycle control, by CDK phosphorylation of wild-type *pRb*. Some of these genes are also involved with DNA repair, or changes in chromatin structure. As expected, a significant fraction of Rb-repressed genes have promoters that are bound/regulated by E2F family members. However, targets were also identified that are distinct from genes known to be stimulated by overexpression of specific E2F proteins, suggesting that some of the multiple pRb effects are not directly related to E2F proteins.

The conformation and activity of pRb is rather complex, and not fully understood. It is widely accepted that the activity of this large tumor suppressor protein is largely dependent upon the phosphorylation status of at least 16 potential CDK phosphorylation sites. But how exactly the phosphorylation of any of these sites changes the full range of activities of pRb remains a matter of intense study. Low-molecular-weight drugs designed to block 'site-specific phosphorylation' of these sites are also under study, as they may ultimately arrest the growth of populations of tumor cells.

Yuen-Kai Fung's laboratory at the University of Southern California has identified all the CDK sites (Thr-356, Ser-807/Ser-811, and Thr-821), the phosphorylation of which drastically modifies the conformation of pRb. The so-called *m89*

structural motif (identified in the m89 mutant of pRb) has greatly enhanced growth suppressing activity, similar to a mutant with alanine substitutions at Ser-807/Ser-811. Moreover, this m89 region is part of a structural domain, p5, conserved antigenically and functionally between pRb and p53.

Rationally designed drugs capable of interacting with these key molecular sites may exploit the coordinated regulation of activity of these two tumor suppressors, or at least block the conformation of the tumor suppressor pRb into its active growth inhibitory hypophosphorylated structure (see also Fig. 3).

One of the seemingly tragic, and yet-unexplained, features of our human genome is that the key sensors that control many of the functional interactions between Rb and p53 are actually linked in the same gene, making them dually vulnerable to the same genetic attack. In general, mutational events that disable the Rb pathway and facilitate cell proliferation are counterbalanced by a p53-dependent response that eliminates, or at least inhibits, incipient cancer cells. Conversely, loss of p53 function enables cells that sustain oncogenic damage to survive and proliferate. Unfortunately for us, as explained before, the INK4A-ARF locus encodes, in the same genetic locus, two distinct tumor suppressor proteins that regulate both the Rb and the p53 pathways. ARF (p19) is a sensor of inappropriate proliferation brought about by loss of Rb. The product of the *p53* gene is part of the intrinsic mechanisms that monitor the cell cycle. For example, inducing the expression of p21, and mutations, deletions or underexpression of p19ARF facilitate MDM2's degradation of p53, leaving the cell unaware of the need to initiate cell death.

To complete the picture, reactivation of telomerase activity, normally suppressed in most normal human tissues, can dramatically contribute to the carcinogenesis process. Telomerase activity is needed to maintain chromosomal stability, particularly at the – tips of chromosomes where bits of DNA are otherwise lost during each round of DNA replication and cell division, because of the way DNA polymerase works and the need for "primers." If it were not for the activity of telomerase, many cancer types would eventually self destroy, because of the cumulative loss of DNA material at each round of cell division.

See also Theoretical Foundations of Cancer Chemotherapy.

Bibliography

Books and Reviews

Aiello, A., Tamborini, E., Frattini, M. et al. (2004) Genetic Markers in Sporadic Tumors, in: Bronchud, M.H., Foote, M.A., Giaccone, G., Olopade, O. and Workman, P. (Eds.) *Principles of Molecular Oncology*, 2nd edition, Humana Press, Totowa, NJ, pp. 73–150.

Baird, R., Workman, P. (2004) Emerging Molecular Therapies: Drugs Interfering with Signal Transduction Pathways, in: Bronchud, M.H., Foote, M.A., Giaccone, G., Olopade, O., Workman, P. (Eds.) *Principles of Molecular Oncology*, 2nd edition, Humana Press, Totowa, NJ, pp. 569–606.

Bronchud, M.H. (2004) Selecting the Right Targets for Cancer Chemotherapy, in: Bronchud, M.H., Foote, M.A., Giaccone, G., Olopade, O., Workman, P. (Eds.) *Principles of Molecular Oncology*, 2nd edition, Humana Press, Totowa, NJ, pp. 3–49.

Bronchud, M.H., Brizuela, L., Gyuris, J., Mansuri, M.M. (2004) Cyclin-dependent Kinases and their Regulators as Potential Targets for Anticancer Therapeutics, in: Bronchud, M.H., Foote, M.A., Giaccone, G., Olopade, O., Workman, P. (Eds.) *Principles of Molecular Oncology*, 2nd edition, Humana Press, Totowa, NJ, pp. 359–410.

Castillo, L., Etienne-Grimaldi, M.C., Fischel, J.L. et al. (2004) Pharmacological background of EGFR targeting, *Ann. Oncol.* **15**, 1007–1012.

Chabner, B.A., Boral, A.L., Multani, P. (1998) Translational research: walking the bridge between idea and cure – Seventeeth Bruce F. Cain Memorial Award lecture, *Cancer Res.* **58**, 4211–4216.

Chu, E., DeVita Jr., V.T. (2002) *Cancer Chemotherapy Drug Manual*, Jones and Bartlett Publishers, Boston, MA.

Conacci-Sorrel, M., Zhurinsky, J., Ben-Ze'ev, A. (2002) The Cadherin-Catenin adhesion system in signaling and cancer, *J. Clin. Invest.* **109**, 987–991.

Davies, A.J., Rohatiner, A.Z.S., Howell, S. et al. (2004) Tositumomab and Iodine I 131 tositumomab for recurrent indolent and transformed B-cell Non Hodgkin's Lymphoma, *J. Clin. Oncol.* **22**(8), 1469–1479.

Hahn, W.C., Weinberg, R.A. (2002) Modelling the molecular circuitry of cancer, *Nat. Rev. Cancer* **2**, 331–341.

Hahn, W.C., Weinberg, R.A. (2002) Rules for making human tumor cells, *N. Engl. J. Med.* **347**, 1593–1603.

Lane, D. (1998) The promise of molecular oncology, *Lancet* **351**(suppl II), SII17–SII20.

Lane, D. (2004) Curing cancer with p53, *N. Engl. J. Med.* **350**, 2711–2712.

Oved, S., Yarden, Y. (2002) Signal transduction: molecular ticket to enter cells, *Nature* **416**, 133–136.

Rich, T.A., Shepard, R.C., Mosley, S.T. (2004) Four decades of continuing innovation with Fluorouracil: current and future approaches to fluorouracil chemoradiation therapy, *J. Clin. Oncol.* **22**(11), 2214–2232.

Stratton, M.S., Stratton, S.P., Dionne, S.O. et al. (2004) Treatment of Carcinogenesis, in: Bronchud, M.H., Foote, M.A., Giaccone, G., Olopade, O., Workman, P. (Eds.) *Principles of Molecular Oncology*, 2nd edition, Humana Press, Totowa, NJ, 607–673.

Weinstein, I.B. (2002) Cancer: addiction to oncogenes- the Achilles heal of cancer, *Science* **297**, 63–64.

Primary Literature

Adams, J. (2002) Proteasome inhibition: a novel approach to cancer therapy, *Trends Mol. Med.* **8**, S49–S54.

Armitage, P., Doll, R. (1954) The age-distribution of cancer and a multistage theory of carcinogenesis, *Br. J. Cancer* **8**, 1–12.

Armitage, P., Doll, R. (1957) A two-stage theory of carcinogenesis in relation to the age distribution of human cancer, *Br. J. Cancer* **11**, 161–169.

Baltimore, D. (1976) Viruses, polymerases and cancer, *Science* **192**, 632–636.

Banerjee, D., Bertino, J.R. (2002) E2F and Cancer Chemotherapy, in: La Thangue, N.B., Bandara, L.R. (Eds.) *Targets for Cancer Chemotherapy: Transcription Factors and other Nuclear Proteins*, Humana Press, Totowa, NJ, 289–298.

Barrie, E., Eno-Amooquaye, E., Hardcastle, A. et al. (2003) High-throughput screening for the identification of small-molecule inhibitors of retinoblastoma protein phosphorylation in cells, *Anal. Biochem.* **320**, 66–74.

Basehoar, A.D. et al. (2004) Identification and distinct regulation of yeast TATA box-containing genes, *Cell* **116**, 699–709.

Bast, R.C., Ravdin, P., Hayes, D.F. et al. (2001) 2000 Update of recommendations for the use of tumor markers in breast and colorectal cancer: clinical practice guidelines of the American Society of Clinical Oncology, *J. Clin. Oncol.* **19**, 1865–1878.

Bates, S., Vousden, K.H. (1996) P53 in signaling checkpoint arrest or apoptosis, *Curr. Opin. Genet. Dev.* **6**, 12–19.

Beer, M.A., Tavazoie, S. (2004) Predicting gene expression from sequence, *Cell* **117**, 185–198.

Bronchud, M.H., Scarffe, J.H., Thatcher, N. et al. (1987) Phase I/II study of recombinant human granulocyte colony-stimulating factor in patients receiving intensive chemotherapy for small cell lung cancer, *Br. J. Cancer* **56**, 809–813.

Brown, R., Strathdee, G. (2002) Epigenomics and epigenetic therapy of cancer, *Trends Mol. Med.* **8**, S43–S48.

Bykov, V.J.N., Issaeva, N., Shilov, A. et al. (2002) Restoration of tumor suppressor function to mutant p53 by a low molecular weight compound, *Nat. Med.* **8**, 282–288.

Carter, P. (2001) Improving the efficacy pf antibody-based cancer therapies, *Nat. Rev. Cancer* **1**, 118–129.

Chin, L., Pomerantz, J., Polsky, D. et al. (1997) Cooperative effects of INK4A and ras in melanoma susceptibility in vivo, *Genes Dev.* **11**, 2822–2834.

Coiffier, B., Lepage, E., Briere, J. et al. (2002) CHOP chemotherapy plus rituximab compared with CHOP alone in elderly patients with diffuse large-B-cell lymphoma, *N. Engl. J. Med.* **346**, 235–242.

Couch, D.B. (1996) Carcinogenesis: basic principles, *Drug Chem. Toxicol.* **19**, 133–148.

Dillman, R.O. (1997) Magic bullets at last! Finally – Approval of a monoclonal antibody for the treatment of cancer!!!, *Cancer Biother. Radiopharm.* **12**, 223–225.

Doll, R. (1996) Nature and nurture:possibilities for cancer control, *Carcinogenesis (Lond.)* **17**, 177–184.

Druker, B.J., Tamura, S., Buchdunger, E. et al. (1996) Effects of a selective inhibitor of the Abl tyrosine kinase on the growth of Bcr-Abl positive cells, *Nat. Med.* **2**, 561–566.

Dy, G.K., Adjei, A.A. (2002) Novel targets for lung cancer therapy: Part I, *J. Clin. Oncol.* **20**, 2881–2894.

Dy, G.K., Adjei, A.A. (2002) Novel targets for lung cancer therapy: Part II, *J. Clin. Oncol.* **20**, 3016–3028.

Early BreastCancer Trialists' Collaborative Group (1998) Tamoxifen for early breast cancer:an overview of the randomised trials, *Lancet* **351**, 1451–1467.

El-Deiry, W.S. (1998) Regulation of p53 downstream genes, *Semin. Cancer Biol.* **8**, 345–357.

Elsayed, Y.A., Sausville, E.A. (2001) Selected novel anticancer treatments targeting cell signaling proteins, *The Oncologist* **6**, 517–537.

Fearon, E.R., Vogelstein, B. (1990) A genetic model for colorectal tumorigenesis, *Cell* **61**, 759–767.

Fisher, J.C. (1958) Multiple-mutation theory of carcinogenesis, *Nature* **181**, 651–652.

Fisher, J.C., Hollomon, J.H. (1951) A hypothesis for the origin of cancer foci, *Cancer* **4**, 916–918.

Fox, E., Curt, G.A., Balis, F.M. (2002) Clinical trial design for target-based therapy, *Oncologist* **7**, 401–409.

Friedewald, W.F., Rous, P. (1944) The initiating and promoting elements in tumor production, *J. Exp. Med.* **80**, 101–126.

Gelmann, E.P. (2002) Molecular biology of the androgen receptor, *J. Clin. Oncol.* **20**, 3001–3015.

Goldie, J.H., Coldman, A.J. (1979) A mathematic model for relating the drug sensitivity of tumors to the spontaneous mutation rate, *Cancer Treat. Rep.* **63**, 1727–1733.

Goldman, J.M. (2000) Tyrosine-kinase inhibition in treatment of chronic myeloid leukaemia, *The Lancet* **355**, 1031–1032.

Goss, P.E., Ingle, J.N., Martino, S. et al. (2003) A randomized trial of letrozole in postmenopausal women after five years of tamoxifen therapy for early-stage breast cancer, *N. Engl. J. Med.* **349**, 1793–1802.

Hancock, J.T. (1997) *Cell Signalling*, Addison Wesley Longman Limited, Harlow, England, UK.

Harbour, J., Dean, D. (2000) The Rb/E2F pathway: expanding roles and emerging paradigms, *Genes Dev.* **14**, 2393–2409.

Harris, C.C. (1996) The Walter Hubert Lecture. Molecular epidemiology of human cancer: insights from the mutational analysis of the p53 tumor suppressor gene, *Br. J. Cancer* **73**, 261–269.

Hernández-Bronchud, M. (1995) Growth factors and cancer, *Br. J. Hosp. Med.* **53**, 20–26.

Hortobagyi, G.N. (2004) What is the role of high-dose chemotherapy in the era of targeted therapies? *J. Clin. Oncol.* **22**(12), 2263–2266.

Huisinga, K.L., Pugh, B.F. (2004) A genome-wide housekeeping role for TFIID and a highly regulated stress-related role for SAGA in Saccharomyces cerevisiae, *Mol. Cell.* **13**, 573–585.

Huron, D., Mizenina, O., Rosen, N., Moasser, M. (2002) A second generation inhibitor of Abl tyrosine kinase with picomolar biologic potency and selective activity against CML cells, *American Association for Cancer Research, 93rd Annual Meeting*, San Francisco CA: abstract 4198.

Innocenti, F., Undevia, S.D., Iyer, L. et al. (2004) Genetic variants in the UDP-glucuronosyltransferase 1A1 gene predict the risk of severe neutropenia of irinotecan, *J. Clin. Oncol.* **22**(8), 1382–1388.

Jain, K.K. (2000) Applications of proteomics in oncology, *Pharmacogenomics* **1**, 385–393.

Johnstone, R.W. (2002) Histone-deacetylase inhibitors: novel drugs for the treatment of cancer, *Nat. Rev. Drug Discov.* **1**, 287–299.

Jonasson, J., Harris, H. (1977) The analysis of malignancy by cell fusion. (8) Evidence for the intervention of an extra-chromosomal element, *J. Cell Sci.* **24**, 255–263.

Kaelin, W.G. Jr. (2002) Cancer Chemotherapy Based on E2F and the Retinoblastoma Pathway, in: La Thangue, N.B., Bandara, L.R. (Eds.) *Targets for Cancer Chemotherapy: Transcription Factors and other Nuclear Proteins*, Humana Press, Totowa, NJ, 1–13.

Karin, M., Hunter, T. (1995) Transcriptional control by protein phosphorylation: signal transmission from the cell surface to the nucleus, *Curr. Biol.* **5**, 747–757.

Kim, H., Kwon, Y.M., Kim, J.S. et al. (2004) Tumor-specific methylation in bronchial lavage for the early detection of non-small-cell lung cancer, *J. Clin. Oncol.* **22**(12), 2363–2370.

Kinzler, K.W., Vogelstein, B. (1996) Lessons from hereditary colorectal cancer, *Cell* **87**, 159–170.

Kinzler, K.W., Vogelstein, B. (1997) Gatekeepers and caretakers, *Nature (London)* **386**, 761–763.

Knudson, A.G. (1973) Mutation and human cancer, *Adv. Cancer Res.* **17**, 317–352.

Kodadek, T. (2001) Protein microarrays: Prospects and problems, *Chem. Biol.* **8**, 105–115.

Li, S. et al. (2004) A map of the interactome network of the metazoan C *elegans*, *Science* **303**, 540–543.

Liggett, W.H., Sidransky, D. (1998) Role of the p16 tumor suppressor gene in cancer, *J. Clin. Oncol.* **16**, 1197–1206.

Lindor, N.M., Greene, M.H. (1998) The concise handbook of family cancer syndromes. Mayo Familial Cancer Program, *J. Natl. Cancer Inst.* **90**, 1039–1071.

Lindor, N.M., Burgart, L.J., Leontovich, O. et al. (2002) Immunohistochemistry versus microsatellite instability testing in phenotyping colorectal tumors, *J. Clin. Oncol.* **20**, 1043–1048.

Loeb, L. (1991) A Mutator phenotype may be required for multistage carcinogenesis, *Cancer Res.* **51**, 3075–3080.

Loeb, L.A. (1998) Cancer cells exhibit a mutator phenotype, *Adv. Cancer Res.* **72**, 25–56.

Lord, B.I., Bronchud, M.H., Owens, S. et al. (1989) The kinetics of human granulopoiesis following treatment with granulocyte colony-stimulating factor "in vivo", *Proc. Natl. Acad. Sci. U.S.A.* **86**, 9499–9503.

Maloney, A., Workman, P. (2002) HSP90 as a new therapeutic target for cancer therapy: the story unfolds, *Expert Opin. Biol. Ther.* **2**, 3–24.

Mao, L., Hurban, R.H., Boyle, J.O. et al. (1994) Detection of oncogene mutations in sputum precedes diagnosis of lung caner, *Cancer Res.* **54**, 1634–1637.

Massagué, J., Polyak, K. (1995) Mammalian antiproliferative signals and their targets, *Curr. Opin. Genet. Dev.* **5**, 91–96.

Melnick, A., Licht, J.D. (1999) Deconstructing a disease: RARalpha, its fusion partners, and their roles in the pathogenesis of acute promyelocytic leukemia, *Blood* **93**, 3167–3215.

Mendelsohn, J. (2002) Targeting the Epidermal Growth Factor Receptor for cancer therapy, *J. Clin. Oncol.* **20**(Sept 15 Suppl.), 1s–13s.

Monks, A., Scudiero, D., Skehan, P. et al. (1991) Feasibility of a high-flux anticancer drug screen using a diverse panel of cultured human tumor cell lines, *J. Natl. Cancer Inst.* **83**, 757–766.

McCormick, F. (2001) Cancer gene therapy: fringe or cutting edge? *Nat. Rev. Cancer* **1**, 130–141.

Nordling, C.O. (1953) A new theory on the cancer-inducing mechanism, *Br. J. Cancer* **7**, 68–72.

Odom, D.T. et al. (2004) Control of pancreas and liver gene expression by HNF transcription factors, *Science* **303**, 1378–1381.

Opalinska, J.B., Gewirtz, A.M. (2002) Nucleic-acid therapeutics: basic principles and recent applications, *Nat. Rev. Drug Discov.* **1**, 503–514.

Palmer, H.G. (2001) Vitamin D promoted the differentiation of colon carcinoma cells by the induction of E-cadherin and the inhibition of beta-catenin signaling, *J. Cell Biol.* **154**, 369–387.

Paull, K.D., Shoemaker, R.H., Hodes, L. et al. (1989) Display and analysis of patterns of differential activity of drugs against human tumor cell lines: development of mean graph and COMPARE algorithm, *J. Natl. Cancer Inst.* **81**, 1088–1092.

Perera, F.P. (1996) Molecular epidemiology: insights into cancer susceptibility, risk assessment, and prevention, *J. Natl. Cancer Inst.* **88**, 496–509.

Ponder, B. (1997) Genetic testing for cancer risk, *Science (Washington DC)* **278**, 1050–1054.

Rosenberg, S.A. (2001) Progress in human tumour immunology and immunotherapy, *Nature* **411**, 380–384.

Rubin, B.P., Schuetze, S.M., Eary, J.F. et al. (2002) Molecular targeting of platelet-derived growth factor B by imatinib mesylate in a patient with metastatic dermatofibrosarcoma protuberans, *J. Clin. Oncol.* **20**, 3586–3591.

Rusch, V., Klimstra, D., Linkov, I. et al. (1995) Aberrant expression of p53 or the epidermal growth factor receptor is frequent in early bronchial neoplasia, and coexpression precedes squamous cell carcinoma development, *Cancer Res.* **55**, 1365–1372.

Sansal, I., Sellers, W.R. (2004) The biology and clinical relevance of the PTEN tumor suppressor pathway, *J. Clin. Oncol.* **22**, 2954–2963.

Senior, K. (1999) Fingerprinting disease with protein chip arrays, *Mol. Med. Today* **5**, 326–327.

Sharp, P.A. (2001) RNA interference-2001, *Genes Dev.* **15**, 485–490.

Sharpless, N., Bardeesy, N., Lee, K.-H. et al. (2001) Loss of p16INK4a with retention of p19Arf predisposes mice to tumorigenesis, *Nature* **413**, 86–91.

Shields, P.G., Harris, C.C. (1991) Molecular epidemiology and the genetics of environmental cancer, *J. Am. Med. Assoc.* **266**, 681–687.

Slamon, D.J., Leyland-Jones, B., Shak, S. et al. (2001) Use of chemotherapy plus a monoclonal antibody against HER2 for metastatic breast cancer that overexpresses HER2, *N. Engl. J. Med.* **344**, 783–792.

Snyder, E.L., Meade, B.R., Saenz, C.C., Dowdy, S.F. (2004) Treatment of terminal peritoneal carcinomatosis by a transducible p53-activating peptide, *PloS Biol.* **2**(2), 186–193.

Sporn, M.B., Roberts, A.B. (1985) Autocrine growth factors and cancer, *Nature* **313**, 745–747.

Sporn, M.B., Todaro, G.H. (1980) Autocrine secretion and malignant transformation of cells, *N. Engl. J. Med.* **303**, 878–880.

Stark, A., Hulka, B.S., Joens, S. et al. (2000) HER-2/neu amplification in benign breast disease and the risk of subsequent breastcancer, *J. Clin. Oncol.* **18**(2), 267–274.

Temin, H.M. (1971) The protovirus hypothesis: speculations on the significance of RNA-directed DNA synthesis for normal development and for carcinogenesis, *J. Natl. Cancer Inst.* **46**, iii–viii.

Tewari, M. et al. (2004) Systematic interactome mapping and genetic perturbation analysis of a C. elegans TGF-ß signaling network, *Mol. Cell.* **13**, 469–482.

Tian, E., Zhan, F., Walker, R., Rasmussen, E. et al. (2003) The role of the Wnt-signaling antagonist DKK1 in the development of osteolytic lesions in multiple myeloma, *N. Engl. J. Med.* **349**, 2483–2494.

Torrance, C.J., Jackson, P.E., Montgomery, E. et al. (2000) Combinatorial chemoprevention of intestinal neoplasia, *Nat. Med.* **6**, 1024–1028.

Visakorpi, T., Hyytinen, E., Koivisto, P. et al. (1995) In vivo amplification of the androgen receptor gene and progression of human prostate cancer, *Nat. Genet.* **9**, 401–406.

Walker, J.W., Hayward, N.K. (2002) P16INK4A and p14ARF tumour suppressors in melanoma: lessons from the mouse, *The Lancet* **359**, 7–8.

Welte, K., Gabrilove, J., Bronchud, M.H. et al. (1996) Filgrastim (r-metHuG-CSF): the first ten years, *Blood* **88**, 1907–1929.

Wiener, F., Klein, G., Harris, H. (1971) The analysis of malignancy by cell fusion (3). Hybrids between diploid fibroblasts and other tumour cells, *J. Cell. Sci.* **8**, 681–692.

Woodford-Richens, K.L., Rowan, A.J., Gorman, P. et al. (2001) SMAD4 mutations in colorectal cancer probably occur before chromosomal instability, but after divergence of the microsatellite instability pathway, *Proc. Natl. Acad. Sci. U.S.A.* **98**, 9719–9723.

Yuan, A., Yu, C.J., Luh, K.T., Kuo, S.H., Lee, Y.C., Yang, P.C. (2002) Aberrant p53 expression correlates with expression of vascular endothelial growth factor mRNA and interleuikin-8 mRNA and neoangiogenesis in non-small cell lung cancer, *J. Clin. Oncol.* **20**, 900–910.

Zhu, H., Snyder, M. (2001) Protein arrays and microarrays, *Curr. Opin. Chem. Biol.* **5**, 40–45.

23

Theoretical Foundations of Cancer Chemotherapy

Nicholas B. La Thangue
Division of Biochemistry and Molecular Biology, Davidson Building,
University of Glasgow, Glasgow, UK

1   Cancer Therapy   757

2   The New Era of Mechanism-based Drug Design   757

3   Gleevec and CML   758

4   The ErbB Family   758

5   Manipulating p53 Tumor Suppressor Activity   760

6   Regulating the Cancer Cell Cycle: E2F and Cdks   761

7   Targeting Chromatin Control in Cancer   763

8   Regulating Hsp90   764

9   Blocking Angiogenesis Through Inhibiting HIF1 Activity   766

10   Regulating Protein Turnover   768

11   Conclusions and Perspectives   768

        Acknowledgment   770

        Bibliography   770
        Books and Reviews   770
        Primary Literature   770

Pharmacology. From Drug Development to Gene Therapy. Edited by Robert A. Meyers.
Copyright © 2008 Wiley-VCH Verlag GmbH & Co. KGaA, Weinheim
ISBN: 978-3-527-32343-2

Keywords

Cancer
One of the most common human diseases.

Drug Design
The process of developing a new medicine.

Therapy
The administration to human subjects of a drug

p53
A tumour suppressor protein seen to be frequently mutated in cancer cells.

Cell Cycle
The process through which cells grow and divide.

Angiogenesis
The formation of new blood vessels.

Hsp90
A ubiquitously expressed protein that acts to protect cells from thermal stress.

Erb B
The epidermal growth factor receptor.

E2F
A key protein transcription regulating protein involved in cell cycle control.

■ The massive research efforts that have been applied to understanding the workings of the cancer cell have provided a wealth of detail on key mechanisms that become abnormal during tumorigenesis. Translating and exploiting this large body of cancer research information in the design and implementation of new drugs should yield better medicines for the cancer patient than those that are currently available. It is an implicit assumption in this objective that mechanism-based agents that target discrete abnormalities in tumor cells will provide improved treatments over conventional therapies. In this respect, we are beginning to witness emerging clinical efficacy in a new generation of cancer drugs designed to target key mechanisms in tumor cells.

1
Cancer Therapy

Cancer remains largely a clinically unmet disease. Statistics tell us that cancer affects one person in three, and in the Western world, it is the cause of about a quarter of all mortality. Worldwide, cancer is the second largest cause of death, and the World Health Organization estimates that by 2020, there will be 20 million new cancer patients each year. Cancer is not a single disease, as there are over 200 different types of diseases that fall into this category. However, four cancers dominate, namely, lung, breast, colon, and prostate, which account for over half of all new cases.

Most current cancer therapies employ one of three approaches, namely, surgery, radiotherapy, or chemotherapy. Surgery and radiotherapy are frequently used to treat localized primary tumors, but have limited application in disseminated disease in which the tumor is not localized, usually as a result of metastasis. Needless to say, disseminated disease is the cause of most cancer deaths. Current cancer chemotherapy is dominated by treatments that use cytotoxic agents or hormone-based therapy, for example, in breast and prostate cancer (Table 1).

Tab. 1 Examples of conventional cancer chemotherapeutic agents.

Drug	Category
Methotrexate	Antimetabolite
Taxol	Spindle modulator
Cyclophosphamide	Alkylating agent
Cisplatin	Platinum-DNA complexes
Doxorubicin	DNA intercalating/topoisomerase inhibitor

Furthermore, while advances have been made in all three approaches to treatment, the impact on mortality rates has been modest. As an example, lung cancer, the leading cause of cancer death worldwide, has a five-year survival rate of only 5%, which hardly differs from the survival that prevailed 30 years ago (www.cancerresearchuk.org). However, there are some notable improvements. Cures are achievable in certain childhood leukemias and testicular cancer, although of the six most common cancers, only breast cancer has a survival rate greater than 50%. Overall, conventional chemotherapy is relatively ineffective in many cancers.

This situation reflects the mechanism of action of most current cancer therapy regimes, which are dominated by cytotoxic chemotherapies (Table 1). In general, these chemotherapies target mechanisms employed by most dividing cells, rather than specific genetic abnormalities associated with tumor cells. Because of this, their normal healthy counterparts are affected almost as severely as the tumor cells, leading to the highly debilitating side effects seen with many therapies, such as myelosuppression, hair loss, and gastrointestinal toxicity. This problem, combined with the poor quality of life and diminishing effectiveness in the patient (usually because of the emergence of drug resistance), means that many late stage cancer treatments provide minimal survival advantage.

2
The New Era of Mechanism-based Drug Design

Because of the limited therapeutic value of many current treatments, major efforts are being applied toward identifying new cancer therapies that target specific mechanisms in tumor cells, in the hope that this approach will yield drugs with increased specificity for cancer. Here, we review progress and provide a snapshot of this rapidly advancing field. Selected examples of mechanism-based drug design programs, which illustrate the guiding principles behind the new era of cancer drug development, are discussed. The success stories are clear; a situation we anticipate will be repeated in the continuing efforts to deliver tailored therapies into the cancer clinic.

3
Gleevec and CML

Gleevec (ST1571) provides a paradigm for a successfully developed, rationally designed, and mechanism-based therapy for the treatment of a specific cancer. In chronic myelogenous leukemia (CML), the consistent chromosomal abnormality, the Philadelphia (Ph) chromosome, is a translocation event between chromosome 9 and 22 that results in the bcr-*abl* fusion product derived from the juxtaposition of c-*abl* oncogene and breakpoint cluster region (bcr). bcr-*abl* is present in over 95% of CML patients and in about 5% of acute lymphoblastic leukemia (ALL) patients in whom it functions as a constitutively active tyrosine kinase that is essential for the oncogenic activity of the fusion protein (Fig. 1).

Originally, Gleevec was identified by high-throughput screening for compounds with kinase inhibitory activity, and was subsequently optimized using rational drug design procedures for activity against Abl tyrosine kinase in CML cells. A successful Phase I study indicated remarkable single agent activity during CML blast crisis (and Ph-positive ALL), although the

responses did not appear to be long term. Nevertheless, the success in Phase I prompted further Phase II clinical analysis, followed by FDA approval.

The appearance of resistance to Gleevec was a surprising clinical outcome: the majority of CML patients that relapse after initial response have reactivated bcr-*abl* kinase. Molecular analysis indicated that in many cases resistant cells carry point mutations in the *abl* kinase gene that rendered the kinase less sensitive to STI571, for example, at a site that would be predicted to contact STI571 from the crystal structure. In another category of patients, relapse was correlated with amplification at the bcr-*abl* translocation. These results suggest that while rationally designed drugs like Gleevec may exhibit promising clinical efficacy, the appearance of resistance could be a significant problem.

Gleevec also inhibits the c-kit tyrosine kinase where activating mutations are found in gastrointestinal stromal tumors (GIST), a tumor frequently refractory to chemotherapy. While a range of other tumors express c-kit, the encouraging results of the Gleevec Phase I study on GIST suggest that its clinical application may be wider than initially anticipated, with the proviso that clinical resistance may also appear in other indications.

4
The ErbB Family

The epidermal growth factor (EGF) family of tyrosine kinase receptors (the ErbB receptors) play a crucial role in regulating proliferation. In tumor cells, a variety of mutagenic events give rise to increased ErbB activity, including gene amplification and mutations that alter protein stability.

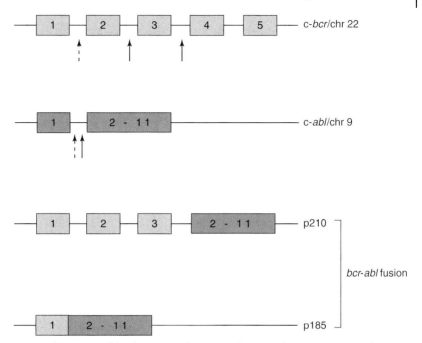

Fig. 1 Chromosomal breakpoints in chronic myelogenous leukemia (CML) and acute lymphoblastic leukemia (ALL). In CML and ALL, a breakpoint occurs between the first exon of c-*abl* on chromosome 9, translocating most of c-*abl* to c-*bcr* on chromosome 22. In CML, the translocations in c-*bcr* occur after exon 2 or 3, to yield the p210 fusion protein, and in Ph-positive ALL, they occur after exon 1 to create p185. The solid arrows indicate CML breakpoints and broken arrows indicate ALL breakpoints.

Both humanized monoclonal antibodies and small molecules have been developed against ErbB1 (also known as EGF receptor and HER1) and ErbB2 (also known as HER2 and Neu). Herceptin (trastuzumab) has received regulatory approval as a single agent for treatment of metastatic breast cancers expressing ErbB2, whereas other humanized antibodies against ErbB1 such as Cetuximab remain in clinical development.

Iressa (ZD1839) is an optimized small molecule ATP competitive antagonist of the ErbB1 tyrosine kinase, originally identified by high-throughput screening and subsequently shown to be active against breast cancer cells. Phase II clinical trials with Iressa demonstrated activity in nonsmall cell lung cancer (NSCLC), squamous cell carcinomas of the head and neck, and hormone refractory prostate cancer. Recently, Iressa was evaluated in a randomized Phase II study for activity in advanced NSCLC, where it was found that it did not provide improvement in survival when added to standard platinum-based chemotherapy.

A significant question regarding the clinical utility of mechanism-based drugs like Iressa relates to how they will be used in the clinical setting. A relevant administration schedule and, as mechanism-based drugs may be cytostatic, identifying an appropriate combination agent and patient population are likely to be critical determinants in reaching optimal clinical efficacy.

5
Manipulating p53 Tumor Suppressor Activity

As one of the most frequently mutated genes in human cancer, the p53 tumor suppressor protein has attracted great interest from drug discoverers. In normal cells, p53 acts as a stress-responsive transcription factor, becoming activated in response to, for example, ionizing radiation, ultraviolet light, and many cancer chemotherapeutic drugs. Once activated, p53 targets genes involved in limiting cellular proliferation, causing either cell cycle arrest or apoptosis (Fig. 2). Its frequent inactivation in cancer has led to many attempts to identify ways of reinstating p53 activity, or approaches that exploit the absence of p53 in tumor cells. However, though it is an intrinsically difficult task for a small molecule to reinstate wild-type activity in a mutant protein, the extensive number of distinct mutations (over 1700 different mutations have been reported) that can occur in the p53 gene provides an additional challenge to this approach.

Despite these significant obstacles, compounds have been identified that reinstate certain wild-type functions on mutant p53 protein. These compounds appear to stabilize p53 in a form that allows some properties of the p53 response to be retained. Relating to this general strategy is the identification of p53-binding peptides, which similarly stabilize mutant p53, providing further support for the idea that the ultimate goal of generating compounds that reinstate p53 activity may be achievable.

In another approach that exploits p53 activity, attempts have been made to generate compounds that block p53 activity. A potential therapeutic application for such inhibitors would be in reducing the level of p53-dependent toxicity in normal healthy tissues that occurs, for example, upon cancer therapy. Pifithrin α, which reduces p53 activity, was identified by high-throughput screening in a cell-based p53 screen. The

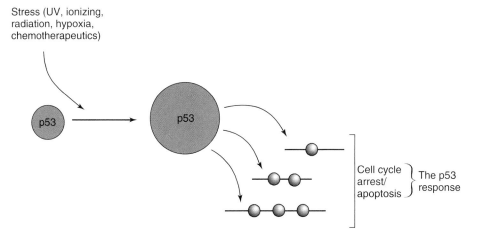

Fig. 2 The p53 response. In normal cells, p53 can be activated by different types of stress, and it then acts to transcriptionally induce target genes that cause cell cycle arrest and apoptosis. In tumor cells, the activity of p53 is lost through mutation in the p53 gene, or in upstream regulators that control p53 activity.

compound is active in mice where it reduces the side effects, such as hair loss and myelosuppression, of the widely used cancer cytotoxic agent doxorubicin.

Although the anticipated clinical utility of p53 inhibitor drugs would be in combination treatments to enhance the efficacy of a conventional cytotoxic, a shortcoming of this approach could lie in the potential mutagenic activity resulting from p53 inhibition. Developing a p53 inhibitor with a sufficiently short half-life may overcome such a concern.

6
Regulating the Cancer Cell Cycle: E2F and Cdks

Abnormal cellular growth and division is a hallmark of tumor cells. It is acquired through a multistep process involving the gradual transformation of a normal cell to a tumor cell, and it involves mutation of critical pathways that act to restrain proliferation, together with the activation of those that promote proliferation.

The retinoblastoma tumor suppressor protein (pRb) provides a perfect example of how a crucial point of growth control can become abnormal in tumor cells, and thereby contribute to tumor cell growth. An important function of pRb is in regulating cell cycle progression through G1 into S phase, particularly passage through the restriction point, where it influences the activity of the E2F family of transcription factors (Fig. 3). E2F coordinates the timely expression of a large body of genes required for cell cycle progression (including DNA synthesis, cyclins, and regulatory proteins), and it is the progressive phosphorylation of pRb that relieves its physical interaction with E2F, thereby enabling E2F to activate target genes (Fig. 3).

Tumor cells employ diverse mechanisms to overcome the tumor suppressor activity of pRb. The Rb gene is mutated in about 25% of human tumors, crippling pRb so that it is not able to bind to E2F. Alternatively, aberrant levels of upstream regulators of pRb, like cyclin D-dependent kinase, occur which leads to the constitutive phosphorylation of pRb and release of E2F. Because of the high frequency of abnormal pRb control, it is believed that deregulation of the pRb/E2F pathway is essential in achieving the transformed state.

In this respect, E2F is an obvious target for therapeutic intervention, and several approaches have been made toward its validation as a cancer target. That E2F plays a crucial role in the cell cycle is supported by E2F knockout cells, in which inactivation of E2F-1, -2 and -3 causes cell cycle arrest. Furthermore, administering short oligonucleotides containing the E2F DNA binding site to sequestor E2F activity away from cellular target genes, the so-called *decoy* approach, prevents cellular proliferation, and short peptides that block E2F function by inhibiting dimerization (with its essential partner protein DP-1) or its interaction with DNA cause apoptosis in tumor cells. Furthermore, a small molecule that is believed to act by modulating the E2F pathway has entered Phase I clinical studies.

Other regulatory factors involved in control of the pRb/E2F pathway, including cyclin-dependent kinases (Cdk) have also attracted considerable attention as a drug target. Though most members of the Cdk family control cell cycle transitions such as cyclin D/Cdk4 and cyclin E/Cdk2 (Fig. 3), other members have been assigned much more specific roles, like cyclinT1/Cdk9, which regulates targets including RNA

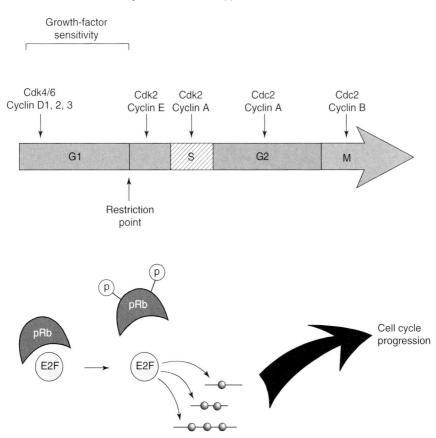

Fig. 3 Regulation of the cell cycle. The four phases of the cell cycle is indicated, together with the nature and the timing of the cyclin-Cdk complexes involved in cell cycle progression. The Restriction point, positioned in G1(R), is the point at which cells become committed to cell cycle progression and no longer require growth factors. The regulation of E2F activity, which controls the early cell cycle, is indicated underneath. In normal cells, the pRb binds to E2F to inactivate E2F activity. As pRb becomes phosphorylated (indicated by p) by Cdk complexes, E2F is released leading to the activation of target genes required for cell cycle progression. Normal control of pRb activity is frequently lost in human tumor cells, either through mutation in pRb or altered levels of its upstream regulators, including Cdk complexes.

polymerase II to influence the expression of a diverse set of genes.

Compounds that act on multiple Cdk enzymes, together with those that are more selective, have been taken into clinical development. UCN-01 is an example of a nonspecific kinase inhibitor active against a variety of kinases including Cdks, protein kinase C, and checkpoint 1 kinase.

In contrast, flavopiridol and R-roscovitine exhibit greater specificity for Cdk targets. Flavopiridol inhibits Cdk1, 2, 4, and 7 (including Cdk2 at nM concentrations) by competing with the ATP binding site, and has reached Phase II clinical trials as a monotherapy for cancer. Roscovitine possesses moderate specificity for Cdk2, but also inhibits other kinases like Cdk7 and Cdk2 at lower potency. In a similar fashion to flavopiridol, roscovitine acts as a competitive inhibitor and induces apoptosis in tumor cells. Roscovitine (also known as CYC 202) has completed a Phase I clinical trial and appears to be well tolerated.

Advances are continuing to be made in improving the selectivity of Cdk inhibitors. For example, a number of oxindole-substituted Cdk inhibitors have greater than tenfold selectivity for Cdk2 against a panel of other Cdks. In this respect, it is hoped that the clinical development of selectively acting Cdk inhibitors will identify molecules with greater efficacy than some of the broad-spectrum agents currently in clinical development.

7
Targeting Chromatin Control in Cancer

Recent advances have highlighted a new and exciting area for therapeutic intervention, namely, the interplay between the cell cycle and chromatin control. Chromatin is the DNA-proteinaceous material in which chromosomal DNA resides in the nucleus. The majority of chromatin proteins is composed of histones that assemble into nucleosomes, and thereby assist in DNA packaging and transcriptional control. The histone tail is subject to a variety of enzymatic modifications, including phosphorylation, acetylation, and methylation, and many of the critical enzymes responsible for these modifications have recently come to light. Histone deacetylases (HDACs) are responsible for removing acetyl groups from lysine residues in histones and many proteins involved in the cell cycle (Fig. 4).

From the perspective of cancer therapy, HDACs have gained recognition as an important target, which, in part, reflects the identification of proteins other than histones that are subject to acetylation control. The activity of cell cycle regulators including E2F, p53, and pRb is influenced by acetylation, and pRb controls E2F activity through the recruitment of chromatin-modifying enzymes, such as HDACs (Fig. 4). Several oncogenic proteins have altered recruitment of HDACs, which leads to aberrant gene transcription. This is exemplified by the fusion protein PML-RARα, which occurs through a chromosomal translocation in acute promyelocytic leukemia (APL). The PML-RARα fusion protein recruits HDAC and represses transcription, causing a block to differentiation and promoting the oncogenic phenotype in APL. Perhaps, not surprisingly, compounds that inhibit HDAC activity cause potent cell cycle effects and frequently induce apoptosis; encouraging results of HDAC inhibitor clinical trials have begun to validate HDAC enzymes as drug targets.

SAHA (suberoylanilide hydroxamic acid) is a small molecule HDAC inhibitor that has reached Phase II clinical trials for the treatment of solid and hematological malignancy, and a range of other HDAC inhibitors are gaining clinical acceptance, for example, PXD101 is a highly potent HDAC inhibitor that blocks proliferation of tumor cells and has entered clinical trials. In addition, a variety of studies have demonstrated the potential for synergy using combinations of HDAC inhibitors with several mechanistically distinct antitumor agents, such as SAHA, which together with radiotherapy, produces an additive effect in human prostate cancer spheroids. While HDAC inhibitors have yet to be completely validated, nevertheless, they do represent

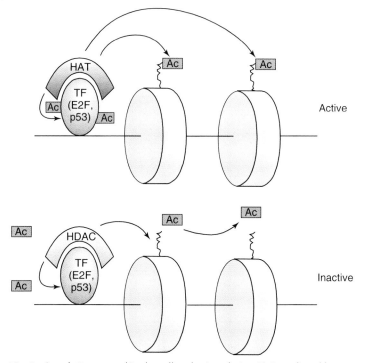

Fig. 4 Acetylation control in the cell cycle. Acetylation (Ac) mediated by acetyltransferases (HATS) can target histone tails in the form of nucleosomes (yellow) or transcription factors (TF) involved in cell cycle control, like E2F and p53. In most cases so far studied, acetylation appears to activate transcription. In contrast, deacetylation mediated by histone deacetylases (HDAC) causes transcriptional inactivity by targeting histones in nucleosomes, leading to a more transcriptionally inert state, together with dampening the activity of transcription factors. (See color plate p. xxi.)

a promising new approach to cancer treatment.

8
Regulating Hsp90

Heat shock protein 90 (Hsp90) is a molecular chaperone that regulates the activity of a variety of cellular proteins, enabling protein folding and preventing denaturation, and perhaps aggregation, of misfolded proteins. Hsp90 is gaining recognition as a cancer target in part because it is overexpressed in a variety of tumor cells and associates with oncoproteins including the tyrosine kinase v-Src, the serine/threonine kinase Raf1, HIF1 (discussed later), and mutated p53. A small molecule inhibitor of Hsp90, geldanamycin, blocks the interaction of Hsp90 with client proteins, including v-Src and Raf1, by interacting with the hydrophobic ATP-binding pocket in the N-terminal region and inhibiting the Hsp90 ATPase activity.

Geldanamycin has been used as a molecular probe to explore the regulation and composition of Hsp90. Two distinct sets of Hsp90 chaperone are endowed with opposing functions, reflecting the nucleotide occupying the binding pocket. When ATP is present, Hsp90 assembles with the cochaperone proteins p23 and p50^{Cdc37}, resulting in the stabilization of client proteins. In contrast, in the presence of ADP, Hsp90 assembles with a different set of proteins, including Hsp70 and p60^{Hop}, to promote client protein ubiquitination and degradation via the proteasome (Fig. 5). Binding of geldanamycin to the nucleotide pocket of Hsp90 locks Hsp90 in the form that favors client protein degradation. The mechanism through which Hsp90 causes the degradation of client proteins remains unclear, although E3 ligases that associate with Hsp90 and ubiquitinate some client proteins have been identified. Thus, Hsp90 complexes have opposing functions, and geldanamycin promotes formation of the degrading Hsp90 chaperone complex.

An interesting property of Hsp90 inhibitors observed in preclinical studies is the induction of cytostasis or apoptosis, depending on the cell-type. This may reflect the nature of the Hsp90 chaperone complex and the variation in target client proteins present in cells. Some evidence suggests that the integrity of pRb may dictate sensitivity to Hsp90 inhibition, as cells lacking pRb appear to be quite sensitive to inhibitor-induced apoptosis.

In preclinical studies, Hsp90 inhibitors have shown promising activity. While geldanamycin exhibits levels of hepato-toxicity

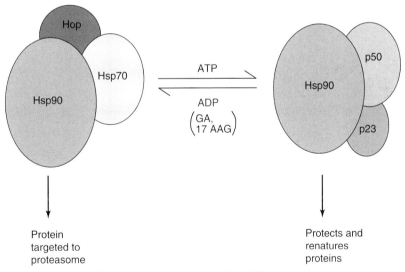

Fig. 5 Regulation of Hsp90 activity. Hsp90 can form different protein chaperone complexes with opposing activities. When ATP is bound to the nucleotide-binding pocket, assembly with p23 and p50^{Cdc37} occurs resulting in a chaperone complex that stabilizes and protects client proteins, whereas ADP in the pocket causes Hsp90 to assemble with Hsp70 and p60^{Hop}, resulting in client protein degradation via the proteasome. With geldanamycin (GA) or its derivative 17-allylaminogeldanamycin (17AAG), the chaperone assembles with Hsp70 and p60^{Hop} to favor client protein degradation.

that are too high for clinical application, the derivative 17-allylaminogeldanamycin (17AAG) exhibits improved efficacy, and has now reached phase I clinical trials.

In the clinical setting, if cytostasis were to be the primary outcome of treating a patient with an Hsp90 inhibitor, then sustained chronic administration of the drug may not be possible because of the associated toxicity profile. Conversely, if Hsp90 inhibition causes apoptosis upon short administration, then efficacy with limited toxicity may be achievable. As suggested by Neckers, this situation may be solved eventually by profiling the patient's tumor for the nature and expression level of Hsp90 client proteins. Combined with further information on the appropriate clinical schedule for Hsp90 inhibitors, it may be possible to identify and treat those tumors that will preferentially enter apoptosis upon inhibition of Hsp90 activity. This general principle could be important for other new agents, such as HDAC inhibitors.

9
Blocking Angiogenesis Through Inhibiting HIF1 Activity

Hypoxia-inducible factor 1 (HIF1) plays an important role in regulating angiogenesis by controlling the expression of genes linking vascular oxygen supply to metabolic demand. Tumor progression is associated with higher levels of vascularization that results from the increased synthesis of proangiogenesis factors and decreased synthesis of antiangiogenic factors, and angiogenesis progresses hand-in-hand with the adaptation of tumor cells to growth in low oxygen levels, by increasing glucose transport and glycolysis. HIF1 controls the activity of a variety of genes involved in

these processes; for example, the gene for vascular endothelial growth factor (VEGF), which is required for tumor angiogenesis, is regulated by HIF1. Similarly, target genes include glucose transporters GLUT1 and 3, together with enzymes involved in glycolysis like aldolase A and C, enolase 1, and hexokinase 1 and 3.

In cells, HIF1 exists as a heterodimer composed of HIF1α and HIF1β; HIF1β is constitutively expressed, whereas HIF1α is maintained at low levels in most cells under normoxic conditions. While HIF1α is regulated through a multistep process, a key event involves the hydroxylation of specific residues in an oxygen-dependent manner (Fig. 6). The modification of two prolyl residues (P402 and P564) mediates the binding of the von Hippel-Lindau (VHL) protein, which is the targeting component of an E3 ubiquitin ligase that confers degradation on HIF1 through the proteasomal pathway. In hypoxic conditions, prolyl hydroxylation becomes rate limiting, allowing HIF1α to escape degradation to favor increased levels of HIF1α. Further, Lando et al. identified a second hydroxylation-dependent control process occurring in the C-terminal transcriptional activation domain, where an asparagine residue (N803) is hydroxylated by an asparaginyl hydroxylase, which blocks the interaction with the p300 co-activator, again downregulating HIF activity (Fig. 6). Collectively, HIF1α activity is regulated by a series of oxygen-dependent posttranslational modifications mediated by three prolyl hydroxylases and one or more asparaginyl hydroxylases.

Increased activity of the HIF pathway is seen in many tumor types, resulting from the intratumoral hypoxia together with genetic alterations that affect HIF1 control. The impact of genetic alterations on the

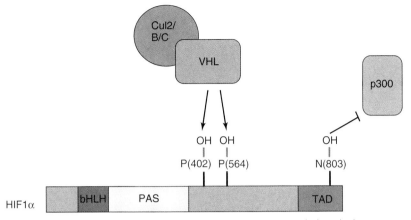

Fig. 6 Regulation of the HIFIα protein. The domains in HIFIα including the basic helix–loop–helix (bHLH) and PAS domains, required for dimerization and DNA binding and the C-terminal trans-activation domain are indicated. Hydroxylation of proline (P) residues at 402 and 564 is required for binding of the von Hippel-Lindau (VHL) tumor suppressor protein, which recruits an E3 ligase (Cul2/B/C complex) that degrades HIFIα. Hydroxylation of the asparagines (N) residue at 803 in the TAD prevents the interaction with p300 and downregulates HIF activity.

activity of HIF1 is influenced by the signal transduction pathway active in the tumor, and may involve pathways regulated by insulin, epidermal growth factor, Ras, or Src. In this respect, VHL is an important component of HIF1 regulation, and inactivation of VHL tumor suppressor activity in VHL hereditary cancer syndrome is characterized by a highly restricted cancer predisposition involving renal cell carcinoma, hemanglioblastoma, and pheochromocytoma. In many other tumors, HIF1α is commonly overexpressed, where its levels sometimes correlate with increased vascular density such as in brain tumors. In other cases, HIF1α overexpression is a marker for aggressive disease, such as cervical cancer. However, it should be borne in mind that HIF1α is not a universal marker for clinical outcome. In ovarian cancer, the overexpression of HIF1α with p53 is correlated with apoptosis, contrasting with the coexpression of HIF1α with mutant p53.

HIF1α is gaining increased acceptance as a potential therapeutic target. The antitumor effect of some chemotherapeutic agents may be derived from effects on the HIF1 pathway. For example, rapamycin inhibits hypoxia-induced HIF1 expression, most likely by blocking the serine/threonine FRAP kinase required for translation of HIF1 mRNA. Agents that target other signaling molecules in the PI3K-AKT-FRAP pathway would similarly be expected to alter HIF1 activity together with many other effects independent of HIF1.

To date, mechanism-based therapeutics that directly target HIF1 are not available. However, a recent Phase III trial supports the therapeutic value of agents that modulate angiogenesis in cancer therapy. The therapeutic antibody, Avastin^{TM}, designed to inhibit VEGF activity, which plays a critical role in tumor angiogenesis, provided a 50% increase in patient survival chance compared to patients receiving chemotherapy alone. While cancer therapies that inhibit angiogenesis remain in their infancy, clinical studies like the Avastin trial emphasize future potential.

10
Regulating Protein Turnover

Increasing evidence suggests that drugs that influence protein degradation may prove to be beneficial in cancer treatment. As we have discussed, protein degradation plays a crucial role in regulating cell viability, not only in the control of damaged proteins but also in controlling key regulatory processes. The turnover of many cell cycle regulatory proteins is required for normal cell cycle control, for example, the Cdk inhibitor p27 whose degradation is enhanced in certain tumor cells. Similarly, signaling to the NFκB transcription factor is dependent upon protein turnover of its specific inhibitor IκB, allowing NF-κB to activate a variety of genes including cytokines (like tumor necrosis factor) and antiapoptotic proteins.

The proteasome plays a central role in regulating protein turnover. The 26S proteasome is a large multiprotein complex composed of a 20S catalytic complex together with two 19S regulatory subunits that degrade proteins targeted by ubiquitination through the addition of ubiquitin to lysine residues. Ubiquitinated proteins are broken down to short peptides by the central subunit rings of the proteasome, which contain multiple active sites recognizing threonine as the catalytic residue (Fig. 7).

It has become increasingly clear that compounds that block proteasome function possess potential as anticancer agents.

The first compounds identified exhibited inappropriate pharmacokinetic properties but ultimately led to the generation of compounds with improved properties, including PS-341 (known as Velcade and developed by Millenium). Velcade has activity across a wide range of tumor cells but appears to act preferentially on tumor cells compared to normal cells. Myeloma cells undergo apoptosis when treated with Velcade, in contrast, for example, to normal bone marrow stromal cells, which exhibit a much reduced sensitivity profile.

Other promising properties of proteasome inhibitors relate to the potential utility in resistant disease. Velcade will arrest the growth of myeloma cells that are resistant to conventional chemotherapies, and overexpression of Bcl2 does not affect the sensitivity of myeloma to Velcade. Velcade was the first proteasome inhibitor to enter clinical trials in hematological malignancy and solid tumors. While the drug is rapidly cleared from plasma (over 90% clearance within 15 min of administration), early indications of efficacy were observed in Phase I trials. Efficacy was subsequently confirmed in a Phase II trial on patients with refractory multiple myeloma. Velcade has successfully completed Phase III clinical trials in multiple myeloma, and is the first proteasome inhibitor to be approved (by the US FDA), for multiple myeloma.

11
Conclusions and Perspectives

We are beginning to see subtle hints that exploiting mechanism-based approaches will deliver improved cancer medicines over many existing chemotherapeutics.

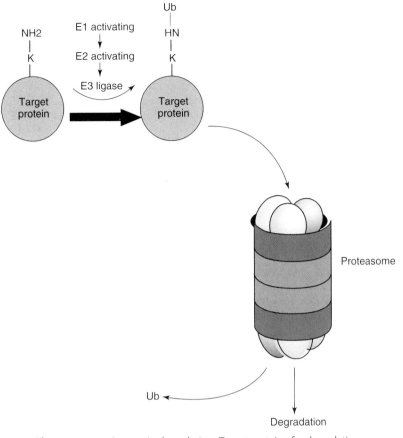

Fig. 7   The proteasome in protein degradation. Target proteins for degradation are ubiquitinated (Ub) at lysine (K) residues through a process involving a ubiquitin-activating enzyme (E1), the transfer of ubiquitin to a conjugating enzyme (E2), which is then transferred to a target protein by an E3 protein ligase. Polyubiquitinated proteins are then recognized and degraded by the 26S proteasome.

Both Gleevec and Valcade directed against the bcr-*abl* tyrosine kinase and the proteasome respectively have shown clinical efficacy. While we await further clinical results with Iressa, HDAC, Cdk, and Hsp90 inhibitor programs, we are left with the compelling view that improved therapies will also arise from these routes of enquiry.

Perhaps, it will be of greater significance to understand the clinical practice with these new cancer agents. Should these compounds be progressed as single agents or, which seems more likely, be applied as combination therapies perhaps with existing cytotoxic agents? It remains a significant hurdle to address this question, and to further provide scientific rationale in considering the array of possible combination options that could be studied. An interrelated question concerns the scheduling regime for administering the drug, particularly in combination therapies, which will reflect knowledge of the critical targets through which the inhibitor regulates cancer cell growth and the expression of these targets in the particular cancer type. In this respect, we have already discussed the different properties of Hsp90 inhibitors in apoptosis and cell cycle arrest, and how these properties could impact on the clinical regimen and perhaps require patient stratification for maximum clinical benefit.

The possibility of resistance to mechanism-based agents remains to be determined. Tumor cells are adept at acquiring drug resistance phenotypes through diverse mechanisms, and we have already seen clinical resistance to Gleevec, but we await further information before this becomes clinically exemplified for other new agents. Of course, if drug resistance does appear as a clinical hurdle, then it may be possible to modulate its progression by altering drug concentration and exposure through a combination therapy approach.

It is clear that many questions remain to be answered. Nevertheless, we are witnessing an exciting era in cancer drug discovery in which newer drugs are beginning to replace conventional cytotoxic approaches. Our views and anticipations, which are shared by many others, reflect the gathering momentum that translating research knowledge about the cancer cell will yield improved and more efficacious drugs for treating the cancer patient.

Acknowledgment

We thank Marie Caldwell for help in preparing the manuscript. Work in our laboratory was supported by the MRC, CRUK, LRF, AICR and EC.

See also Disposition and Clearance Prediction of Drug Bioavailability.

Bibliography

Books and Reviews

Adams, J., Palombella, V.J., Elliott, P.J. (2000) Proteasome inhibition: a new strategy in cancer treatment, *Invest. New Drugs* **18**, 109–121.

Brooks, G., La Thangue, N.B. (1999) The cell cycle and drug discovery: the promise and the hope, *Drug Discovery Today*, **4**, 455.

Demonacos, C., La Thangue, N.B. (2002) p53 and drug discovery, *PCCR* **5**, 375–382.

Faderl, S., Talpaz, M., Estrov, Z., Kantarjian, H.M. (1999) Chronic myelogenous leukaemia: biology and therapy, *Ann. Intern. Med.* **131**, 207–219.

Hanahan, D., Weinberg, R. (2000) The hallmarks of cancer, *Cell* **100**, 57–70.

McLaughlin, F., Finn, P., La Thangue, N.B. (2003) The cell cycle, chromatin and cancer: mechanism-based therapeutics come of age, *Drug Discovery Today* **8**, 793–802.

Neckers, L. (2002) Hsp90 inhibitors as novel cancer chemotherapeutic agents, *Trends Mol. Med.* **84** Suppl., S55–S61.

Semenza, G.L. (2001) Hypoxia-inducible factor 1: oxygen homeostasis and disease pathophysiology, *Trends Mol. Med.* **7**, 345–350.

Simon, M.A. (2000) Receptor tyrosine kinases: specific outcomes from general signals, *Cell* **103**, 13–15.

Workman, P., Kaye, S. (2002) Translating basic cancer research into new cancer therapeutics, *Trends Mol. Med.* **8**(()4 Suppl.), S1–S9.

Primary Literature

Agnew, E.B., Wilson, R.H., Grem, J.L. et al. (2001) Measurement of the novel anti-tumour agent 17-(allylamino)-17-demethoxygeldanamycin in human plasma by high-performance liquid chromatography, *J. Chromatogr., B.: Biomed. Sci. Appl.* **755**, 237–243.

Akiyama, T., Yoshida, T., Tsujita, T., et al. (1997) G1 phase accumulation induced by UCN-01 is associated with dephosphorylation of Rb and CDK2 proteins as well as induction of CDK inhibitor p21/Cip1/WAF1/Sdl1 in p53-mutated human epidermoid carcinoma A431 cells, *Cancer Res.* **576**, 1495–1501.

An, W.G., Schulte, T.W., Neckers, L.M. (2000) The heat-shock protein 90 antagonist geldanamycin alters chaperone association with p210bcr-abl and v-src proteins before their degradation by the proteasome, *Cell Growth Differ.* **11**, 355–360.

Anderson, P.G.A. (2003) A Phase 2 study of bortezomib in relapsed, refractory myeloma, *N. Engl. J. Med.* **348**, 2609–2617.

Bandara, L.R., Girling, R., LaThangue, N.B. (1997) Apoptosis induced in mammalian cells by small peptides that functionally antagonise the Rb-regulated E2F transcription factor, *Nat. Biotech.* **15**, 896–901.

Baselga, J. (2000) Continuous administration of ZD1839 (Iressa), a novel oral epidermal growth factor receptor tyrosine kinase inhibitor, in patients with five selected-tumour types: evidence of activity and good tolerability, *Proc. Am. Soc. Oncol.* **19**, 177a.

Baselga, J. (2001) The EGFR as a target for anticancer therapy-focus on cetuximab, *Eur. J. Cancer* **37**, S16–S22.

Birner, P., Schindl, M., Obermair, A., et al. (2000) Over-expression of hypoxia-inducible factor 1α is a marker for an unfavourable prognosis in early-stage invasive cervical cancer, *Cancer Res.* **60**, 4693–4696.

Birner, P., Schindl, M., Obermair, A., Breitenecker, G., Oberhuber, G. (2001a) Expression of hypoxia-inducible factor 1α in epithelial ovarian tumours: its impact on prognosis and on response to chemotherapy, *Clin. Cancer Res.* **7**, 1661–1668.

Birner, P., Gatterbauer, B., Oberhuber, G., et al. (2001b) Expression of hypoxia-inducible factor 1α in oligodendrogliomas: its impact on prognosis and on neoangiogenesis, *Cancer* **92**, 165–171.

Chan, H.-M., La Thangue, N.B. (2001) p300/CBP proteins: HATS for transcriptional bridges and scaffolds, *J. Cell Sci.* **114**, 2363–2373.

Chiarle, R., Budel, L.M., Skolnik, J., et al. (2000) Increased proteasome degradation of cyclin-dependent kinase inhibitor p27 is associated with a decreased overall survival in mantle cell lymphoma, *Blood* **95**, 619–626.

Ciardiello, F., Tortora, G. (2001) A novel approach in the treatment of cancer: targeting the epidermal growth factor receptor, *Clin. Cancer Res.* **7**, 2958–2970.

Connell, P., Ballinger, C.A., Jiang, J., et al. (2001) The co-chaperone CHIP regulates protein triage decisions mediated by heat-shock proteins, *Nat. Cell Biol.* **3**, 93–96.

Deininger, M.W., Goldman, J.M., Lydon, N., Melo, J.V. (1997) The tyrosine kinase inhibitor CGP57148B selectively inhibits the growth of BCR-ABL-positive cells, *Blood* **90**, 3691–3698.

Deininger, M.W., Goldman, J.M., Melo, J.V. (2000) The molecular biology of chronic myeloid leukaemia, *Blood* **96**, 3343–3356.

Druker, B.J., Lydon, N.B. (2000) Lessons learned from the development of an abl tyrosine inhibitor for chronic myelogenous leukaemia, *J. Clin. Invest.* **105**, 3–7.

Dyson, N. (1998) The regulation of E2F by pRB-family proteins, *Genes Dev.* **12**, 2245–2262.

Feinman, R., Gangurde, P., Miller, S., et al. (2001) Proteasome inhibitor PS-341 inhibits constitutive NF-KB activation and bypass the anti-apoptotic Bcl2 signal in human multiple myeloman cells, *Blood* **98**, 640a.

Foster, B.A. (1999) Pharmacological rescue of mutant p53 conformation and function, *Science* **286**, 2507–2510.

Friedler, A., Hansson, L.O., Veprintsev, D.B., et al. (2002) A peptide that binds and stabilizes p53 core domain: chaperone strategy for rescue of oncogenic mutants, *Proc. Natl. Acad. Sci. U.S.A.* **99**, 937–942.

Gorre, M.E., Mohammed, M., Ellwood, K., et al. (2001) Clinical resistance to STI-571 cancer therapy caused by BCR-ABL gene mutation or amplification, *Science* **293**, 876–880.

Hainaut, P. (2002) Tumour-specific mutations in p53: the acid test, *Nat. Med.* **8**, 21–23.

Hideshima, T., Richardson, P., Chauhan, D., et al. (2001) The proteasome inhibitor PS-341 inhibits growth, induces apoptosis, and overcomes drug resistance in human multiple myeloma cells, *Cancer Res.* **61**, 3071–3076.

Hochhaus, A., Kreil, S., Corbin, A., et al. (2001) Roots of clinical resistance to ATI-571 cancer therapy, *Science* **293**, 2136.

Hockel, M., Vaupel, P. (2001) Tumour hypoxia: definitions and current clinical, biologic, and molecular aspects, *J. Natl. Cancer Inst.* **93**, 266–276.

Hollstein, M., Hergennahn, M., Yang, Q. et al. (1999) New approaches to understanding p53 gene tumour mutation spectra, *Mutat. Res.* **431**, 199–209.

Honma, T., Yoshizumi, T., Hashimoto, N., et al. (2001) A novel approach for the development of selective cdk4 inhibitors: library design based on location of cdk4 specific amino acid residues, *J. Med. Chem.* **44**, 4628–4640.

Hostein, I., Robertson, D., DiStefano, F., Workman, P., Clarke, P.A. (2001) Inhibition of signal transduction by the Hsp90 inhibitor 17-allylamino-17-demethoxygeldanamycin results in cytostasis and apoptosis, *Cancer Res.* **61**, 4003–4009.

Ivan, M., Kondo, K., Yang, H., et al. (2001) HIFα targeted for VHL-mediated destruction by proline hydroxylation: implications for O_2 sensing, *Science* **292**, 464–468.

Jaakkola, P., Mole, D.R., Tian, Y.M., et al. (2001) Targeting of HIF-α to the von Hippel-Lindau ubiquitylation complex by O_2-regulated prolyl hydroxylation, *Science* **292**, 468–472.

Kantarjian, H. (2000) Phase II study of ST1571, a tyrosine kinase inhibitor, in patients with resistant or refractory Philadelphia chromosome positive chronic myeloid leukaemia, *Blood* **96**, 470a.

Ko, L., Prives, C. (1996) p53: puzzle and paradigm, *Genes Dev.* **10**, 1054–1072.

Komarov, P.G., Komarova, E.A., Kondratov, R.V., et al. (1999) A chemical inhibitor of p53 that protects mice from the side effects of cancer therapy, *Science* **285**, 1733–1737.

Kouzarides, T. (1999) Histone acetylases in cell proliferation, *Curr. Opin. Genet. Dev.* **9**, 40–48.

Lando, D., Peet, D.J., Whelan, D.A., Gorman, J.J., Whitelaw, M.L. (2002) Asparagine hydroxylation of the HIF transactivation domain: a hypoxic switch, *Science* **295**, 858–861.

Laughner, E., Taghavi, P., Chiles, K., Mahon, P.C., Semenza, G.L. (2001) HER2 (neu) signalling increases the rate of hypoxia-inducible factor 1α (HIF1α) synthesis: novel mechanism for HIF-1 mediated vascular endothelial growth factor expression, *Mol. Cell. Biol.* **21**, 3995–4004.

Laurence, V., Faivre, S., Vera, K., et al. (2002) Preliminary results of an ongoing phase 1 and pharmacokinetic study of CYC202, a novel oral cyclin-dependent kinases inhibitor, in patients with advanced malignancies, *Eur. J. Cancer* **38**, S49.

Li, Y., Sun, X., Lamout, J.T., Pardee, A.B., Li, C.J. (2003) Selective killing of cancer cells by beta-lapachone; direct checkpoint activation as a strategy against cancer, *Proc. Natl. Acad. Sci. U.S.A.* **100**, 2674–2678.

Lin, R.J., Nagy, L., Inoue, S., Shao, W., Miller, W.H. Jr., Evans, R.M. (1998) Role of the histone deacetylase complex in acute promyelocytic leukaemia, *Nature* **391**, 811–814.

Manegold, C. (2003) Gefitinib (Iressa, ZD 1839) for non-small cell lung cancer (NSCLC): recent results and further strategies, *Adv. Exp. Med. Biol.* **532**, 247–252.

Mann, M.J., Whittemore, A.D., Donaldson, M.D., et al. (2001) Ex-vivo gene therapy of human vascular bypass grafts with E2F decoy: the PREVENT single centre, randomised, controlled trial, *Lancet* **354**, 1493.

Marks, P.A., Rifkind, R.A., Richon, V.M., Breslow, R. (2001) Inhibitors of histone deacetylases are potentially effective anticancer agents, *Clin. Cancer Res.* **7**, 759–760.

McCarthy, M. (2003) Anti-angiogenesis drug promising for metastatic colorectal cancer, *Lancet* **361**, 1959.

McClue, S.J., Blake, D., Clarke, R., et al. (2002) *In vitro* and *in vivo* anti-tumour properties of the cyclin-dependent kinase inhibitor CYC202 (R-Roscovitine), *Int. J. Cancer* **102**, 463–468.

Montigiani, S., Müller, R., Kontermann, R.E. (2003) Inhibition of cell proliferation and induction of apoptosis by novel tetravalent peptides inhibiting DNA binding of E2F, *Oncogene* **22**, 4943–4952.

Moulder, S.L., Yakes, F.M., Muthuswamy, S.K., Bianco, R., Simpson, J.F., Arteaga, C.L. (2001) Epidermal growth factor receptor (HER1) tyrosine kinase inhibitor ZD1839 (Iressa) inhibits HER2/neu (erbB2)-over-expressing breast cancer cells *in vitro* and *in vivo*, *Cancer Res.* **61**, 8887–8895.

Nguyen, V.T., Kiss, T., Michels, A.A., Bensaude, O. et al. (2001) The 7SK small nuclear RNA inhibits the CDK9/cyclinT1 kinase to control transcription, *Nature* **414**, 322–325.

Nimmanapalli, R., O'Bryan, E., Bhalla, K. (2001) Geldanamycin and its analogue 17-allylamino-17-demethoxygeldanamycin lowers Bcr-Abl levels and induces apoptosis and differentiation of Bcr-Abl-positive human leukaemic blasts, *Cancer Res.* **61**, 1799–1804.

Nix, D., Pien, C., Newman, R., et al. (2001) Clinical development of a proteasome inhibitor, PS-341, for the treatment of cancer, *Proc. Am. Soc. Clin. Oncol.* **20**, 86a.

Papandreou, C., Daliani, D., Millikan, R.E., et al. (2001) Phase I study of intravenous (I.V.) proteasome inhibitor PS-341 in patients (Pts) with advanced malignancies, *Proc. Am. Soc. Clin. Oncol.* **20**, 86a.

Plumb, J.A., Finn, P.W., Williams, R.J., et al. (2003) Inhibition of human tumour cell growth by the novel histone deacetylase inhibitor PXD101, *Mol. Cancer Ther.* **2**, 721–728.

Scheibel, T., Buchner, J. (1998) The Hsp90 complex – a super-chaperone machine as a novel drug target, *Biochem. Pharmacol.* **56**, 675–682.

Seidman, A.D., Fornier, M.N., Esteva, F.J., et al. (2001) Weekly trastuzumab and paclitaxel therapy for metastatic breast cancer with analysis of efficacy by HER2 immunophenotype and gene amplification, *J. Clin. Oncol.* **19**, 2587–2595.

Selivanova, G., Ryabchenko, L., Jansson, E., Iotsova, V., Wiman, K.G. (1998) Reactivation of mutant p53: a new strategy for cancer therapy, *Semin. Cancer Biol.* **8**, 369–378.

Sgouros, G., Yang, W.-H., Richon, V.M., Kelly, W.K., Rifkind, R.A., Marks, P.A. (2002) Synergistic interaction of suberoylanillde hydroxamic acid (SAHA) and radiation in human prostate tumour spheroids, *Proc. Am. Soc. Clin. Oncol.* **2**, 105.

Sherr, C.J., Roberts, J.M. (1999) CDK inhibitors: positive and negative regulators of cyclin-dependent regulators of G1-phase progression, *Genes Dev.* **13**, 1501–1512.

Slamon, D.J., Leyland-Jones, B., Shak, S., et al. (2001) Use of chemotherapy plus a monoclonal antibody against HER2 for metastatic breast cancer that over-expresses HER2, *N. Engl. J. Med.* **344**, 783–792.

Stancato, L.F., Silverstein, A.M., Owens-Grillo, J.K., Chow, Y.H., Jove, R., Pratt, W.B. (1997). The hsp90-binding antibiotic geldanamycin decreases Raf levels and epidermal growth factor signaling without disrupting formation of signaling complexes or reducing the specific enzymatic activity of Raf kinase, *J. Biol. Chem.* **272**, 4013–4020.

Stinchcombe, T.E., Mitchell, B.S., Depcik-Smith, N., et al. (2000) PS-341 is active in multiple myeloma: preliminary report of a phase I trial of the proteasome inhibitor PS-341 in patients with hematologic malignancies, *Blood* **96**, 516a.

Strahl, B.D., Allis, C.D. (2000) The language of covalent histone modifications, *Nature* **403**, 41–45.

Srethapakdi, M., Liu, F., Tavorath, R., Rosen, N. (2000) Inhibition of Hsp90 function by ansamycins causes retinoblastoma gene product-dependent G1 arrest, *Cancer Res.* **60**, 3940–3946.

Stebbins, C.E., Russo, A.A., Schneider, C., Rosen, N., Hartl, F.U., Pavletich, N.P. (1997) Crystal structure of an Hsp90-geldanamycin complex: targeting of a protein chaperone by an antitumour agent, *Cell* **89**, 239–250.

Thomas, J.P., Tutsch, K.D., Cleary, J.F., et al. (2002) Phase I clinical and pharmacokinetic trial of the cyclin-dependent kinase inhibitor flavopiridol, *Cancer Chemother. Pharmacol.* **50**, 465–472.

Van Oosterom, A.T., Judson, I., Verweij, J., et al. (2001) STI571, an active drug in metastatic gastrointestinal stromal tumours (GIST), an EORTC Phase 1 study, *Proc. Am. Soc. Clin. Oncol.* **20**, 1a.

Xu, Y., Lindquist, S. (1997) Heat-shock protein hsp90 governs the activity of pp60v-src kinase, *Proc. Natl. Acad. Sci. U.S.A.* **90**, 7074–7078.

Wang, C.Y., Mayo, M.W., Korneluk, R.G., Goeddel, D.V., Baldwin, A.S. Jr. (1998) NF-KB anti apoptosis: induction of TRAF1 and TRAF2 and c-IAP1 and c-IAP2 to suppress caspase 8 activation, *Science* **281**, 1680–1683.

Wu, L., Timmers, C., Maiti, B., et al. (2001) The E2F1-3 transcription factors are essential for cellular proliferation, *Nature* **414**, 457–462.

Zagzag, D., Zhong, H., Scalzitti, J.M., Laughner, E., Simons, J.W., Semenza, G.L. (2000) Expression of hypoxia inducible factor 1α in brain tumours: association with angiogenesis, invasion, and progression, *Cancer* **88**, 2606–2618.

Zhong, H., Chiles, K., Feldser, D., et al. (1999) Over-expression of hypoxia-inducible factor 1α in common human cancers and their metastases, *Cancer Res.* **59**, 5830–5835.

Zhong, H., De Marzo, A.M., Laughner, E., et al. (2000) Modulation of HIF1α expression by the epidermal growth factor phosphatidylinositol 3 kinase/PTEN/AKT/FRAP pathway in human prostate cancer cells: implications for tumour angiogenesis and therapeutics, *Cancer Res.* **60**, 1541–1545.

24
Antitumor Steroids

Guy Leclercq
Institut J. Bordet, Université Libre de Bruxelles, Brussels, Belgium

1   **Background   776**

2   **Steroid Hormone Receptors   777**
2.1   Structure and Conformation of the Hormone Binding Domains   777
2.2   Conformational Changes of Ligand-binding Domains Induced by
         Agonists or Antagonists   778

3   **Restrictive Conditions for Efficient Targeting of Antitumor Estrogens   781**
3.1   Main Structural Requirements for Estradiol Binding   782
3.1.1   A-ring   782
3.1.2   B-ring   782
3.1.3   C-ring   782
3.1.4   D-ring   783
3.2   Nucleocytoplasmic Shuttle of Estrogen Receptors   783
3.3   Ligand-induced Regulation of Estrogen Binding Capacity   784
3.4   Ligand-induced Regulation of Estrogen Receptor Level   785

4   **Antitumor Estrogens   785**
4.1   Organometallic Estradiol Derivatives   786
4.1.1   A-ring Complexion   786
4.1.2 7α and 11β Derivatives   787
4.1.3 17α Derivatives   787
4.2   Radiolabeled Estradiol Derivatives   789
4.2.1 ^{123}I and ^{125}I Labeled Compounds   790
4.2.2 α-Emitting Compounds   791
4.3   Electrophilic 11β Derivative   792

         Bibliography   793
         Books and Reviews   793
         Primary Literature   793

Pharmacology. From Drug Development to Gene Therapy. Edited by Robert A. Meyers.
Copyright © 2008 Wiley-VCH Verlag GmbH & Co. KGaA, Weinheim
ISBN: 978-3-527-32343-2

Keywords

Steroid Hormones
Lipophilic hormones (lipid-soluble) which derive from cholesterol and act through association with their cognate receptors (specific nuclear receptors for each class of hormones, i.e. estrogens, androgens, progestins, gluco- and mineralocorticoids).

Nuclear Receptor
Large family of ligand-dependent transcription factors (peptides able to modulate the expression of genes).

Targeting
Modality to selectively deliver a compound to a given cell type or tissue to produce a biological effect only at his level.

1
Background

Steroid hormones once secreted are transported through the blood by proteins such as albumin or sex hormone binding globulin to be delivered to specific receptors located in various tissues, including tumors. Hence, steroid hormones appear as attractive vectors that might be used to achieve a selective targeting of anti-neoplastic drugs, at least in hormone-dependent cancer, which contains high amounts of receptors (i.e. breast, prostate etc.). While association of these drugs with receptors is obviously of major importance, their binding ability to transport proteins may also play a role (i.e. albumin localize at the tumor due to enhanced vascular permeability).

Such a concept is obviously not new. High doses of steroid hormones are indeed routinely used for the treatment of various endocrine disorders. Synthetic antagonists aimed to specifically block the action of their receptors or/and metabolic enzymes have also been in clinical practice since a long time. With specific regard to neoplasia, antiestrogens, antiprogestins, as well as aromatase inhibitors (enzymes that convert androgens to estrogens) are drugs of prominent importance for the treatment of breast cancer. Therapeutic effectiveness as well as mechanism of action of such compounds has been the subject of a large number of reviews and will therefore not be addressed here. Potential utility of steroidal derivatives aimed to selectively kill tumor cells (i.e. "antitumor steroids") will solely be analyzed.

In fact, during the last 30 years, several investigators prepared a large number of steroids bearing cytotoxic molecules (e.g. alkylating agents, nitrosoureas, *cis*-platinum complexes, intercalating agents, etc.). Unfortunately, such syntheses led almost always to drugs devoid of therapeutic interest primarily due to the fact that their cytotoxic groups were not linked in appropriate positions onto the steroids, leading to a drastic loss of the binding affinity of the latter for their cognate receptors with concomitant decrease of cellular uptake. Moreover, for the few compounds that overpass this limiting step, specific killing of tumor cells was rarely observed in cell culture

Fig. 1 Chemical formula of estramustine phosphate (Estracyt).

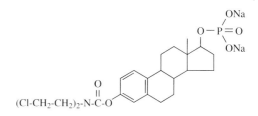

(receptor-positive vs receptor-negative cell lines) precluding their potential testing in clinical trials. Metabolistic instability of compounds also precludes their use. In fact, out of the hundreds of compounds synthesized, estramustine phosphate (Estracyt) (Fig. 1) is the only one having a place in the therapeutic arsenal (treatment of advanced prostatic cancer).

The growing number of experimentally determined crystal structures of ligand-binding domains of steroid hormone receptors provided a theoretical basis for the synthesis of a new generation of cytotoxic-linked steroids having a chance to associate with their cognate receptor. It is our purpose to focus on this topic. First, we will rapidly describe the structural determinants that govern the interactions of a ligand with its receptor, with special emphasis on estrogens and antiestrogens. Major advances in the synthesis of cytotoxic-linked estrogens in comparison with other classes of steroids justify this option. Next, we will move to the description of estrogen derivatives with potential antitumor activity.

2
Steroid Hormone Receptors

2.1
Structure and Conformation of the Hormone Binding Domains

Steroid hormone receptors are members of a superfamily of nuclear receptors, which regulate the expression of gene involved in cell proliferation and/or differentiation. All these receptors encode various domains with specific functions (A/B, C, D, E, and F; Fig. 2). The N-terminal A/B domain of each receptor contains a ligand-independent activation function (AF-1) required for the transcriptional activation of target genes. The adjacent C-domain contains two zinc fingers, which play an important role in DNA sequence-specific bindings (association with specific response elements). The D-domain is a hinge region, which separates ABC domains from the hormone binding domain (HBD; domain E). This binding domain contains a ligand-dependent activation function (AF-2) located in its carboxy-terminal part, a third additional AF-site located on the amino-terminal part of the HBD has been reported in the gluco and estrogen receptors (AF-2b). The C-terminal part of the receptors (end of domain E and F) is involved in the regulation of their half-life (proteolysis) and transcriptional activity.

Binding of a steroidal hormone to its receptor always provokes a conformational change in the latter that allows, ultimately, the transcription of target genes. Receptor molecules, in homo- and heterodimeric associations, exert their transcriptional effect through interaction with response elements located in the promoter region of these genes; alternatively, they may operate via their interaction with other classes of DNA-bound transcription factors (i.e. AP1,

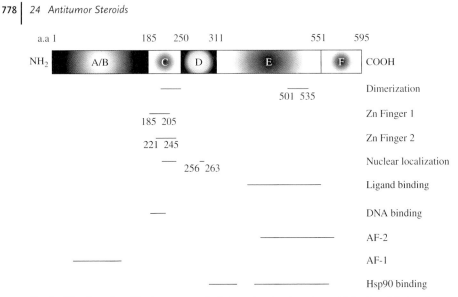

Fig. 2 ERα domains. ERα is composed of six molecular domains, which allow it to localize into the nucleus, dimerize, bind to ligand and DNA, and regulate the transcription through hormone-independent (AF-1) and hormone-dependent (AF-2) mechanisms.

Sp1 etc.). Transcription requires nuclear proteins (coactivators) that are recruited by the DNA-bound receptors. Coactivators vary among tissues eventually giving rise to tissue-specific responses to a given hormonal stimulation. Antagonists repress transcription by a reverse process (blockade of association with response elements and/or recruitment of corepressors).

AF1 expression is regulated by growth factors via classical signal transduction cascades while AF2 (and apparently AF-2b) is entirely dependent on the association of the receptor with the ligand. Under most conditions, the ligand induces a functional synergism between AF1 and AF2 due to major reorganization in the tertiary structure of the receptor. HBD contains 12α-helices (H1–H12) folded into a 3-layered antiparallel α-helical sandwich. The central core of the HBD layer contains 3α-helixes (H5/6, H9, and H10) sandwiched between 2 additional layers of helices composed of H1–4, H7, H8,

and H11; it is flanked by H12, which contains the core region of AF2. Agonists elicit a receptor conformation of the HBD so that H12 is aligned over the hormone binding cavity; the formation of a salt bridge between H4 and H12 stabilizes the reposition of the latter. This main conformational change results in the emergence of a specific binding site (a groove) for a consensus α-helical motif (LxxLL, "NR" box) found in coactivators. Antagonists sterically interfere with H12 positioning thereby preventing recruitment of coactivators and favoring binding of corepressors.

2.2
Conformational Changes of Ligand-binding Domains Induced by Agonists or Antagonists

HBD structure of each steroidal hormone receptor has been established by amino acid labeling with reactive ligands, site-directed mutageneses, hydrophobic cluster analyses, motif-based searches for homology with other proteins of known structures, and crystallographic studies. All HBDs are hydrophobic pockets, except at subsites corresponding to polar centers of cognate hormones; virtually, amino acids of these binding pockets surround the steroids. HBDs are somehow flexible in order to accommodate various ligands. Enlargement of a subsite results from the conformational reorganization of the whole HBD upon ligand binding: occupation of one subsite may modify the flexibility at a second subsite indicating that they respond to the ligand as a whole entity. Subsites are flexible because HBDs are composed of polypeptide segments rich in amino acid residues with mobile side chains (e.g. lysine, methionine, etc.).

Interaction of a steroidal hormone (or any synthetic ligand) with its cognate receptor depends upon several parameters (size, shape, polarity of atoms within the steroidal rings, etc.). Polar functions located at the extremities of the steroidal core (pos. 3 et 17) are of prominent

importance for the onset of a biological function, as illustrated hereunder by the binding of estradiol (E_2) and the partial antiestrogen hydroxytamoxifen (OH-Tam) to the estrogen receptor (α-isoform).

Most important amino acids involved in the binding of E_2 to the ER-HBD are Glu353 and Arg394 on the one hand, His524 on the other hand: Glu353 and Arg394 interact with the C_3 phenolic group of the hormone (H-bridge, participation of an H_2O molecule) while His524 interacts with 17β oxygen (Fig. 3). As stated above, location of E_2 within the HBD leads to a displacement of H12 favoring the access of coactivators to their binding site; virtually H12 surrounds E_2 and shields the pocket where it is locked from the environment ("closed conformation").

OH-Tam (Fig. 4) is a triphenylethylenic derivative of prominent importance for the treatment of ER-positive breast cancer; aminoalkyl side chain of the compound is responsible for its antiestrogenic (and cytostatic/cytotoxic) activity. Phenolic group of the drug (pos. 4) interacts with Glu353 and Arg394, as the C_3 phenolic group of E_2.

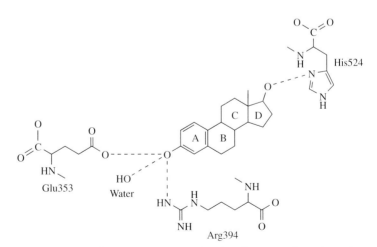

Fig. 3 Docking of E_2 in the ERα-HBD. The phenolic A-ring of E_2 is located in the HBD by Glu353 and Arg394 and tethered by His524.

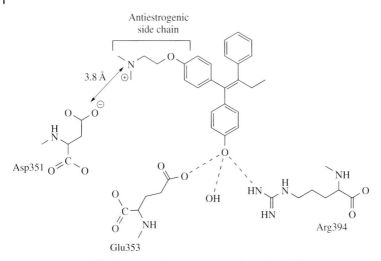

Fig. 4 Docking of OH-Tam (partial antiestrogen) in the ERα-HBD. The phenolic ring of OH-Tam is located in the HBD by Glu353 and Arg394, in analogy with the A-ring of E_2 (see Fig. 3). The nitrogen atom of the amino alkyl side chain of OH-Tam weakly interacts with Asp351. This interaction seems to be the key to the antagonistic activity of the compound.

However, in the hormone binding pocket, binding of OH-Tam to ER promotes a conformational change differing from that driven by E_2 inasmuch as the orientation of H12 appears essentially different. In the OH-Tam–ER complex, H12 is oriented in such a way that it maintains the pocket wide open, allowing the specific interaction of the nitrogen atom of the side chain of OH-Tam with a residue of the binding pocket (Asp351). In this "open conformation", which is stabilized by the side chain of the antiestrogen, H12 occupies a part of a coactivator binding site, which normally becomes accessible upon E_2 exposure. As a consequence, OH-Tam-associated H12 reorientation abrogates the recruitment of coactivators perhaps in favor of corepressors (AF-2 silencing). Hence, interaction between the side chain of OH-Tam and Asp351 seems to be the key to the antagonistic activity of the compound. Note that this open conformation of the HBD allows

the expression of other transcriptional activating sites (AF-1 and to some extent AF-2b) explaining the partial estrogenicity of OH-Tam.

OH-Tam belongs to an important class of clinically relevant compounds, recognized now as *selective estrogen receptor modulators* (SERMs). These compounds act as antagonists or agonists, depending on the cellular type promoters and coregulators (ER isoform is also of importance). A second class of antagonists, (ICI 182,780, ICI 164,384 and RU 58,668; Fig. 5) are capable of completely blocking the transcriptional activity of ER via the inhibition of both AF1 and AF2 action. One may speculate that these "pure antiestrogens" could play an important role as a second-line therapy against advanced breast cancer in patients who develop resistance to tamoxifen treatment. They correspond to 7α or 11β derivatives of E_2 in which specific reactive groups are linked to the steroidal moiety

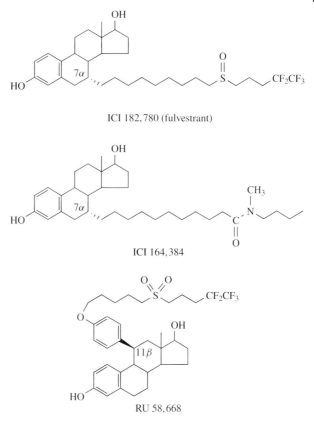

Fig. 5 Chemical formulas of pure antiestrogens.

through a long alkyl side chain intended to protrude out of the HBD when bound to the receptor (as the side chain of OH-Tam and related SERMs). The resulting conformational state of the receptor is, however, slightly different from that elicited by all investigated SERMs, although their long alkyl side chain similarly abrogate the alignment of H-12 onto the steroidal core.

3
Restrictive Conditions for Efficient Targeting of Antitumor Estrogens

To utilize steroid hormones as effective delivery vector of cytotoxic drugs to the tumor cells, several conditions should be satisfied. Concerning the association of the compounds with their receptors, we stress the need for the following four conditions:

1. It is important to link the cytotoxic agent in such a way as to not interfere with the recognition of the steroidal vector.
2. The cytotoxic moiety should be shipped to its target. Since receptors focalize their action at the genomic level, drugs to be linked to the steroid are restricted to those producing damage at the DNA level or associated nuclear proteins.

3. The compounds should not produce a rapid loss of binding ability of their steroidal vector.
4. The concentration of receptors should be sufficiently high to produce an effective cellular uptake of the cytotoxic moiety. This concentration should be maintained until this cytotoxic moiety has reached its target, potential degradation of the receptor (downregulation) induced by the steroidal vector should be limited.

The following paragraphs analyze how such conditions could be satisfied for (anti)estrogenic conjugates.

3.1
Main Structural Requirements for Estradiol Binding

The main and unique characteristic of E_2 is its lack of binding affinity for steroid hormone receptors other than its own receptor. The phenolic group in C_3, not recorded in the other steroid hormone, generates this big difference. Binding data of E_2 and derivatives led to the following conclusions.

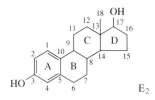

3.1.1 **A-ring**
C_1 is intolerant of both hydrophobic and polar substituents, suggesting close contacts with the HBD. The hydroxy group in C_3 donates a proton to Glu353 and Arg394 (see above), and this bond is donated *syn* to the C_2–C_3 bond. C_4 may be in close proximity to a

cysteine residue, based on inactivation assays of the receptor by 4-mercuri-E_2. The A-ring electron cloud may be engaged in a weak polar interaction with a slightly positively charged receptor residue, situated on the β-face of the steroid.

3.1.2 **B-ring**
C_6 seems to be intolerant for both polar and nonpolar substituents, once again suggesting close interaction of this area to the receptor essential spatial volume. Large aliphatic chains at $C_{7\alpha}$ are well tolerated (i.e. pure antiestrogens ICI 164,384 and ICI 182,780; Fig. 5), they localize within a subsite of the HBD accepting 11β nonpolar substituents (rotation of the E_2 core around a virtual symmetry axis that runs roughly through C_3 and C_{17}). Positions in $C_{7\beta}$ and $C_{8\alpha}$ are unexplored and $C_{9\alpha}$ has low steric tolerance.

3.1.3 **C-ring**
A preformed hydrophobic subsite of the HBD has a high steric tolerance for 11β residues. It can accommodate aromatic substituents bearing aliphatic side chains (pure antiestrogen RU 58,668; Fig. 5) while still retaining high affinity; it is intolerant of polar groups. The covalent binding of tamoxifen aziridine has suggested an accessible receptor nucleophile in $C_{11\beta}$ vicinity; such a hypothesis was rejected since 11β-methyl aziridine estradiol does not covalently label ER. Moreover, 11β-chloromethyl and bromoacetyl analogs also fail to covalently label the receptor. The 11β-chloromethyl substituent of E_2 produces, however, a *quasi*-irreversible binding of the hormone with the receptor. Interaction of the chloride atom with a putative

Zn^{++} ion located within the receptor has been proposed to explain this extremely high binding affinity; hydrophobic interaction with a tryptophane or phenylalanine has been advocated as an alternative hypothesis. The 12β-site accommodates small nonpolar groups as methyl; otherwise, C_{12} has been scarcely investigated.

3.1.4 D-ring

C_{14} can accept small, nonpolar groups at the α- or β-sites without appreciable loss of binding affinity. C_{15} is intolerant of small hydrophobic substituents (methyl) or replacement with oxygen. $C_{16\alpha}$ accommodates large nonpolar groups (e.g. iodine), but $C_{16\beta}$ is sterically less accessible, and even fluorine substitution decreases the binding affinity substantially. ER accepts small nonpolar groups in $C_{17\alpha}$ or groups in which the extended bulk should be directed in an endo manner, for example, $Z-CH{=}CHI$ binds more effectively than the corresponding E-isomer. Spatial tolerances of this area are precise, because even an ethyl group at this position results in significant loss of binding affinity; this effect may be secondary to alteration of rotation of the 17β-hydroxyl group. The 17β-hydroxyl group acts as a H-bond acceptor from His524. There may be a lysine and two cysteine residues (one positioned on each face of the steroid) in the vicinity of C_{15}-C_{16}-C_{17}, based on the reactivity of E_2 derivatives bearing covalently labeling groups. The 18-methyl group is not a significant contributor to binding, indicating no productive contact with the receptor at this site.

Data summarized here define localizations for grafting of a cytotoxic compound onto estradiol.

1. Positions 7α and 11β appear especially appropriate for large substituents without provoking a dramatic loss of binding affinity. In fact, this has been proved by linkage of a porphyrin in position 11β through a side chain. Linkage on 7α or 11β would localize the substituent within the same region of the receptor: the steroid may indeed rotate around a virtual symmetry axis between C_3 and C_{17}. Hence, 7α and 11β seem quite equivalent for grafting a side chain bearing a cytotoxic compound. Flexibility of such chains does not appear of prime importance as revealed by the study of mobile $[(CH_2)_n]$ or inflexible $[(CF_2)_n]$ spacers.

2. Substitution in 17α may also be recommended, provided that a short spacer is introduced between E_2 and the cytotoxic compound to maintain an effective binding affinity. Ethynyl and vinyl groups are especially accurate since they give an effective separation without excessive conformational flexibility. Directing these substituents away from the β-face of the steroid (side of the 17 OH) is required to limit steric interference with the binding pocket.

3.2
Nucleocytoplasmic Shuttle of Estrogen Receptors

Nuclear receptors are "translocating binding proteins," which continuously move between the cytoplasm and the cell nucleus (shuttling mechanism). The nuclear localization, however, always dominates especially under agonist stimulation (a dynamic event resulting from the continuous active transport of the receptor into the nucleus, slightly counterbalanced by its diffusion into the cytoplasm). Receptor detection in the cytosol of extracts from unstimulated cells may derive from its nuclear release at the time of homogenization.

Conveyance of ER into the cell nucleus is governed by specific amino acid sequences and nuclear localization signals (NLSs) situated between its DNA and hormone binding domains (HBDs) (hinge region). The existence of nuclear export signals (NESs) has also been reported; both NESs and NLSs play an important role in nuclear export of the steroid receptors. Nuclear uptake of receptors requires ATP, while nuclear export apparently occurs in the absence of energy production.

Investigations performed on ER-transfected cells revealed an additional subnuclear movement of the receptor under ligand stimulations. E_2 changes the receptor pattern from a diffuse nucleoplasmic aspect to a hyper-speckled distribution, suggesting that the ligand-dependent organization of the receptors within the nuclear matrix involves more complex events than a simple recognition of DNA-binding sites and coregulators. Interestingly, such a hyper-speckled distribution also occurs with the partial antiestrogen OH-Tam, while a substantial effect is solely detected with the pure antagonist ICI 182,780. In this context, it should be stressed that several other investigations localize the receptor within the cytoplasm under exposure to pure antiestrogens. Hence, the cellular localization of the receptor under pure antiestrogens is still not established, although the tendency for a major distribution within the cytoplasm dominates (when downregulation does not occur, see Sect. 3.4).

Concepts outlined here suggest that linkage of cytotoxic residues aimed at altering DNA and associated proteins should be restricted to estrogens (and SERM), pure antiestrogen having only a chance to strongly associate to the nuclear matrix.

3.3
Ligand-induced Regulation of Estrogen Binding Capacity

Shuttling of ER between the cytoplasm and the nucleus influences its ligand-binding ability. The nuclear localization of a receptor is associated with a loss of ligand-binding ability, which is restored by its return into the cytoplasm (dephosphorylation/phosphorylation cycle). After several cycles, ER is degraded by the proteasomal pathway, most probably into the cytoplasm (half-life 3 ~ 4 h); ubiquitination of the receptor favors its shipment to the proteasome. Inhibitors of protein synthesis (cycloheximide, puromycin) interfere with this mechanism leading to a stabilization of the receptor within the cell nucleus in a form devoid of strong ligand-binding ability.

As stated above (Sect. 2.2), E_2 is stably incorporated within the HBD, decreasing the chance of exchange with unbound ligands (closing of the binding pocket). Such a property fixes the majority of the receptor molecules into a conformation appropriate for a specific anchorage within the cell nucleus (hyper-specked pattern) to accomplish functions imposed by the hormone. A progressive decrease of estrogen binding capacity subsequently occurs. As expected, this decrease is closely related to the binding affinity of the estrogen for the receptor, which is a major determinant of its nuclear stabilization. One may anticipate that this receptor form, unable to bind the hormone is subjected to a return into the cytoplasm to be recycled or degraded.

Partial antiestrogens (OH-Tam and related SERMs), which maintain the HBD in an open conformation, accumulate the receptor within the nucleus in which it progressively loses its ability to bind estradiol. Blockade of the proteasomal degradation of ER by these antagonists associated with maintenance of its synthesis (see Sect. 3.4), explains this accumulation process.

3.4
Ligand-induced Regulation of Estrogen Receptor Level

Ligands strongly influence the turnover rate of ER, by regulating its production and ubiquitin-dependent proteolysis. Estrogens block ER synthesis (decrease of ER mRNA level) while antiestrogens do not. Maintenance of ER synthesis under antiestrogen treatment may therefore upregulate the receptor when its proteasomal degradation is weak, as observed with OH-Tam and related SERMs. Estrogens and pure antiestrogens induce a strong and rapid ubiquitination of the receptor, leading to its rapid proteolysis; SERMs are largely less effective in this regard. As a consequence of these regulatory processes, estrogens, and pure antiestrogens downregulate the receptor while SERMs may lead to its accumulation.

The ability of cycloheximide and puromycin to stabilize the activated receptor within the cell nucleus suggests the induction of a protein favoring its return into the cytoplasm where it would be degraded. This concept of cytoplasmic degradation is supported by the observation that cycloheximide and puromycin fail to block the ER elimination when it is provoked by pure antiestrogens, which fail to stabilize the receptor within the nucleus.

In fact, only 10% of ER molecules should be saturated by a ligand to produce the proteasomal degradation of the whole population. Moreover, receptors of which the HBD has been blocked by a covalent binding (i.e. tamoxifen aziridine) are similarly eliminated. The mechanism underlying this amplification process is not known. Secretion of unidentified hydrophobic compounds by early-stimulated cells may play a role. Such compounds, the existence of which has been detected in conditioned media from ligand-treated cells, may act by themselves or in synergy with undetectable concentration of ligands.

4
Antitumor Estrogens

ER content is extremely variable among breast cancer. Median concentrations vary among studies reaching a maximum of 100 fmoles mg^{-1} proteins, which correspond roughly to 10 000 receptors per cell. Only a limited number of cytotoxic drugs would be able to exert significant antitumor effect with such a low concentration of vectors. The high reactivity of alkylating agents (1000 DNA interstrand cross-links is lethal) led to their selection for the synthesis of antitumor estrogens. Numerous compounds were synthesized in the 1970s and 1980s. However, as stated above, most of them failed to display a sufficient binding affinity for ER, or any unambiguous specificity of action, leading to a progressive disinterest to this approach. Other cytotoxic agents such as vinca alkaloids and intercalating agents (like ellipticin and daumomycin) also failed to show any potential therapeutic interest. Note that this remark also holds for nonsteroidal cytotoxic derivatives (i.e. diphenyl and triphenylethylene (anti)estrogens).

In the following years, accumulation of data concerning the receptor's structure, binding requirement, and mode of action (previous sections) dictated new guidelines for syntheses. Research axes of the last decade are overviewed in the following paragraphs.

4.1
Organometallic Estradiol Derivatives

The advance in organometallic chemistry associated with the discovery of the antitumor activity of cisplatin led to the analysis of the potential use of metal-conjugated estrogens. Since cisplatin is unsuitable for breast cancer treatment, the search concentrates mainly on non-platinum metal complexes such as cyclopentadienyl cycles of Ru, Ti, Fe, Co, and so on, which appear attractive in cancer chemotherapy. Nonetheless, cisplatin was also linked with the hope of extending its therapeutic use. While DNA is the expected target of such drugs, some of them were found

to irreversibly associate with the receptor, a behavior that may produce unusual biological properties.

Unfortunately, endocrine and therapeutic activity of most of the metal-conjugated estrogens has not yet been explored. Investigations mainly concern their binding to the receptor. The effect of ER-positive and ER-negative cell lines has been assessed in only a few cases.

4.1.1 A-ring Complexion
An important feature displayed by organometallic clusters is the possibility of their complexion on either the α- or β- side of the steroid A-ring (Fig. 6). Studies conducted with chromium and ruthenium complexes reveal that a π-organometallic adduct on the β-face prevents the binding of E_2 to the receptor while its addition on the α-face maintains some binding affinity. Of these compounds, the neutral chromium complex displayed the highest binding affinity ($\sim$30% of E_2). Although the cationic species Cp^*Ru^+ failed to seriously alter the binding of the hormone, as demonstrated

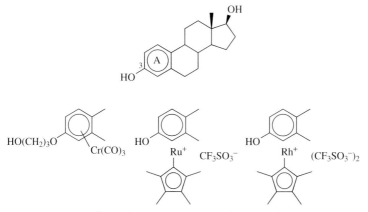

Fig. 6 Organometallic E$_2$ derivatives – chemical formulas of A-ring substituted derivatives described in Sect. 4.1.1. Binding affinity for ER of the organometallic abduct is higher on the α face of A-ring those on its β face.

by α-[Cp*Ru(17β-estradiol)][CF$_3$SO$_3$], an increase in the positive charge of the organic moiety (i.e. Rh^{++}) appears detrimental. This effect may be attributed to an increase in acidity; the complexion of the phenolic A-ring increases its acidity. In a basic medium, the complexed phenolic rings are transformed into the corresponding dienonylic rings with the concomitant loss of 3-OH function required for strong association with the receptor.

4.1.2   *7α and 11β Derivatives*

Grafting of organometallic clusters in these strategic regions is expected to be relatively well tolerated (Sect. 3.1). Hence, various compounds have been synthesized.

Nonradioactive Re systems are analogous to corresponding nonradioactive systems containing ^{99m}Tc, ^{186}Re or ^{188}Re. For this reason, they may be viewed as prototypes for the production of drugs to be used in imaging and radiotherapy. Attempts to produce 7α derivatives in which the rhenium moiety is remote from E$_2$ by a long side chain led to the identification of a few compounds with high binding affinity ($\sim$15% of E$_2$; Fig. 7). The polarity of these complexes was modified to improve biodistribution without loss of binding affinity by introducing (poly)ether linkages into the 7α side chains. Attachment of a rhenium complex in position 11β (Fig. 7) was also relatively well tolerated (binding affinity $\sim$1/10 of E$_2$). Tested on a reported gene, this compound displayed an agonist activity almost as strong as E$_2$.

Linkage of a cobalt cluster in 11β (i.e. 11β-[(ethynyl) Co$_2$(CO)$_6$]estradiol; Fig. 7) strongly increases the stability of the association of the parent-free ligand with the receptor. This behavior is reminiscent of the high performance of 11β-chloromethylestradiol in ER binding (almost irreversible binding in buffered solution). Tested *in vitro* in MVLN cells (MCF-7 cells stably transfected with an estrogen responsive luciferase gene), this cobalt conjugate displays a strong estrogenicity (as effective as E$_2$); no cytotoxicity was recorded.

4.1.3   **17α Derivatives**

Various organometallic moeities (rhenium, cobalt, ruthenium, tungsten, etc.) fail to strongly affect the binding affinity of E$_2$ for ER when linked in its 17α position at the end of a rigid ethynyl spacer (Fig. 8). In contrast, the affinity largely decreases when the spacer is shortened to a simple sp^3 carbon atom confirming that the ER-HBD possesses a subsite able to accommodate rigid narrow substituents. Affinity also decreases when the organometallic moiety is moved toward the D-ring of the steroid, even on a rigid spacer. Moreover, neutral species (ferrocenyl) are relatively well tolerated while cationic species (ruthenium) decrease the binding affinity indicating that the HBD does not accept a positive change in the 17α position of E$_2$. Hence, bulky organometallic moiety may be tolerated if they localize outside a zone of steric/electronic constraint.

Coordination of selected transition-metal moeities to 17α-alkynylestradiol may induce an irreversible (covalent) binding with the receptor (Fig. 8). Nucleophilic sulfur residues within or in the close vicinity of the HBD are good candidates for the establishment of such a covalent bond. The key step in this chemical reaction is the loss of the 17β-OH functionality for the generation of a carbenium ion; this electron-deficient center stabilized by the organometallic

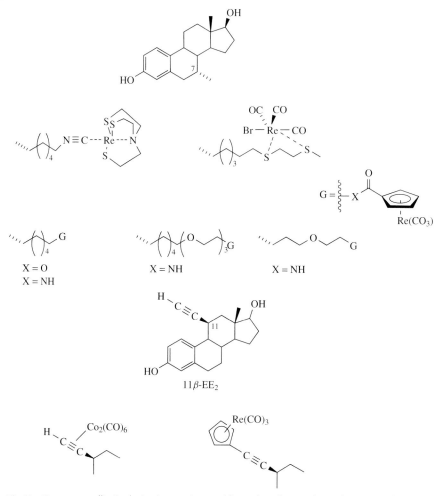

Fig. 7 Organometallic E_2 derivatives – chemical formulas of 7α and 11β derivatives described in Sect. 4.1.2.

fragment promotes an interaction with a vicinal nucleophilic residue. Among E_2 transition-metal complexes examined, dicobalt clusters $[Co_2(CO)_6]$ were found to be the most active affinity markers. Of note, FeCo-$(CO)_6(17\alpha$-ethynyl-17β-dehydroxyestradiol) in which the hetero-bimetallic fragment is sterically similar to the $Co_2(CO)_6$ homolog, prevents the formation of a carbenium-ion-like species confirming the requirement at the 17-position of an OH group and an organometallic unit capable of dissipating the positive charge of the transient carbocation.

Potential influence of covalent binding of these dicobalt clusters on the ER level and transcriptional activity is unknown, and therefore, to be investigated. Potential therapeutic activity should also be assessed. Note in this regard that alkyne $Co_2(CO)_6$ itself shows no cytotoxic effect.

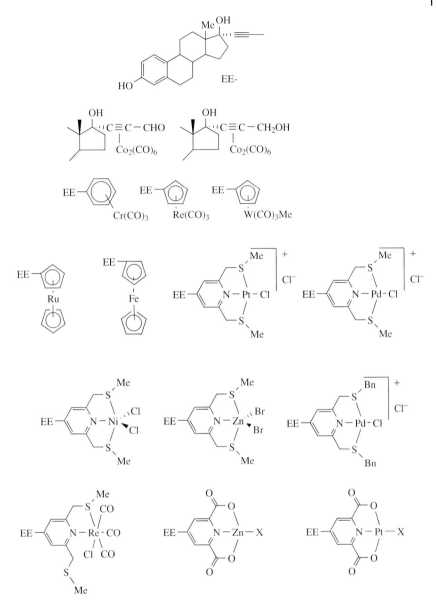

Fig. 8 Organometallic E_2 derivatives – chemical formulas of 17α ethynyl E_2 (EE) derivatives described in Sect. 4.1.3.

4.2
Radiolabeled Estradiol Derivatives

The presence of ER-positive and -negative cells in all tumors led to the concept of using receptor-directed radiochemicals of which the range of radiation is larger than one cell diameter. Compounds of this type would be of great interest since their action would not restrict solely to

ER-positive cells (as for antiestrogens) but also to ER-negative cells located in their neighborhood.

4.2.1 ^{123}I and ^{125}I Labeled Compounds

Several [^{125}I] labeled E$_2$ derivatives have been synthesized for *in vivo* imaging of ER-positive tumors. Utility of this approach in cancer diagnostic has, however, never been demonstrated. Nevertheless, biodistribution as well as imaging investigations performed on both animals and humans suggest some uptake selectivity, especially for 17α-iodovinyl derivatives. Stereochemistry of such compounds appears of prime importance for ER binding; Z-isomers bind more effectively than corresponding E-isomers. These data confirm the concept that the HBD possesses a hydrophobic subsite able to accept

lipophilic moieties linked in position 17α of E$_2$ (see Sect. 3.1.4). In an effort to utilize this concept, a series of 17α-substituted E$_2$ derivatives were synthesized, four of them bearing iodine-123 (Fig. 9). The binding of these four compounds depends on the nature of their substituents with an alkene linkage being greatly preferred over alkynyl and alkyl. Preference for the Z-alkene geometry confirms the conclusion from studies on parent iodovinyls. Additional biodistribution studies performed with the Z-alkene suggested some uptake selectivity (uterus/ovary) and metabolic instability (accumulation of free iodine within the thyroid).

16α-[^{125}I]iodo-estradiol has been shown to produce a receptor-mediated cyto-toxicity on MCF-7 breast cancer cells. The decrease of survival rate provoked

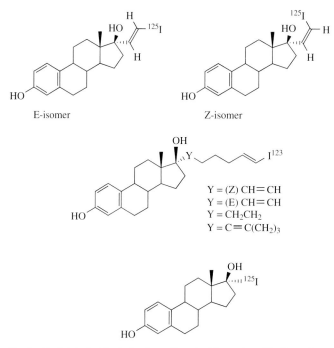

Fig. 9 Radiolabeled E$_2$ derivatives. Chemical formulas of iodinated (^{123}I and ^{125}I) derivatives described in Sect. 4.2.1.

by this radioligand was associated with chromosomal aberrations; of note, an excess of diethylstilbestrol, used as potential competitor, prevented the decrease of survival rate as well as chromosomal aberrations. Despite the promising aspect of these data, estimated residence times of ^{125}I-labeled estrogens in ER-positive cells (ER half-life: less than 3 h) appear be too low for an efficient cell killing. In this regard, the Auger electron-emitting nucleotides such as iodine-123 that release their energy within a short period of time would be more powerful to selectively kill ER-positive cells (i.e. half-life of ^{123}I = 4.4 h vs ^{125}I = 60 days). Testing of 17α-[^{123}I]iodovinyl-11β methoxy-estradiol on Chinese hamster ovary cells expressing or not high level of ER provided credence to this concept.

4.2.2 α-Emitting Compounds

Auger electron emitter agents would only affect ER-positive cells due to their weak distance of irradiation potency. α-particle emitting radionucleotides such as astatine-211 are attractive candidates to palliate this gap and affect neighboring ER-negative cells (range of radiation in tissue is 10 to 100 μm); astatine-211 can substitute iodine in many syntheses making the production of ^{211}At-labeled E$_2$ easily feasible. In fact, [^{211}At]astatinovinylestradiol (as well as its 11β methoxylated derivative) has been established. One may hope that such compounds produce a cytotoxic effect as their ^{125}I-labeled analogs.

The possibility to generate α-emitting isotopes by boron capture therapy is another approach under exploration. Boron-10, when irradiated with low energy thermal neutrons, yields α-particles and ^{7}Li-nuclei. The success of this therapy is dependant on the quantity of boron-10 and thermal neutrons to deliver to the cancer cells to sustain an α-lethal radiation. Carboranes (dicarba-closo-dodecaboranes) are a class of carbon-containing polyhedral-boron clusters having remarkable thermal stability and exceptional hydrophobic character; they have been utilized to incorporate a large number of boron atoms into tumor cells. Remarkably, hydrophobic interactions between carboranes and ER may occur when linked to a phenol. This finding led to the design of several compounds sharing high binding affinity for the receptor as well as estrogenic and/or antiestrogenic activity on an ER-dependent reporter gene (i.e. analogs of E$_2$, OH-Tam or RU 39,411; Fig. 10). One may speculate that such drugs may play a role in cancer therapy since they combine suitable endocrine and radiotoxic properties.

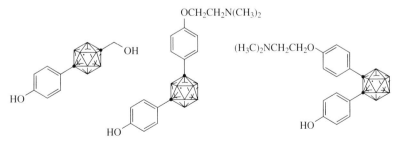

Fig. 10 Chemical formulas of phenolic carboranes with structural and ER binding properties to (a) E$_2$, (b) OH-Tam, and (c) RU 39,411 (Sect. 4.2.2).

4.3
Electrophilic 11β Derivative

Estrogenic and antiestrogenic activity of a few 11β-ethyl, butyl, and decyl derivatives of E_2 bearing various electrophilic functionalities (i.e. bromide, bromo-acetamido, (methylsulfonyl)oxy, and (*p*-tolylsulfonyl)oxy) were determined with MVLN cells (ER-dependent luciferase expression). Ethyl derivatives were mainly estrogenic, whereas butyl and decyl essentially antiestrogenic (most compounds share a significant binding affinity for ER).

Long-term treatment of MVLN cells with OH-Tam progressively abolishes the ability of cells to express luciferase in response to estrogens. This irreversible effect seems to result from an epigenetic mechanism, such as methylation or chromatin remodeling rather than gene mutation. It progressively affects the whole-cell population and occurs by a first-order process, with

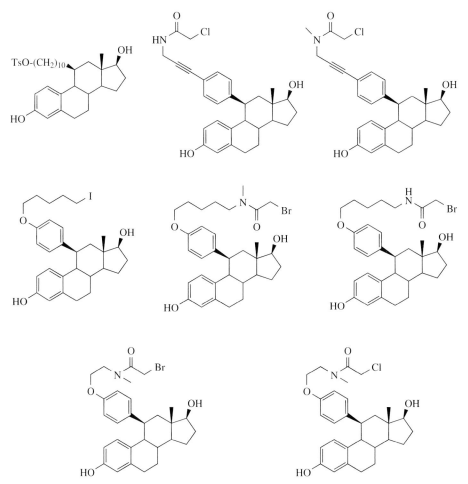

Fig. 11 Electrophilic derivatives of E_2 described in Sect. 4.3.

a half-inactivation time of $\sim$10 days. 11β electrophile conjugates described here, similarly suppresses the expression of the luciferase gene; antiestrogenic electrophiles were more potent than the estrogenic ones but less efficient than OH-Tam. Of note, these antiestrogenic electrophiles decrease cell proliferation with potency less than OH-Tam.

These effects could not be ascribed to an irreversible binding of the compounds to ER since 11β-[(tosyloxy)decyl]E$_2$ (Fig. 11) solely shared such a property. A cysteine residue does not seem to be involved in the covalent attachment of this compound since it was not prevented by a thiol-specific alkylating reagent (MMTS). In fact, length and mobility of the *N*-decyl side chain precluded the identification of the anchorage site. To overcome this drawback, 11β aryl analogs aimed to restrict the localization of the electrophilic carbon to the β-side of the steroid were synthesized (Fig. 11). Both cysteinyl (probably C381 and/or C530) and non-cysteinyl residues located on the β-side and remote from C11 of the steroid (distance > "seven bonds") appear to be potential electrophile covalent attachment sites for such E$_2$ derivatives.

As for most other estrogens bearing reactive groups, no data were reported upon their potential use in antitumor therapy.

Bibliography

Books and Reviews

Blickenstaff, R.T. (1992) *Antitumor Steroids*, Academic Press, New York.

von Angerer, E. (1995) The estrogen receptor as a target for rational drug design, *Molecular Biology Intelligence Unit*, Springer-Verlag, Heidelberg, Germany.

Primary Literature

Aliau, S., Delettre, G., Mattras, H., El Garrouj, D., Nique, F., Teutsch, G., Borgna, J.L. (2000) *J. Med. Chem.* **43**, 613–628.

Aliau, S., Mattras, H., Richard, E., Bonnafous, J.-C., Borgna, J.-L. (2002) *Biochemistry* **41**, 7979–7988.

Anstead, G.M., Carlson, K.E., Katzenellenbogen, J.A. (1997) *Steroids* **62**, 268–303.

Brzozowski, A.M., Pike, A.C.W., Dauter, Z., Hubbard, R.W., Bonn, T., Angström, O., Öhman, L., Greene, G.L., Gustafsson, J.Ä., Carlquist, M. (1997) *Nature* **389**, 753–758.

Cummins, C.H. (1993) *Steroids* **58**, 245–259.

DeFranco, D.B. (2002) *Mol. Endocrinol.* **16**, 1449–1455.

DeSombre, E.R., Shafii, B., Hanson, R.N., Kuivanen, P.C., Hughes, A. (1992) *Cancer Res.* **52**, 5752–5758.

Endo, Y., Iijima, T., Yamakoshi, Y., Yamaguchi, M., Fukasawa, H., Shudo, K. (1999) *J. Med. Chem.* **42**, 1501–1504.

Endo, Y., Yoshimi, T., Iijima, T., Yamakoshi, Y. (1999) *Bioorg. Med. Chem. Lett.* **9**, 3387–3392.

El Hamouri, H., Vessières, A., Vichard, D., Top, S., Gruselle, M., Jaouen, G. (1992) *J. Med. Chem.* **35**, 3130–3135.

El Khissiin, A., Journé, F., Laïos, I., Seo, H.-S., Leclercq, G. (2000) *Steroids* **65**, 903–913.

Hart, L.L., Davie, J.R. (2002) *Biochem. Cell Biol.* **80**, 335–341.

Jaouen, G., Vessières, A. (1993) *Acc. Chem. Res.* **26**, 361–369.

Jackson, A., Davis, J., Pither, R.J., Rodger, A., Hannon, M.J. (2001) *Inorg. Chem.* **40**, 3964–3973.

Kabalka, G.W., Shoup, T.M., Daniel, G.B., Goodman, M.M. (2000) *Nucl. Med. Biol.* **27**, 279–287.

Lobaccaro, C., Pons, J.-F., Duchesne, M.-J., Auzou, G., Pons, M., Nique, F., Teutsch, G., Borgna, J.-L. (1997) *J. Med. Chem.* **40**, 2217–2227.

Morel, P., Top, S., Vessières, A., Stéphan, E., Laïos, I., Leclercq, G., Jaouen, G. (2001) *C. R. Acad. Sci., Paris, Chem.* **4**, 201–205.

Osella, D. (2002) *Second Workshop on Pharmaco-Bio-Metallics*; Communication in Sienna, Italy.

Osella, D., Cavigiolio, G., Vincenti, M., Vessières, A., Laïos, I., Leclercq, G., Napolitano, E., Fiaschi, R., Jaouen, G. (2000) *J. Organomet. Chem.* **596**, 242–247.

Reid, G., Denger, S., Kos, M., Gannon, F. (2002) *Cell. Mol. Life Sci.* **59**, 1–11.

Shiau, A.K., Barstad, D., Loria, P.M., Chang, L., Kushner, P.J., Agard, D.A., Greene, G.L. (1998) *Cell* **95**, 927–937.

Skaddan, M.B., Wüst, F.R., Katzenellenbogen, J.A. (1999) *J. Org. Chem.* **64**, 8108–8121.

Top, S., El Hafa, H., Vessières, A., Huché, M., Vaissermann, J., Jaouen, G. (2002) *Chem. Eur. J.* **8**, 5241–5249.

Tsai, M.J., O'Malley, B.W. (1994) *Annu. Rev. Biochem.* **63**, 451–486.

25

Immunotoxins and Recombinant Immunotoxins in Cancer Therapy

Yoram Reiter and Avital Lev
Technion-Israel Institute of Technology, Haifa, Israel

1   Introduction   797

2   First- and Second-generation Immunotoxins   800

3   The Development of Recombinant DNA-based Immunotoxins: Design of
        Recombinant Immunotoxins   801
3.1   The Toxin Moiety   801
3.1.1   Plant Toxins   801
3.1.2   Bacterial Toxins: DT and DT Derivatives   802
3.1.3   Bacterial Toxins: PE and PE Derivatives   803
3.2   The Targeting Moiety – Recombinant Antibody Fragments   804

4   Construction and Production of Recombinant Immunotoxins   805

5   Preclinical Development of Recombinant Immunotoxins   808

6   Application of Recombinant Immunotoxins   809
6.1   Recombinant Immunotoxins against Solid Tumors   809
6.2   Recombinant Immunotoxins against Leukemias and Lymphomas   810

7   Isolation of New and Improved Antibody Fragments as Targeting Moieties:
        Display Technologies for the Improvement of Immunotoxin Activity   812

8   Improving The Therapeutic Window of Recombinant Immunotoxins:
        The Balance of Toxicity, Immunogenicity, and Efficacy   815
8.1   Immune Responses and Dose-limiting Toxicity   816
8.2   Specificity Dictated by the Targeting Moiety   817

9   Conclusions and Perspectives   818

Pharmacology. From Drug Development to Gene Therapy. Edited by Robert A. Meyers.
Copyright © 2008 Wiley-VCH Verlag GmbH & Co. KGaA, Weinheim
ISBN: 978-3-527-32343-2

Bibliography   818
Books and Reviews   818
Primary Literature   818

Keywords

Cancer Therapy
Strategies to kill and eliminate transformed malignant cells using various approaches such as chemotherapy, immunotherapy, gene therapy, and others.

Immunotoxins
A form of targeted therapy approach in which a potent toxin is conjugated or genetically fused to an anitbody or other targeting moiety to specifically target the toxin to the malignant cell.

Recombinant Antibodies
Antibody molecules or their fragments generated and produced by recombinant DNA technology.

Targeted Therapy
Therapeutic strategy in which a cytotoxic drug or an effector function is delivered specifically to the malignant transformed cell by using a specific marker related to the cancerous phenotype.

Targeted cancer therapy in general and immunotherapy in particular, combines rational drug design with the progress in understanding cancer biology. This approach takes advantage of our recent knowledge of the mechanisms by which normal cells are transformed into cancer cells, thus, using the special properties of cancer cells to device novel therapeutic strategies.

Recombinant immunotoxins are excellent examples for such processes, combining the knowledge of antigen expression by cancer cells with the enormous developments in recombinant DNA technology and antibody engineering. Recombinant immunotoxins are composed of a very potent protein toxin fused to a targeting moiety such as recombinant antibody fragment or growth factor.

These molecules bind to surface antigens specific for cancer cells and kill the target cells by catalytic inhibition of protein synthesis. Recombinant immunotoxins are developed for solid tumors and hematological malignances and have been characterized intensively for their biological activity *in vitro* on cultured tumor cell lines as well as *in vivo* in animal models of human tumor xenografts. The excellent *in vitro* and *in vivo* activities of recombinant immunotoxins have lead to their preclinical development and to the initiation of clinical trial protocols. Recent trial results have demonstrated potent clinical efficacy in patients with malignant diseases that are refractory to traditional modalities of cancer treatment; surgery, radiation therapy, and chemotherapy.

1
Introduction

The rapid progress in understanding the molecular biology of cancer cells has made a large impact on the design and development of novel therapeutic strategies. These have been developed because treatment of cancer by chemotherapy is limited by a number of factors, and usually fails in patients whose malignant cells are not sufficiently different from normal cells in their growth and metabolism. Other limiting factors are the low therapeutic index of most chemotherapeutic agents, the emergence of drug-resistant populations, tumor heterogeneity, and the presence of metastatic disease.

The concept of targeted cancer therapy is thus an important means of improving the therapeutic potential of anticancer agents and lead to the development of novel approaches such as immunotherapy. The approach of cancer immunotherapy and targeted cancer therapy combines rational drug design with the current advances in our understanding of cancer biology. This approach takes advantage of some special properties of cancer cells – many of them contain mutant or overexpressed oncogenes on their surface and these proteins are attractive antigens for targeted therapy. The first cell surface receptor to be linked to cancer was the epidermal growth factor (EGF) receptor present in lung, brain, kidney, bladder, breast, and ovarian cancer. Several other members of the EGF receptor family, that is, *erb*B2, *erb*B3, and *erb*B4 receptors, appear to be abundant on breast and ovary tumors, and *erb*B2, for example, is the target for phase I and II immunotherapy clinical trials.

Other promising candidates for targeted therapy are differentiation antigens that are expressed on the surface of mature cells, but not on the immature stem cells. The most widely studied examples of differentiation antigens currently being used for targeted therapy are expressed by hematopoietic malignancies, and include CD19, CD20, and CD22 on B-cell lymphomas and leukemias, and the interleukin (IL-)-2 receptor on T-cell leukemias. Differentiation antigens have also been found on ovarian, breast, and prostate cancer.

Another class of antigen, termed *tumor-associated antigens* (TAAs), is made up of molecules that are tightly bound to the surface of cancer cells and are associated with the transformed cancer cells. An example is the carbohydrate antigen Lewis Y (LeY) that is found in many types of solid tumors. Another class of TAAs includes cancer peptides that are presented by class I MHC molecules on the surface of tumor cells.

It should be possible to use these molecular cell surface markers as targets to eliminate the cancer cells while sparing the normal cells. For this approach to be successful, we must generate a targeting moiety that will bind very specifically to the antigen or receptor expressed on the cancer cell surface and arm this targeting moiety with an effector cytotoxic moiety. The targeting moiety can be a specific antibody directed toward the cancer antigen or a ligand for a specific overexpressed receptor. The cytotoxic arm can be a radioisotope, a cytotoxic drug, or a toxin. One strategy to achieve this is to arm antibodies that target cancer cells with powerful toxins that can originate from both plants and bacteria. The molecules generated are termed *recombinant immunotoxins*.

The goal of immunotoxin therapy is to target a very potent cytotoxic agent to cell surface molecules, which will then internalize the cytotoxic agent, resulting in cell death. Developing this type of therapy has gained much interest in recent years. Since immunotoxins differ greatly from chemotherapy in their mode of action and toxicity profile, it is hoped that immunotoxins will have the potential to improve the systemic treatment of tumors incurable with existing modes of therapy.

As shown in Fig. 1, immunotoxins can be divided into two groups: chemical conjugates (or first-generation immunotoxins) and second-generation (or recombinant)

immunotoxins. They both contain toxins that have their cell binding domains either mutated or deleted to prevent them from binding to normal cells and are either fused or chemically conjugated to a ligand or an antibody specific for cancer cells (Table 1).

This article will summarize our current understanding of the design and application of second-generation recombinant Fv–immunotoxins, which utilize recombinant antibody fragments as the targeting moiety, in the treatment of cancer, and will also discuss briefly the use of recombinant

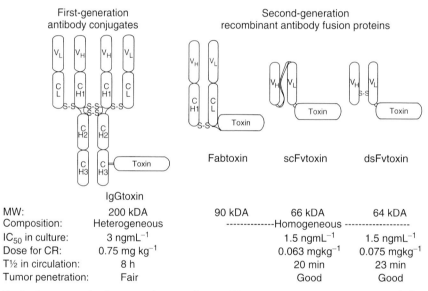

Fig. 1 Immunotoxins for targeted cancer therapy. First-generation immunotoxins are whole mAbs to which the toxin is chemically conjugated. Second-generation immunotoxins are made by recombinant DNA technology by fusing recombinant antibody fragments to the toxin (usually a truncated or mutated form of the toxin). Three types of recombinant antibody fragments are used as the targeting moiety in recombinant immunotoxins. Fabs are composed of the light-chain and the heavy-chain Fd fragment (V_H and C_H1), connected to each other via the interchain disulfide bond between C_L and C_H1. scFv fragments are stabilized by a peptide linker, which connects the C-terminus of V_H or V_L with the N-terminus of the other domain. The V_H and V_L heterodimer in dsFv is stabilized by engineering a disulfide bond between the two domains. The biochemical and biological properties described in the lower part of the figure are depicted for B3–lysPE38 (LMB-1) (a first-generation antibody–PE chemical conjugate), B3(Fv)–PE38 (LMB-7) (second-generation recombinant scFv–immunotoxin for an scFv–immunotoxin) and B3(dsFv)–PE38 (LMB-9) (for a second-generation recombinant dsFv–immunotoxin).

Tab. 1 Examples of recombinant immunotoxins against cancer.

Immunotoxin	Antigen	Toxin	Cancer	Clinical Trial
Anti-CD7-dgA	CD7	Ricin	Non-Hodgkin's lymphoma	Phase I
DAB$_{389}$-IL2	IL-2R	DT	T-cell lymphoma Hodgkin's disease	Phase III
Anti-Tac (Fv)-PE38 (LMB-2)	CD25	PE	B and T lymphoma, leukemias	Phase I
DT-Anti-Tac(Fv)	CD25	DT	Leukemias, lymphoma	–
RFB4(dsFv)-PE38	CD22	PE	B leukemias	Phase I
Di-dgA-RFB4	CD22	Ricin	Leukemias, non-Hodgkin's lymphoma	–
B3-lysPE38 (LMB-1)	Lewis Y	PE	Carcinomas	Phase I
B3(Fv)-PE38 (LMB-7)	Lewis Y	PE	Carcinomas	Phase I
B3(dsFv)-PE38 (LMB-9)	Lewis Y	PE	Carcinoma	Phase I
BR96(sFv)-PE40	Lewis Y	PE	Carcinoma	–
e23(Fv)-PE38	erbB2/HER2	PE	Breast cancer	Phase I
FRP5(scFv)ETA	erbB2/HER2	PE	Breast cancer	–
Tf-CRM107	Transferrin-R	DT	Glioma	Phase I
HB21(Fv)-PE40	Transferrin-R	PE	Various	–
MR1(Fv)-PE38	Mutant EGF-R	PE	Liver, brain tumors	–
SS1(Fv)-PE38	Mesothelin	PE	Ovarian cancer	–

antibody fragments for other modes of cancer therapy and diagnosis.

2
First- and Second-generation Immunotoxins

First-generation immunotoxins were made in the early 1970s and were composed of cancer-specific monoclonal antibodies (mAbs) to which native bacterial or plant toxins were chemically conjugated. The understanding of toxin structure–function properties and the advancement in recombinant DNA technology and antibody engineering led to important breakthroughs in the late 1980s to construct second-generation recombinant immunotoxins that are composed of recombinant antibody fragments derived from cancer-specific antibodies or phage-display libraries and truncated forms of toxins. These molecules are produced in large amounts, needed for preclinical and clinical studies, in bacteria and feature better clinical properties.

As shown in Fig. 1, first- and second-generation immunotoxins contain toxins that have their cell binding domains either mutated or deleted to prevent them from binding to normal cells, and are either chemically conjugated or fused to a ligand or an antibody specific for cancer cells.

First-generation immunotoxins, composed of whole antibodies chemically conjugated to toxins, demonstrated the feasibility of this concept. Cancer cells cultured *in vitro* could be killed under conditions in which the immunotoxin demonstrated low toxicity toward cultured normal cells. Clinical trials with these agents had some success; however, they also revealed several problems, such as nonspecific toxicity toward some normal cells, difficulties

in production and, particularly for the treatment of solid tumors, poor tumor penetration due to their large size.

Second-generation immunotoxins have overcome many of these problems. Progress in the elucidation of the toxin's structure and function combined with the techniques of protein engineering facilitated the design and construction of recombinant molecules with a higher specificity for cancer cells and reduced toxicity to normal cells. At the same time, advances in recombinant DNA technology and antibody engineering enabled the generation of small antibody fragments. Thus, it was possible to decrease the size of immunotoxins significantly and to improve their tumor-penetration potential *in vivo*. The development of advanced methods of recombinant protein production enabled the large-scale production of recombinant immunotoxins of high purity and quality for clinical use in sufficient quantities to perform clinical trials.

Another strategy to target cancer cells is to construct chimeric toxins in which the engineered truncated portion of the toxin [*Pseudomonas* exotoxin (PE) or diphtheria toxin (*DT*)] gene is fused to cDNA encoding growth factors or cytokines. These include transforming growth factor (TGF)-β, insulin-like growth factor (IGF)-1, acidic and basic fibroblast growth factor (FGF), IL-2, IL-4, and IL-6. These recombinant toxins (oncotoxins) are designed to target specific tumor cells that overexpress these receptors (Fig. 1).

In the following sections, we will summarize the rationale and current knowledge on the design and application of second-generation recombinant Fv–immunotoxins that utilize recombinant antibody fragments as the targeting moiety. Recent results of clinical trials are summarized. We will also discuss the powerful new technologies for selecting new antibodies with unique specificities and improved properties.

3
The Development of Recombinant DNA-based Immunotoxins: Design of Recombinant Immunotoxins

3.1
The Toxin Moiety

The toxins that are most commonly used to make immunotoxins are ricin, DT, and PE. These toxins belong to a group of polypeptide enzymes that catalytically inactivate protein synthesis leading to cell death. Some of these toxins have been shown to induce apoptosis.

The genes for these toxins have been cloned and expressed in *Escherichia coli*, and the crystal structures of all three proteins have been solved. This information, in combination with mutational studies, has elucidated which toxin subunits are involved in their biological activity and, most importantly, the different steps of the cytocidal process. DT, PE, ricin, and their derivatives have all been successfully used to prepare immunotoxin conjugates, but only PE- and DT-containing fusion proteins generate active recombinant immunotoxins. This is because the toxic moiety must be separated from the binding moiety after internalization. PE and DT fusion proteins generate their free toxic moieties by proteolytic processing. Ricin does not possess such a proteolytic processing site and therefore cannot be attached to the targeting moiety with a peptide bond without losing cytotoxic activity. Recently, proteolytic processing sites were introduced into ricin

by recombinant DNA techniques to try to overcome this problem.

3.1.1 Plant Toxins

Ricin, or the ricin A-chain fragment, has been a commonly used toxin for conjugation to antibodies. Ricin is synthesized as single polypeptide chains and processed posttranslationally into two subunits A and B linked through a disulfide bond. Ricin is a 65-kDa glycoprotein purified from the seeds of the castor bean (*Ricinus communis*). It is composed of an A subunit, which kills cells by catalytically inactivating ribosomes. The A subunit is linked by a disulfide bond to a B subunit, which is responsible for cell binding. The B chain is a galactose-specific lectin that binds to galactose residues present on cell surface glycoproteins and glycolipids. Once the B subunit of ricin binds to the cell membrane, the protein enters the cell through coated pits and endocytic vesicles. The A and B subunits of ricin are separated by a process involving disulfide bond reduction. The A subunit of ricin translocates across an intracellular membrane to the cell cytosol, probably with the assistance of the B subunit. In the cytosol, it arrests protein synthesis by enzymatically inactivating the 28S subunit of eukaryotic ribosomes. Because native ricin is highly toxic and lacks specificity, several modified forms of ricin have been developed to prepare immunotoxins that are better tolerated by patients.

To decrease the nonspecific binding of whole ricin, the A chain alone has been coupled to antibodies. The A chain is obtained by reducing the disulfide bond that links it to the B chain. Immunotoxins composed of the ricin A chain coupled to well-internalized antibodies can be highly cytotoxic. In the absence of the B chain (the binding subunit), however, immunotoxins made with poorly internalized antibodies are not cytotoxic.

Immunotoxins containing the ricin A chain are rapidly cleared from the circulation by the liver by the binding of mannose and fucose residues of the A chain to receptors present on the reticuloendothelial system and hepatocytes. To circumvent this problem, these carbohydrate residues were chemically modified, resulting in a deglycosylated A chain (dgA) molecule. In preclinical studies, dgA-containing immunotoxins were found to have longer half-lives in the circulation and better antitumor efficacy *in vivo*. Also, recombinant A chain produced in *E. coli* can be used in place of dgA because it is devoid of carbohydrate and is not rapidly cleared by the liver.

Another strategy to decrease the non-specific toxicity of native ricin is to block the galactose binding sites of the B chain by cross-linking with glycopeptide or to use short cross-linkers to connect the antibody to the toxin so that the galactose binding site is sterically blocked by the antibody. Blocked ricin retains a low affinity for galactose binding sites, which enhances internalization and cytotoxicity of an antibody that binds to a poorly internalized antigen.

Other plant toxins commonly used for clinical immunotoxin construction are saporin and pokeweed antiviral protein, which are single polypeptide chains that inactivate ribosomes in a similar fashion to ricin. Because these toxins lack the binding chain (B chain), they are relatively nontoxic to cells and are used for immunotoxin production.

3.1.2 Bacterial Toxins: DT and DT Derivatives

DT is a 58-kDa protein, secreted by pathogenic *Corynebacterium diphtheria*, which contains a lysogenic β phage. DT ADP-ribosylates eukaryotic elongation factor (EF)-2 at a "diphthamide" residue located at His415, using NAD^+ as a cofactor. This modification arrests protein synthesis and subsequently leads to cell death. Only a few, and perhaps only one, DT molecules need to reach the cytosol in order to kill a cell. When DT is isolated from the culture medium of *C. diphtheria*, it is composed of an N-terminal 21-kDa A subunit and a C-terminal 37-kDa B subunit held together by a disulfide bond. DT is the expression product of a single gene, which when secreted into the medium is processed into two fragments by extracellular proteases. When DT is produced as a recombinant single-chain protein in *E. coli*, it is not cleaved by the bacteria, but is instead cleaved by a protease in the target cells. The A domain of DT contains its enzymatic activity. The N-terminus of the B subunit of DT (or the region between A and B in single-chain DT) mediates translocation of the A subunit into the cytoplasm. The B domain, especially its C-terminus, is responsible for the binding of DT to target cells. Deletions or mutations in this part of the molecule abolish or greatly diminish the binding and toxicity of DT. DT enters cells via coated pits and is proteolytically cleaved within the endocytic compartment, if it is not already in the two-chain form, and reduced. It also undergoes a conformational change at the acidic pH present in endosomes, which probably assists translocation of the A chain into the cytosol, perhaps via a porelike structure mediated by the B chain. Derivatives of DT that are used to make immunotoxins have the C-terminus altered by mutations or partially deleted (DAB486, DAB389, and DT388), but retain the translocation and ADP-ribosylation activity of DT. Recombinant antibody fusion proteins with such derivatives target only cells that bind the antibody moiety of the immunotoxin.

3.1.3 Bacterial Toxins: PE and PE Derivatives

Two major research studies have enabled the use and genetic manipulation of PE for the design of immunotoxins: (1) the elucidation of the crystal structure of PE, showing the toxin to be composed of three major structural domains, and (2) the finding that these domains are different functional modules of the toxin.

PE is a single-chain 66-kDa molecule secreted by *Pseudomonas aeruginosa* that, like DT, irreversibly ADP-ribosylates the diphthamide residue of EF-2, using NAD^+ as cofactor. As a consequence, protein synthesis is inhibited and cell death ensues. PE is composed of three major domains. Different functions have been assigned to each domain by mutational analysis. The N-terminal domain Ia mediates binding to the α_2-macroglobulin receptor. Domain Ib is a small domain that lies between domains II and III, and has no known function. Domain II mediates translocation of domain III, the C-terminal ADP-ribosylating domain, into the cytosol of target cells (Fig. 2). Translocation occurs after internalization of the toxin and after a variety of other steps including a pH-induced conformational change, proteolytic cleavage at a specific site in domain II, and a reductive step that separates the amino and carboxyl fragments. Ultimately, the C-terminal portion of PE is translocated from the endoplasmic reticulum into the cytosol. Despite a similar mode of action of PE and DT, which is ADP-ribosylation, and a similar initial pathway of cell entry (internalization via coated pits and endocytic vesicles) and of processing (proteolytic cleavage and a reductive step), they share almost no sequence homology.

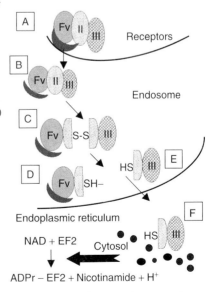

Fig. 2 The biological activity of PE A. The Fv portion of the immunotoxin targets domains II and III of PE to a cell surface receptor or other target molecule on the tumor cell (A). The immunotoxin enters the cell by internalization and is transferred into the endosome (B). Within the endosome, the molecule unfolds owing to a fall in pH. The conformational change exposes a proteolytic site, and a proteolytic cleavage occurs in the translocation domain between amino acids 279 and 280 (C). A disulfide bond is then broken, thus creating two fragments: the Fv moiety and a small part of domain II, and the rest of domain II connected to domain III (D). The C-terminal fragment containing the ADP-ribosylation domain (domain III) and most of the translocation domain (domain II) is carried into the endoplasmic reticulum (E), and translocation occurs from the endoplasmic reticulum into the cytosol (F). The enzymatically active domain ADP-ribosylates EF-2 at a diphthamide residue located at His415, using NAD^+ as a cofactor. This modification arrests protein synthesis and subsequently leads to cell death by apoptosis. In DT, the proteolytic processing occurs between residues 193 and 194. The catalytic A chain (amino acids 1–193) then translocates to the cytosol through the endosome with the help of translocation domain residues 326–347 and 358–376, which form an ion channel.

The only similarity is the spatial arrangement of key residues in their active sites that are arranged around residue Glu553 in PE and Glu145 in DT.

When the whole toxin is used to make an immunotoxin, nonspecific toxicity occurs mainly because of binding of the toxin portion to cells, mediated by the binding domain. Consequently, the goal of making improved derivatives of PE-based immunotoxins has been to inactivate or remove the binding domain. Molecules in which the binding domain has been retained but inactivated by mutations were made; however, a better alternative to inactivating the cell binding domain by mutations is to remove it from PE. The prototype molecule with this sort of deletion is PE40 (amino acids 253–613, MW 40 kDa]. Because PE40 and its derivatives described below lack the binding domain (amino acids 1–252), they have very low nonspecific toxicity, but make very active and specific immunotoxins when fused to recombinant antibodies. Currently, almost all PE-derived recombinant immunotoxins are constructed with PE38 (MW 38 kDa), a PE40 derivative that has, in addition to the deletion of domain Ia, a second deletion encompassing a portion of domain Ib (amino acids 365–379). Another useful mutation is to change the C-terminal sequence of PE from REDLK to KDEL. This improves the cytotoxicity of PE and its derivatives, presumably by increasing their delivery to the endoplasmic reticulum where translocation takes place.

3.2
The Targeting Moiety – Recombinant Antibody Fragments

The antibody moiety of the recombinant immunotoxin is responsible for specifically directing the immunotoxin to the target cell; thus, the usefulness of the immunotoxin depends on the specificity of the antibody or antibody fragment that is connected to the toxin. Consequently, for the construction of recombinant immunotoxins, the only antibodies that should be used are those that recognize antigens that are expressed on target cancer cells and are not present on normal cells, present at very low levels, or are only present on less-essential cells (Table 1). Receptors for growth factors like EGF, IL-2, IL-4, IL-6, or *erb*B2 are common targets for targeted cancer therapy because they are highly expressed on many cancer cells. Other carcinoma-related antigens include developmental antigens such as complex carbohydrates, which are often highly abundant on the surface of cancer cells.

The use of antibodies for immunotoxin production also requires that the antibody–antigen complex be internalized, because the mechanism of PE-toxin killing requires endocytosis as a first step in the entry of the toxin into the cell.

Recombinant immunotoxins contain antibody fragments as the targeting moiety. These fragments can be produced in *E. coli*, and are the result of intensive research and development in recombinant antibody technologies. Several antibody fragments have been used to construct recombinant immunotoxins (Fig. 1). One type contains Fab fragments in which the light chain and the heavy chain Fd fragment (V_H and C_H1) are connected to each other via an interchain disulfide bond between C_L and C_H1. The toxin moiety can be fused to the carboxyl end of either C_L or C_H1. Fabs can be produced in *E. coli*, either by secretion, with coexpression of light chains and Fd fragments or by expression of the chains in intracellular inclusion bodies in separate cultures; in the latter case, they are reconstituted by a refolding reaction using a redox-shuffling buffer system. Several immunotoxins with Fab fragments have been constructed and produced in this way.

The smallest functional modules of antibodies required for antigen binding are Fv fragments. This makes them especially useful for clinical applications, not only for generating recombinant immunotoxins but also for tumor imaging, because their small size improves tumor penetration. Fv fragments are heterodimers of the variable heavy chain (V_H) and the variable light chain (V_L) domains. Unlike whole IgG or Fab, in which the heterodimers are held together and stabilized by interchain disulfide bonds, the V_H and V_L of Fvs are not covalently connected and are consequently unstable; this instability can be overcome by making recombinant Fvs that have the V_H and V_L covalently connected by a peptide linker that fuses the C-terminus of the V_L or V_H to the N-terminus of the other domain (Fig. 1). These molecules are termed *single-chain Fvs* (scFvs), and many retain the specificity and affinity of the original antibody. The cloning, construction, and composition of recombinant Fv fragments of antibodies and Fv–immunotoxins are described in Fig. 3.

Many recombinant immunotoxins have been constructed using scFvs, in which molecules, the *scFv* gene is fused to PE38 to generate a potent cytotoxic agent with targeted specificity (Figs. 1 and 3).

Until recently, the construction of scFvs was the only general method available to make stable Fvs. However, many scFvs are unstable or have reduced affinity for the antigen compared with the parent antibody or Fab fragment. This is because the linker interferes with binding or because the linker does not sufficiently stabilize the Fv structure, leading to aggregation and loss of activity. This is particularly true

at physiological temperatures (37 °C). To overcome these problems, an alternative strategy has been developed that involves generating stable Fvs by connecting the V_H and V_L domains by an interchain disulfide bond engineered between structurally conserved framework residues of the Fv; these molecules are termed *disulfide-stabilized Fvs* (dsFvs). The positions at which the cysteine residues were to be placed were identified by computer-based molecular modeling; as they are located in the framework of each V_H and V_L, this location can be used as a general method to stabilize almost all Fvs without the need for any structural information. Many dsFvs have been constructed in the past three years (mainly as dsFv–immunotoxins, in which the dsFv is fused to PE38) and they show several advantages over scFvs. In addition to their increased stability (due to a decreased tendency to aggregate), they are often produced in higher yields than scFvs; in several cases, the binding affinity of the dsFv was significantly improved over that of the scFv.

4
Construction and Production of Recombinant Immunotoxins

In the recombinant immunotoxins derived from PE, the recombinant antibody fragments are fused to the N-terminus of the truncated derivative of PE (with the cell binding domain deleted, for example, PE40 or PE38). This restores the original domain arrangement of PE, which consists of an N-terminal binding domain followed by the translocation domain and the C-terminal ADP-ribosylation domain.

Only fusions of an antigen binding domain (Fv) to the N-terminus of truncated PE are active; C-terminal fusions are not active because the bulky antigen binding domain blocks translocation of the C-terminal fragment into the cytoplasm.

DT immunotoxins are fusions of mutated DT with antigen binding regions of a recombinant antibody. However, in this case the antigen binding domain must be fused to the C-terminus of DT. This corresponds to the inverse arrangement of the functional modules of PE and DT (see Fig. 3). DT immunotoxins are active only when the enzymatically active N-terminal domain is free to translocate into the cytosol.

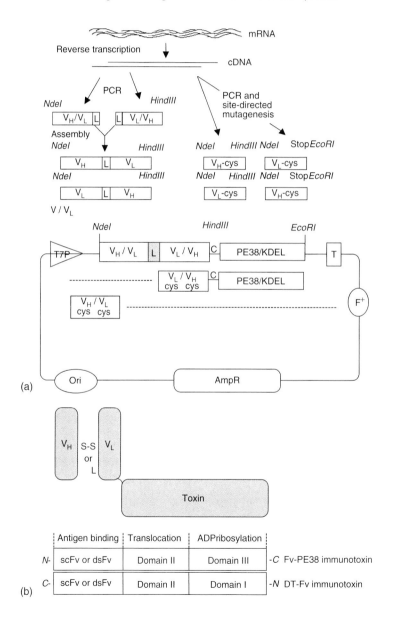

(a)

(b)

	Antigen binding	Translocation	ADPribosylation	
N-	scFv or dsFv	Domain II	Domain III	-C Fv-PE38 immunotoxin
C-	scFv or dsFv	Domain II	Domain I	-N DT-Fv immunotoxin

The expression vectors used for DT immunotoxins are very similar to those used with PE with the exception that the DNA fragments encoding the binding moiety are ligated to the 3′-end of the DT coding region. The cloning of the antibody variable regions is performed using cloning techniques that are now well established (Fig. 3). The plasmid vector for the expression of scFv–immunotoxins or the components of dsFv–immunotoxins is a high copy–number plasmid derived from vectors made and described by Studier and Moffatt. These contain the T7 promoter, translation initiation signals, and a transcription terminator, as well as an F+ phage replication origin to generate single-stranded DNA to be used for site-directed mutagenesis.

When these plasmids are transformed into *E. coli* BL21/DE3 (which contain the *T7 RNA* polymerase gene under the control of the *lac*UV5 promoter) they generate large amounts of recombinant protein upon IPTG induction. The recombinant scFv–immunotoxin or the components of the dsFv–immunotoxin accumulate in insoluble intracellular inclusion bodies. [dsFv–immunotoxins require two cultures, one expressing the V_H and one expressing the V_L; the toxin moiety (PE38) can be fused to either the V_H or the V_L.] The inclusion bodies are then isolated, purified, solubilized, reduced, and subsequently used in a refolding reaction that is controlled for oxidation (redox shuffling). In the case of dsFv–immunotoxins, solubilized inclusion bodies of V_H and V_L

Fig. 3 Cloning, construction, and composition of scFv–and dsFv–immunotoxins. (a) Cloning and construction of recombinant scFv–and dsFv–immunotoxins. The genes encoding the V_H and V_L variable domains are cloned usually from hybridoma mRNA by reverse transcription, cDNA synthesis, and subsequent PCR amplification using degenerate primers that are complementary to the 5′ or 3′ end of the V_H and V_L genes, or by primers that are designed according to the N-terminal amino acid sequence of the mAb to be cloned and conserved sequences at the N-terminal of the heavy and light constant regions. The variable genes can be also cloned by constant domains primers and using the RACE rapid amplification of cDNA ends (method). Restriction sites for assembling the peptide linker sequence that connects the V_H and V_L domains and for cloning into the expression vector are also introduced by PCR. Construction of dsFv involves the generation of two expression plasmids that encode the two components of the dsFv V_H-Cys and V_L-Cys. The cysteines are introduced in position 44 in FR2 of V_H and position 100 of FR4 of V_L or position 105 of FR4 in V_H and position 43 of FR2 in V_L (numbering system of Kabat et al.) by site-directed mutagenesis using as a template a uracil-containing single-stranded DNA of the scFv construct from the F+ origin present in the expression plasmid and cotransfection with M13 helper phage. In addition to the cysteines, cloning sites, ATG translation initiation codons and stop codons are introduced at the 5′ and 3′ ends and of the V_H and V_L genes as shown by site-directed mutagenesis or PCR. The antibody variable genes are subcloned into an expression vector, which contains the gene for a truncated form of PE. This expression vector is controlled by the T7 promoter and upon induction of the T7 RNA polymerase, which is under the control of the *lac*UV5 promoter, in *E. coli* BL21λDE3 by IPTG, large amounts of recombinant protein are produced. (b) Composition of recombinant immunotoxins. In PE-derived recombinant Fv–immunotoxins, the Fv region of the targeting antibody is fused to the N-terminus of a truncated form of PE, which contains the translocation domain (domain II) and enzymatically active ADP-ribosylation domain (domain III). The cell binding domain of whole PE (domain I) is replaced by the Fv targeting moiety thus preserving the relative position of the binding domain function to the other functional domains of PE. In the dsFv–immunotoxins, there are two components. In one, the V_H or V_L domains are fused to the N-terminus of the truncated PE and, in the other, the variable domain is covalently linked by the engineered disulfide bond. DT-derived immunotoxins are fused to the C-terminus due to the inverse arrangement of the functional modules of PE and DT.

(with the toxin fused to either) are mixed in a 1:1 molar ratio into the refolding solution. The formation of the interchain disulfide bond between the V_H and V_L domains is promoted by inducing oxidation using excess oxidized glutathione or by refolding at high pH. The immunotoxins are then purified from the refolding mixtures by ion-exchange and size-exclusion chromatography. Approximately 20 mg of clinical-grade active immunotoxin can be obtained from 1 L of a fermentor culture induced with IPTG.

5
Preclinical Development of Recombinant Immunotoxins

A wide variety of recombinant immunotoxins have been made and tested against cancer target cells. If found to be active and are considered to be tested in clinical trials, they undergo several years of preclinical

development to determine their efficacy and toxicity in several *in vitro* and *in vivo* experimental models (Table 2).

The initial phase is the characterization of the biological activity of the immunotoxin on cultured tumor cells. These assays include measurement of cell free enzymatic activity, that is, ADP-ribosylation activity in the case of bacterial toxins, and the binding affinity of the immunotoxin to the target antigen, which can be determined on purified antigen, on cells by binding displacement assays or by surface plasmon resonance assays. Cytotoxicity assays are performed on antigen-bearing cells and measure either inhibition of protein synthesis, proliferation, colony counts or cell viability.

Cytotoxicity assays on malignant, single-cell suspensions directly obtained from patients are a very useful test, if available, since such cells contain the physiological numbers of receptor or target density, which, in many cases is lower than

Tab. 2 Functional properties *in vitro* and *in vivo* of PE-based recombinant Fv-immunotoxins.

Immunotoxin	Specificity	Activity in vitro (IC$_{50}$) [ng mL^{-1}]	Binding affinity (Kd) [nM]	Antitumor activity in vivo (xenograft model)
Anti-Tac(Fv)-PE38 (LMB-2)	CD25	0.15	1.4	Complete regressions/ cures (ATAC4)
B3(Fv)-PE38 (LMB-7)	Lewis Y	1.5	1300	Complete regressions/ cures (A431)
B3(dsFv)-PE38 (LMB-9)	Lewis Y	1.5	24000	Complete regressions/ cures (A431)
e23(Fv)-PE38 (erb-38)	erbB2/HER2	0.3	40	Partial regressions (A431)
RFB4(dsFv)-PE38 (BL22)	CD22	10	10	Partial and some complete regressions (CA46)
SS1(Fv)-PE38	Mesothelin	0.5	11	Complete regressions/ cures (A431-K5)
MR1(Fv)-PE38	Mutant EGF-R	3.0	11	Partial regressions (glioblastoma)
55.1(Fv)-PE38	Mucin carbohydrate	0.3	80	Complete regressions (Colo205)

established cell lines. The stability of recombinant immunotoxins *in vitro* in various physiological buffers or human serum is also an important test to predict their stability *in vivo*. *In vivo* efficacy of recombinant immunotoxins is usually demonstrated in immunodeficient mice bearing xenografts of human tumor cells. The tumor xenografts can be established as subcutaneous solid tumors, orthotopic implants, or disseminated leukemia.

Initial toxicity and pharmacokinetics studies have also been performed in mice; however, many target antigens are present at some level on some normal tissues, and thus toxicology and pharmacokinetics studies should be tested in an animal that has normal cells capable of binding the target antigen. For most immunotoxins, this requires studies in monkeys to test for targeted damage to normal tissues to predict whether such damage will occur in humans.

6
Application of Recombinant Immunotoxins

6.1
Recombinant Immunotoxins against Solid Tumors

The treatment of solid tumors with immunotoxins is challenging because of their physiological nature of tight junctions between tumor cells, high interstitial pressure within tumors and heterogeneous blood supply, and also antigen expression. The greatest need for new therapies is in the treatment of metastatic epithelial cancers, and immunotoxins can be a useful addition to the standard procedures of surgery, radiation, and chemotherapy.

As already described, the use of recombinant fragments of antibodies for making

recombinant immunotoxins is especially useful for the treatment of solid tumors because their small size improves tumor penetration. Over recent years, several recombinant immunotoxins that target solid tumors have been developed (Table 2); targets include breast, lung, gastric, bladder, and central nervous system cancers. They are at different stages of clinical development and some are already employed in clinical trials.

mAb B3 is an antibody that reacts with the LeY antigen present on cancers of the colon, breast, stomach, lung, and bladder. Early trials with a first-generation immunotoxin (LMB-1) in which an antibody to LeY (mAb B3) was used to make a chemical conjugate with PE38 showed significant clinical activity, with responses in colon and breast cancer. The one complete response and one partial response observed in this trial were the first major responses to immunotoxins documented for metastatic breast and colon cancer respectively.

The B3 antibody was then used to make a single-chain immunotoxin termed *B3(Fv)–PE38* or *LMB-7*. LMB-7 has shown good activity against human cancer xenografts growing in mice and it is also able to cure carcinomatous meningitis in rats when given by the intrathecal route. A phase I clinical trial with LMB-7 began in 1995 and is nearing completion. During the trial, it became evident that LMB-7 lost activity when incubated at 37 °C because of aggregation, which greatly limited its ability to penetrate solid tumors.

B3(dsFv)–PE38 (LMB-9) is the dsFv version of LMB-7 with stability improved over that of LMB-7. This improved stability also allowed it to be used in a continuous-infusion mode in mice bearing human tumor xenografts; this route of administration showed an improved therapeutic window over a bolus injection. Clinical trials with LMB-9 started in the middle of 1998. A different recombinant single-chain immunotoxin, BR96(scFv)–PE40 was derived from the anti-LeY mAb BR96 and is also currently undergoing clinical testing.

Monoclonal antibody e23 is directed at *erb*B2 (Her2/*neu*), which is highly expressed in many breast, lung, ovarian, and stomach cancers. e23(dsFv)–PE38 is a dsFv–immunotoxin composed of the Fv portion of the e23 antibody and PE38. This dsFv–immunotoxin has a significantly improved binding affinity and stability compared with its scFv analog, e23(Fv)–PE38. FRP5scFv–ETA is also a recombinant immunotoxin targeting *erb*B2. Clinical trials with e23(Fv)–PE38 were initiated in early 1998. In a phase I study on breast cancer patients, hepatotoxicity was observed in all patients. Immunohistochemistry showed the presence of *erb*B2 on hepatocytes, explaining the liver toxicity of the immunotoxin. This study demonstrated that targeting of tumors with antibodies to *erb*B2 armed with toxic agents or radioisotopes may result in unexpected organ toxicity due to the expression of the target antigen on normal cells.

Other recombinant immunotoxins that have been constructed and have antitumor activities *in vitro* and in mouse models *in vivo* include: B1(Fv)–PE38, also directed against the LeY antigen; 55.1(Fv)–PE38 and 55.1(dsFv)–PE38, which are directed at a carbohydrate mucin antigen overexpressed in colon cancers; MR1(Fv)–PE38, constructed by antibody phage-display technology and directed to a mutant EGF receptor overexpressed in liver and brain tumors; and SS(Fv)–PE38, a new recombinant immunotoxin specific for mesothelin, a differentiation antigen present on the surface of ovarian cancers, mesotheliomas, and several other types of human cancers.

SS(Fv)–PE38 was constructed from an Fv fragment that was isolated by antibody-phage display from mice that underwent DNA immunization with a plasmid expressing the cloned antigen. This approach to antibody formation eliminates the need for the production of proteins for immunization.

Immunotoxins were also used to target tumors of the central nervous system. Since the transferrin receptor is expressed on tumor and normal hepatic cells but not in normal brain, several trials have targeted antitransferrin receptor immunotoxins to brain tumors. These include a conjugate of mAb 454A12 with a recombinant form of ricin-A (plant toxin), a conjugate of human transferrin with a mutant form of DT and chimeric toxin of recombinant IL-4–PE38 fusion.

6.2
Recombinant Immunotoxins against Leukemias and Lymphomas

Conventional immunotoxins, in which IgGs or Fabs are coupled to toxins, have also been used to target leukemias and lymphomas. This approach should be quite effective because many of the tumor cells are in the blood and bone marrow, where they are readily accessible to the drug. Moreover, fresh cells from patients may be easily tested for immunotoxin binding and cytotoxic activity.

Immunotoxins have also been developed for indirect treatment of malignancies by their killing of T cells that mediate graft-versus-host disease (GvHD) in the setting of allogeneic transplantation. Clinical trials using ricin-based immunoconjugates for treatment of leukemias have shown some promising results, but dose escalation has been limited by the side effects of the toxin. In addition, it is important to eliminate not only easily accessible tumor cells but also malignant cells that are less accessible. Therefore, even for leukemias, there is a need to develop small recombinant immunotoxins that will reach cells outside the circulation. Recombinant immunotoxins targeted at leukemia and lymphoma antigens have been made with antibody fragments specific for the subunit of the IL-2 receptor (CD25) and for CD22. In addition, growth factor fusion proteins have been made that target the IL-2, IL-4, IL-6, and granulocyte macrophage colony stimulating factor (GM-CSF) receptors.

The most potent immunotoxin produced against leukemia cells is anti-Tac(Fv)−PE38 (LMB-2); this targets CD25, which is overexpressed on many T-cell leukemias. LMB-2 is very active against leukemia cell lines *in vitro* and has very good activity in animal models. It also selectively kills cells *in vitro* obtained from patients with adult T-cell leukemia without harming hematopoietic stem cells. Phase I clinical trials with LMB-2 are showing promising results. The immunotoxin was administered to 35 patients for a total of 59 treatment cycles. One hairy cell leukemia (HCL) patient achieved a complete remission, which is ongoing at 20 months. Seven partial responses were observed in cutaneous T-cell lymphoma, HCL, chronic lymphocytic leukemia, Hodgkin's disease and adult T-cell leukemia. Responding patients had a 2 to 5 log reduction of circulating malignant cells, improvement in skin lesions, and regression of lymphomatous mass and splenomegally. All four patients with HCL responded to the treatment (one with complete responses and three had 98−99.8% reductions in malignant circulating cells). A phase II trial is planned in patients with CD25$^+$ hematologic malignancies and phase I trials are planned

for the prevention of GvHD in patients undergoing high-risk allotransplantation.

The conventional immunotoxin RFT5−SMPT−dgA has also been developed to target CD25 and has resulted in several responses in Hodgkin's disease, one of which lasted over two years. It is already undergoing testing for the prevention of GvHD in patients undergoing allotransplantation and has recently been shown *ex vivo* to remove alloreactive donor T cells while preserving antileukemia and antiviral T-cell responses.

A new agent, RFB4(dsFv)−PE38 (BL22), is a dsFv−immunotoxin directed at the CD22 differentiation antigen present on most B-cell leukemias. It has high cytotoxic activity on cultured tumor cells as well as in animal models and preclinical tests have been completed. This recombinant immunotoxin recently entered clinical trials in patients with leukemias. Initial phase I trials in 16 chemotherapy-resistant HCL patients resulted in 11 complete responses and two partial responses, including two partial responses in patients ineligible for LMB-2 because of CD25$^-$ HCL cells. Responses to BL22 were associated with at least a 99.5% reduction in circulating HCL cells. BL22 also induced responses in chronic lymphocytic leukemia. These recent results demonstrate that recombinant Fv−immunotoxins containing truncated PE are particularly effective in patients with chemotherapy-refractory HCL and other hematological malignancies. Other targets for the development of B-cell leukemia−specific recombinant immunotoxins include the CD19 and CD20 differentiation antigens in B-cell tumors, and CD30 in Hodgkin's lymphoma.

The B-cell lymphoma markers CD22 and CD19 were also targeted using conventional first-generation immunotoxins with dgA – IgG – RFB4 – dgA (targeting CD22) and IgG – HD37 – dgA (targeting CD19). Leukemias and lymphomas were also targeted with recombinant fusions of IL-2 with truncated DT.

7
Isolation of New and Improved Antibody Fragments as Targeting Moieties: Display Technologies for the Improvement of Immunotoxin Activity

The generation of mAbs made by immunizing animals and allowing *in vivo* processes, such as immune tolerance and somatic hypermutation, to shape the antigen-combining site is a key issue for the generation of specific antibodies. The unique features required from these molecules were already described in Sect. 1 of this article. These antibodies created *in vivo* can be used for many research and diagnostic applications. Mouse mAbs might be made less immunogenic and more effective for human therapy by reformatting the binding site into chimeric or complementary-determining region (CDR)-grafted antibodies. The advances in recombinant DNA technology and antibody engineering have also led to the ability to manipulate the size of the antigen binding domain as described in this article. The two variable domains of the binding site can be cloned and arranged into a large array of possible molecular formats and sizes, and expressed in a variety of hosts, ranging from bacteria, lower eukaryotes such as yeast and fungi, to the higher eukaryotes, including mammalian cells, transgenic animals and plants. Extraordinary progress in engineering and selecting small antibody fragments for immunotherapeutic approaches has been made over the past

decade, when molecular display technologies have been developed that allow us to create very large repertoires of mouse or fully human antibodies that are displayed on filamentous phage or other molecular display systems. These technologies are now revolutionizing the way in which we can build high-affinity binding sites from scratch, from any species (including humans) and use them for clinical applications such as the targeting of a drug or toxin to cancer cells as in recombinant Fv – immunotoxins.

The concept of molecular display technology relays on the physical linkage between the genotype (the antibody variable region genes) and the phenotype (antigen-binding capability) to allow simultaneous selection of the genes that encode a protein with the desired binding function. This concept can be viewed as an *in vitro* mimicking system for the natural antibody response function of the immune system. This concept was first applied by George Smith in 1985 to small peptides. The display of functional antibody repertoires on phages required several additional discoveries. First, a procedure for accessing large collections of antibody variable domains was needed; this was first described in 1989, when partially degenerate oligonucleotides priming to the 5′ and 3′ end of variable region genes and the polymerase chain reaction (PCR) were used to amplify hybridoma or large collections of variable genes. Second, as whole antibodies cannot yet be functionally expressed in bacteria, a crucial discovery was that antibody fragments (Fab or scFv) were functionally expressed in *E. coli* when they were secreted into the periplasm of the bacteria, which simulated the naturally oxidizing environment of the endoplasmic reticulum. By providing restriction sites in the oligonucleotides used for PCR amplification, antibody libraries could thus be cloned for expression in *E. coli*. Initially, such antibody libraries were expressed from phage-λ vectors; a plaque-screening assay with labeled antigen was then used to identify antigen-specific binding sites. Such time-consuming procedures were rapidly replaced by the third seminal development: the provision of a link between the phenotype and the genotype using phages. In 1990, McCafferty et al. showed that antibody fragments could be displayed on the surface of filamentous phage particles by fusion of the antibody variable genes to one of the phage coat proteins. Multiple rounds of affinity selection could subsequently enrich antigen-specific phage antibodies, because the phage particle carries the gene encoding the displayed antibody. This was originally reported for scFv fragments, and later for Fab fragments and other antibody derivatives such as diabodies, as well as extended to various display systems. With these advances in place, it became possible to make phage antibody libraries by PCR cloning of large collections of variable region genes expressing each of the binding sites on the surface of a different phage particle and harvesting the antigen-specific binding sites by *in vitro* selection of the phage mixture on a chosen antigen. In the early 1990s, Clackson et al. showed for the first time that phage-display technology could be used to select antigen-specific antibodies from libraries made from the spleen B cells of immunized mice, thereby bypassing the requirement to immortalize the antigen-specific B cells, as in the hybridoma technology. Similarly, libraries were made from human B cells taken from animals or individuals immunized with antigen, exposed to infectious agents, with autoimmune diseases or with cancer. Thus, phage-display technology in

the early 1990s had already shown the potential to replace hybridoma technology by rescuing *V* genes from immune B cells. Further advances were reported in the mid-1990s that would bypass the use of immunization and animals altogether. First, it was shown that antibodies against many different antigens could be selected from nonimmune libraries, made from the naive light-chain and heavy-chain *IgM* *V*-gene pools of B cells of a non-immunized, healthy individual. Second, libraries of synthetic antibody genes, with variable genes not harvested from immune sources but consisting of germline segments artificially provided with diversity by oligonucleotide cloning, were shown to behave in a similar way to naive antibody libraries. It thus became possible to use primary antibody libraries, with huge collections of binding sites with different specificities, to select *in vitro* binding sites against most antigens, including nonimmunogenic molecules, toxic substances, and targets conserved between species.

Since these key discoveries, there have been numerous reports on applications of phage antibody libraries, ranging from basic research to drug development. In addition, many novel, related molecular display methods for antibodies have been described, including display systems on ribosomes, bacteria, and yeast cells. These technologies follow similar concepts for *in vitro* selection and improvement of binding sites. Novel selection strategies of phage-display libraries and other molecular display systems are being developed for the identification of novel antigen-binding fragments. These include selection for binding using purified or nonpurified antigen, selection for function, selection based on display capability and phage infectivity, subtractive selection procedures, and also using high-throughput selection and screening. The use of phage-display systems will revolutionize the field of targeted drug therapy in general and the recombinant immunotoxin field in particular, because advances in this field are dependent not only on the identification of new targets on cancer cells but also on the development of new and very specific targeting moieties such as antibody fragments (scFvs). Phage-display technology now enables one to select such molecules against unique targets, especially when hybridoma technology fails to produce antibodies against an antigen or when nonimmunogenic or conserved targets between species are being used. Alternatives to phage display for making fully human antibodies are technologies developed using transgenic mice (xenomice). These transgenic mice have been engineered to lack the native murine immune repertoire and instead harbor most of the human immune system *V* genes in the germline. Injection of these "humanized" animals with a foreign antigen or hapten effectively evokes an immune response and a humanlike antibody is produced in the B cells. The antibody genes can be recovered from B cells either by PCR and library selection or by fusion into a monoclonal cell line by classic hybridoma technology. Several examples of recombinant Fv–immunotoxins that were constructed from scFvs isolated by phage display have already been reported and are being considered for use in clinical trials.

The phage-display approach has been used to isolate an scFv that binds with high affinity to a mutant form of the EGF receptor in which a deletion of a portion of the extracellular domain of the receptor generates a tumor-specific antigen. Another novel target for cancer therapy could be cancer-specific peptides presented on human leukocyte antigen (HLA) molecules on the surface of tumor cells. To accomplish this, it will be necessary to isolate antibodies that recognize tumor-specific peptides associated with class I MHC molecules on tumor cells. As a first step in this direction, a recombinant immunotoxin has been constructed using an antibody that was isolated by phage display and that binds specifically to peptide/MHC complexes found on virally infected cells. This recombinant immunotoxin was cytotoxic only to cells specifically expressing hemagglutinin peptide HA255–262 in complex with H-2K^k (mouse class I MHC) and was not cytotoxic to cells that express other peptides associated with H-2K^k or to cells not expressing H-2K^k. These studies indicate that, if antibodies that recognize tumor-specific peptides in the context of class I MHC molecules can be developed, they should be very useful agents for targeted cancer immunotherapy. Recently, the isolation of a human antibody directed against a peptide encoded by the melanoma-associated antigen MAGE-A1 presented by HLA-A1 molecules was reported. A large phage-Fab antibody repertoire was selected on a recombinant version of the complex. One of the selected phage antibodies shows binding to HLA-A1 complexed with the MAGE-A1 peptide, but does not show binding to HLA-A1 complexed with a peptide encoded by gene *MAGE-A3* and differing from the MAGE-A1 peptide by only three residues. Phages carrying this recombinant antibody bind to HLA-A1$^+$ cells only after *in vitro* loading with MAGE-A1 peptide. It remains now to see if such human anti-MHC/peptide complexes may prove useful for monitoring the cell surface expression of these complexes and, eventually, as a targeting reagent for the specific killing of tumor cells expressing tumor peptide/MHC complexes. The isolation of such rare antibodies against unique tumor targets is a proof of the powerful abilities of antibody phage-display technology for the development of new generations of targeting molecules for cancer therapy and diagnosis.

Phage-display technology can be used not only to create new scFv antibodies but also to improve the properties of existing scFvs. Improvements in antibody stability, expression, and binding affinity can be achieved by using a combination of strategies including random and directed mutagenesis of CDR regions, DNA shuffling, and error-prone PCR. These mutagenesis strategies combined with the powerful selection methods available to *screen* antibody phage-display libraries can yield scFv molecules with significantly improved properties for clinical applications. For example, phage display was used to improve antibody affinity by mimicking somatic hypermutation *in vitro*. *In vivo* affinity maturation of antibodies involves mutation of hot spots in the DNA encoding the variable regions. This information was used to develop a strategy to improve antibody affinity *in vitro* using phage-display technology. The anti-mesothelin scFv, SS(scFv), was used to identify DNA sequences in the variable regions that are naturally prone to hypermutations. In a few selected hot spot regions encoding nonconserved amino acids, random mutations were introduced to make libraries with a size requirement between 10^3 and 10^4 independent clones. Panning of the hot spot libraries yielded several mutants with a 15- to 55-fold increase in affinity compared with a single clone with a 4-fold increased affinity from a library in which mutagenesis was done outside the hot spots (Table 2). This is an example of a powerful phage-display-based strategy that should be generally applicable for the rapid isolation of higher-affinity mutants

of Fvs, Fabs, and other recombinant antibodies from antibody-phage libraries that are smaller in size.

In another example, random CDR mutagenesis to obtain mutants of MR1(Fv)−PE38, a single-chain recombinant immunotoxin that targets a mutant form of the EGF receptor, EGFRvIII, that is frequently overexpressed in malignant glioblastomas, was performed (Table 2). Initially, nine residues of heavy chain CDR3 were randomly mutagenized and several mutants with increased binding affinity were isolated. All mutations were in regions that correspond to a DNA hot spot. The mutant MR1Fvs with an increased affinity for EGFRvIII had an increased activity when converted to recombinant immunotoxins. A specific region of the variable region of the antibody light chain CDR3 that corresponded to a hot spot was mutagenized, and a mutant antibody with an additional increase in affinity and cytotoxic activity was isolated. These studies further show that targeting hot spots in the CDRs of Fvs is an effective approach for obtaining Fvs with increased affinity.

8
Improving The Therapeutic Window of Recombinant Immunotoxins: The Balance of Toxicity, Immunogenicity, and Efficacy

Although some of the problems, including design, large-scale production and stability, associated with the initial recombinant immunotoxins have been solved, other fundamental problems need to be addressed that are relevant to much of the immunotherapy field. Specificity, toxicity, and immunogenicity are major factors that will determine the usefulness and success of recombinant immunotoxins.

8.1
Immune Responses and Dose-limiting Toxicity

As with any cytotoxic agent, side effects such as nonspecific toxicity and immunogenicity can occur when multiple injections of immunotoxins are given. One class of side effects is due to inappropriate targeting of the immunotoxin to normal cells because of the poor specificity of the antibody. In addition, the toxin or the Fv portion of the antibody can bind nonspecifically to various tissues. For example, in mice, which usually do not contain target antigens, liver damage occurs when large amounts of immunotoxins are given. Molecular modeling combined with site-directed mutagenesis may help in the design of new versions of the toxin with decreased toxicity caused by nonspecific binding.

The development of neutralizing antibodies usually occurs after 10 days and limits the therapeutic application of immunotoxins to this 10-day period. Recent data from clinical trials indicate that patients with solid tumors develop antibodies much more readily then those with hematologic tumors. It is speculated that some hematologic tumors may be associated with less immunogenicity than others. For example, none of 14 patients with chronic lymphocytic leukemia treated with LMB-2 or BL22 have shown any evidence of antibodies.

Several approaches have been taken to reduce immunogenicity. One is to make small molecules, which appear to be less immunogenic; another is to use immunosuppressive agents such as deoxyspergualin or CTLA-4–Ig, an inhibitor of the costimulation pathways required for T-cell help and activation through the CD28/CTLA-4–CD80/CD86

complex. Another approach is to use the anti-CD20 mAb, Rituximab, which induces B-cell depletion in the majority of patients and is itself nonimmunogenic.

The dose-limiting toxicity of many immunotoxins is vascular leak syndrome (VLS). Recent studies indicate that recombinant toxins, including those containing mutated forms of PE, produce VLS in rats and that inflammation, which can be suppressed by steroids or nonsteroidal anti-inflammatory agents, mediates the VLS. VLS can also be mediated indirectly by the activation of endothelial cells and/or macrophages via cytokines such as tumor necrosis factor-α and interferon-γ. The activated cells produce nitric oxide (NO), which then can mediate oxidative damage to the endothelial cells and result in increased permeability.

Some studies demonstrate direct endothelial cell damage caused by binding the toxin to the cells. The direct damage to the cell is mediated by the enzymatic activity of the toxin, while others show an indirect damage that is mediated by binding of the targeting moiety. For example, experiments with human umbilical vein endothelial cells exposed to LMB-1 (antibody conjugate with truncated PE38) indicated that the mAb B3 rather than PE38 was binding to the LeY antigen on endothelial cells. Recent experiments using an *in vivo* model composed of human neonatal foreskin xenografts in severe combined immuno-deficient (SCID) mice identified a 3-amino acid motif present in protein toxins and in IL-2 that causes VLS without other toxin activity. Thus, VLS can be blocked in future trials with anti-inflammatory agents to block cytokine action, or by mutations or peptide inhibitors that will prevent the binding of the toxin or the targeting moiety to endothelial cells.

Toxicity can also be reduced by modifications in the scFv-targeting moiety. For example, reduction of the nonspecific animal toxicity of recombinant Fv–immunotoxin anti-Tac(Fv)–PE38 (which targets the IL-2 receptor) was achieved by introducing mutations in the framework regions of the Fv, which lower the isoelectric point (pI). The dose escalation with this recombinant Fv–immunotoxin (that has produced eight responses, including a durable clinically complete remission in a recently completed phase I trial of leukemias and lymphomas) was limited by liver toxicity. It was noted that the Fv of anti-Tac has a pI of 10.2, which brought about the hypothesis that the overall positive charge on the Fv portion of anti-Tac(Fv)–PE38 contributes to nonspecific binding to liver cells and results in dose-limiting liver toxicity. A mouse model was used to investigate the basis of this toxicity, and it was found that lowering the pI of the Fv of anti-Tac from 10.2 to 6.82 by selective mutation of surface residues causes a 3-fold decrease in animal toxicity and hepatic necrosis. This change in pI did not significantly alter the CD25 binding affinity, the cytotoxic activity toward target cells, or antitumor activity, resulting in a 3-fold improvement in the therapeutic index. If this decreased toxicity occurs in humans, it should greatly increase the clinical utility of this immunotoxin.

Another strategy to overcome the problems of nonspecific toxicity and antigenicity is by the chemical modification of the recombinant Fv–immunotoxins. An example of this was also demonstrated recently in which site-specific chemical modification with polyethylene glycol (PEGylation) of anti-Tac(Fv)–PE38 (LMB-2) improved its antitumor activity, and reduced animal toxicity and immunogenicity. PEGylation

can increase plasma half-lives, stability, and therapeutic potency. To produce a PEGylated recombinant immunotoxin with improved therapeutic properties, a mutant form of anti-Tac(Fv)–PE38 (LMB-2) in which one cysteine residue was introduced into the peptide connector (ASGCGPE) between the Fv and the toxin was constructed. This mutant LMB-2 (Cys1-LMB-2), which retained full cytotoxic activity, was then site-specifically conjugated with 5 or 20 kDa of polyethylene glycol–maleimide. When compared with unmodified LMB-2, both PEGylated immunotoxins showed similar cytotoxic activities *in vitro*, but superior stability at 37 °C in mouse serum, a 5- to 8-fold increase in plasma half-lives in mice and a 3- to 4-fold increase in antitumor activity. This was accompanied by a substantial decrease in animal toxicity and immunogenicity. Site-specific PEGylation of recombinant immunotoxins may thus increase their therapeutic potency in humans.

8.2
Specificity Dictated by the Targeting Moiety

Specificity of the recombinant immunotoxin is determined by the distribution of the target antigens; several target antigens are relatively cancer specific, but are present on some normal cells in small amounts. For example, *erb*B2, although overexpressed on tumor cells, is also expressed on a limited number of normal cells. This reactivity with normal cells may cause side effects during immunotoxin therapy. It was discovered during a clinical trial that small amounts of the LeY antigen are expressed on the surface of endothelial cells and damage to these cells caused VLS. To overcome such problems, new specific targets and new reagents against the cancer antigens that will recognize only the tumor-associated molecules must be identified and developed. The construction of large phage-display antibody libraries may result in the isolation and characterization of new reagents with improved specificity and affinity for cancer-targeted therapy.

9
Conclusions and Perspectives

Over the past decade, several second-generation recombinant immunotoxins with improved properties have been developed and are currently being evaluated in clinical trials. Several of these show clinical activity and promising results in phase I trials. The outcome of these clinical trials demonstrates that the promising preclinical results with these new agents can be translated into more substantial clinical responses, and that similar agents that target other cancer antigens merit further clinical development. These accumulating results suggest that Fv–immunotoxins merit further development as a new modality for targeted cancer treatment.

See also Molecular Oncology.

Bibliography

Books and Reviews

Kreitman, R.J. (1999) Immunotoxins in cancer therapy, *Curr. Opin. Immunol.* **11**, 570–8.
Kreitam, R.J., Pastan, I. (1998) Immunotoxins for targeted cancer therapy, *Adv. Drug Deliv. Rev.* **31**, 53–88.
Pastan, I., Chaudhary, V., FitzGerald, D.J. (1992) Recombinant toxins as novel therapeutic agents, *Annu. Rev. Biochem.* **61**, 331–54.

Vitteta, E.S. (1994) From the basic science of B cells to biological missiles at the bedside, *J. Immunol.* **153**, 1407–20.

Primary Literature

Allured, V.S., Collier, R.J., Carroll, S.F., McKay, D.B. (1986) Structure of exotoxin A of *Pseudomonas aeruginosa* at 3.0 Angstrom resolution, *Proc. Natl. Acad. Sci. U. S. A.* **83**, 1320–4.
Amlot, P.L., Stone, M.L., Cunningham, D. et al. (1993) A phase I study of an anti-CD22–deglycosylated ricin A chain immunotoxin in the treatment of B-cell lymphomas resistant to conventional therapy, *Blood* **82**, 2624–33.
Andersen, P.S., Stryhn, A., Hansen, B.E., Fugger, L., Engberg, J., Buus, S.A. (1996) Recombinant antibody with the antigen-specific, major histocompatibility complex-restricted specificity of T cells, *Proc. Natl. Acad. Sci. U. S. A.* **93**, 1820–4.
Baluna, R., Vitetta, E.S. (1997) Vascular leak syndrome: a side effect of immunotherapy, *Immunopharmacology* **37**, 117–32.
Baluna, R., Vitetta, E.S. (1999) An *in vivo* model to study immunotoxin-induced vascular leak in human tissue, *J. Immunother.* **22**, 41–47.
Baluna, R., Rizo, J., Gordon, B.E., Ghetie, V., Vitetta, E.S. (1999) Evidence for a structural motif in toxins and interleukin-2 that may be responsible for binding to endothelial cells and initiating vascular leak syndrome, *Proc. Natl. Acad. Sci. U. S. A.* **96**, 3957–62.
Barbas, C.F. III, Bain, J.D., Hoekstra, D.M., Lerner, R.A. (1992) Semisynthetic combinatorial antibody libraries: a chemical solution to the diversity problem, *Proc. Natl. Acad. Sci. U. S. A.* **89**, 4457–61.
Batra, J.K., Kasprzyk, P.G., Bird, R.E., Pastan, I., King, C.R. (1992) Recombinant anti-erbB2 immunotoxins containing *Pseudomonas* exotoxin, *Proc. Natl. Acad. Sci. U. S. A.* **89**, 5867–71.
Batra, J.K., Jinno, Y., Chaudhary, V.K. et al. (1989) Antitumor activity in mice of an immunotoxin made with anti-transferrin receptor and a recombinant form of *Pseudomonas* exotoxin, *Proc. Natl. Acad. Sci. U. S. A.* **86**, 8545–9.
Beers, R., Chowdhury, P., Bigner, D., Pastan, I. (2000) Immunotoxins with increased activity

against epidermal growth factor receptor vIII-expressing cells produced by antibody phage display, *Clin. Cancer Res.* **6**, 2835–43.

Benhar, I., Pastan, I. (1995) Characterization of B1(Fv)PE38 and B1(dsFv)PE38: single-chain and disulfide-stabilized Fv–immunotoxins with increased activity that cause complete remissions of established human carcinoma xenografts in nude mice, *Clin. Cancer Res.* **1**, 1023–9.

Benhar, I., Reiter, Y., Pai, L.H., Pastan, I. (1995) Administration of disulfide-stabilized Fv–immunotoxins B1(dsFv)–PE38 and B3(dsFv)–PE38 by continuous infusion increases their efficacy in curing large tumor xenografts in nude mice, *Int. J. Cancer* **62**, 351–5.

Better, M., Chang, C.P., Robinson, R.R., Horwitz, A.H. (1988) *Escherichia coli* secretion of an active chimeric antibody fragment, *Science* **240**, 1041–3.

Bird, R.E., Hardman, K.D., Jacobson, J.W. et al. (1988) Single-chain antigen-binding proteins, *Science* **242**, 423–6.

Blakey, O.S., Watson, G.J., Knowles, P.P. et al. (1987) Effect of chemical deglycosylation of ricin A-chain on the *in vivo* fate and cytotoxic activity of an immunotoxin composed of ricin A-chain and anti-Thy 1. 1 antibody, *Cancer Res.* **47**, 947–52.

Boder, E.T., Wittrup, K.D. (1997) Yeast surface display for screening combinatorial polypeptide libraries, *Nat. Biotechnol.* **15**, 553–7.

Bolognesi, A., Tazzari, P.L., Olivieri, F. et al. (1996) Induction of apoptosis by ribosome-inactivating proteins and related immunotoxins, *Int. J. Cancer* **68**, 349–55.

Brandhuber, B.J., Allured, V.S., Falbel, T.G., McKay, D.B. (1988) Mapping the enzymatic active site of *Pseudomonas aeruginosa* exotoxin A, *Proteins* **3**, 146–54.

Brinkmann, U., Pastan, I. (1995) Recombinant immunotoxins: from basic research to cancer therapy, *Methods Enzymol.* **8**, 143–56.

Brinkmann, U., Pai, L.H., FitzGerald, D.J., Willingham, M., Pastan, I. (1991) B3(Fv)–PE38KDEL, a single-chain immunotoxin that causes complete regression of a human carcinoma in mice, *Proc. Natl. Acad. Sci. U. S. A.* **88**, 8616–20.

Brinkmann, U., Reiter, Y., Jung, S.H., Lee, B., Pastan, I. (1993) A recombinant immunotoxin containing a disulfide-stabilized Fv fragment, *Proc. Natl. Acad. Sci. U. S. A.* **90**, 7538–42.

Burton, D.R., Barbas, C.F. III, Persson, M.A., Koenig, S., Chanock, R.M., Lerner, R.A. (1991) A large array of human monoclonal antibodies to type 1 human immunodeficiency virus from combinatorial libraries of asymptomatic seropositive individuals, *Proc. Natl. Acad. Sci. U. S. A.* **88**, 10134–7.

Cai, X., Garen, A. (1995) Anti-melanoma antibodies from melanoma patients immunized with genetically modified autologous tumor cells: selection of specific antibodies from single-chain Fv fusion phage libraries, *Proc. Natl. Acad. Sci. U. S. A.* **92**, 6537–41.

Carroll, S.F., Collier, R.J. (1987) Active site of *Pseudomonas aeruginosa* exotoxin A. Glutamic acid 553 is photolabeled by NAD and shows functional homology with glutamic acid 148 of diphtheria toxin, *J. Biol. Chem.* **262**, 8707–11.

Carroll, S.F., Collier, R.J. (1988) Amino acid sequence homology between the enzymic domains of diphtheria toxin and *Pseudomonas aeruginosa* exotoxin A, *Mol. Microbiol.* **2**, 293–6.

Chames, P., Hufton, S.E., Coulie, P.G., Uchanska-Ziegler, B., Hoogenboom, H.R. (2000) Direct selection of a human antibody fragment directed against the tumor T-cell epitope HLA-A1–MAGE-A1 from a nonimmunized phage-Fab library, *Proc. Natl. Acad. Sci. U. S. A.* **97**, 7969–74.

Chang, C.N., Landolfi, N.F., Queen, C. (1991) Expression of antibody Fab domains on bacteriophage surfaces. Potential use for antibody selection, *J. Immunol.* **147**, 3610–4.

Chang, K., Pastan, I. (1996) Molecular cloning of mesothelin, a differentiation antigen present on mesothelium, mesotheliomas, and ovarian cancers, *Proc. Natl. Acad. Sci. U. S. A.* **93**, 136–40.

Chang, K., Pai, L.H., Batra, J.K., Pastan, I., Willingham, M.C. (1992) Characterization of the antigen (CAK1) recognized by monoclonal antibody K1 present on ovarian cancers and normal mesothelium, *Cancer Res.* **52**, 181–6.

Chaudhary, V.K., FitzGerald, D.J., Pastan, I. (1991) A proper amino terminus of diphtheria toxin is important for cytotoxicity, *Biochem. Biophys. Res. Commun.* **180**, 545–51.

Chaudhary, V.K., FitzGerald, D.J., Adhya, S., Pastan, I. (1987) Activity of a recombinant fusion protein between transforming growth factor type α and *Pseudomonas* toxin, *Proc. Natl. Acad. Sci. U. S. A.* **84**, 4538–42.

Chaudhary, V.K., Gallo, M.G., FitzGerald, D.J., Pastan, I. (1990) A recombinant single-chain immunotoxin composed of anti-Tac variable regions and a truncated diphtheria toxin, *Proc. Natl. Acad. Sci. U. S. A.* **87**, 9491–4.

Chaudhary, V.K., Jinno, Y., FitzGerald, D., Pastan, I. (1990) *Pseudomonas* exotoxin contains a specific sequence at the carboxyl terminus that is required for cytotoxicity, *Proc. Natl. Acad. Sci. U. S. A.* **87**, 308–12.

Chaudhary, V.K., Queen, C., Junghans, R.P., Waldmann, T.A., FitzGerald, D.J., Pastan, I. (1989) A recombinant immunotoxin consisting of two antibody variable domains fused to *Pseudomonas* exotoxin, *Nature* **339**, 394–7.

Chiang, Y.L., Sheng-Dong, R., Brow, M.A., Larrick, J.W. (1989) Direct cDNA cloning of the rearranged immunoglobulin variable region, *Biotechniques* **7**, 360–6.

Choe, M., Webber, K.O., Pastan, I. (1994) B3(Fab)–PE38M: a recombinant immunotoxin in which a mutant form of *Pseudomonas* exotoxin is fused to the Fab fragment of monoclonal antibody B3, *Cancer Res.* **54**, 3460–7.

Choe, S., Bennett, M.J., Fujii, G. et al. (1992) The crystal structure of diphtheria toxin, *Nature* **357**, 216–22.

Chowdhury, P.S., Pastan, I. (1999) Improving antibody affinity by mimicking somatic hypermutation *in vitro*, *Nat. Biotechnol.* **17**, 568–72.

Chowdhury, P.S., Viner, J.L., Beers, R., Pastan, I. (1998) Isolation of a high-affinity stable single-chain Fv specific for mesothelin from DNA-immunized mice by phage display and construction of a recombinant immunotoxin with anti-tumor activity, *Proc. Natl. Acad. Sci. U. S. A.* **95**, 669–74.

Clackson, T., Hoogenboom, H.R., Griffiths, A.D., Winter, G. (1991) Making antibody fragments using phage display libraries, *Nature* **352**, 624–8.

Conry, R.M., Khazaeli, M.B., Saleh, M.N. et al. (1995) Phase I trial of an anti-CD19 deglycosylated ricin A chain immunotoxin in non-Hodgkin's lymphoma: effect of an intensive schedule of administration, *J. Immunother.* **18**, 231–41.

Crameri, A., Cwirla, S., Stemmer, W.P. (1996) Construction and evolution of antibody-phage libraries by DNA shuffling, *Nat. Med.* **2**, 100–2.

Dall'Acqua, A., Carter, P. (1998) Antibody engineering, *Curr. Opin. Struct. Biol.* **8**, 443–50.

de Haard, H.J., van Neer, N., Reurs, A. et al. (1999) A large non-immunized human Fab

fragment phage library that permits rapid isolation and kinetic analysis of high affinity antibodies, *J. Biol. Chem.* **274**, 18218–30.

Debinski, W., Pastan, I. (1995) Recombinant F(ab') C242–*Pseudomonas* exotoxin, but not the whole antibody-based immunotoxin, causes regression of a human colorectal tumor xenograft, *Clin. Cancer Res.* **1**, 1015–22.

Debinski, W., Puri, R.K., Kreitman, R.J., Pastan, I. (1993) A wide range of human cancers express interleukin 4 (IL-4) receptors that can be targeted with chimeric toxin composed of IL-4 and *Pseudomonas* exotoxin, *J. Biol. Chem.* **268**, 14065–70.

Eiklid, K., Olsnes, S., Pihl, A. (1980) Entry of lethal doses of abrin, ricin and modeccin into the cytosol of HeLa cells, *Exp. Cell Res.* **126**, 321–9.

Endo, Y., Tsurigi, K. (1987) RNA *N*-glycosidase activity of ricin A-chain. Mechanism of action of the toxic lectin ricin on eukaryotic ribosomes, *J. Biol. Chem.* **262**, 8128–30.

Engberg, J., Krogsgaard, M., Fugger, L. (1999) Recombinant antibodies with the antigen-specific, MHC restricted specificity of T cells: novel reagents for basic and clinical investigations and immunotherapy, *Immunotechnology* **4**, 273–8.

Engert, A., Marlin, G., Amlot, P., Wijdenes, J., Diehl, V., Thorpe, P. (1991) Immunotoxins constructed with anti-CD25 monoclonal antibodies and deglycosylated ricin A-chain have potent anti-tumor effects against human Hodgkin cells *in vitro* and solid Hodgkin tumors in mice, *Int. J. Cancer* **49**, 450–6.

Engert, A., Oiehl, V., Schnell, R. et al. (1997) A phase-1 study of an anti-CD25 ricin A-chain immunotoxin (RFT5–SMPT–dgA) in patients with refractory Hodgkin's lymphoma, *Blood* **89**, 403–410.

Flavell, O.J. (1998) Saporin immunotoxins, *Curr. Topics Microbiol. Immunol.* **234**, 57–61.

Frankel, A.E., Laver, J.H., Willingham, M.C., Burns, L.J., Kersey, J.H., Vallera, D.A. (1997) Therapy of patients with T-cell lymphomas and leukemias using an anti-CD7 monoclonal antibody–ricin A chain immunotoxin, *Leuk. Lymph.* **26**, 287–98.

Garrard, L.J., Yang, M., O'Connell, M.P., Kelley, R.F., Henner, D.J. (1991) Fab assembly and enrichment in a monovalent phage display system, *Biotechnology* **9**, 1373–7.

Georgiou, G., Stathopoulos, C., Daugherty, P.S., Nayak, A.R., Iverson, B.L., Curtiss, R. III (1997)

Display of heterologous proteins on the surface of microorganisms: from the screening of combinatorial libraries to live recombinant vaccines, *Nat. Biotechnol.* **15**, 29–34.

Ghetie, M-A., Richardson, J., Tucker, T., Jones, D., Uhr, J.W., Vitetta, E.S. (1991) Antitumor activity of Fab' and IgG-anti-CD22 immunotoxins in disseminated human B lymphoma grown in mice with severe combined immunodeficiency disease: effect on tumor cells in extranodal sites, *Cancer Res.* **51**, 5876–80.

Giannini, G., Rappuoli, R., Ratti, G. (1984) The amino-acid sequence of two non-toxic mutants of diphtheria toxin: CRM45 and CRM197, *Nucleic Acids Res.* **12**, 4063–9.

Glockshuber, R., Malia, M., Pfitzinger, I., Pluckthun, A. (1990) A comparison of strategies to stabilize immunoglobulin Fv-fragments, *Biochemistry* **29**, 1362–7.

Gram, H., Marconi, L.A., Barbas, C.F. III, Collet, T.A., Lerner, R.A., Kang, A.S. (1992) In vitro selection and affinity maturation of antibodies from a naive combinatorial immunoglobulin library, *Proc. Natl. Acad. Sci. U. S. A.* **89**, 3576–80.

Graus, Y.F., de Baets, M.H., Parren, P.W. et al. (1997) Human anti-nicotinic acetylcholine receptor recombinant Fab fragments isolated from thymus-derived phage display libraries from myasthenia gravis patients reflect predominant specificities in serum and block the action of pathogenic serum antibodies, *J. Immunol.* **158**, 1919–29.

Greenfield, L., Johnson, V.G., Youle, R.J. (1987) Mutations in diphtheria toxin separate binding from entry and amplify immunotoxin selectivity, *Science* **238**, 536–9.

Greenfield, L., Bjorn, M.J., Horn, G. et al. (1983) Nucleotide sequence of the structural gene for diphtheria toxin carried by corynebacteriophage β, *Proc. Natl. Acad. Sci. U. S. A.* **80**, 6853–7.

Grossbard, M.L., Lambert, J.M., Goldmacher, V.S. et al. (1993) Anti-B4-blocked ricine: a phase I trial of 7-day continuous infusion in patients with B-cell neoplasms, *J. Clin. Oncol.* **11**, 726–737.

Hanes, J., Pluckthun, A. (1997) *In vitro* selection and evolution of functional proteins by using ribosome display, *Proc. Natl. Acad. Sci. U. S. A.* **94**, 4937–42.

Hoogenboom, H.R. (1997) Designing and optimizing library selection strategies for generating high-affinity antibodies, *Trends Biotechnol.* **15**, 62–70.

Hoogenboom, H.R., Chames, P. (2000) Natural and designer binding sites made by phage display technology, *Immunol. Today* **21**, 371–8.

Hoogenboom, H.R., Griffiths, A.D., Johnson, K.S., Chiswell, D.J., Hudson, P., Winter, G. (1991) Multi-subunit proteins on the surface of filamentous phage: methodologies for displaying antibody (Fab) heavy and light chains, *Nucleic Acids Res.* **19**, 4133–7.

Hudson, P.J. (1999) Recombinant antibody constructs in cancer therapy, *Curr. Opin. Immunol.* **11**, 548–57.

Hudson, P.J. (2000) Recombinant antibodies: a novel approach to cancer diagnosis and therapy, *Exp. Opin. Invest. Drugs* **9**, 1231–42.

Hung, M.C., Lau, Y.K. (1999) Basic science of HER-2/neu: a review, *Semin. Oncol.* **26**(4 Suppl 12), 51–9.

Huse, W.D., Sastry, L., Iverson, S.A. et al. (1989) Generation of a large combinatorial library of the immunoglobulin repertoire in phage lambda, *Science* **246**, 1275–81.

Huston, J.S., Levinson, D., Mudgett-Hunter, M. et al. (1988) Protein engineering of antibody binding sites: recovery of specific activity in an anti-digoxin single-chain Fv analogue produced in *Escherichia coli*, *Proc. Natl. Acad. Sci. U. S. A.* **85**, 5879–83.

Hwang, J., FitzGerald, D.J., Adhya, S., Pastan, I. (1987) Functional domains of *Pseudomonas* exotoxin identified by deletion analysis of the gene expressed in *E. coli*, *Cell* **48**, 129–36.

Idziorek, T., FitzGerald, D., Pastan, I. (1990) Low pH-induced changes in *Pseudomonas* exotoxin and its domains: increased binding of Triton X-114, *Infect. Immun.* **58**, 1415–20.

Iglewski, B.H., Kabat, D. (1975) NAD-dependent inhibition of protein synthesis by *Pseudomonas aeruginosa* toxin, *Proc. Natl. Acad. Sci. U. S. A.* **72**, 2284–8.

Irvin, J.O., Uckun, F.M. (1992) Pokeweed antiviral protein: ribosome inactivation and therapeutic applications, *Pharmacol. Ther.* **55**, 279–302.

Jain, R.K. (1996) Delivery of molecular medicine to solid tumors, *Science* **271**, 1079–80.

Jakobovits, A. (1998) Production and selection of antigen-specific fully human monoclonal antibodies from mice engineered with human Ig loci, *Adv. Drug. Deliv. Rev.* **31**, 33–42.

Jiang, J.X., London, E. (1990) Involvement of denaturation-like changes in *Pseudomonas* exotoxin a hydrophobicity and membrane penetration determined by characterization of pH and thermal transitions. Roles of two distinct conformationally altered states, *J. Biol. Chem.* **265**, 8636–41.

Jinno, Y., Chaudhary, V.K., Kondo, T., Adhya, S., FitzGerald, D.J., Pastan, I. (1988) Mutational analysis of domain I of *Pseudomonas* exotoxin. Mutations in domain I of *Pseudomonas* exotoxin which reduce cell binding and animal toxicity, *J. Biol. Chem.* **263**, 13203–7.

Jinno, Y., Ogata, M., Chaudhary, V.K., Willingham, M.C., Adhya, S., FitzGerald, D., Pastan, I. (1989) Domain II mutants of *Pseudomonas* exotoxin deficient in translocation, *J. Biol. Chem.* **264**, 15953–9.

Johnson, V.G., Youle, R.J. (1989) A point mutation of proline 308 in diphtheria toxin B chain inhibits membrane translocation of toxin conjugates, *J. Biol. Chem.* **264**, 17739–44.

Kiyokawa, T., Shirono, K., Hattori, T. et al. (1989) Cytotoxicity of interleukin 2–toxin toward lymphocytes from patients with adult T-cell leukemia, *Cancer Res.* **49**, 4042–6.

Komatsu, N., Oda, T., Muramatsu, T. (1998) Involvement of both caspase-like proteases and serine proteases in apoptotic cell death induced by ricin, modeccin, diphtheria toxin, and *Pseudomonas* toxin, *J. Biol. Chem.* **124**, 1038–44.

Kondo, T., FitzGerald, D., Chaudhary, V.K., Adhya, S., Pastan, I. (1988) Activity of immunotoxins constructed with modified *Pseudomonas* exotoxin A lacking the cell recognition domain, *J. Biol. Chem.* **263**, 9470–5.

Kounnas, M.Z., Morris, R.E., Thompson, M.R., FitzGerald, D.J., Strickland, D.K., Saelinger, C.B. (1992) The α_2-macroglobulin receptor/low density lipoprotein receptor-related protein binds and internalizes *Pseudomonas* exotoxin A, *J. Biol. Chem.* **267**, 12420–3.

Kreitman, R.J., Pastan, I. (1995) Targeting *Pseudomonas* exotoxin to hematologic malignancies, *Semin. Cancer Biol.* **6**, 297–306.

Kreitman, R.J., Puri, R.K., Paslan, I. (1994) A circularly permuted recombinant interleukin 4 toxin with increased activity, *Proc. Natl. Acad. Sci. U. S. A.* **91**, 6889–93.

Kreitman, R.J., Bailon, P., Chaudhary, V.K., FitzGerald, D.J.P., Pastan, I. (1994) Recombinant immunotoxins containing anti-Tac(Fv) and derivatives of *Pseudomonas* exotoxin produce complete regression in mice of an interleukin-2 receptor-expressing human carcinoma, *Blood* **83**, 426–34.

Kreitman, R.J., Chang, C.N., Hudson, D.V., Queen, C., Bailon, P., Pastan, I. (1994) Anti-Tac(Fab)–PE40, a recombinant double-chain immunotoxin which kills interleukin-2-receptor-bearing cells and induces complete remission in an *in vivo* tumor model, *Int. J. Cancer* **57**, 856–64.

Kreitman, R.J., Chaudhary, V.K., Kozak, R.W., FitzGerald, D.J.P., Waldmann, T.A., Pastan, I. (1992) Recombinant toxins containing the variable domains of the anti-Tac monoclonal antibody to the interleukin-2 receptor kill malignant cells from patients with chronic lymphocytic leukemia, *Blood* **80**, 2344–52.

Kreitman, R.J., Chaudhary, V.K., Waldmann, T., Willingham, M.C., FitzGerald, D.J., Pastan, I. (1990) The recombinant immunotoxin anti-Tac(Fv)–*Pseudomonas* exotoxin 40 is cytotoxic toward peripheral blood malignant cells from patients with adult T-cell leukemia, *Proc. Natl. Acad. Sci. U. S. A.* **87**, 8291–5.

Kreitman, R.J., Wilson, W.H., Robbins, D. et al. (1999) Responses in refractory hairy cell leukemia to a recombinant immunotoxin, *Blood* **94**, 3340–8.

Kreitman, R.J., Wilson, W.H., Whie, J.D. et al. (2000) Phase I trial of recombinant immunotoxin anti-tac(Fv)–PE38 (LMB-2) in patients with hematological malignancies, *J. Clin. Oncol.* **18**, 1622–36.

Kreitman, R.J., Wyndham, H., Bergeron, K. et al. (2001) Efficacy of the anti-CD22 recombinant immunotoxin BL22 in chemotherapy-resistant hairy cell leukemia, *N. Engl. J. Med.* **345**, 241–7.

Kuan, C., Pai, L.H., Pastan, I. (1995) Immunotoxins containing *Pseudomonas* exotoxin targeting Ley damage human endothelial cells in an antibody-specific mode: relevance to vascular leak syndrome, *Clin. Cancer Res.* **1**, 1589–94.

Kuan, C.T., Pastan, I. (1996) Improved antitumor activity of a recombinant anti-Lewis(Y) immunotoxin not requiring proteolytic activation, *Proc. Natl. Acad. Sci. U. S. A.* **93**, 974–8.

Laske, D.W., Youle, R.J., Oldfield, E.H. (1997) Tumor regression with regional distribution of the targeted toxin TF-CRM1 07 in patients with malignant brain tumors, *Nat. Med.* **3**, 1362–8.

Laske, D.W., Muraszko, K.M., Oldfield, E.H. et al. (1997) Intraventricular immunotoxin therapy for leptomeningeal neoplasia, *Neurosurgery* **41**, 1039–49.

Lau, J.L., Fowler, J., Ghosh, L. (1988) Epidermal growth factor in normal and neoplastic kidney and bladder, *J. Urol.* **139**, 170–5.

LeMaistre, C.F., Saleh, M.N., Kuzel, T.M. et al. (1998) Phase I trial of a ligand fusion-protein (DAB389IL-2) in lymphomas expressing the receptor for interleukin-2, *Blood* **91**, 399–405.

Lindstrom, A.L., Erlandsen, S.L., Kersey, J.H., Pennell, C.A. (1997) An *in vitro* model for toxin-mediated vascular leak syndrome: ricin toxin A chain increases the permeability of human endothelial cell monolayers, *Blood* **90**, 2323–34.

Lorberboum-Galski, H., FitzGerald, D., Chaudhary, V., Adhya, S., Pastan, I. (1988) Cytotoxic activity of an interleukin 2–*Pseudomonas* exotoxin chimeric protein produced in *Escherichia coli*, *Proc. Natl. Acad. Sci. U. S. A.* **85**, 1922–6.

Lorimer, I.A., Keppler-Hafkemeyer, A., Beers, R.A., Pegram, C.N., Bigner, D.D., Pastan, I. (1996) Recombinant immunotoxins specific for a mutant epidermal growth factor receptor: targeting with a single chain antibody variable domain isolated by phage display, *Proc. Natl. Acad. Sci. U. S. A.* **93**, 14815–20.

Mansfield, E., Amlot, P., Pastan, I., FitzGerald, D.J. (1997) Recombinant RFB4 immunotoxins exhibit potent cytotoxic activity for CD22-bearing cells and tumors, *Blood* **90**, 2020–6.

Marks, J.D., Hoogenboom, H.R., Bonnert, T.P., McCafferty, J., Griffiths, A.D., Winter, G. (1991) By-passing immunization. Human antibodies from V-gene libraries displayed on phage, *J. Mol. Biol.* **222**, 581–97.

Mavroudis, O.A., Jiang, Y.Z., Hensel, N. et al. (1996) Specific depletion of alloreactivity against haplotype mismatched related individuals: a new approach to graft-versus-host disease prophylaxis in haploidentical bone marrow transplantation, *Bone Marrow Transplant.* **17**, 793–9.

McCafferty, J., Griffiths, A.D., Winter, G., Chiswell, D.J. (1990) Phage antibodies: filamentous phage displaying antibody variable domains, *Nature* **348**, 552–4.

McGuinness, B.T., Walter, G., FitzGerald, K. et al. (1996) Phage diabody repertoires for selection of large numbers of bispecific antibody fragments, *Nat. Biotechnol.* **14**, 1149–54.

McLaughlin, P., Grillo-Lopez, A.J., Link, B.K. et al. (1998) Rituximab chimeric anti-CD20 monoclonal antibody therapy for relapsed indolent lymphoma: half of patients respond to a four-dose treatment program, *J. Clin. Oncol.* **16**, 2825–33.

Montagna, O., Yvon, E., Calcaterra, V. et al. (1999) Depletion of alloreactive T cells by a specific anti-interleukin-2 receptor p55 chain immunotoxin does not impair *in vitro* antileukemia and antiviral activity, *Blood* **93**, 3550–7.

Moroney, S.E., O'Alarcao, L.J., Goldmacher, V.S. et al. (1987) Modification of the binding site(s) of lectins by an affinity column carrying an activated galactose-terminated ligand, *Biochemistry* **26**, 8390–8.

Moskaug, J.O., Sletten, K., Sandvig, K., Olsnes, S. (1989) Translocation of diphtheria toxin A-fragment to the cytosol. Role of the site of interfragment cleavage, *J. Biol. Chem.* **264**, 15709–13.

Multani, P.S., O'Oay, S., Nadler, L.M., Grossbard, M.L. (1998) Phase II clinical trial of bolus infusion anti-B4 blocked ricin immunoconjugate in patients with relapsed B-cell non-Hodgkin's lymphoma, *Clin. Cancer Res.* **4**, 2599–604.

Myers, D.A., Villemez, C.L. (1988) Specific chemical cleavage of diphtheria toxin with hydroxylamine. Purification and characterization of the modified proteins, *J. Biol. Chem.* **263**, 17122–7.

Ogata, M., Pastan, I., FitzGerald, D. (1991) Analysis of *Pseudomonas* exotoxin activation and conformational changes by using monoclonal antibodies as probes, *Infect. Immun.* **59**, 407–14.

Ogata, M., Chaudhary, V.K., Pastan, I., FitzGerald, D.J. (1990) Processing of *Pseudomonas* exotoxin by a cellular protease results in the generation of a 37,000-Da toxin fragment that is translocated to the cytosol, *J. Biol. Chem.* **265**, 20678–85.

Olsnes, S., Pihl, A. (1982) Toxic Lectins and Related Proteins, in: Cohen, P. van Heyningen, S. (Eds.) *Molecular Action of Toxins and Viruses*, Elsevier Science, New York, pp. 51.

Omura, F., Kohno, K., Uchida, T. (1989) The histidine residue of codon 715 is essential for function of elongation factor 2, *Eur. J. Biochem.* **180**, 1–8.

Onda, M., Kreitman, R.J., Vasmatzis, G., Lee, B., Pastan, I. (1999) Reduction of the nonspecific animal toxicity of anti-Tac(Fv)−PE38 by mutations in the framework regions of the Fv which lower the isoelectric point, *J. Immunol.* **163**, 6072−7.

Orlandi, R., Gussow, D.H., Jones, P.T., Winter, G. (1989) Cloning immunoglobulin variable domains for expression by the polymerase chain reaction, *Proc. Natl. Acad. Sci. U. S. A.* **86**, 3833−7.

Ouvic, M., Kuzel, T., Olsen, E. et al. (1998) Quality of life is significantly improved in CTCl patients who responded to DAB389l-2 (ONTAK) fusion protein, *Blood* **92**(Suppl. 1), 2572.

Pai, L.H., Pastan, I. (1998) Clinical trials with *Pseudomonas* exotoxin immunotoxins, *Curr. Topics Microbiol. Immunol.* **234**, 83−96.

Pai, L.H., Wittes, R., Setser, A., Willingham, M.C., Pastan, I. (1996) Treatment of advanced solid tumors with immunotoxin LMB-1: an antibody linked to *Pseudomonas* exotoxin, *Nat. Med.* **2**, 350−3.

Pai-Scherf, L.H., Vill, J., Pearson, D. et al. (1999) Hepatotoxicity in cancer patients receiving erb-38, a recombinant immunotoxin that targets the erbB2 receptor, *Clin. Cancer Res.* **5**, 2311−5.

Pasqualucci, L., Wasik, M., Teicher, B.A. et al. (1995) Antitumor activity of anti-CD30 immunotoxin (Ber-H2/saporin) *in vitro* and in severe combined immunodeficiency disease mice xenografted with human CD30$^+$ anaplastic large-cell lymphoma, *Blood* **85**, 2139−46.

Pastan, I., FitzGerald, D. (1991) Recombinant toxins for cancer treatment, *Science* **254**, 1173−7.

Pastan, I., Lovelace, E., Rutherford, A.V., Kunwar, S., Willingham, M.C., Peehl, D.M. (1993) PR1−a monoclonal antibody that reacts with an antigen on the surface of normal and malignant prostate cells, *J. Natl. Cancer Inst.* **85**, 1149−54.

Pastan, I., Lovelace, E.T., Gallo, M.G., Rutherford, A.V., Magnani, J.L., Willingham, M.C. (1991) Characterization of monoclonal antibodies B1 and B3 that react with mucinous adenocarcinomas, *Cancer Res.* **51**, 3781−7.

Pastan, I.H., Pai, L.H., Brinkmann, U., Fitzgerald, D.J. (1995) Recombinant toxins: new therapeutic agents for cancer, *Ann. N.Y. Acad. Sci.* **758**, 345−54.

Pastan, I.H., Archer, G.E., McLendon, R.E. et al. (1995) Intrathecal administration of single-chain immunotoxin, LMB-7 [B3(Fv)−PE38], produces cures of carcinomatous meningitis in a rat model, *Proc. Natl. Acad. Sci. U. S. A.* **92**, 2765−9.

Persson, M.A., Caothien, R.H., Burton, D.R. (1991) Generation of diverse high-affinity human monoclonal antibodies by repertoire cloning, *Proc. Natl. Acad. Sci. U. S. A.* **88**, 2432−6.

Prior, T.I., Helman, L.J., FitzGerald, D.J., Pastan, I. (1991) Cytotoxic activity of a recombinant fusion protein between insulin-like growth factor I and *Pseudomonas* exotoxin, *Cancer Res.* **51**, 174−80.

Puri, R.K., Leland, P., Kreilman, R.J., Paslan, I. (1994) Human neurological cancer cells express interleukin-4 (IL-4) receptors which are targets for the toxic effects of IL-4−*Pseudomonas* exotoxin chimeric protein, *Int. J. Cancer* **58**, 574−81.

Puri, R.K., Hoon, D.S., Leland, P. et al. (1996) Preclinical development of a recombinant toxin containing circularly permuted interleukin 4 and truncated *Pseudomonas* exotoxin for therapy of malignant astrocytoma, *Cancer Res.* **56**, 5631−7.

Raag, R., Whitlow, M. (1995) Single-chain Fvs, *FASEB J.* **9**, 73−80.

Re, G.G., Waters, C., Poisson, L., Willingham, M.C., Sugamura, K., Frankel, A.E. (1996) Interleukin 2 (lL-2) receptor expression and sensitivity to diphtheria fusion toxin DAB(389) lL-2 in cultured hematopoietic cells, *Cancer Res.* **56**, 2590−5.

Reiter, Y., Pastan, I. (1996) Antibody engineering of recombinant Fv−immunotoxins for improved targeting of cancer: disulfide-stabilized Fv−immunotoxins, *Clin. Cancer Res.* **2**, 245−52.

Reiter, Y., Brinkmann, U., Lee, B., Pastan, I. (1996) Engineering antibody Fv fragments for cancer detection and therapy: disulfide-stabilized Fv fragments, *Nat. Biotechnol.* **14**, 1239−45.

Reiter, Y., Wright, A.F., Tonge, D.W., Pastan, I. (1996) Recombinant single-chain and disulfide-stabilized Fv−immunotoxins that cause complete regression of a human colon cancer xenograft in nude mice, *Int. J. Cancer* **67**, 113−23.

Reiter, Y., Di Carlo, A., Fugger, L., Engberg, J., Pastan, I. (1997) Peptide-specific killing of antigen-presenting cells by a recombinant antibody–toxin fusion protein targeted to major histocompatibility complex/peptide class I complexes with T cell receptor-like specificity, *Proc. Natl. Acad. Sci. U. S. A.* **94**, 4631–6.

Reiter, Y., Pai, L.H., Brinkmann, U., Wang, Q.C., Pastan, I. (1994) Antitumor activity and pharmacokinetics in mice of a recombinant immunotoxin containing a disulfide-stabilized Fv fragment, *Cancer Res.* **54**, 2714–8.

Reiter, Y., Brinkmann, U., Jung, S.H., Lee, B., Kasprzyk, P.G., King, C.R., Pastan, I. (1994) Improved binding and antitumor activity of a recombinant anti-erbB2 immunotoxin by disulfide stabilization of the Fv fragment, *J. Biol. Chem.* **269**, 18327–31.

Rosenberg, S.A. (1999) A new era for cancer immunotherapy based on the genes that encode cancer antigens, *Immunity* **10**, 281–7.

Ross, J.S., Fletcher, J.A. (1999) HER-2/*neu* (c-erb-B2) gene and protein in breast cancer, *Am. J. Clin. Pathol.* **112**(1 Suppl 1), S53–67.

Rozemuller, H., Rombouts, W.J., Touw, I.P., FitzGerald, D.J., Kreitman, R.J., Pastan, I., Hagenbeek, A., Martens, A.C. (1996) Treatment of acute myelocytic leukemia with interleukin-6 *Pseudomonas* exotoxin fusion protein in a rat leukemia model, *Leukemia* **10**, 1796–803.

Sandvig, K., Olsnes, S. (1980) Diphtheria toxin entry into cells is facilitated by low pH, *J. Cell. Biol.* **87**, 828–32.

Sausville, E.A., Headlee, D., Stetler-Stevenson, M. et al. (1995) Continuous infusion of the anti-CD22 immunotoxin IgG–RFB4–SMPT–dgA in patients with B-cell lymphoma: a phase I study, *Blood* **85**, 3457–65.

Scheuermann, R.H., Racila, E. (1995) CD19 antigen in leukemia and lymphoma diagnosis and immunotherapy, *Leuk. Lymph.* **18**, 385–97.

Schnell, R., Vitetta, E., Schindler, J. et al. (1998) Clinical trials with an anti-CD25 ricin A-chain experimental and immunotoxin (RFT5–SMPT–dgA) in Hodgkin's lymphoma, *Leuk. Lymph.* **30**, 525–37.

Seetharam, S., Chaudhary, V.K., FitzGerald, D., Pastan, I. (1991) Increased cytotoxic activity of *Pseudomonas* exotoxin and two chimeric toxins ending in KDEL, *J. Biol. Chem.* **266**, 17376–81.

Senderowicz, A.M., Vitetta, E., Headlee, D. et al. (1997) Complete sustained response of a refractory post-transplantation, large B-cell lymphoma to an anti-CD22 immunotoxin, *Ann. Intern. Med.* **126**, 882–5.

Shen, G-L., Li, J-L., Ghetie, M.A., Ghetie, V. et al. (1988) Evaluation of four C022 antibodies as ricin A-chain containing immunotoxins for the *in vivo* therapy of human B-cell leukemias and lymphomas, *Int. J. Cancer* **42**, 792–7.

Siegall, C.B., Chaudhary, V.K., FitzGerald, D.J., Pastan, I. (1989) Functional analysis of domains II, Ib, and III of *Pseudomonas* exotoxin, *J. Biol. Chem.* **264**, 14256–61.

Siegall, C.B., Liggitt, D., Chace, D., Tepper, M.A., Fell, H.P. (1994) Prevention of immunotoxin-mediated vascular leak syndrome in rats with retention of antitumor activity, *Proc. Natl. Acad. Sci. U. S. A.* **91**, 9514–8.

Siegall, C.B., Schwab, G., Nordan, R.P., FitzGerald, D.J., Pastan, I. (1990) Expression of the interleukin 6 receptor and interleukin 6 in prostate carcinoma cells, *Cancer Res.* **50**, 7786–8.

Siegall, C.B., Liggitt, D., Chace, D., Mixan, B., Sugai, J., Davidson, T., Steinitz, M. (1997) Characterization of vascular leak syndrome induced by the toxin component of *Pseudomonas* exotoxin-based immunotoxins and its potential inhibition with nonsteroidal anti-inflammatory drugs, *Clin. Cancer Res.* **3**, 339–45.

Siegall, C.B., Chace, D., Mixan, B. et al. (1994) *In vitro* and *in vivo* characterization of BR96 sFv–PE40. A single-chain immunotoxin fusion protein that cures human breast carcinoma xenografts in athymic mice and rats, *J. Immunol.* **152**, 2377–84.

Siegall, C.B., Epstein, S., Speir, E. et al. (1991) Cytotoxic activity of chimeric proteins composed of acidic fibroblast growth factor and *Pseudomonas* exotoxin on a variety of cell types, *FASEB J.* **13**, 2843–9.

Skerra, A., Pluckthun, A. (1988) Assembly of a functional immunoglobulin Fv fragment in *Escherichia coli*, *Science* **240**, 1038–41.

Skrepnik, N., Zieske, A.W., Robert, E., Bravo, J.C., Mera, R., Hunt, J.D. (1998) Aggressive administration of recombinant oncotoxin AR209 (anti-ErbB-2) in athymic nude mice implanted with orthotopic human non-small cell lung tumours, *Eur. J. Cancer* **34**, 1628–33.

Smith, G.P. (1985) Filamentous fusion phage: novel expression vectors that display cloned antigens on the virion surface, *Science* **228**, 1315–7.

Stone, M.J., Sausville, E.A., Fay, L.W. et al. (1996) A phase I study of bolus versus continuous infusion of the anti-CD19 immunotoxin, IgG–HD37–dgA, in patients with B-cell lymphoma, *Blood* **88**, 1188–97.

Studier, F.W., Moffatt, B.A. (1986) Use of bacteriophage T7 polymerase to direct selective expression of cloned genes, *J. Mol. Bio1.* **189**, 113–30.

Thorpe, P.E., Ross, W.C.J., Brown, A.N.F. et al. (1984) Blockade of the galactose-binding sites of ricin by its linkage to antibody. Specific cytotoxic effects of the conjugates, *Eur. J. Biochem.* **140**, 63–71.

Thorpe, P.E., Wallace, P.M., Knowles, P.P. et al. (1988) Improved anti-tumor effects of immunotoxins prepared with deglycosylated ricin-A chain and hindered disulfide linkages, *Cancer Res.* **48**, 6396–403.

Tsutsumi, Y., Onda, M., Nagata, S., Lee, B., Kreitman, R.J., Pastan, I. (2000) Site-specific chemical modification with polyethylene glycol of recombinant immunotoxin anti-Tac(Fv)–PE38 (LMB-2) improves antitumor activity and reduces animal toxicity and immunogenicity, *Proc. Natl. Acad. Sci. U. S. A.* **97**, 8548–53.

Uckun, F.M., Reaman, G.H. (1995) Immunotoxins for treatment of leukemia and lymphoma, *Leuk. Lymph.* **18**, 195–201.

Veale, D., Kerr, N., Gibson, G.J., Harris, A.L. (1989) Characterization of epidermal growth factor receptor in primary human non-small cell lung cancer, *Cancer Res.* **49**, 1313–7.

Vitetta, E.S., Fulton, R.J., May, R.D., Till, M., Uhr, J.W. (1987) Redesigning nature's poisons to create anti-tumor reagents, *Science* **238**, 1098–104.

Vitteta, E.S., Sonte, M., Amlot, P. et al. (1991) Phase I immunotoxin trial in patients with B-cell lymphoma, *Cancer Res.* **51**, 4052–8.

Waldmann, T.A., Pastan, I., Gansow, O.A. et al. (1992) The multichain interleukin-2 receptor: a target for immunotherapy, *Ann. Intern. Med.* **116**, 148–60.

Wang, R.F., Rosenberg, S.A. (1999) Human tumor antigens for cancer vaccine development, *Immunol. Rev.* **170**, 85–100.

Ward, E.S., Gussow, D., Griffiths, A.D., Jones, P.T., Winter, G. (1989) Binding activities of a repertoire of single immunoglobulin variable domains secreted from *Escherichia coli*, *Nature* **341**, 544–6.

Waters, C.A., Schimke, P.A., Snider, C.E. et al. (1990) Interleukin 2 receptor-targeted cytotoxicity. Receptor binding requirements for entry of a diphtheria toxin-related interleukin 2 fusion protein into cells, *Eur. J. Immunol.* **20**, 785–91.

Waurzyniak, B., Schneider, E.A., Tumer, N. et al. (1997) *In vivo* toxicity, pharmacokinetics, and antileukemic activity of TXU (anti-CD7)–pokeweed antiviral protein immunotoxin, *Clin. Cancer Res.* **3**, 881–90.

Wels, W., Harwerth, I.M., Mueller, M., Groner, B., Hynes, N.E. (1992) Selective inhibition of tumor cell growth by a recombinant single-chain antibody-toxin specific for the erbB-2 receptor, *Cancer Res.* **52**, 6310–7.

Williams, D.P., Wen, Z., Watson, R.S., Boyd, J., Strom, T.B., Murphy, J.R. (1990) Cellular processing of the interleukin-2 fusion toxin DAB486–IL-2 and efficient delivery of diphtheria fragment A to the cytosol of target cells requires Arg194, *J. Biol. Chem.* **265**, 20673–7.

Williams, D.P., Parker, K., Bacha, P. et al. (1987) Diphtheria toxin receptor binding domain substitution with interleukin-2: genetic construction and properties of a diphtheria toxin-related interleukin-2 fusion protein, *Protein Eng.* **1**, 493–8.

Wilson, B.A., Collier, R.J. (1992) Diphtheria toxin and *Pseudomonas aeruginosa* exotoxin A: active-site structure and enzymic mechanism, *Curr. Topics Microbiol. Immunol.* **175**, 27–41.

Winter, G., Milstein, C. (1991) Man-made antibodies, *Nature* **349**, 293–9.

Winter, G., Griffiths, A.D., Hawkins, R.E., Hoogenboom, H.R. (1994) Making antibodies by phage display technology, *Annu. Rev. Immunol.* **12**, 433–55.

Wozniak, D.J., Hsu, L.Y., Galloway, D.R. (1988) His-426 of the *Pseudomonas aeruginosa* exotoxin A is required for ADP-ribosylation of elongation factor II, *Proc. Natl. Acad. Sci. U. S. A.* **85**, 8880–4.

Yang, X.D., Jia, X.C., Corvalan, J.R., Wang, P., Davis, C.G., Jakobovits, A. (1999) Eradication of established tumors by a fully human monoclonal antibody to the epidermal growth factor receptor without concomitant chemotherapy, *Cancer Res.* **59**, 1236–43.

Part IV
Gene Therapy

26
Liposome Gene Transfection

Nancy Smyth Templeton
Department of Molecular and Cellular Biology, Baylor College of Medicine,
Houston, TX, USA

1   Introduction   831

2   Optimization of Cationic Liposome Formulations for Use *in vivo*   833

3   Liposome Morphology and Effects on Gene Delivery and Expression   834

4   Optimal Lipids and Liposome Morphology: Effects on Gene Delivery
        and Expression   837

5   Liposome
        Encapsulation, Flexibility, and Optimal Colloidal Suspensions   837

6   Overall Charge of Complexes and Entry into the Cell   839

7   Ligands Used for Targeted Delivery   840

8   Attachment of Ligands   841

9   Serum Stability of Optimized Nucleic Acid–Liposome Complexes
        for Use *in vivo*   842

10   Optimized Half-life in the Circulation   843

11   Broad Biodistribution of Optimized Liposome Formulations   844

12   Optimization of Targeted Delivery   844

Pharmacology. From Drug Development to Gene Therapy. Edited by Robert A. Meyers.
Copyright © 2008 Wiley-VCH Verlag GmbH & Co. KGaA, Weinheim
ISBN: 978-3-527-32343-2

13   Efficient Dissemination Throughout Target Tissues and Migration
          Across Tight Barriers   845

14   Optimization of Plasmids for *in vivo* Gene Expression   846

15   Optimization of Plasmid DNA Preparations   848

16   Detection of Gene Expression   849

17   Optimization of Dose and Frequency of Administration   850

18   Summary   850

          Acknowledgment   850

          Bibliography   851
          Books and Reviews   851
          Primary Literature   851

Keywords

Colloidal Suspensions
The density of complexes in a specific volume.

Formulation
Procedures used to make liposomes and complexes.

Gene Therapy
Treatments that are mediated by either the addition of needed genes or the destruction
of transcripts encoding unwanted gene products.

Lamellar Structures
Alternation of a lipid bilayer and a water layer.

Liposomes
Bilayers made from lipids.

Nonviral Delivery
Delivery vehicles that are not viruses or any other live organism.

Optimization
Creation of optimal conditions.

Serum Stability
Complexes that do not precipitate in specific percentage of serum.

Systemic Delivery
Delivery in the bloodstream.

■ Varied results have been obtained using cationic liposomes for *in vivo* delivery. Furthermore, optimization of cationic liposomal complexes for *in vivo* applications is complex involving many diverse components. These components include nucleic acid purification, plasmid design, formulation of the delivery vehicle, administration route and schedule, dosing, detection of gene expression, and others. This chapter will also focus on optimization of the delivery vehicle formulation. These formulation issues include morphology of the complexes, lipids used, flexibility versus rigidity, colloidal suspension, overall charge, serum stability, half-life in circulation, biodistribution, delivery to and dissemination throughout target tissues. Broad assumptions have been frequently made on the basis of the data obtained from focused studies using cationic liposomes. However, these assumptions do not necessarily apply to all delivery vehicles and, most likely, do not apply to many liposomal systems when considering these other key components that influence the results obtained *in vivo*. Optimizing all components of the delivery system is pivotal and will allow broad use of liposomal complexes to treat or cure human diseases or disorders. This chapter will highlight the features of liposomes that contribute to successful delivery, gene expression, and efficacy.

1

Introduction

Many investigators are focused on the production of effective nonviral gene therapeutics and on creating improved delivery systems that mix viral and nonviral vectors. Use of improved liposome formulations for delivery *in vivo* is valuable for gene therapy and would avoid several problems associated with viral delivery. Delivery of nucleic acids using liposomes is promising as a safe and nonimmunogenic approach to gene therapy. Furthermore, gene therapeutics composed of artificial reagents can be standardized and regulated as drugs rather than as biologics. Cationic lipids have been used for efficient delivery of nucleic acids to cells in tissue culture

for several years. Much effort has also been directed toward developing cationic liposomes for efficient delivery of nucleic acids in animals and in humans. Most frequently, the formulations that are best to use for transfection of a broad range of cell types in culture are not optimal for achieving efficacy in small and large animal disease models.

Much effort has been devoted to the development of nonviral delivery vehicles due to the numerous disadvantages of viral vectors that have been used for gene therapy. Following viral delivery *in vivo*, immune responses are generated to expressed viral proteins that subsequently kill the target cells required to produce the therapeutic gene product. An innate humoral immune response can be produced to certain viral vectors due to previous exposure to the naturally occurring virus. Random integration of some viral vectors into the host chromosome could occur and cause activation of proto-oncogenes, resulting in tumor formation. Clearance of viral vectors delivered systemically by complement activation can also occur. Viral vectors can be inactivated upon readministration by the humoral immune response. Potential for recombination of the viral vector with DNA sequences in the host chromosome that generates a replication-competent infectious virus also exists. Specific delivery of viral vectors to target cells can be difficult because two distinct steps in engineering viral envelopes or capsids must be achieved. First, the virus envelope or capsid must be changed to inactivate the natural tropism of the virus to enter specific cell types. Then, sequences must be introduced that allow the new viral vector to bind and internalize through a different cell surface receptor. Other disadvantages of viral vectors include the inability to administer certain viral vectors more than once, the high costs for producing large amounts of high-titer viral stocks for use in the clinic, and the limited size of the nucleic acid that can be packaged and used for viral gene therapy. Attempts are being made to overcome the immune responses produced by viral vectors after administration in immune competent animals and in humans, such as the use of gutted adenoviral vectors or encapsulation of viral vectors in liposomes. However, complete elimination of all immune responses to viral vectors may be impossible.

Use of liposomes for gene therapy provides several advantages. A major advantage is the lack of immunogenicity after *in vivo* administration, including systemic injections. Therefore, the nucleic acid-liposome complexes can be readministered without harm to the patient and without compromising the efficacy of the nonviral gene therapeutic. Improved formulations of nucleic acid–liposome complexes can also evade complement inactivation after *in vivo* administration. Nucleic acids of unlimited size can be delivered ranging from single nucleotides to large mammalian artificial chromosomes. Furthermore, different types of nucleic acids can be delivered including plasmid DNA, RNA, oligonucleotides, DNA–RNA chimeras, synthetic ribozymes, antisense molecules, RNAi, viral nucleic acids, and others. Certain cationic formulations can also encapsulate and deliver viruses, proteins or partial proteins with a low isoelectric point (pI), and mixtures of nucleic acids and proteins of any pI. Creation of nonviral vectors for targeted delivery to specific cell types, organs, or tissues is relatively simple. Targeted delivery involves elimination of nonspecific charge interactions with nontarget cells and addition of ligands for binding and internalization through target cell surface receptors. Other advantages of nonviral vectors include the low cost and relative ease in producing nucleic acid-liposome complexes in large scale for use in the clinic. In addition, greater safety for patients is provided using nonviral delivery vehicles due to few or no viral sequences present in the nucleic acids used for delivery, thereby precluding generation of an infectious virus. The disadvantage of nonviral delivery systems had been the low levels of delivery and gene expression produced by ''first-generation'' complexes. However, recent advances have dramatically improved transfection efficiencies and efficacy of liposomal vectors. Reviews of other *in vivo* delivery systems and improvements using cationic liposomes have been published recently.

Cationic liposome–nucleic acid complexes can be administered via numerous delivery routes *in vivo*. Routes of delivery include direct injection (e.g. intratumoral), intravenous, intraperitoneal, intra-arterial, intrasplenic, mucosal (nasal, vaginal, rectal), intramuscular, subcutaneous, transdermal, intradermal, subretinal, intratracheal, intracranial, and others. Much interest has focused on noninvasive intravenous administration because many investigators believe that this route of delivery is the "holy grail" for the treatment or cure of cancer, cardiovascular, and other inherited or acquired diseases. Particularly for the treatment of metastatic cancer, therapeutics must reach not only the primary tumor but also the distant metastases.

Optimization of cationic liposomal complexes for *in vivo* applications and therapeutics is complex, involving many distinct components. These components include nucleic acid purification, plasmid design, formulation of the delivery vehicle, administration route and schedule, dosing, detection of gene expression, and others. Often I make the analogy of liposome optimization to a functional car. Of course, the engine of the car, analogous to the liposome delivery vehicle, is extremely important. However, if the car does not have wheels, adequate tyres, and so on, the motorist will not be able to drive the vehicle to its destination. This chapter will focus on optimization of these distinct components for use in a variety of *in vivo* applications. Optimizing all components of the delivery system will allow broad use of liposomal complexes to treat or cure human diseases or disorders.

2
Optimization of Cationic Liposome Formulations for Use *in vivo*

Much research has been directed toward the synthesis of new cationic lipids. Some new formulations led to the discovery of more efficient transfection agents for cells in culture. However, their efficiency measured *in vitro* did not correlate with their ability to deliver DNA after administration in animals. Functional properties defined *in vitro* do not assess the stability of the complexes in plasma or their pharmacokinetics and biodistribution, all of which are essential for optimal activity *in vivo*. Colloidal properties of the complexes, in addition to the physicochemical properties of their component lipids, also determine these parameters. In particular, in addition to efficient transfection of target cells, nucleic acid–liposome complexes must be able to traverse tight barriers *in vivo* and penetrate throughout the target tissue to produce efficacy for the treatment of disease. These are not issues for achieving efficient transfection of cells in culture with the exception of polarized tissue culture cells. Therefore, we are not surprised that optimized liposomal delivery vehicles for use *in vivo* may be different than those used for efficient delivery to cells in culture.

In summary, *in vivo* nucleic acid–liposome complexes that produce efficacy in animal models of disease have extended half-life in the circulation, are stable in serum, have broad biodistribution, efficiently encapsulate various sizes of nucleic acids, are targetable to specific organs and cell types, penetrate across tight barriers in several organs, penetrate evenly throughout the target tissue, are optimized for nucleic acid:lipid ratio and colloidal suspension *in vivo*, can be size fractionated to produce a totally homogenous population of complexes prior to injection, and can be repeatedly administered. Recently, we demonstrated efficacy of a robust liposomal delivery system in small and large animal models for lung, breast, head and neck, and pancreatic cancers, and for Hepatitis B and C (Clawson and Templeton, unpublished data). On the basis of efficacy in these animal studies, this liposomal delivery system will be used in upcoming clinical trials to treat these cancers. Our studies have demonstrated broad efficacy in the use of liposomes to treat disease and have dispelled several myths that exist concerning the use of liposomal systems.

3
Liposome Morphology and Effects on Gene Delivery and Expression

Efficient *in vivo* nucleic acid–liposome complexes have unique features including their morphology, mechanisms for crossing the cell membrane and entry into the nucleus, ability to be targeted for delivery to specific cell surface receptors, and ability to penetrate across tight barriers and throughout target tissues. Liposomes have different morphologies based upon their composition and the formulation method. Furthermore, the morphology of complexes can contribute to their ability to deliver nucleic acids *in vivo*. Formulations frequently used for the delivery of nucleic acids are lamellar structures including small unilamellar vesicles (SUVs), multilamellar vesicles (MLVs), or bilamellar invaginated vesicles (BIVs) recently developed in our laboratory (Fig. 1). Several investigators have developed liposomal delivery systems using hexagonal structures; however, they have demonstrated efficiency primarily for the transfection of some cell types in culture and not for *in vivo* delivery. SUVs condense nucleic acids on the surface and form "spaghetti and meatballs" structures. DNA–liposome complexes made using SUVs produce little or no gene expression upon systemic delivery, although these complexes transfect

Types of lamellar vesicles

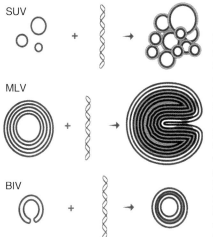

Fig. 1 Diagrams drawn from cryoelectron micrographs of cross sections through vitrified films of various types of liposomes and DNA–liposome complexes. SUVs are small unilamellar vesicles that condense nucleic acids on the surface and produce "spaghetti and meatballs" structures. MLVs are multilamellar vesicles that appear as "Swiss Rolls" after mixing with DNA. BIVs are bilamellar invaginated vesicles produced using a formulation developed in our laboratory. Nucleic acids are efficiently encapsulated between two bilamellar invaginated structures (BIVs).

numerous cell types efficiently *in vitro*. Furthermore, SUV liposome–DNA complexes cannot be targeted efficiently. SUV liposome–DNA complexes also have a short half-life within the circulation, generally about 5 to 10 min. Polyethylene glycol (PEG) has been added to liposome formulations to extend their half-life; however, PEGylation created other problems that have not been resolved. PEG seems to hinder delivery of cationic liposomes into cells due to its sterically hindering ionic interactions, and it interferes with optimal condensation of nucleic acids onto the cationic delivery vehicle. Furthermore, extremely long half-life in the circulation, for example, several days, has caused problems for patients because the bulk of the PEGylated liposomal formulation doxil that encapsulates the cytotoxic agent, doxorubicin, accumulates in the skin, hands, and feet. For example, patients contract mucositis and "Hand and Foot Syndrome" that cause extreme discomfort to the patient. Attempts to add ligands to doxil for delivery to specific cell surface receptors has not resulted in much cell-specific delivery, and the majority of the injected targeted formulation still accumulates in the skin, hands, and feet. Addition of PEG into formulations developed in our laboratory also caused steric hindrance in the bilamellar invaginated structures that did not encapsulate DNA efficiently, and gene expression was substantially diminished.

Some investigators have loaded nucleic acids within SUVs using a variety of methods; however, the bulk of the DNA does not load or stay within the liposomes. Furthermore, most of the processes used for loading nucleic acids within liposomes are extremely time-consuming and not cost effective. Therefore, SUVs are not the ideal liposomes for creating nonviral vehicles for targeted delivery.

Complexes made using MLVs appear as "Swiss rolls" when viewing cross-sections by cryoelectron microscopy. These complexes can become too large for systemic administration or deliver nucleic acids inefficiently into cells due to the inability to "unravel" at the cell surface. Addition of ligands onto MLV liposome–DNA complexes further aggravates these problems. Therefore, MLVs are not useful for the development of targeted delivery of nucleic acids.

Using a formulation developed in our laboratory, nucleic acids are efficiently encapsulated between two bilamellar invaginated vesicles, BIVs. We created these unique structures using 1,2-bis(oleoyloxy)-3-(trimethylammino)propane (DOTAP) and cholesterol (Chol) and a novel formulation procedure. This procedure is different because it includes a brief, low frequency sonication followed by manual extrusion through filters of decreasing pore size. The 0.1 and 0.2 µm filters used are made of aluminum oxide and not polycarbonate that is typically used by other protocols. Aluminum oxide membranes contain more pores per surface area, evenly spaced and sized pores, and pores with straight channels. During the manual extrusion process, the liposomes are passed through each of the four different sized filters only once. This process produces 88% invaginated liposomes. Use of high-frequency sonication and/or mechanical extrusion produces only SUVs.

The BIVs produced condense, unusually large amounts of nucleic acids of any size Fig. 2 or viruses Fig. 3. Furthermore, addition of other DNA condensing agents including polymers is not necessary. For example, condensation of plasmid DNA onto polymers first before encapsulation in the BIVs did not increase condensation or subsequent gene

Assembly of complexes

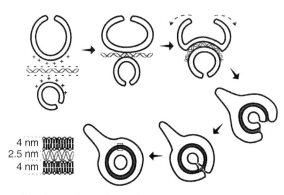

4 nm
2.5 nm
4 nm

Fig. 2 Proposed model showing cross sections of extruded DOTAP: Chol liposomes (BIVs) interacting with nucleic acids. Nucleic acids adsorb onto a BIV via electrostatic interactions. Attraction of a second BIV to this complex results in further charge neutralization. Expanding electrostatic interactions with nucleic acids cause inversion of the larger BIV and total encapsulation of the nucleic acids. Inversion can occur in these liposomes because of their excess surface area, which allows them to accommodate the stress created by the nucleic acid–lipid interactions. Nucleic acid binding reduces the surface area of the outer leaflet of the bilayer and induces the negative curvature due to lipid ordering and reduction of charge repulsion between cationic lipid headgroups. Condensation of the internalized nucleic acid–lipid sandwich expands the space between the bilayers and may induce membrane fusion to generate the apparently closed structures. The enlarged area shows the arrangement of nucleic acids condensed between two 4 nm bilayers of extruded DOTAP:Chol.

Assembly of BIV + adenovirus complexes

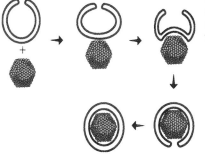

Fig. 3 Proposed model showing cross sections of an extruded DOTAP:Chol liposome (BIV) interacting with adenovirus. Adenovirus interacts with a BIV causing negative curvature and wrapping around the virus particle.

expression after transfection *in vitro* or *in vivo*. Encapsulation of nucleic acids by these BIVs alone is spontaneous and immediate, and, therefore, cost effective, requiring only one step of simple mixing. The extruded DOTAP:Chol–nucleic acid complexes are also large enough so that they are not cleared rapidly by Kupffer cells in the liver and yet extravasate across tight barriers, including the endothelial cell barrier of the lungs in a normal mouse, and diffuse through target organs efficiently. Our recent work demonstrating efficacy for treatment of nonsmall cell lung cancer showed that only BIV DOTAP:Chol-p53 DNA–liposome complexes produced efficacy, and SUV DOTAP:Chol-p53 DNA–liposome complexes produced no efficacy. Therefore, the choice of lipids alone is not sufficient for optimal DNA delivery, and the morphology of the complexes is essential.

4
Optimal Lipids and Liposome Morphology: Effects on Gene Delivery and Expression

Choosing the best cationic lipids and neutral lipids is also essential for producing the optimal *in vivo* formulation. For example, using our novel manual extrusion procedure does not produce BIVs using the cationic lipid dimethyldioctadecylammonium bromide (DDAB). Furthermore, DOTAP is biodegradable, whereas DDAB is not biodegradable. Use of biodegradable lipids is preferred for use in humans. Furthermore, only DOTAP- and not DDAB-containing liposomes produced highly efficient gene expression *in vivo*. DDAB did not produce BIVs and was unable to encapsulate nucleic acids. Apparently, DDAB- and DOTAP-containing SUVs produce similar efficiency of gene delivery *in vivo*; however, these SUVs are not as efficient as BIV DOTAP:Chol. In addition, use of L-α dioleoyl phosphatidylethanolamine (DOPE) as a neutral lipid creates liposomes that cannot wrap or encapsulate nucleic acids. Several investigators have reported efficient transfection of cells in culture using DOPE in liposomal formulations. However, our data showed that formulations consisting of DOPE were not efficient for producing gene expression *in vivo*.

Investigators must also consider the source and lot of certain lipids purchased from companies. For example, different lots of cholesterol from the same vendor can vary dramatically and will affect the formulation of liposomes. Currently, we are using synthetic cholesterol (Sigma, St. Louis, MO). The Food and Drug Administration prefers synthetic cholesterol instead of natural cholesterol that is purified from the wool of sheep for use in producing therapeutics for injection into humans.

Our BIV formulations are also stable for a few years as liquid suspensions. Freeze-dried formulations can also be made that are stable indefinitely even at room temperature. Stability of liposomes and liposomal complexes is also essential, particularly for the commercial development of human therapeutics.

5
Liposome Encapsulation, Flexibility, and Optimal Colloidal Suspensions

A common belief is that artificial vehicles must be 100 nm or smaller to be effective for systemic delivery. However, this belief is most likely true only for large, inflexible delivery vehicles. Blood cells are several microns (up to 7000 nm) in size, and yet have no difficulty circulating in the blood, including through the smallest capillaries. However, sickle cell blood cells, that are rigid, do have problems in the circulation. Therefore, we believe that flexibility is a more important issue than small size. In fact, BIV DNA–liposome complexes in the size range of 200 to 450 nm produced the highest levels of gene expression in all tissues after intravenous injection. Kupffer cells in the liver quickly clear delivery vehicles (including nonviral vectors and viruses) that are not PEGylated and are smaller than 200 nm. Therefore, increased size of liposomal complexes could extend their circulation time, particularly when combined with injection of high colloidal suspensions. BIVs were able to encapsulate nucleic acids and viruses apparently due to the presence of cholesterol in the bilayer (Fig. 4). Whereas, formulations including DOPE instead of cholesterol could not assemble nucleic acids by a "wrapping

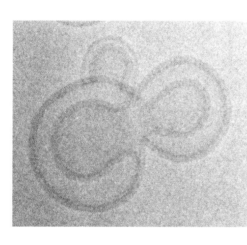

Fig. 4 Cryoelectron micrograph of BIV DOTAP:Chol–DNA–liposome complexes. The plasmid DNA is encapsulated between two BIVs.

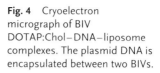

Fig. 5 Cryoelectron micrograph of extruded DOTAP:DOPE liposomes complexed to plasmid DNA. Although these liposomes were prepared by the same protocol that produces BIV DOTAP:Chol, these vesicles cannot wrap and encapsulate nucleic acids. The DNA condenses on the surfaces of the liposomes shown.

type" of mechanism (Fig. 5), and produced little gene expression in the lungs and no expression in other tissues after intravenous injections. Because the extruded DOTAP:Chol BIV complexes are flexible and not rigid, are stable in high concentrations of serum, and have extended half-life, they do not have difficulty circulating efficiently in the bloodstream.

We believe that colloidal properties of nucleic acid–liposome complexes also determine the levels of gene expression produced after *in vivo* delivery. These properties include the DNA:lipid ratio that determines the overall charge density of the complexes and the colloidal suspension that is monitored by its turbidity. Complex size and shape, lipid composition and formulation, and encapsulation efficiency of nucleic acids by the liposomes also contribute to the colloidal properties of the complexes. The colloidal properties affect serum stability, protection from nuclease degradation, blood circulation time, and biodistribution of the complexes.

Our *in vivo* transfection data showed that an adequate amount of colloids in suspension was required to produce efficient gene expression in all tissues examined. The colloidal suspension is assessed by measurement of adsorbance at 400 nm using a spectrophotometer optimized to measure turbidity. Our data showed that transfection efficiency in all tissues corresponded to OD400 of the complexes measured prior to intravenous injection.

6
Overall Charge of Complexes and Entry into the Cell

In addition, our delivery system is efficient because the complexes deliver DNA into cells by fusion with the cell membrane and avoid the endocytic pathway (Fig. 6). Cells are negatively charged on the surface, and specific cell types vary in their density of negative charge. These differences in charge density can influence the ability of cells to be transfected. Cationic complexes have nonspecific ionic charge interactions with cell surfaces. Efficient transfection of cells by cationic complexes is, in part, contributed by adequate charge interactions. In addition, recent publications report that certain viruses have a partial positive charge around key subunits

of viral proteins on the virus surface responsible for binding to and internalization through target cell surface receptors. Therefore, this partial positive charge is required for virus entry into the cell. Thus, maintenance of adequate positive charge on the surface of targeted liposome complexes is essential for optimal delivery into the cell. Different formulations of liposomes interact with cell surfaces via a variety of mechanisms. Two major pathways for interaction are by endocytosis or by direct fusion with the cell membrane. Preliminary data suggest that nucleic acids delivered *in vitro* and *in vivo* using complexes developed in our lab enter the cell by direct fusion (Fig. 6). Apparently, the bulk of the nucleic acids do not enter endosomes, and, therefore, far more nucleic acid enters the nucleus. Cell transfection by direct fusion produces orders of magnitude increased levels of gene expression and numbers of cells transfected versus cells transfected through the endocytic pathway.

We believe that maintenance of adequate positive charge on the surface of complexes is essential to drive cell entry by direct fusion. Therefore, we create targeted delivery of our complexes *in vivo* without

Cell entry of complexes

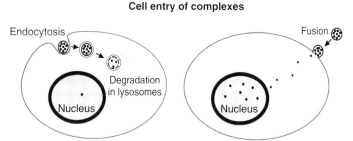

Fig. 6 Mechanisms for cell entry of nucleic acid–liposome complexes. Two major pathways for interaction are by endocytosis or by direct fusion with the cell membrane. Complexes that enter the cell by direct fusion allow delivery of more nucleic acids to the nucleus because the bulk of the nucleic acids do not enter endosomes.

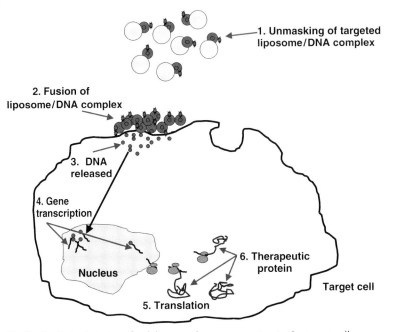

Fig. 7 Optimized strategy for delivery and gene expression in the target cell. Optimization of many steps is required to achieve targeted delivery, deshielding, fusion with the cell membrane, entry of nucleic acids into the cell and to the nucleus, and production of gene expression of a cDNA cloned in a plasmid.

the use of PEG. These ligand-coated complexes also reexpose the overall positive charge of the complexes as they approach the target cells. Through ionic interactions or covalent attachments, we have added monoclonal antibodies, Fab fragments, proteins, partial proteins, peptides, peptide mimetics, small molecules, and drugs to the surface of our complexes after mixing. These ligands efficiently bind to the target cell surface receptor, and maintain entry into the cell by direct fusion. Using novel methods for addition of ligands to the complexes for targeted delivery results in further increased gene expression in the target cells after transfection. Therefore, we design targeted liposomal delivery systems that retain predominant entry into cells by direct fusion versus the endocytic pathway. Figure 7 shows our

optimized strategy to achieve targeted delivery, deshielding, fusion with the cell membrane, entry of nucleic acids into the cell and to the nucleus, and production of gene expression of a cDNA cloned in a plasmid.

7
Ligands Used for Targeted Delivery

Using liposomes that encapsulate nucleic acids, ligands can be coated onto the surface of the complexes formed (Fig. 8). We have added monoclonal antibodies, Fab fragments, proteins, partial proteins, peptides, peptide mimetics, small molecules, and drugs to the surface of the complexes after mixing. Ligands are chosen by their ability to efficiently bind to a

Attachment of ligands for targeted delivery

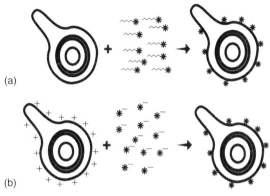

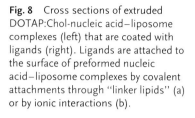

Fig. 8 Cross sections of extruded DOTAP:Chol-nucleic acid–liposome complexes (left) that are coated with ligands (right). Ligands are attached to the surface of preformed nucleic acid–liposome complexes by covalent attachments through "linker lipids" (a) or by ionic interactions (b).

target cell surface receptor while maintaining entry into the cell by direct fusion. Entry into the cell will be discussed further below. The ligands most useful for gene therapeutics in humans will be those that are smallest and possess high affinity for the target receptor. Nonviral systems are desirable because they can be repeatedly administered. Therefore, immune responses may be generated in animals or people upon repeated administration of complexes containing too much ligand or too large a ligand on the surface. These immune responses could cause the targeted therapeutics to be unsafe and/or ineffective for treatments in the clinic.

However, often the "best ligand" is not always available immediately. An investigator could also wait for years for the most appropriate ligand to be generated or produced in the amounts required for large experiments. Our experience shows that much useful information can be generated concerning targeting of a particular cell surface receptor of interest using the "less-than-ideal ligand" *in vitro* and *in vivo* in pilot experiments while creating the best ligand concurrently.

8
Attachment of Ligands

Generally, investigators attach ligands to PEG for incorporation into liposomes and other conjugates or for coating onto the surface of complexes after mixing. After extensive work with PEG in our lab, we have chosen or created alternative methods to use for the attachment of ligands, and have avoided the use of PEG due to its numerous disadvantages discussed above and below in this chapter.

Alternative strategies to the use of PEG include attachment of ligands through ionic interactions or by covalent attachment to "linker lipids". The ligands listed in the section above are generally negatively charged. Therefore, the ligands can simply be adsorbed onto the surface of complexes with encapsulated nucleic acids after mixing (Fig. 8b). Additional moieties can be added to the ligand to increase the amount of negative charge, and yet do not interfere with the ability of the modified ligand to efficiently bind to the appropriate cell surface receptor. For example, we used succinylated asialofetuin to target delivery of DNA–liposome complexes to the asialoglycoprotein receptor on hepatocytes in the liver. The succinic acid amides provided greater negative charge to asialofetuin, and, therefore, bound to the surface of complexes more efficiently than asialofetuin alone. The amount used for adsorption onto the surface of complexes is ligand dependent. Titration studies must be performed to determine the optimal amount of ligand to coat onto the surface of complexes. Ultimately, *in vivo* transfection experiments must be performed to verify the optimal amount of ligand to use to provide delivery to the target cells and the highest levels of gene expression in these cells with no generation of an immune response.

Ligands or modified ligands containing reactive groups can be covalently attached to linker lipids (Fig. 8a). These ligand–lipid conjugates must be checked for optimal activity of the ligand to bind to its receptor. Furthermore, the covalent linkage must not be immunogenic in animals or people after repeated administration. Ligand–lipid conjugates can be spontaneously inserted into the outside membrane of complexes in which the nucleic acids are encapsulated within liposomes (Figure 8b). The amount of ligand–lipid used for insertion into the surface of complexes is also ligand dependent. Titration studies must be performed to determine the optimal amount of ligand–lipid to insert into the surface of complexes. Again, *in vivo* transfection experiments must be performed to verify the optimal amount of ligand–lipid to use to provide delivery to the target cells and the highest levels of gene expression in these cells with no generation of an immune response.

Using the alternative approaches described above, we have produced complexes that provide delivery of nucleic acids to target cells. Furthermore, the gene expression in the target cells using the targeted complexes is higher than that using the "generic" extruded DOTAP:Chol complexes.

9
Serum Stability of Optimized Nucleic Acid–Liposome Complexes for Use *in vivo*

Serum stability of cationic complexes is complicated and cannot be assessed by simply performing studies at a random concentration of serum. Figure 9 shows results from serum stability studies of DNA–liposome complexes that have been optimized in our laboratory for systemic delivery. Serum stability of these complexes was studied at $37\,^\circ$C out to 24 h at concentrations of serum ranging from 0 to 100%. Two different serum stability assays were performed. The first assay measured the OD400 of BIV DOTAP:Chol–DNA–liposome complexes added into tubes containing a different concentration of serum in each tube, ranging from 0 to 100%. The tubes were incubated at $37\,^\circ$C, and small aliquots from each tube were removed at various time points out to 24 h. The OD400 of each aliquot was measured on a spectrophotometer calibrated to accurately measure turbidity. Previous work in our laboratory demonstrated that the OD400 predicted both the stability of the complexes and the transfection efficiency results obtained for multiple organs after intravenous injections. Percent stability for this assay is defined as the transfection efficiency that is obtained at a particular OD400 of the complexes used for intravenous injections. Therefore, this assay is rigorous because slight declines in OD400 of these complexes result in obtaining

Serum stability of complexes

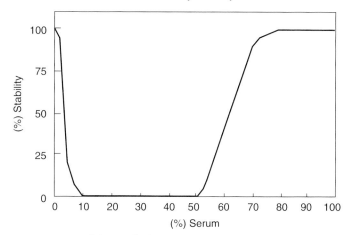

Fig. 9 Serum stability profile for DNA–liposome complexes optimized for systemic delivery. Serum stability of these complexes was studied at 37 °C out to 24 h at concentrations of serum ranging from 0 to 100%. Serum stability at the highest concentrations of serum, about 70 to 100%, that are physiological concentrations of serum found in the bloodstream is required.

no transfection *in vivo*. Declines in the OD400 also measure precipitation of the complexes.

A second assay was performed to support the results obtained from the OD400 measurements described above. A different concentration of serum, ranging from 0 to 100%, was placed into each well of a 96-well micro titer dish. BIV DOTAP:Chol–DNA–liposome complexes were added to the serum in the wells, and the plate was incubated at 37 °C. The plate was removed at various time points out to 24 h and complexes in the wells were observed under the microscope. Precipitation of complexes in the wells was assessed. 100% stability was set at no precipitation observed. Results from this assay were compared with those obtained in the first assay. 100% stability of complexes was set at no decline of OD400 in assay #1 and no observed precipitation in assay #2 at each % serum

concentration, and the results were plotted (Fig. 9).

The results showed serum stability at the highest concentrations of serum, about 70 to 100%, that are physiological concentrations of serum found in the bloodstream. In addition, these complexes were also stable in no or low concentrations of serum. The complexes were unstable at 10 to 50% serum, perhaps due to salt bridging. Therefore, *in vitro* optimization of serum stability for formulations of cationic complexes must be performed over a broad range of serum concentration to be useful for applications *in vivo*.

10
Optimized Half-life in the Circulation

As stated above, the extruded BIV DOTAP:Chol–nucleic acid complexes are large enough so that they are not cleared rapidly by Kupffer cells in the liver and yet extravasate across tight barriers and diffuse through the target organ efficiently. Further addition of ligands to the surface of extruded BIV DOTAP:Chol–nucleic acid complexes does not significantly increase the mean particle size. Extravasation and penetration through the target organ and gene expression produced after transfection are not diminished. These modified formulations are positively charged and deliver nucleic acids efficiently into cells *in vitro* and *in vivo*. Because extruded BIV DOTAP:Chol–nucleic acid complexes with or without ligands have a 5-h half-life in the circulation, these complexes do not accumulate in the skin, hands, or feet. Extended half-life in the circulation is provided primarily by the formulation, preparation method, injection of optimal colloidal suspensions, and optimal nucleic acid:lipid ratio used for mixing complexes, serum stability, and size (200 to 450 nm). Therefore, these BIVs are ideal for use in the development of effective, targeted non-viral delivery systems that clearly require encapsulation of nucleic acids.

11
Broad Biodistribution of Optimized Liposome Formulations

Our "generic" BIV nucleic acid–liposome formulation transfects many organs and tissues efficiently after intravenous injection, and has demonstrated efficacy in animal models for lung cancer, pancreatic cancer, breast cancer, Hepatitis B and C (Clawson and Templeton, unpublished data), and cardiovascular diseases. Therefore, optimization of the morphology of the complexes, the lipids used, flexibility of the liposomes and complexes, colloidal suspension, overall charge, serum stability,

and half-life in circulation allows for efficient delivery and gene expression in many organs and tissues other than the lung. Apparently, these extruded DOTAP:Chol BIV nucleic acid–liposome complexes can overcome the tendency to be adsorbed only by the endothelial cells lining the circulation surrounding the lungs described by other investigators. However, as discussed above and below, we can further direct delivery to specific target tissues or cells by our targeted delivery strategies in combination with reversible masking used to bypass nonspecific transfection.

12
Optimization of Targeted Delivery

Much effort has been made to specifically deliver nucleic acid–liposome complexes to target organs, tissues, and/or cells. Ligands that bind to cell surface receptors are usually attached to PEG and then attached to the cationic or anionic delivery vehicle. Owing to the shielding of the positive charge of cationic complexes by PEG, delivery to the specific cell surface receptor can be accomplished by only a small fraction of complexes injected systemically. Furthermore, delivery of PEGylated complexes into the cell occurs predominantly through the endocytic pathway, and subsequent degradation of the bulk of the nucleic acid occurs in the lysosomes. Thus, gene expression is generally lower in the target cell than when using the nonspecific delivery of highly efficient cationic complexes.

As discussed above, the vast majority of the injected PEGylated complexes bypasses the target cell. Apparently, the PE-Gylated complexes cannot utilize critical charge interactions for optimal transfection into cells by direct fusion. Inability to expose positive charge on the surface of optimized complexes results in the trans-fection of fewer cells. PEGylation was first used to increase the half-life of complexes in the circulation and to avoid uptake in the lung. However, this technology also destroys the ability to efficiently transfect cells. We were able to increase the half-life in circulation of BIVs to 5 h without the use of PEG. Because the extended half-life of BIVs is not too long, this delivery system does not result in the accumulation of com-plexes in nontarget tissues that circulate for one to three days. Some investigators have now reported targeted delivery that produces increased gene expression in the target cell over their nontargeted com-plexes. However, these nontargeted and targeted delivery systems are inefficient compared to efficient delivery systems such as the BIVs.

In using the extruded BIV DOTAP: Chol–nucleic acid:liposome complexes, we produced an optimal half-life in the cir-culation without the use of PEG. Extended half-life was produced primarily by the for-mulation, preparation method, injection of optimal colloidal suspensions, serum sta-bility, and optimal nucleic acid:lipid ratio used for mixing complexes, and size (200 to 450 nm). Furthermore, we avoided up-take in the lungs using the negative charge of the ligands and "shielding/deshielding compounds" that can be added to the complexes used for targeting just prior to injection or administration *in vivo*. Our strategy to bypass nonspecific transfection is called *reversible masking*. Addition of lig-ands using the novel approaches that we developed, adequate overall positive charge on the surface of complexes is preserved. In summary, we achieve optimal circu-lation time of the complexes, reach and deliver to the target organ, avoid uptake in nontarget tissues, and efficiently interact with the cell surface to produce optimal transfection.

13
Efficient Dissemination Throughout Target Tissues and Migration Across Tight Barriers

A primary goal for efficient *in vivo* delivery is to achieve extravasation into and pene-tration throughout the target organ/tissue ideally by noninvasive systemic adminis-tration. Without these events, therapeutic efficacy is highly compromised for any treatment, including gene and drug ther-apies. Achieving this goal is difficult be-cause of the many tight barriers that exist in animals and people. Furthermore, many of these barriers become tighter in the tran-sition from neonates to becoming adults. Penetration throughout an entire tumor is further hindered because of the increased interstitial pressure within most tumors. We believe that nonviral systems can play a pivotal role in achieving target organ extravasation and penetration needed to treat or cure certain diseases. Our prelim-inary studies have shown that extruded BIV DOTAP:Chol–nucleic acid:liposome complexes can extravasate across tight barriers and penetrate evenly through-out entire target organs, and viral vectors cannot cross identical barriers. These bar-riers include the endothelial cell barrier in a normal mouse, the posterior blood retinal barrier in adult mouse eyes, com-plete and even diffusion throughout large tumors, and penetration through several tight layers of smooth muscle cells in the arteries of pigs. Diffusion throughout large tumors was measured by expres-sion of ß-galactosidase or the proapoptotic gene *p*53 in about half of the *p*53-null tumor cells after a single injection of BIV DOTAP:Chol – DNA–liposome complexes into the center of a tumor. Transfected cells were evenly spread throughout the tumors. Tumors injected with complexes encapsulating plasmid DNA encoding p53 showed apoptosis in almost all of the tumor cells by TUNEL staining. Tumor cells expressing p53 mediate a bystander effect on neighboring cells perhaps due to upregulation by Fas ligand that causes nontransfected tumor cells to undergo apoptosis. Currently, we are investigating the mechanisms used by extruded DOTAP:Chol–nucleic acid:liposome complexes to cross barriers and penetrate throughout target organs. By knowing more about these mechanisms, we hope to develop more robust nonviral gene therapeutics.

14
Optimization of Plasmids for *in vivo* Gene Expression

Delivery of DNA and subsequent gene expression may be poorly correlated. Investigators may focus solely on the delivery formulation as the source of poor gene expression. In many cases, however, the delivery of DNA into the nucleus of a particular cell type may be efficient, although little or no gene expression is achieved. The causes of poor gene expression can be numerous. The following issues should be considered independent of the delivery formulation, including suboptimal promoter-enhancers in the plasmid, poor preparation of plasmid DNA, and insensitive detection of gene expression.

Plasmid expression cassettes typically have not been optimized for animal studies. For example, many plasmids lack a full-length CMV promoter-enhancer. Over one hundred variations of the CMV promoter-enhancer exist, and some variations produce greatly reduced or no gene expression in certain cell types. Even commercially available plasmids contain suboptimal CMV promoters-enhancers, although these plasmids are advertised for use in animals. Furthermore, upon checking the company data for these plasmids, one would discover that these plasmids have never been tested in animals and have been tested in only one or two cultured cell lines. Conversely, plasmids that have been optimized for overall efficiency in animals may not be best for transfection of certain cell types *in vitro* or *in vivo*. For example, many investigators have shown that optimal CMV promoters-enhancers produce gene expression at levels several orders of magnitude less in certain cell types. In addition, one cannot assume that a CMV promoter that expresses well within the context of a viral vector, such as adenovirus, will function as well in a plasmid-based transfection system for the same cell context. Virus proteins produced by the viral vector are required for producing high levels of mRNA by the CMV promoter in specific cell nuclei.

Ideally, investigators design custom promoter-enhancer chimeras that produce the highest levels of gene expression in their target cells of interest. Recently, we designed a systematic approach for customizing plasmids used for breast cancer gene therapy using expression profiling. Gene therapy clinical trials for cancer frequently produce inconsistent results. We believe that some of this variability could result from differences in transcriptional regulation that limit expression of therapeutic genes in specific cancers. Our systemic liposomal delivery of a nonviral plasmid DNA showed efficacy in animal models for several cancers. However, we observed large differences in the levels of gene expression from a CMV promoter-enhancer between lung and breast cancers. To optimize gene expression in breast cancer cells *in vitro* and *in vivo*, we created a new promoter-enhancer chimera to regulate gene expression. Serial analyses of gene expression (SAGE) data from a panel of breast carcinomas and normal breast cells predicted promoters that are highly active in breast cancers, for example, the glyceraldehyde 3-phosphate dehydrogenase (GAPDH) promoter. Furthermore, GAPDH is upregulated by hypoxia, which is common in tumors. We added the GAPDH promoter, including the hypoxia enhancer sequences, to our *in vivo* gene expression plasmid. The novel CMV-GAPDH promoter-enhancer showed up to 70-fold increased gene expression in breast tumors compared to the optimized CMV promoter-enhancer alone. No significant increase in gene expression was observed in other tissues. These data demonstrate tissue-specific effects on gene expression after nonviral delivery, and suggest that gene delivery systems may require plasmid modifications for the treatment of different tumor types. Furthermore, expression profiling can facilitate the design of optimal expression plasmids for use in specific cancers.

Several reviews have stated that nonviral systems are intrinsically inefficient compared to viral systems. However, as discussed above, one must separate issues of the delivery vehicle versus the plasmid that is delivered. Case in point, we have shown that our extruded liposomes optimized for systemic delivery could outcompete delivery using a lentivirus. For example, we have compared SIVmac239, a highly noninfectious virus, with nonviral delivery of SIVmac239 DNA complexed to BIVs in adult rhesus macaques after injection into the saphenous vein of the leg. Our data showed that the monkeys injected with SIV DNA encapsulated in DOTAP:Chol BIVs were infected four days postinjection, and high levels of infection were produced in these monkeys at 14 days postinjection. Furthermore, higher levels of SIV RNA in the blood were produced using our BIV liposomes for delivery versus that using the SIV virus. CD4 counts were measured before and after injections. CD4 levels dropped in all monkeys to the lowest levels ever detected in the macaques in any experiment by 28 days postinjection, the first time point at which these counts were measured postinjection. All monkeys had clinical SIV infections and lost significant weight by day 28. These results were surprising because SIVmac239 is not highly infectious, and monkeys become sick with SIV infection only after several months or years postinjection with SIVmac239 virus. Therefore, we were able to induce SIV infection faster using our nonviral delivery of SIV plasmid DNA. In this case, we delivered a replication-competent plasmid so that gene expression increased over time posttransfection. Our delivery system was highly efficient and exceeded that of the lentivirus. The critical feature in this nonviral experiment was the plasmid DNA that was delivered.

Plasmids can be engineered to provide for specific or long-term gene expression, replication, or integration. Persistence elements, such as the inverted terminal repeats from adenovirus or adeno-associated virus, have been added to plasmids to prolong gene expression *in vitro* and *in vivo*. Apparently, these elements bind to the nuclear matrix thereby retaining the plasmid in cell nuclei. For regulated gene expression, many different inducible promoters are used that promote expression only in the presence of a positive regulator or in the absence of a negative regulator. Tissue specific promoters have been used for the production of gene expression exclusively in the target cells. As discussed in the previous paragraph, replication-competent plasmids or plasmids containing sequences for autonomous replication can be included that provide prolonged gene expression. Other plasmid-based strategies produce site-specific integration or homologous recombination within the host cell genome. Integration of a cDNA into a specific "silent site" in the genome could provide long-term gene expression without disruption of normal cellular functions. Homologous recombination could correct genetic mutations upon integration of wild-type sequences that replace mutations in the genome. Plasmids that contain fewer bacterial sequences and that produce high yield upon growth in *Escherichia coli* are also desirable.

15
Optimization of Plasmid DNA Preparations

The transfection quality of plasmid DNA is dependent on the preparation protocol and training of the person preparing the DNA. For example, we performed a blinded study asking three people to make DNA preparations of the same plasmid from the same box of a Qiagen Endo-Free Plasmid Preparation kit. One person then mixed all of the DNA–liposome complexes on the same morning using a single vial of liposomes. One person performed all tail vein injections, harvesting of tissues, preparation of extracts from tissues, and reporter gene assays on the tissue extracts. *In vivo* gene expression differed 30-fold among these three plasmid DNA preparations.

One source for this variability is that optimized methods to detect and remove contaminants from plasmid DNA preparations have not been available. We have identified large amounts of contaminants that exist in laboratory and clinical grade preparations of plasmid DNA. These contaminants copurify with DNA by anion exchange chromatography and by cesium chloride density gradient centrifugation. Endotoxin removal does not remove these contaminants. HPLC cannot detect these contaminants. Therefore, we developed three proprietary methods for the detection of these contaminants in plasmid DNA preparations. We can now make clinical grade good manufacturing practices (GMP) DNA that does not contain these contaminants. To provide the greatest efficacy and levels of safety, these contaminants must be assessed and removed from plasmid DNA preparations. These contaminants belong to a class of molecules known to inhibit both DNA and RNA polymerase activities. Therefore, gene expression posttransfection can be increased by orders of magnitude if these contaminants are removed from DNA preparations. The presence of these contaminants in DNA also precludes high dose delivery of DNA–liposome complexes intravenously. Our group and other investigators have shown that intravenous injections of high doses of improved liposomes alone cause no adverse effects in small and large animals.

Some investigators have removed the majority of CpG sequences from their plasmids and report reduced toxicity after intravenous injections of cationic liposomes complexed to these plasmids. However, only low doses containing up to 16.5 μg of DNA per injection into each mouse were shown to reduce toxicity. Therefore, no significant dose response to CpG motifs in plasmid DNA was demonstrated. To achieve efficacy for cancer metastases, particularly in mice bearing aggressive tumors, most investigators are interested in injecting higher doses in the range of 50 to 150 µg of DNA per mouse. Therefore, removal of CpG sequences from plasmid-based gene therapy vectors will not be useful for these applications because no difference in toxicity was shown after intravenous injections of these higher doses of plasmids, with or without reduced CpG sequences, complexed to liposomes. Therefore, we believe that removal of the other contaminants in current DNA preparations, discussed above, is the major block to the safe intravenous injection of high doses of DNA–liposome complexes.

16
Detection of Gene Expression

Thought should also be given to choosing the most sensitive detection method for every application of nonviral delivery rather than using the method that seems most simple. For example, detection of ß-galactosidase expression is far more sensitive than that for the green fluorescent protein (GFP). Specifically, 500 molecules of ß-galactosidase (ß-gal) per cell are required for detection using X-gal staining. Whereas, about one million molecules of GFP per cell are required for direct detection. Furthermore, detection of GFP may be impossible if the fluorescence background of the target cell or tissue is too high. Detection of chloramphenicol acetyltransferase (CAT) is extremely sensitive with little or no background detected in untransfected cells. Often, assays for CAT expression can provide more useful information than using ß-gal or GFP as reporter genes.

Few molecules of luciferase in a cell can be detected by luminescence assays of cell or tissue extracts posttransfection. The sensitivity of these assays is highly dependent on the type of instrument used to measure luminescence. However, luciferase results may not predict the therapeutic potential of a nonviral delivery system. For example, if several hundred or thousand molecules per cell of a therapeutic gene are required to produce efficacy for a certain disease, then production of only few molecules will not be adequate. If only few molecules of luciferase are produced in the target cell using a specific nonviral delivery system, then the investigator may be misled in using this system for therapeutic applications.

Furthermore, noninvasive detection of luciferase expression *in vivo* is not as sensitive as luminescence assays of cell or tissue extracts posttransfection. Recently, some colleagues of mine tried cooled charge coupled device (CCD) camera imaging on live mice after intravenous injection of other cationic liposomes complexed to plasmid DNA encoding luciferase, and they were not able to detect any transfection. However, these liposomal delivery systems had been used to detect luciferase by luminescence assays of organ extracts. My colleagues detected luciferase expression by CCD imaging after intravenous injections of BIV DOTAP:Chol-luciferase DNA–liposome complexes. Using the same CCD imaging system following intravenous injections of PEI-DNA complexes, extremely poor transfection efficiency was observed in all tissues. Because the luciferase protein is short-lived, maximal expression was detected at 5 h posttransfection. Whereas, detection of HSV-TK gene expression using microPET imaging in the same mice was highest at 24 h posttransfection. In contrast to luciferase, the CAT protein accumulates over time, and, therefore, the investigator is not restricted to a narrow time frame for assaying gene expression. Furthermore, detection of CAT seems to be more sensitive than CCD imaging of luciferase following intravenous injections of DNA–liposome complexes. However, the animals must be sacrificed in order to perform CAT assays on tissue or organ extracts. In summary, further work is still needed to develop *in vivo* detection systems that have high sensitivity and low background.

17
Optimization of Dose and Frequency of Administration

To establish the maximal efficacy for the treatment of certain diseases or for the creation of robust vaccines, injections, or administrations of the nonviral gene therapeutic, and so on via different routes may be required. For particular treatments, one should not assume that one delivery route is superior to others without performing the appropriate animal experiments. In addition, people with the appropriate expertise should perform the injections and administrations. In our experience, only a minority of people who claim expertise in performing tail vein injections can actually perform optimal injections.

The optimal dose should be determined for each therapeutic gene or other nucleic acid that is administered. The investigator should not assume that the highest tolerable dose is optimal for producing maximal efficacy. The optimal administration schedule should also be determined for each therapeutic gene or other nucleic acid. To progress faster, some investigators have simply used the same administration schedule that they used for chemotherapeutics, for example. The investigator should perform *in vivo* experiments to determine when gene expression and/or efficacy drops significantly. Most likely, readministration of the nonviral gene therapeutic is not necessary until this drop occurs. Loss of the therapeutic gene product will vary with the half-life of the protein produced. Therefore, if a therapeutic protein has a longer half-life, then the gene therapy could be administered less frequently.

18
Summary

Overcoming some hurdles remains in the broad application of nonviral delivery; however, we are confident that we will successfully accomplish the remaining challenges soon. Furthermore, we predict that eventually the majority of gene therapies will utilize artificial reagents that can be standardized and regulated as drugs rather than biologics. We will continue to incorporate the molecular mechanisms of viral delivery that produce efficient delivery to cells into artificial systems. Therefore, the artificial systems, including liposomal delivery vehicles, will be further engineered to mimic the most beneficial parts of the viral delivery systems while circumventing their limitations. We will also maintain the numerous benefits of the liposomal delivery systems discussed in this chapter.

Acknowledgment

I thank Dr. David D. Roberts at the National Cancer Institute, National Institutes of Health, Bethesda, MD for preparation of the figures.

Bibliography

Books and Reviews

Templeton, N.S. *Gene Targeting Protocols*, (2000) Vol. 133, Humana Press, Totowa, NJ, pp. 1–244.

Jain, R.K. (1994) Barriers to drug delivery in solid tumors, *Sci. Am.* **271**, 58–65.

Jain, R.K. (1999) Transport of molecules, particles, and cells in solid tumors, *Annu. Rev. Biomed. Eng.* **1**, 241–263.

Li, S., Ma, Z., Tan, Y., Liu, F., Dileo, J., Huang, L. (2002) Targeted Delivery Via Lipidic Vectors, in: Curiel, D.T., Douglas, J.T. (Eds.) *Vector Targeting for Therapeutic Gene Delivery*, Wiley-Liss Inc., Hoboken, NJ, pp. 17–32.

Marshall, E. (2003) Second child in French trial is found to have leukemia, *Science* **299**, 320.

Pirollo, K.F., Xu, L., Chang, E.H. (2002) Immunoliposomes: A Targeted Delivery Tool for Cancer Treatment, in: Curiel, D.T., Douglas, J.T. (Eds.) *Vector Targeting for Therapeutic Gene Delivery*, Wiley-Liss Inc., Hoboken, NJ, pp. 33–62.

Templeton, N.S., Lasic, D.D. (1999) New directions in liposome gene delivery, *Mol. Biotechnol.* **11**, 175–180.

Primary Literature

Aksentijevich, I., Pastan, I., Lunardi-Iskandar, Y., Gallo, R.C., Gottesman, M.M., Thierry, A.R. (1996) In vitro and in vivo liposome-mediated gene transfer leads to human MDR1 expression in mouse bone marrow progenitor cells, *Hum. Gene Ther.* **7**, 1111–1122.

Behr, J.-P., Demeneix, B., Loeffler, J.P., Perez-Mutul, J. (1989) Efficient gene transfer into mammalian primary endocrine cells with lipopolyamine-coated DNA, *Proc. Natl. Acad. Sci. U.S.A.* **86**, 6982–6986.

Felgner, P.L., Ringold, G.M. (1989) Cationic liposome-mediated transfection, *Nature* **337**, 387–388.

Felgner, J.H., Kumar, R., Sridhar, C.N., Wheeler, C.J., Tsai, Y.J., Border, R., Ramsey, P., Martin, M., Felgner, P.L. (1994) Enhanced gene delivery and mechanism studies with a novel series of cationic lipid formulations, *J. Biol. Chem.* **269**, 2550–2561.

Felgner, P.L., Gadek, T.R., Holm, M., Roman, R., Chan, H.W., Wenz, M., Northrop, J.P., Ringold, G.M., Danielson, H. (1987) Lipofection: a highly efficient lipid-mediated DNA transfection procedure, *Proc. Natl. Acad. Sci. U.S.A.* **84**, 7413–7417.

Gabizon, A., Catane, R., Uziely, B., Kaufman, B., Safra, T., Cohen, R., Martin, F., Huang, A., Barenholz, Y. (1994) Prolonged circulation time and enhanced accumulation in malignant exudates of doxorubicin encapsulated in polyethylene-glycol coated liposomes, *Cancer Res.* **54**, 987–992.

Gordon, K.B., Tajuddin, A., Guitart, J., Kuzel, T.M., Eramo, L.R., VonRoenn, J. (1995) Hand-foot syndrome associated with liposome-encapsulated doxorubicin therapy, *Cancer* **75**, 2169–2173.

Gustafsson, J., Arvidson, G., Karlsson, G., Almgren, M. (1995) Complexes between cationic liposomes and DNA visualized by cryo-TEM, *Biochim. Biophys. Acta* **1235**, 305–312.

Handumrongkul, C., Zhong, W., Debs, R.J. (2002) Distinct sets of cellular genes control the expression of transfected, nuclear-localized genes, *Mol. Ther.* **5**, 186–194.

Hildebrandt, I.J., Iyer, M., Wagner, E., Gambhir, S.S. (2003) Optical imaging of transferrin targeted PEI/DNA complexes in living subjects, *Gene Ther.* **10**, 758–764.

Hood, J.D., Bednarski, M., Frausto, R., Guccione, S., Reisfeld, R.A., Xiang, R., Cheresh, D.A. (2002) Tumor regression by targeted gene delivery to the neovasculature, *Science* **296**, 2404–2407.

Iyer, M., Berenji, M., Templeton, N.S., Gambhir, S.S. (2002) Noninvasive imaging of cationic lipid-mediated delivery of optical and PET reporter genes in living mice, *Mol. Ther.* **6**, 555–562.

Jain, R.K. (1991) Haemodynamic and transport barriers to the treatment of solid tumours, *Int. J. Radiat. Biol.* **60**, 85–100.

Leventis, R., Silvius, J.R. (1990) Interactions of mammalian cells with lipid dispersions containing novel metabolizable cationic amphiphiles, *Biochim. Biophys. Acta* **1023**, 124–132.

Liu, F., Qi, H., Huang, L., Liu, D. (1997) Factors controlling the efficiency of cationic lipid-mediated transfection in vivo via intravenous administration, *Gene Ther.* **4**, 517–523.

Liu, Y., Liggitt, D., Zhong, W., Tu, G., Gaensler, K., Debs, R. (1995) Cationic liposome-mediated intravenous gene delivery, *J. Biol. Chem.* **270**, 24864–24870.

Liu, Y., Mounkes, L.C., Liggitt, H.D., Brown, C.S., Solodin, I., Heath, T.D., Debs, R.J. (1997) Factors influencing the efficiency of cationic-liposome mediated intravenous gene delivery, *Nat. Biotechnol.* **15**, 167–173.

Loeffler, J.P., Behr, J.-P. (1993) Gene transfer into primary and established mammalian cell lines with lipopolyamine-coated DNA, *Methods Enzymol.* **217**, 599–618.

Lu, H., Zhang, Y., Roberts, D.D., Osborne, C.K., Templeton, N.S. (2002) Enhanced gene expression in breast cancer cells in vitro and tumors in vivo, *Mol. Ther.* **6**, 783–792.

Mislick, K.A., Baldeschwieler, J.D. (1996) Evidence for the role of proteoglycans in cation-mediated gene transfer, *Proc. Natl. Acad. Sci. U.S.A.* **93**, 12349–12354.

Papahadjopoulos, D., Allen, T.M., Gabizon, A., Mayhew, E., Matthay, K., Huang, S.K., Lee, K., Woodle, M.C., Lasic, D.D., Redemann, C., Martin, F.J. (1991) Sterically stabilized liposomes: improvements in pharmacokinetics and antitumor therapeutic efficacy, *Proc. Natl. Acad. Sci. U.S.A.* **88**, 11460–11464.

Philip, R., Liggitt, D., Philip, M., Dazin, P., Debs, R. (1993) In vivo gene delivery: efficient transfection of T lymphocytes in adult mice, *J. Biol. Chem.* **268**, 16087–16090.

Pinnaduwage, P., Huang, L. (1989) The role of protein-linked oligosaccharide in the bilayer stabilization activity of glycophorin A for dioleoylphosphatidylethanolamine liposomes, *Biochim. Biophys. Acta* **986**, 106–114.

Ramesh, R., Saeki, T., Templeton, N.S., Ji, L., Stephens, L.C., Ito, I., Wilson, D.R., Wu, Z., Branch, C.D., Minna, J.D., Roth, J.A. (2001) Successful treatment of primary and disseminated human lung cancers by systemic delivery of tumor suppressor genes using an improved liposome vector, *Mol. Ther.* **3**, 337–350.

Rose, J.K., Buonocore, L., Whitt, M.A. (1991) A new cationic liposome reagent mediating nearly quantitative transfection of animal cells, *Biotechniques* **10**, 520–525.

Senior, J., Delgado, C., Fisher, D., Tilcock, C., Gregoriadis, G. (1991) Influence of surface hydrophilicity of liposomes on their interaction with plasma protein and clearance from the circulation: studies with poly(ethylene glycol)-coated vesicles, *Biochim. Biophys. Acta* **1062**, 77–82.

Shi, H.Y., Liang, R., Templeton, N.S., Zhang, M. (2002) Inhibition of breast tumor progression by systemic delivery of the maspin gene in a syngeneic tumor model, *Mol. Ther.* **5**, 755–761.

Solodin, I., Brown, C.S., Bruno, M.S., Ching-Yi, C., Eun-Hyun, J., Debs, R., Heath, T.D. (1995) A novel series of amphiphilic imidazolinium compounds for in vitro and in vivo gene delivery, *Biochemistry* **34**, 13537–13544.

Sternberg, B. (1996) Morphology of cationic liposome/DNA complexes in relation to their chemical composition, *J. Liposome Res.* **6**, 515–533.

Templeton, N.S., Lasic, D.D., Frederik, P.M., Strey, H.H., Roberts, D.D., Pavlakis, G.N. (1997) Improved DNA: liposome complexes for increased systemic delivery and gene expression, *Nat. Biotechnol.* **15**, 647–652.

Templeton, N.S., Alspaugh, E., Antelman, D., Barber, J., Csaky, K.G., Fang, B., Frederik, P., Honda, H., Johnson, D., Litvak, F., Machemer, T., Ramesh, R., Robbins, J., Roth, J.A., Sebastian, M., Tritz, R., Wen, S.F., Wu, Z. (1999) Non-viral Vectors for the Treatment of Disease, *Keystone Symposia on Molecular and Cellular Biology of Gene Therapy*, Salt Lake City, UT.

Thierry, A.R., Lunardi-Iskandar, Y., Bryant, J.L., Rabinovich, P., Gallo, R.C., Mahan, L.C. (1995) Systemic gene therapy: biodistribution and long-term expression of a transgene in mice, *Proc. Natl. Acad. Sci. U.S.A.* **92**, 9742–9746.

Tirone, T.A., Fagan, S.P., Templeton, N.S., Wang, X.P., Brunicardi, F.C. (2001) Insulinoma induced hypoglycemic death in mice is prevented with beta cell specific gene therapy, *Ann. Surg.* **233**, 603–611.

Tsukamoto, M., Ochiya, T., Yoshida, S., Sugimura, T., Terada, M. (1995) Gene transfer and expression in progeny after intravenous DNA injection into pregnant mice, *Nat. Genet.* **9**, 243–248.

Uziely, B., Jeffers, S., Isacson, R., Kutsch, K., Wei-Tsao, D., Yehoshua, Z., Libson, E., Muggia, F.M., Gabizon, A. (1995) Liposomal doxorubicin: antitumor activity and unique toxicities during two complementary phase I studies, *J. Clin. Oncol.* **13**, 1777–1785.

Xu, Y., Szoka, F.C. (1996) Mechanism of DNA release from cationic liposome/DNA complexes used in cell transfection, *Biochemistry* **35**, 5616–5623.

Yew, N.S., Zhao, H., Przybylska, M., Wu, I.-H., Tousignant, J.D., Scheule, R.K., Cheng, S.H. (2002) CpG depleted plasmid DNA vectors with enhanced safety and long-term gene expression in vivo, *Mol. Ther.* **5**, 731–738.

Yotnda, P., Chen, D.-H., Chiu, W., Piedra, P.A., Davis, A., Templeton, N.S., Brenner, M.K. (2002) Bilamellar cationic liposomes protect adenovectors from preexisting humoral immune responses, *Mol. Ther.* **5**, 233–241.

Zhu, N., Liggitt, D., Liu, Y., Debs, R. (1993) Systemic gene expression after intravenous DNA delivery in adult mice, *Science* **261**, 209–211.

27
Genetic Vaccination

Joerg Reimann[1], Martin Schleef[2], and Reinhold Schirmbeck[1]
[1] *University of Ulm, Ulm, Germany*
[2] *Plasmid Factory, Bielefeld, Germany*

1   **Principles   857**
1.1   The Emerging Technique of DNA Vaccination   857
1.2   The Novel Aspect of DNA Vaccination   857

2   **Techniques   859**
2.1   Basic Structure of a Eukaryotic Expression Vector   859
2.2   Increasing the Antigenic Information Delivered by DNA Vaccines   860
2.3   Strategies to Enhance the Immunogenicity of DNA Vaccines   861
2.3.1   Synthetic Genes   861
2.3.2   Promoter/Enhancer Sequences   861
2.3.3   Enhancing Transfection Efficiency of DNA Vaccines   861
2.3.4   Subcellular Targeting of Antigen Expression   862
2.3.5   Targeting Antigens to APCs   862
2.3.6   Codelivery of Antigen with Immune-stimulating/modulating
             Cytokines and Chemokines   862
2.3.7   Codelivery of Transcription Factors   863
2.3.8   CpG-containing Oligodeoxynucleotides (ODN)   863
2.3.9   Stress Proteins   863
2.3.10   Copriming Specific "Help"   864
2.4   Production and Quality Control of DNA Vaccines   864
2.4.1   Quality Control and Safety in Plasmid DNA Vaccine Production   864
2.4.2   Plasmid Identity   864
2.4.3   Animal-free DNA Production   865
2.4.4   Genomic DNA   865
2.4.5   Host Cell Impurities   866
2.4.6   Importance of Supercoiled Forms   866
2.5   Stability of DNA Vaccines   868
2.5.1   Storage Stability of Plasmid DNA   868

Pharmacology. From Drug Development to Gene Therapy. Edited by Robert A. Meyers.
Copyright © 2008 Wiley-VCH Verlag GmbH & Co. KGaA, Weinheim
ISBN: 978-3-527-32343-2

2.5.2   Stability in Plasmid Vector Applications   868
2.6   Delivery of DNA Vaccines   868
2.6.1   Combining DNA Vaccines and Protein Vaccines   869
2.6.2   Routes of DNA Vaccine Delivery   869

3   Applications   869
3.1   Priming Immune Responses by DNA Vaccination   869
3.1.1   Priming T-cell Responses   869
3.1.2   Priming B-cell (Antibody) Responses   870
3.2   DNA Vaccination as an Experimental Tool   870
3.3   Potential Advantages of DNA Vaccination   870

4   Perspectives   871
4.1   Achievement and Unresolved Issues of the Technology   871
4.2   Preclinical and Clinical Trials that Test Potential Applications of DNA
             Vaccination in Clinical Practice   871
4.3   Risks and Safety Issues Raised by DNA Vaccination   872

             Acknowledgment   873

             Bibliography   873
             Books and Reviews   873
             Primary Literature   873

Keywords

DNA (genetic or nucleic acid) vaccination
Stimulating an immune response to antigen(s) produced *in vivo* by cells transfected
with injected expression plasmid DNA.

In genetic or nucleic acid (DNA or RNA) vaccination, antigenic information
is delivered by *in vivo* expression of antigen from inoculated vector DNA (or
RNA). Combining different antigen-encoding sequences, modifying their sequence
and/or codelivering them with sequences encoding immune-stimulating factors
(readily achieved through recombinant DNA technologies) strikingly enhances and
modulates the immunogenicity of genetic vaccines and extends the repertoire of
epitopes to which different compartments of the adaptive immune system can be
specifically primed. Large-scale production of DNA vaccines, their formulation and
alternative modes of delivery are currently optimized. Experimental DNA vaccines
have demonstrated efficacy in priming antibody and/or cellular immune responses
that protect against a variety of pathogens or transplantable tumors in animal models.

Genetic vaccination has therefore become an unrivaled tool in preclinical research. Although highly attractive in principle, the practical development of DNA vaccination for clinical applications is at an early and experimental stage, and will have to resolve different issues before entering widespread use.

1
Principles

1.1
The Emerging Technique of DNA Vaccination

Active immune prophylaxis (vaccination) has been undeniably one of the greatest achievements in medicine. Vaccine development started centuries ago with the identification and large-scale production of attenuated pathogens. As these induced only limited clinically apparent disease after infection but expressed many of the immunogenic determinants of the pathogenic strain, they could elicit specific, protective immunity with a low burden of clinical disease after deliberate infection. This vaccination strategy evolved into the use of defined products of pathogens feasible after their molecular identification, inactivation (if they displayed a pathogenic potential like toxins, for e.g.), and formulation (to enhance their often weak intrinsic immunogenicity).

Genetic (nucleic acid) vaccination is a recently developed immunization technique in which antigen is expressed in immunogenic form (i.e. able to specifically prime an immune response) from inoculated nucleic acid fragments containing antigen-encoding sequences. The nucleic acid fragments are engineered to efficiently support expression of the respective antigen(s) *in situ*. Nucleic acid fragments used as genetic vaccines can be either plasmid DNA (DNA vaccines), or messenger (m) RNA (RNA vaccines). If cloned into suitable expression vectors, and delivered in an appropriate formulation at a suitable dose by a suitable route, these vaccines efficiently prime humoral and cellular immune responses to a large spectrum of protein antigens. The different steps in developing and testing a DNA vaccine are outlined in Table 1.

1.2
The Novel Aspect of DNA Vaccination

Genetic vaccination introduced new prospects into the field of vaccinology, which remain to be fully explored. Antigens produced *in situ* from DNA or RNA vaccines undergo all posttranslational modifications, such as folding, glycosylation, and oligomerizations (with host cell-derived or pathogen-derived molecules). This is a key issue in eliciting protective, neutralizing antibody (B cell) responses to many pathogens, as these usually bind only conformational epitopes. This is difficult to achieve by recombinant protein vaccines (expressed in a heterologous source and subjected to extensive purification procedures), but comparatively easy to achieve by genetic vaccines. Furthermore, genetic immunization has been shown to be exceptionally potent in stimulating cellular (T cell) responses. Antigenic peptides are generated from proteins produced from the DNA or RNA vaccine within a cell of the host. These can be introduced into

Tab. 1 The objectives of consecutive steps in DNA vaccination and the issues that have to be addressed.

Step	Objective	Issues to be addressed
1.	Construction of DNA vaccine	• Type of vector • Selection of antigen, antigenic domains, epitopes • Choice of costimulator (cytokine) to be codelivered
2.	Evaluate antigen expression from DNA vaccine	• Test amount, integrity, longevity of antigen expressed from the DNA vaccine in transient transfection assays
3.	Large-scale DNA vaccine production	• Production and isolation of supercoiled plasmid DNA on a large scale • Quality control (quantitative assessment of contaminants) • Define storage and shipment conditions
4.	Formulation of DNA vaccine	• Nonpackaged ("naked") plasmid DNA • Plasmid DNA packaged into liposomes, lipoplexes, polymers, cationic peptides, aluminum phosphate • Particle-coated plasmid DNA • Transformation of bacteria
5.	Delivery of DNA vaccine	• Intramuscular, subcutaneous, intradermal injection • Directly "shooting" DNA-coated gold microprojectiles into cells of the skin or the mucosa with the "gene gun" • Electroporation • Oral infection with DNA vaccine-carrying bacteria
6.	*In vivo* expression of antigen from a DNA vaccine	• *In situ* production of secreted antigen for priming antibody responses (humoral immunity) • Production and processing of antigen to (cross) prime T-cell responses (cellular immunity)
7.	Evaluate the vaccine-induced, specific immunity	• Follow over weeks postvaccination the specific serum antibody titers elicited • Measure numbers and functional properties of specifically primed CD4 and CD8 T-cell responses • Test response to boost injections • Test longevity of specific immunological memory • Test protective efficacy of the specific immunity
8.	Evaluate long-term safety issues	• Persistence of integrated plasmid DNA in the vaccinated individual • Autoimmune reactions

different processing pathways to generate presentation-competent major histocompatibility complex (MHC) (class I or class II) molecules, an essential prerequisite to prime cellular (T cell) responses. Modifications introduced into the antigen expressed by a DNA vaccine can facilitate its processing, thereby enhancing its antigenicity for T cells. Hence, both compartments of the specific immune system can be specifically stimulated by genetic vaccines.

Large numbers of vaccine candidates have been identified in different pathogens through sequencing of their genomes. DNA vaccination is an attractive tool to evaluate this expanding repertoire of potentially interesting antigens to experimentally identify vaccine candidates, and to evaluate and modulate their immunogenicity. This can be achieved through either expression library immunization, or genomic vaccination. DNA vaccines opened new ways to produce (native, variant, or chimeric) antigens in heterologous expression systems including complex, chimeric antigens that prime multivalent responses to different proteins of the same or different pathogens. Genetic vaccination has been shown to efficiently prime immune responses to viral, bacterial, parasitic, and tumor antigens in informative, preclinical animal models (including e.g. mice, rats, woodchuck, pig, rabbit, sheep, cattle, dogs, monkeys, chimps, fish, and chicken). Some of these vaccines demonstrated protective value, that is, either induced specific resistance to pathogens, or primed immunity that specifically rejected transplantable tumors. DNA vaccination contributed to the rational design of adjuvants by defining factors that modulate the immunogenicity and/or the polarization of an immune response (i.e. the repertoire of immune effector functions specifically activated).

Though similar to vaccines based on recombinant viruses, genetic vaccination has distinct advantages. The antigen load delivered by a genetic vaccine is restricted and readily controlled. DNA or RNA vaccines do not replicate, thus avoiding the complications of uncontrolled infections in immunodeficiency conditions. Many viral proteins selectively and efficiently interfere with distinct steps of antigen-processing pathways that generate and/or present antigenic peptides. They thereby inhibit immune responses. This does not operate in genetic vaccines, which can focus the response to selected determinants and exclude suppressive interfering determinants or molecules. This stresses the value of genetic vaccination as an attractive candidate for prophylactic or therapeutic immunization against intracellular and extracellular (viral, bacterial, or parasitic) pathogens and cancer.

2
Techniques

2.1
Basic Structure of a Eukaryotic Expression Vector

A "DNA vaccine" is a nonreplicative, closed circular, double-stranded plasmid DNA often 2 to 10 kb in size. Plasmids >10 kb in size are often ineffective as DNA vaccines. The vector contains 2 units. In the *transcription unit*, the target antigen-encoding sequence is cloned downstream from appropriate promoter/enhancer sequences that control transcription in human cells. Additional sequences regulating transcription (e.g. intron sequences, termination, and polyadenylation signals) are usually inserted into this unit. The *bacterial backbone* is required to produce the recombinant DNA in bacteria. It contains a bacterial origin of replication and a prokaryotic selection marker. These sequences are not essential constituents of DNA vaccines as minimal expression constructs with a transcription unit (as a covalently closed, linear DNA fragment) but no bacterial backbone have been successfully used as DNA vaccines. Plasmids used for DNA vaccination should be designed to minimize chances for integration into the host cell genome although it is difficult to exclude integration events.

Most genetic vaccines are DNA vectors because work with DNA is easier than work with RNA. However, successful vaccination with antigen-encoding mRNA has been reported. The half-life of antigen expression, the persistence of the vaccine (and the related safety issues), and the intrinsic adjuvant effect differ between RNA- and DNA-based vaccines.

2.2
Increasing the Antigenic Information Delivered by DNA Vaccines

A key objective in vaccinology is the development of multivalent vaccines. This facilitates acceptance and logistics of the vaccine, and decreases its cost. It is furthermore desirable to include different antigens of the same pathogen to increase the chance to prime protective immunity in an outbred population. DNA vaccine technology offers different options to achieve this goal. The technology comprises expression strategies that range from the expression of "minigenes" encoding only a single epitope (at the one extreme), to the coexpression of different, large antigens at stoichiometrically defined ratios (at the other extreme).

Minigenes inserted into DNA vaccines focus the immune response to only a single epitope. This allows selective priming of a monospecific response, excluding interferences from coprimed and potentially suppressive (regulatory or immunodominant) responses. Although an interesting tool to study the requirements for the induction and regulation of monospecific immune responses, the approach has limited practical value. Combining different minigenes into a single sequence leads to polytope vaccines. Different short sequences encoding only a single epitope

inserted into a DNA vaccine like "pearls on a string" are coexpressed by these vaccines that have been shown to successfully prime multispecific responses in inbred animal species. By fusing sequences encoding large antigens (or antigenic domains), DNA vaccines that produce chimeric antigens can be generated. Such constructs specifically stimulate multispecific T-cell responses. Coexpression of different antigens by either polycistronic expression constructs or bidirectional promoters, or a combination of both, generates complex expression vectors in which up to four complete antigens can be coexpressed at stoichiometrically defined ratios in immunogenic form. The large size of such vectors limits their usefulness as DNA vaccines. Expression of different antigens from alternative reading frames of the same nucleotide sequence is another way to increase the antigenic information delivered by a DNA vaccine of limited size. Coinjection of mixtures of DNA plasmid vectors encoding different antigens can prime multispecific antibody and T-cell responses. Extreme cases of mixing different expression plasmids are the immunization with mixtures of plasmids containing either large numbers of transcripts generated in expression libraries, or genomic fragments representing the complete genome of a pathogen. These studies showed that as few as one plasmid in 10^5 can give rise to an immune response. Rapidly evolving strategies for expressing antigens in DNA vaccines thus cover a broad range, from a strictly monospecific T-cell response, to a single epitope (present in a minigene), to multispecific T- and B-cell responses, to epitopes on independent antigens coexpressed by complex expression constructs.

2.3
Strategies to Enhance the Immunogenicity of DNA Vaccines

Immune responses to DNA vaccines alone have been weak, especially in humans. To be immunogenic (i.e. to prime a specific immune response), an antigen has to be produced by a DNA vaccine *in situ* in sufficient quantity with "costimulatory signals" mostly provided by antigen-presenting cells (APC). DNA vaccines can be designed to optimize antigen expression (through the choice of promoter sequences and optimization of codon usage) in the relevant tissues (secondary lymphoid tissues, i.e. lymph nodes) by appropriate APCs (macrophages, B cells, or dendritic cells). "Costimulatory signals" are ligands that activate receptors expressed by cells of the innate immune system or APC. Some of the molecularly defined "costimulatory factors" are of microbial origin while others are produced early in infection as "danger signals" by the host. Codelivery of such factors is often essential to prime a specific response, but can sometimes be bypassed by copriming responses in different compartments of the specific immune system (e.g. eliciting CD4$^+$ T-cell and CD8$^+$ T-cell responses to different epitopes of the same antigen). Here, the specific interaction of APCs with two different T-cell subsets allows initiation of both T-cell responses through mutual "help."

2.3.1 Synthetic Genes
Recently, synthetic genes have been designed with optimized codon usage that can strikingly enhance translation efficiency of antigens from some vector constructs. This technology is particularly interesting for expressing bacterial antigens in eukaryotic cells.

2.3.2 Promoter/Enhancer Sequences
To support optimal translation of the protein antigen from a DNA vaccine, the antigen-encoding sequence in the transcription unit has to be inserted downstream from strong promoter/enhancer sequences. Different promoter sequences can be used to construct effective DNA vaccines. Viral sequences (e.g. from cytomegalo, papova, or retroviruses), especially those from the immediate early region of the human cytomegalovirus (HCMV), have been favored as they drive high-level production of proteins in many cell types. Control sequences from other viruses (e.g. retrovirus or papova virus) or bacteria (e.g. borrelia) have been demonstrated to support high-level antigen expression from DNA vaccines that efficiently prime humoral and cellular immune responses. Alternatives to this viral control element have been developed because interferons (released early in an immune response) suppress many viral promoters. Mammalian cell–derived promoter sequences (controlling e.g. desmin, elongation factor-1α or metallothionein expression) have therefore been used to drive antigen production in DNA vaccine. Attempts to selectively express antigen from DNA vaccines in APCs (e.g. dendritic cells) through tissue-specific promoter/enhancer sequences have been less successful, presumably because tissue specificity of expression requires large, discontinuous sequence elements that are not yet correctly defined and are difficult to accommodate into a small DNA vaccine plasmid.

2.3.3 Enhancing Transfection Efficiency of DNA Vaccines
The DNA vaccine has to be delivered to the cytosol of the cell. The most critical process in transfection is the transport

of DNA from the cytosol to the nucleus. Tagging DNA vector constructs with viral sequences, or coupling DNA to nuclear localization signal peptides can facilitate the delivery of vector DNA to nuclei where transcription can take place.

2.3.4 Subcellular Targeting of Antigen Expression

To facilitate B-cell priming (antibody responses), antigen is usually expressed as a membrane-anchored or secreted protein because antibodies recognize cell surface or extracellular antigens in their native conformation. Antigens (or its fragments) should be expressed as intracellular proteins to facilitate T-cell priming because the T-cell receptor for antigen recognizes peptides generated by partial proteolytic degradation of antigens within cells. Antigen produced in the cytosol is degraded by proteasomes into peptides that are translocated into the endoplasmic reticulum by specialized transported molecules, where they are loaded to MHC class I molecules before trafficking to the cell surface. This is the prerequisite for priming $CD8^+$ T-cell responses. Priming $CD4^+$ T-cell responses is facilitated if antigens (or their antigenic fragments or epitopes) are targeted to a vesicular pathway. This allows their degradation in a specialized endolysosomal compartment. The generated peptides are "loaded" to MHC class II molecules that are transported to the cell surface. This is a prerequisite for priming $CD4^+$ T-cell responses. Subcellular targeting of antigen traffic by appropriate engineering of the DNA vaccine can thus be used to prime selected compartments of the specific immune system.

2.3.5 Targeting Antigens to APCs

Uptake of secreted antigen produced from a DNA vaccine can be targeted to professional APCs to enhance its immunogenicity. This can be achieved by fusing the antigen-encoding sequence to a ligand of a receptor expressed (preferentially or exclusively) by APCs. Ligands binding CD58, CD40, or CD80/CD86 have been used for this purpose. Such strategies also facilitate uptake of antigen by APC through receptor-mediated endocytosis, an efficient way to deliver antigen directly to some antigen-processing compartments. Similarly, antigen released at the site of DNA vaccine inoculation can be targeted to lymph nodes (the site of priming of immune responses) by fusion with CD62L (L-selectin) that binds to a receptor selectively expressed by high endothelia of venules of these tissues.

2.3.6 Codelivery of Antigen with Immune-stimulating/modulating Cytokines and Chemokines

Short-range humoral mediators regulate most steps of the immune response, that is, specific activation (priming), clonal expansion, effector cell differentiation, and memory cell generation. The factors exert their function *in situ* in a paracrine or autocrine manner at the right site (often in synapse-like contact areas between cells) at the right time (often as a short pulse at a critical stage of the process) in the right dose (often at very low concentrations). It is difficult to develop a DNA vaccine that codelivers a cytokine or chemokine signal together with the antigen and can fulfill all these requirements. Nevertheless, many cytokines have been reported to enhance priming of humoral and/or cellular immune responses when codelivered with DNA vaccines. In addition to enhancing the immunogenicity of an antigen, codelivered cytokines modulate the spectrum of immune effector functions that are specifically stimulated.

Cytokines reported to enhance and modulate DNA vaccine-induced immune responses include GM-CSF, IL-2, IL-15, IL-6, interferon-α, IL-10, or IL-12/IL-23. Expression plasmids encoding chemokines act as strong adjuvant for eliciting Th1-derived immunity when inoculated together with DNA vaccines. In these experimental settings, cytokines were codelivered by DNA vaccines as fusion constructs with the antigen, as plasmid mixtures, or as polycistronic constructs. Delivery of cytokines or chemokines (that are autoantigens) by DNA vaccination can prime autoreactive immune reactivities that neutralize the bioactivity of these factors. Repeated administration of DNA vaccines containing chemokine-encoding genes inhibited the development and progression of arthritis through the development of chemokine-neutralizing autoantibodies, even when administered after the onset of disease. However, the appearance of autoantibodies binding cytokines or chemokines is also a regular phenomenon in many chronic infections. It is unexpected that such a wide variety of cytokines with very different modes of action enhance priming of specific immunity by DNA vaccines. It is uncertain whether the reported findings have general validity for vaccination protocols in species other than the mouse. However, they certainly provided information on the molecular basis of "adjuvant effects" that until recently were largely empirically defined.

2.3.7 Codelivery of Transcription Factors

Proteins produced from DNA vaccines by transfected cells can include transcription factors or antiapoptotic molecules. An example is the codelivery of interferon regulatory factors (IRFs). Using an experimental DNA vaccination model, it

was shown that IRF-3 had good activity for T cells, IRF-7 had good activity for both antibody and T cells, and IRF-1 had good activity for antibody. This opens a new field of manipulating intracellular signaling pathways to induce, enhance, or modulate inflammatory reactions to create a supportive milieu for the initiation of an adaptive immune response. A further option is to extend the life span of antigen-bearing APCs by codelivering antiapoptotic signals that prolong the period they can specifically stimulate T-cell responses. These strategies target the differentiation and the functional life span of APC, the key regulators at the interface between the innate and adaptive immune system that regulate priming, magnitude, and polarization of an immune response.

2.3.8 CpG-containing Oligodeoxynucleotides (ODN)

Motifs in DNA sequences containing cytosine/guanine (CpG) nucleotides flanked by 2 to 3 other nucleotides exert potent immune-stimulating signals through binding to the toll-like receptor (TLR) 9. Such motifs are present in many plasmid DNAs used for genetic immunization. It has been proposed that they provide a critical contribution to the immunogenicity of these constructs. This is not supported by the observation that TLR9-deficient mice are perfectly able to respond to DNA vaccines. The role of CpG-containing motifs in the immunogenicity of DNA vaccines is thus unresolved.

2.3.9 Stress Proteins

Heat shock or stress proteins (hsp) have been incorporated into DNA-, protein-, or peptide-based vaccines as either antigens, chaperones, or adjuvant. T- cell reactivities to many bacterial and protozoan pathogens (e.g. mycobacteria, chlamydia, yersinia, malaria plasmodia, or leishmania) are directed against hsp epitopes. An immunogenicity-potentiating role of hsp is apparent in DNA vaccines in which antigen and hsp molecules are linked, either by fusing sequence encoding antigens to hsp-encoding sequences, or by fusing hsp-capturing domains to antigen-encoding sequences. This strikingly enhances the potency of the vaccine to elicit, for example, tumor-rejecting T-cell responses indicating a potent adjuvant effect of hsp molecules.

2.3.10 Copriming Specific "Help"

DNA vaccines can deliver large protein antigens that either contain naturally or are engineered to contain epitopes that stimulate $CD4^+$ T-cell "help." This specific T-cell reactivity can "help" prime either B cells (enhancing antibody responses), or $CD8^+$ T cells (cell-mediated cytolytic and/or cytokine response). This has been used to increase the potency of DNA vaccines for priming antibody or cytotoxic T-cell responses.

2.4
Production and Quality Control of DNA Vaccines

Traditional production methods used sophisticated methodology to separate DNA from contaminating organic components. In contrast, new processes for manufacturing plasmid DNA pharmaceuticals have been significantly improved and are shorter but also fulfill established GMP (*good manufacturing practices*) guidelines. The core elements used in manufacturing and quality control are nearly identical (generic) for plasmids <10 kb in size, but require modifications for the manufacturing and formulation process of larger

plasmids. The first step in plasmid production is the stable transformation of a defined *Escherichia coli* host strain with the plasmid DNA vector, followed by cultivation in a bioreactor, alkaline lysis of the bacterial biomass, followed by several filtration and chromatography steps to obtain DNA pharmaceuticals of the required quality. The most important requirements for the plasmid purification process are:

1. separation of plasmid DNA from substances derived from the DNA isolation process or the bacterial host cell;
2. purification of the "supercoiled" (ccc) form from other plasmid DNA forms to obtain a homogeneous product; and
3. protection of the ccc form throughout the manufacturing, formulation, storage, and delivery process.

2.4.1 Quality Control and Safety in Plasmid DNA Vaccine Production

Plasmid DNA quality depends on manufacturing, storage, and application. Its safety depends on vector construction, characterization, and testing by toxicology before clinical trials. These parameters are well defined but subjected to ongoing improvements regarding analytical techniques. Table 2 shows relevant quality control tests for in-process-control (IPC) and product release. A safe, state-of-the-art manufactured, well-controlled product is usually requested, the relevant guidelines for the specification for clinical material are currently subject to continuous improvements.

2.4.2 Plasmid Identity

Plasmid DNA is tested for identity by digestion with a panel of restriction enzymes followed by agarose gel electrophoresis (AGE) to determine the length of the digestion fragments obtained. These have to

Tab. 2 Important physical and microbial specifications for quality assurance and quality control of plasmid DNA vaccines.

	Test	Analytical method
1.	DNA concentration	UV Absorption (260 nm)
2.	General purity	UV Scan (220–320 nm)
3.	Homogeneity (ccc content)	CGE (*capillary gel electrophoresis*)
4.	Purity (visible)	Visual inspection
5.	Purity (genomic DNA)	Agarose gel (visual); Southern blot, Quantitative PCR
6.	Purity (RNA)	Agarose gel (visual); fluorescence assay, quantitative PCR
7.	Purity (protein)	BCA test
8.	Purity (LPS)	LAL test
9.	Purity (microorganisms)	Bioburden test; sterility test
10.	Identity (vector structure)	Restriction fragment lengths conforms to reference in AGE (3–4 enzymes)
11.	Identity (sequence)	Sequencing (double strand)

Notes: AGE: agarose gel electrophoresis; BCA: Bicinchoninic acid; ccc: covalently closed circular or supercoiled; CGE: capillary gel electrophoresis; LAL: *Limulus* amebocyte lysate; LPS: lipopolysaccharide.
Source: Schleef, M., Schmidt, T. (2004) Animal-free production of ccc-supercoiled plasmids for research and clinical applications, *J. Gene Med.* **6**, S45–S53.

conform to the calculated lengths of the fragments. The nucleotide sequence of the plasmid is determined by sequencing the plasmid DNA.

2.4.3 Animal-free DNA Production

Because RNA from *E. coli* is the major contaminant of the plasmid DNA produced, a typical and critical process in its purification is usually the treatment with ribonucleases (e.g. RNase A from bovine pancreas) to destroy RNA molecules. Current pharmaceutical DNA manufacturing technology avoids bovine RNase treatment to increase the quality of the product, even in large-scale production of GMP-grade DNA. To ensure product purity and safety, no enzymes should be used in the purification and cultivation processes that thus should be carried out without animal-derived substances.

2.4.4 Genomic DNA

A major impurity in plasmid DNA preparations is chromosomal and genomic DNA (gDNA) from plasmid-producing bacterial cells. The most critical step is alkaline lysis, in which gDNA as well as plasmid DNA are denatured by alkaline pH shift. As chromosomal DNA is extremely sensitive to shearing, this can result in its fragmentation. Some gDNA fragments can migrate as distinct bands in AGE while smaller fragments can be detected as undefined smears in overloaded AGE analyses. Sensitive assays, for example, Southern blot hybridization or quantitative PCR, are often used to quantify gDNA contamination. While contaminations of gDNA in plasmid DNA preparations were often in the range of 5 to 10% in the past, novel purification technologies allowed a significant reduction.

DNA species must be completely removed from the manufacturing environments at product change. This aspect of changeover is important if different DNAs are produced within the same facility.

2.4.5 Host Cell Impurities

Host cell–derived contaminants (e.g. proteins, RNA, lipopolysaccharides) should be reduced to minimal concentrations in the plasmid DNA purification process. Proteins can be detected by colorimetric assays. Quantification of residual RNA is performed by fluorescence assays after digestion of plasmid DNA with DNase. Lipopolysaccharides can be detected in the *Limulus polyphemus* lysate assay. A striking reduction of these impurities has to be achieved before the manufactured DNA can be used in research or clinics.

2.4.6 Importance of Supercoiled Forms

Structural homogeneity of plasmid DNA is usually determined by AGE. Different forms of plasmid DNA with an identical nucleotide sequence are present within a given DNA preparation from *E. coli* cells and can be assigned to different AGE bands. However, the assignment of bands to different plasmid topologies is complicated because the electrophoretic mobility of plasmids of different shapes changes with the electrophoretic operating conditions. In addition, the quantification of DNA plasmid forms based on signal intensity of stained bands in AGE may not be reliable due to nonlinear responses. It is well known that typically only one band (the ccc form) is observed when only a small amount of plasmid DNA is applied to AGE while two prominent bands (ccc and a slower migrating, nicked, open (oc) form), are usually revealed by standard AGE. Capillary gel electrophoresis (CGE) allows the

identification and more reliable quantification of all forms of plasmid DNA. CGE is performed using thin (diameter 100 μm), coated capillaries with a length of 40 to 60 cm, filled with a liquid polymer, for example, a solution of hydroxypropylmethylcellulose. Electrophoretic separation takes place by applying a high 5 to 30 kV voltage followed by high-resolution detection using special intercalating dyes. This allows quantitative detection of all plasmid forms by laser-induced fluorescence. This automated system offers high reproducibility, reliable quantification, and short analysis time. In contrast to AGE, quantification of plasmid forms by CGE is possible in a wide range of linearity and needs only 50-ng plasmid DNA.

The ccc plasmid topology is the most compact structure and is expected to be the most active topology. Other plasmid topologies also appear often and have to be eliminated from the product. If one strand is broken (nicked), the oc form results. This is caused either naturally by processes within the plasmid-producing bacteria or during processing (enzymatic or mechanic degradation) of the biomass. Linear forms are generated if both strands are cleaved once at approximately the same position. In addition, plasmids may appear as oligomeric forms (e.g. concatemers) detectable in different topologies (Fig. 1a,b). The only intact, nondamaged form is the ccc supercoil DNA because linear forms and oc forms are randomly damaged at different gene locations and may be inactive if promoter- or antigen-encoding regions are destroyed. Any process development must therefore be subjected to IPC systems to assess the characteristics of the produced plasmid molecules. In particular, methods are required for obtaining supercoiled ccc plasmid DNA in pure form.

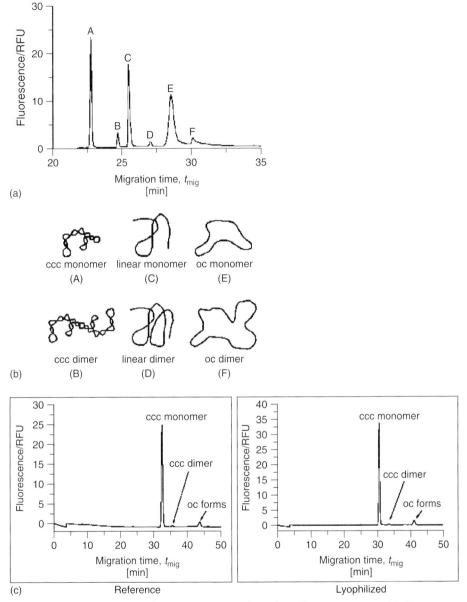

(a)

(b)

(c)

Fig. 1 (a) Electropherogram indicating individual peaks of (b) various plasmid topologies, (c) visualized in the corresponding graph (a and b from Schleef, M., Schmidt, T. (2004) Animal-free production of ccc-supercoiled plasmids for research and clinical applications, *J. Gene Med.* **6**, S45–S53). The comparison of the plasmid topology pattern in DNA before (reference) and after lyophilization indicated no difference ((c) from Schmidt, T., Voß, C., Schleef, M. (2005) From Bulk to Delivery: Plasmid Manufacturing and Storage, in: Schleef, M. (Ed.) *Plasmid Pharmaceuticals*, Wiley-VCH, Weinheim).

2.5
Stability of DNA Vaccines

Manufacturing, formulation, storage, and application of DNA vaccines should be easy and cost efficient. Physical and chemical stability of plasmid DNA is required for DNA-based pharmaceuticals that can be stored, shipped, and applied even under critical environmental conditions. DNA delivery sometimes requires protection of the active pharmaceutical ingredient, which is an issue of DNA formulation.

2.5.1 Storage Stability of Plasmid DNA
Recent studies have shown alterations of plasmid DNA stored at different temperatures (e.g. -80, -20, or $+4\,^{\circ}C$) over 13 to 30 months. Plasmid DNA stored at -20 or $-80\,^{\circ}C$ shows no degradation of the intact ccc into the damaged oc form. In contrast, ccc plasmid DNA stored at $+4\,^{\circ}C$ is degraded into damaged oc and linear forms within months. Hence, storage conditions are critical to maintain the bioactivity of plasmid DNA pharmaceuticals. An attractive option in plasmid DNA storage and shipment is lyophilization, a technology often applied to other vaccines or pharmaceuticals. Although lyophilization of plasmid DNA has been accompanied by damage to its ccc supercoil topology and insufficient reconstitution, recent improvements in lyophilization could be shown not to damage ccc supercoil plasmid DNA (Fig. 1c).

2.5.2 Stability in Plasmid Vector Applications
Very little is known about the *in vivo* fate of a formulated DNA vaccine after its injection. Complexing DNA with cationic agents provides some physical protection *in vivo* but raises the question whether plasmid topology is maintained during formulation. This can be determined by CGE analysis of small samples reextracted from the complexes.

2.6
Delivery of DNA Vaccines

DNA vaccines can be delivered either as nonpackaged ("naked") plasmid DNA, or as formulated or "packaged" plasmid DNA. A single (intramuscular, subcutaneous, or intradermal) injection of a fairly high dose (50–100 µg/mouse) of "naked" plasmid DNA into mice usually primes an immune response. Unfortunately, this is not reproducible in other species, including man. Many formulations have therefore been used to formulate plasmid DNA in an effort to facilitate *in vivo* its half-life, its transfection efficacy, and the expression of an immunogenic product from the vector. These included incorporation into cationic liposomes, virosomes or lipoplexes; binding to cationic polymers, peptides or proteins; mixing with aluminum phosphate; *in vivo* electroporation; or treatment with chloroquine (to reduce plasmid DNA degradation in an acid endolysosomal compartment after uptake). Plasmid DNA vaccines can be introduced into invasive bacterial cells (from strains that are used for vaccination). Following infection after oral vaccination, the DNA vaccine is directly delivered to the cell. Another promising delivery technique is a biolistic system in which DNA-coated gold microprojectiles are directly propelled into cells in the living animal ("gene gun"). This technique has been successful in genetic vaccination of many animal species, and has been employed in clinical trials. The plethora of alternatives in this rapidly evolving field of delivery techniques is an indicator that the issue is not yet resolved in a practical way. This is a major drawback in introducing this technique into clinical practice.

2.6.1 Combining DNA Vaccines and Protein Vaccines

Traditional protein antigen vaccines and DNA vaccines can be combined. Protein antigens and DNA vaccines emulsified together in aluminum phosphate can prime multivalent immune responses to both components of the vaccine. DNA vaccines, delivered as a complex with antigenic, cationic peptides, or proteins can prime immune responses to epitopes in the DNA vaccines and in the cationic antigens. These preliminary data suggest that DNA vaccines could be a part of multicomponent vaccines.

2.6.2 Routes of DNA Vaccine Delivery

Similar to the many formulation protocols, many different routes of plasmid DNA delivery have been described. These include intramuscular, subcutaneous, or intradermal injection of "naked" or formulated plasmid DNA, or intradermal and mucosal delivery of plasmid DNA by the gene gun. Finding a reliable, easy, safe, and accepted route for delivering DNA vaccines in clinical practice is a high priority in the field.

3 Applications

3.1 Priming Immune Responses by DNA Vaccination

DNA vaccines effectively prime and boost immune responses, which is evident by the generation of specific (B and/or T cell) reactivity and/or the specific induction of protective memory against pathogens. An immune response primed by a conventional (e.g. protein-based) vaccine can be boosted by DNA vaccination. A response primed by DNA vaccination can be boosted by alternative vaccine formulations of the relevant antigen (e.g. a protein antigen or a recombinant virus), a protocol apparently eliciting superior protective immunity to some clinically important pathogens. Most experimental studies have been performed on the mouse, in which immune responses can be readily primed by different DNA vaccination protocols and in which many specific readout assays are available. In contrast, DNA vaccination had mixed successes in species other than the mouse, including man.

3.1.1 Priming T-cell Responses

In contrast to most alternative vaccines, DNA vaccines are particularly potent in priming MHC class I-restricted CD8 T-cell responses and MHC class II-restricted CD4 T-cell responses. Priming CD8 T-cell responses by genetic vaccination can be indirect or direct. Antigens produced from a DNA vaccine by transiently transfected cells (myocytes, keratinocytes) seem to be transferred to professional APC that present their epitopes in an immunogenic way. This indirect way of antigen expression, processing, and presentation is called *cross-priming*. In contrast, resident dendritic cells (DC) in the targeted tissue may be directly transfected by a DNA vaccine and process the antigen it produces for immunogenic presentation. Direct priming may operate after intradermal delivery of low amounts of plasmid DNA with the gene gun. It is complicated by the finding that resident DC usually are immature and tend to elicit tolerogenic or regulatory rather than effector/memory T-cell responses. Engineering antigenic constructs in DNA vaccines to target APC in lymph nodes, codelivery of factors that enhance their immunogenicity, and an increase of antigenic information they carry offer attractive prospects for optimizing potent T cell–stimulating vaccines. DNA vaccination could prime T-cell responses to nonstructural viral antigens that support cross-strain protection, and could override nonresponder status. The exceptional potency of DNA vaccines to elicit specific T-cell responses has generated the hope that it might contribute to solve some major current health issues, such as the development of vaccines to be used against, for example, HIV, mycobacteria, papillomaviruses, or cancer.

3.1.2 Priming B-cell (Antibody) Responses

DNA vaccines expressing secreted antigen readily prime antibody responses. In mice, injection of a high dose of a DNA vaccine induces high titers of specific IgG2a antibodies (indicating Th1 priming), while injection of a low dose of the same DNA vaccine induces preferentially specific IgG1 antibodies (indicating Th2 priming). Antibody responses have been elicited after DNA vaccination to subdominant (cryptic) epitopes of antigen fragments that were difficult to detect by conventional vaccination strategies. *In situ* production of native antigen with all post-translational modifications allows priming of neutralizing antibodies to conformational epitopes that are usually CD4 T-cell ''help''-dependent.

3.2 DNA Vaccination as an Experimental Tool

Expression library immunization is a DNA vaccine–based tool to identify vaccine candidates out of a large number of gene products expressed by a pathogen. Although its usefulness has only been demonstrated in a few systems, it may gain in interest as more genomes of pathogens are sequenced. Owing to the ease of deleting or recombining fragments of open reading frames, DNA vaccines are furthermore useful in identifying antigenic domains or epitopes of complex antigens. Once identified, these antigenic determinants can be combined into polyvalent, chimeric vaccines that contain immunodominant domains from different antigens and/or different pathogens. The selective incorporation of an antigenic domain or epitope into a DNA vaccine has been used to generate monospecific immunological probes, either monoclonal antibodies, or T-cell clones.

3.3 Potential Advantages of DNA Vaccination

Genetic vaccination can provide long-lived immunity, and multivalent vaccines can be given by a single inoculation. As DNA vaccines to different pathogens are produced using similar or identical generic production techniques, the development of formulation, delivery, and safety issues are greatly simplified. A particular feature of DNA vaccination is its exceptional potency to prime T-cell responses. DNA vaccines have been shown to override low responder status in preclinical animal models to subdominant T-cell epitopes. It can prime T cells to nonstructural virus proteins, thereby extending the repertoire of vaccine candidates that can be used to control virus infections. Priming T-cell immunity to (nonvariant) internal viral antigens can establish cross-strain protection against pathogenic viruses, a goal difficult to obtain with conventional vaccines that rely on the induction of neutralizing antibody responses against variant envelope proteins. Newborn mice immunized with DNA vaccines develop balanced Th1/Th2 immune responses. DNA vaccination is thus an attractive option to prime antiviral Th1 immunity in neonates or young children, overcoming the bias for specific tolerance induction of the neonatal immune system. Hence, this type of vaccine may have advantages for protection early in life, an objective difficult to achieve with most conventional vaccines currently available.

4
Perspectives

4.1
Achievement and Unresolved Issues of the Technology

The technology introduced only a decade ago has made striking progress in vector design, large-scale DNA production, and optimizing the antigenic information and the immunogenicity of antigens, their domains or selected epitopes. Major unresolved issues are the efficient delivery of the vaccine in man and the critical assessment of safety issues. While the former needs an easy, safe, and reliable technique soon, the latter will only be resolved with clinical experience accumulating over extended time spans.

4.2
Preclinical and Clinical Trials that Test Potential Applications of DNA Vaccination in Clinical Practice

In informative preclinical animal models of *infectious diseases*, DNA vaccination proved effective as a *prophylactic* vaccine against a broad spectrum of pathogens including, for example; influenza, malaria plasmodia, leishmania, mycobacteria, simian immunodeficiency virus, papilloma virus, and herpes viruses. Even more challenging is the development of therapeutic vaccines against HIV, hepatitis B and C virus, and malaria plasmodia or mycobacteria. DNA vaccine-based specific immunotherapy protocols against these and other pathogens that cause chronic infection are under investigation in various informative animal species.

The specific *immunotherapy of cancer* relies on induction of efficient cellular immunity to tumor-associated antigens by therapeutic vaccination. Because it efficiently primes T cells, DNA vaccination has played a prominent role in designing treatment schemes for the treatment of growing tumors in preclinical models.

DNA vaccination primes potent Th1 immunity. An established Th2 bias of an immune response can be specifically converted into a Th1 phenotype by boosting with the relevant antigen in conjunction with a strong Th1-driving stimulus. DNA vaccination has been successfully used in a preclinical model to specifically suppress established *allergy* by converting the pathogenic Th2 response into a harmless Th1 response.

These are some of the many potential areas of interest where DNA vaccination may find clinical applications. Clinical trials using either DNA vaccination alone, or DNA vaccine priming and boosting with recombinant viruses have been initiated. These include vaccination of uninfected volunteers to assess safety and immunogenicity, and therapeutic vaccination of chronically infected or cancer-bearing patients to assess safety and therapeutic efficacy. An infectious disease targeted with high priority is AIDS caused by the human immunodeficiency virus (HIV). DNA vaccines containing >20 CD8 T cell–defined epitopes (polytope vaccines) of HIV, its envelope (gp160, gp40, gp120) protein or its antigenic fragments, its nucleocapsid gag (p17, p24), a fusion protein containing gag and polymerase, or its small regulator proteins (tat, nef) from different HIV clades have been tested in Phase I clinical trials using different formulations and different constructs, sometimes with selected cytokine adjuvants (e.g. IL-2). In addition, some clinical trials have been initiated to assess the efficacy of DNA-based vaccination for the specific control of herpes viruses; human papilloma virus, Ebola virus; *Plasmodium falciparum* (causing malaria), or mycobacteria. The therapeutic value of DNA vaccines is currently tested in melanomas, renal and prostate cancers, hepatocellular carcinoma, chronic lymphatic leukemia, and colon cancer. It is expected that these studies will generate a wealth of information on the safety, immunogenicity, and therapeutic efficacy of DNA vaccination strategies.

4.3
Risks and Safety Issues Raised by DNA Vaccination

Only limited experience on the long-term safety of DNA vaccination has been derived from preclinical animal models and their validity for the critical assessment of the risks under clinical conditions is uncertain. The following potential risks of DNA vaccination have been discussed.

Integration of plasmid DNA into coding or regulatory sequences of cellular DNA could lead to *insertional mutagenesis*. It is conceivable that insertion into the genome of the germline could occur as a rare event. The integrated "foreign" DNA could contribute to tumor development by activating oncogenes, inactivating tumor suppressor genes, or inducing chromosomal instability through the induction of chromosomal breaks or rearrangements. DNA vaccines usually produce only low amounts of antigen that may induce low zone tolerance rather than immunity. This possibility has not been verified experimentally up to now. In contrast, it has been shown that DNA vaccine-primed responses that were undetectable post-priming could be readily boosted. Some DNA vaccines were exceptionally potent raising the concern that they could induce autoimmunity specific for either codelivered, autologous costimulator molecules (cytokines, chemokines), or for the transfected cell. As autoantibody responses against cytokines regularly occur during tissue damage in the course of chronic infections, it is uncertain whether this is a complication typical for DNA vaccination. Anti-DNA antibodies have been only rarely induced by DNA vaccines in experimental animal models. As the *in vivo* transfection of cells by injected plasmid DNA of the vaccine is not controlled, and destructive Th1 immune responses are elicited, immune-mediated tissue lesions could occur. Whether this is an advantageous (deleting genetically altered cells) or deleterious event is uncertain. Antibiotic resistance genes are usually transferred with the DNA vaccine, but the stable induction of this resistance in vaccinated individuals is an unlikely event because resistance genes are expressed under prokaryotic promoter control in the bacterial backbone, and not expected to be expressed at high levels for extended periods of time by human cells. Furthermore, most of the antibiotics used for selection are not of clinical importance.

Acknowledgment

We greatly appreciate the helpful comments of Drs. M.L. Michel (Institut Pasteur, Paris, France) and D.M. Klinman (FDA, Bethesda, USA).

See also Medicinal Chemistry; Molecular Oncology; Somatic Gene Therapy; Vector System: Plasmid DNA.

Bibliography

Books and Reviews

Barry, M.A., Johnston, S.A. (1997) Biological features of genetic immunization, *Vaccine* **15**, 788–791.

Donnelly, J.J., Ulmer, J.B., Liu, M.A. (1994) Immunization with DNA, *J. Immunol. Methods* **176**, 145–152.

Donnelly, J.J., Ulmer, J.B., Shiver, J.W., Liu, M.A. (1997) DNA vaccines, *Annu. Rev. Immunol.* **15**, 617–648.

Ertl, H.C., Xiang, Z. (1996) Novel vaccine approaches, *J. Immunol.* **156**, 3579–3582.

Gurunathan, S., Klinman, D.M., Seder, R.A. (2000) DNA vaccines: immunology, application and optimization, *Annu. Rev. Immunol.* **18**, 927–974.

Johnston, S.A., Tang, D.C. (1994) Gene gun transfection of animal cells and genetic immunization, *Methods Cell Biol.* **43**, 353–365.

Krieg, A.M. (2002) CpG motifs in bacterial DNA and their immune effects, *Annu. Rev. Immunol.* **20**, 709–760.

Mor, G., Singla, M., Steinberg, A.D., Hoffman, S.L., Okuda, K., Klinman, D.M. (1997) Do DNA vaccines induce autoimmune disease? *Hum. Gene Ther.* **8**, 293–300.

Roman, M., Spiegelberg, H.L., Broide, D., Raz, E. (1997) Gene immunization for allergic disorders, *Springer Semin. Immunopathol.* **19**, 223–232.

Schleef, M. (1999) Issues of Large Scale Plasmid DNA Manufacturing, in: Rehm, H.-J., Reed, G., Puehler, A., Stadler, P. (Eds.) *Recombinant Proteins, Monoclonal Antibodies and Therapeutic Genes*, Wiley-VCH, Weinheim, pp. 443–469.

Schleef, M., Schmidt, T. (2004) Animal-free production of ccc-supercoiled plasmids for research and clinical applications, *J. Gene Med.* **6**, S45–S53.

Schmidt, T., Friehs, K., Flaschel, E. (2001) Structures of Plasmid DNA, in: Schleef, M. (Ed.) *Plasmids for Therapy and Vaccination*, Wiley-VCH, Weinheim, pp. 29–42.

Schmidt, T., Voß, C., Schleef, M. (2005) From Bulk to Delivery: Plasmid Manufacturing and Storage, in: Schleef, M. (Ed.) *Plasmid Pharmaceuticals*, Wiley-VCH, Weinheim.

Siegrist, C.-A. (1997) Potential advantages and risks of nucleic acid vaccines for infant immunization, *Vaccine* **15**, 798–800.

Stevenson, F.K. (2004) DNA vaccines and adjuvants, *Immunol. Rev.* **199**, 5–278.

Primary Literature

Amara, R.R., Villinger, F., Altman, J.D., Lydy, S.L., O'Neil, S.P., Staprans, S.I., Montefiori, D.C., Xu, Y., Herndon, J.G., Wyatt, L.S., Candido, M.A., Kozyr, N.L., Earl, P.L., Smith, J.M., Ma, H.L., Grimm, B.D., Hulsey, M.L., Miller, J., McClure, H.M., McNicholl, J.M., Moss, B., Robinson, H.L. (2001) Control of a mucosal challenge and prevention of AIDS by a multiprotein DNA/MVA vaccine, *Science* **292**, 69–74.

Arichi, T., Saito, T., Major, M.E., Belyakov, I.M., Shirai, M., Engelhard, V.H., Feinstone, S.M., Berzofsky, J.A. (2000) Prophylactic DNA vaccine for hepatitis C virus (HCV) infection: HCV-specific cytotoxic T lymphocyte induction and protection from HCV-recombinant vaccinia infection in an HLA-A2.1 transgenic mouse model, *Proc. Natl. Acad. Sci. U.S.A.* **97**, 297–302.

Barouch, D.H., Craiu, A., Kuroda, M.J., Schmitz, J.E., Zheng, X.X., Santra, S., Frost, J.D., Krivulka, G.R., Lifton, M.A., Crabbs, C.L., Heidecker, G., Perry, H.C., Davies, M.E., Xie, H., Nickerson, C.E., Steenbeke, T.D., Lord, C.I., Montefiori, D.C., Strom, T.B., Shiver, J.W., Lewis, M.G., Letvin, N.L. (2000) Augmentation of immune responses to HIV-1 and simian immunodeficiency virus DNA vaccines by IL-2/Ig plasmid administration in rhesus monkeys, *Proc. Natl. Acad. Sci. U.S.A.* **97**, 4192–4197.

Boyer, J.D., Ugen, K.E., Chattergoon, M., Wang, B., Shah, A., Agadjanyan, M.G., Bagarazzi, M.L., Javadian, A., Carrano, R., Coney, L., Williams, W.V., Weiner, D.B. (1997) DNA vaccination as anti-human immunodeficiency virus immunotherapy in infected chimpanzees, *J. Infect. Dis.* **176**, 1501–1509.

Boyer, J.D., Cohen, A.D., Vogt, S., Schumann, K., Nath, B., Ahn, L., Lacy, K., Bagarazzi, M.L., Higgins, T.J., Baine, Y., Ciccarelli, R.B., Ginsberg, R.S., MacGregor, R.R., Weiner, D.B. (2000) Vaccination of seronegative volunteers with a human immunodeficiency virus type 1 env/rev DNA vaccine induces antigen-specific proliferation and lymphocyte production of β-chemokines, *J. Infect. Dis.* **181**, 476–483.

Boyle, J.S., Brady, J.L., Lew, A.M. (1998) Enhanced responses to a DNA vaccine encoding a fusion antigen that is directed to sites of immune induction, *Nature* **392**, 408–411.

Broide, D., Schwarze, J., Tighe, H., Gifford, T., Nguyen, M.D., Malek, S., van Uden, J.H., Martin, O.E., Gelfand, E.W., Raz, E. (1998) Immunostimulatory DNA sequences inhibit IL-5, eosinophilic inflammation, and airway hyperresponsiveness in mice, *J. Immunol.* **161**, 7054–7062.

Calarota, S.A., Leandersson, A.C., Bratt, G., Hinkula, J., Klinman, D.M., Weinhold, K.J., Sandstrom, E., Wahren, B. (1999) Immune responses in asymptomatic HIV-1-infected patients after HIV-DNA immunization followed by highly active antiretroviral treatment, *J. Immunol.* **163**, 2330–2338.

Casares, S., Inaba, K., Brumeanu, T.D., Steinman, R.M., Bona, C.A. (1997) Antigen presentation by dendritic cells after immunization with DNA encoding a major histocompatibility complex class II-restricted viral epitope, *J. Exp. Med.* **186**, 1481–1486.

Charo, J., Ciupitu, A.M., Le-Chevalier-De-Preville, A., Trivedi, P., Klein, G., Hinkula, J., Kiessling, R. (1999) A long-term memory obtained by genetic immunization results in full protection from a mammary adenocarcinoma expressing an EBV gene, *J. Immunol.* **163**, 5913–5919.

Coon, B., An, L.L., Whitton, J.L., von-Herrath, M.G. (1999) DNA immunization to prevent autoimmune diabetes, *J. Clin. Invest.* **104**, 189–194.

Cornell, K.A., Bouwer, H.G., Hinrichs, D.J., Barry, R.A. (1999) Genetic immunization of mice against Listeria monocytogenes using plasmid DNA encoding listeriolysin O, *J. Immunol.* **163**, 322–329.

Darji, A., Guzman, C.A., Gerstel, B., Wachholz, P., Timmis, K.N., Wehland, J., Chakraborty, T., Weiss, S. (1997) Oral somatic transgene vaccination using attenuated *S. typhimurium*, *Cell* **91**, 765–775.

Dupuis, M., Denis, M.K., Woo, C., Goldbeck, C., Selby, M.J., Chen, M., Otten, G.R., Ulmer, J.B., Donnelly, J.J., Ott, G., McDonald, D.M. (2000) Distribution of DNA vaccines determines their immunogenicity after intramuscular injection in mice, *J. Immunol.* **165**, 2850–2858.

Feltquate, D.M., Heaney, S., Webster, R.G., Robinson, H.L. (1997) Different T helper cell types and antibody isotypes generated by saline and gene gun DNA immunization, *J. Immunol.* **158**, 2278–2284.

Fennelly, G.J., Khan, S.A., Abadi, M.A., Wild, T.F., Bloom, B.R. (1999) Mucosal DNA vaccine immunization against measles with a highly attenuated *Shigella flexneri* vector, *J. Immunol.* **162**, 1603–1610.

Fissolo, N., Riedl, P., Reimann, J., Schirmbeck, R. (2004) DNA vaccines prime $CD8^+$ T cell responses to epitopes of viral antigens produced from overlapping reading frames of a single coding sequence, *Eur. J. Immunol.* **35**, 117–127.

Fournillier, A., Nakano, I., Vitvitski, L., Depla, E., Vidalin, O., Maertens, G., Trepo, C., Inchauspe, G. (1998) Modulation of immune responses to hepatitis C virus envelope E2 protein following injection of plasmid DNA using single or combined delivery routes, *Hepatology* **28**, 237–244.

Fu, T.M., Friedman, A., Ulmer, J.B., Liu, M.A., Donnelly, J.J. (1997) Protective cellular immunity: cytotoxic T-lymphocyte responses against dominant and recessive epitopes of influenza virus nucleoprotein induced by DNA immunization, *J. Virol.* **71**, 2715–2721.

Gurunathan, S., Sacks, D.L., Brown, D.R., Reiner, S.L., CHarest, H., Glaichenhaus, N., Seder, R.A. (1997) Vaccination with DNA encoding the immunodominant LACK parasite antigen confers protective immunity to mice infected with *Leishmania major*, *J. Exp. Med.* **186**, 1137–1147.

Hassett, D.E., Zhang, J., Whitton, J.L. (1997) Neonatal DNA immunization with a plasmid encoding an internal viral protein is effective in the presence of maternal antibodies and protects against subsequent viral challenge, *J. Virol.* **71**, 7881–7888.

Iwasaki, A., Torres, C.A., Ohashi, P.S., Robinson, H.L., Barber, B.H. (1997) The dominant role of bone marrow-derived cells in CTL induction following plasmid DNA immunization at different sites, *J. Immunol.* **159**, 11–14.

Klavinskis, L.S., Barnfield, C., Gao, L., Parker, S. (1999) Intranasal immunization with plasmid DNA-lipid complexes elicits mucosal immunity in the female genital and rectal tracts, *J. Immunol.* **162**, 254–262.

Kodihalli, S., Haynes, J.R., Robinson, H.L., Webster, R.G. (1997) Cross-protection among lethal H5N2 influenza viruses induced by DNA vaccine to the hemagglutinin, *J. Virol.* **71**, 3391–3396.

Kuhröber, A., Wild, J., Pudollek, H.P., Chisari, F.V., Reimann, J. (1997) DNA vaccination with plasmids encoding the intracellular (HBcAg) or secreted (HBeAg) form of the core protein of hepatitis B virus primes T cell responses to two overlapping K^b- and K^d-restricted epitopes, *Int. Immunol.* **9**, 1203–1212.

Kuklin, N., Daheshia, M., Karem, K., Manickan, E., Rouse, B.T. (1997) Induction of mucosal immunity against herpes simplex virus by plasmid DNA immunization, *J. Virol.* **71**, 3138–3145.

Kwissa, M., Lindblad, E.B., Schirmbeck, R., Reimann, J. (2003) Codelivery of a DNA vaccine and a protein vaccine with aluminum phosphate stimulates a potent and multivalent immune response, *J. Mol. Med.* **81**, 502–510.

Kwissa, M., Unsinger, J., Schirmbeck, R., Hauser, H., Reimann, J. (2000) Polyvalent DNA vaccines with bidirectional promoters, *J. Mol. Med.* **78**, 495–506.

Lai, W.C., Pakes, S.P., Ren, K., Lu, Y.S., Bennett, M. (1997) Therapeutic effect of DNA immunization of genetically susceptible mice infected with virulent mycoplasma pulmonis, *J. Immunol.* **158**, 2513–2516.

Lee, A.Y., Manning, W.C., Arian, C.L., Polakos, N.K., Barajas, J.L., Ulmer, J.B., Houghton, M., Paliard, X. (2000) Priming of hepatitis C virus-specific cytotoxic T lymphocytes in mice following portal vein injection of a liver-specific plasmid DNA, *Hepatology* **31**, 1327–1333.

Letvin, N.L., Montefiori, D.C., Yasutomi, Y., Perry, H.C., Davies, M.E., Lekutis, C., Alroy, M., Freed, D.C., Lord, C.I., Handt, L.K., Liu, M.A., Shiver, J.W. (1997) Potent, protective anti-HIV immune responses generated by bimodal HIV envelope DNA plus protein vaccination, *Proc. Natl. Acad. Sci. U.S.A.* **94**, 9378–9383.

Li, X., Sambhara, S., Li, C.X., Ewasyshyn, M., Parrington, M., Caterini, J., James, O., Cates, G., Du, R.P., Klein, M. (1998) Protection against respiratory syncytial virus infection by DNA immunization, *J. Exp. Med.* **188**, 681–688.

Lin, Y.L., Chen, L.K., Liao, C.L., Yeh, C.T., Ma, S.H., Chen, J.L., Huang, Y.L., Chen, S.S., Chiang, H.Y. (1998) DNA immunization with Japanese encephalitis virus nonstructural protein NS1 elicits protective immunity in mice, *J. Virol.* **72**, 191–200.

Livingston, B., Crimi, C., Newman, M., Higashimoto, Y., Appella, E., Sidney, J., Sette, A. (2002) A rational strategy to design multiepitope immunogens based on multiple Th lymphocyte epitopes, *J. Immunol.* **168**, 5499–5506.

Lodmell, D.L., Ray, N.B., Parnell, M.J., Ewalt, L.C., Hanlon, C.A., Shaddock, J.H., Sanderlin, D.S., Rupprecht, C.E. (1998) DNA immunization protects nonhuman primates against rabies virus, *Nat. Med.* **4**, 949–952.

Lowrie, D.B., Tascon, R.E., Bonato, V.L., Lima, V.M., Faccioli, L.H., Stavropoulos, E., Colston, M.J., Hewinson, R.G., Moelling, K., Silva, C.L. (1999) Therapy of tuberculosis in mice by DNA vaccination, *Nature* **400**, 269–271.

MacGregor, R.R., Boyer, J.D., Ugen, K.E., Lacy, K.E., Gluckman, S.J., Bagarazzi, M.L., Chattergoon, M.A., Baine, Y., Higgins, T.J., Ciccarelli, R.B., Coney, L.R., Ginsberg, R.S., Weiner, D.B. (1998) First human trial of a DNA-based vaccine for treatment of human immunodeficiency virus type 1 infection: safety and host response, *J. Infect. Dis.* **178**, 92–100.

Macklin, M.D., McCabe, D., McGregor, M.W., Neumann, V., Meyer, T., Callan, R., Hinshaw, V.S., Swain, W.F. (1998) Immunization of pigs with a particle-mediated DNA vaccine to influenza a virus protects against challenge with homologous virus, *J. Virol.* **72**, 1491–1496.

Maloy, K.J., Erdmann, I., Basch, V., Sierro, S., Kramps, T.A., Zinkernagel, R.M., Oehen, S., Kundig, T.M. (2001) Intralymphatic immunization enhances DNA vaccination, *Proc. Natl. Acad. Sci. U.S.A.* **98**, 3299–3303.

Mancini, M., Hadchouel, M., Tiollais, P., Michel, M.L. (1998) Regulation of hepatitis B virus mRNA expression in a hepatitis B surface antigen transgenic mouse model by IFN-g-secreting T cells after DNA-based immunization, *J. Immunol.* **161**, 5564–5570.

Mancini-Bourgine, M., Fontaine, H., Scott-Algara, D., Pol, S., Brechot, C., Michel, M.L. (2004) Induction or expansion of T-cell responses by a hepatitis B DNA vaccine administered to chronic HBV carriers, *Hepatology* **40**, 874–882.

Manickan, E., Yu, Z., Rouse, B.T. (1997) DNA immunization of neonates induces immunity despite the presence of maternal antibody, *J. Clin. Invest.* **100**, 2371–2375.

Martinez, X., Brandt, C., Saddallah, F., Tougne, C., Barrios, C., Wild, F., Dougan, G., Lambert, P.H., Siegrist, C.-A. (1997) DNA immunization circumvents deficient induction of T helper type 1 and cytotoxic T lymphocyte responses in neonates and during early life, *Proc. Natl. Acad. Sci. U.S.A.* **94**, 8726–8731.

Murphey, C.M., Wilson, L.A., Trichel, A.M., Roberts, D.E., Xu, K., Ohkawa, S., Woodson, B., Bohm, R., Blanchard, J. (1999) Selective induction of protective MHC class I-restricted CTL in the intestinal lamina propria of rhesus monkeys by transient SIV infection of the colonic mucosa, *J. Immunol.* **162**, 540–549.

Piedrafita, D., Xu, D., Hunter, D., Harrison, R.A., Liew, F.Y. (1999) Protective immune responses induced by vaccination with an expression genomic library of *Leishmania major*, *J. Immunol.* **163**, 1467–1472.

Pilon, S.A., Piechocki, M.P., Wei, W.Z. (2001) Vaccination with cytoplasmic erbb-2 DNA protects mice from mammary tumor growth without anti-erbb-2 antibody, *J. Immunol.* **167**, 3201–3206.

Robinson, H.L., Montefiori, D.C., Johnson, R.P., Manson, K.H., Kalish, M.L., Lifson, J.D., Rizvi, T.A., Lu, S., Hu, S.L., Mazzara, G.P., Panicali, D.L., Herndon, J.G., Glickman, R., Candido, M.A., Lydy, S.L., Wyand, M.S., McClure, H.M. (1999) Neutralizing antibody-independent containment of immunodeficiency virus challenges by DNA priming and recombinant pox virus booster immunizations, *Nat. Med.* **5**, 526–534.

Rosenecker, J., Naundorf, S., Gersting, S.W., Hauck, R.W., Gessner, A., Nicklaus, P., Muller, R.H., Rudolph, C. (2003) Interaction of bronchoalveolar lavage fluid with polyplexes and lipoplexes: analysing the role of proteins and glycoproteins, *J. Gene Med.* **5**, 49–60.

Schirmbeck, R., Fissolo, N., Chaplin, P., Reimann, J. (2003) Enhanced priming of multispecific, murine CD8$^+$ T cell responses by DNA vaccines expressing stress protein-binding polytope peptides, *J. Immunol.* **171**, 1240–1246.

Schirmbeck, R., Kwissa, M., Fissolo, N., Elkholy, S., Riedl, P., Reimann, J. (2002) Priming polyvalent immunity by DNA vaccines expressing chimeric antigens with a stress protein-capturing, viral J-domain, *FASEB J.* **16**, 1108–1110.

Schirmbeck, R., Zheng, X., Roggendorf, M., Geissler, M., Chisari, F.V., Reimann, J., Lu, M. (2001) Targeting murine immune responses to selected T cell- or antibody-defined determinants of the hepatitis B surface antigen by plasmid DNA vaccines encoding chimeric antigen, *J. Immunol.* **166**, 1405–1413.

Schmidt, T., Friehs, K., Flaschel, E. (1996) Rapid determination of plasmid copy number, *J. Biotechnol.* **49**, 219–229.

Schmidt, T., Friehs, K., Schleef, M., Voss, C., Flaschel, E. (2002) Quantitative analysis of plasmid forms by agarose and capillary gel electrophoresis, *Anal. Biochem.* **274**, 235–240.

Sedegah, M., Jones, T.R., Kaur, M., Hedstrom, R., Hobart, P., Tine, J.A., Hoffman, S.L. (1998) Boosting with recombinant vaccinia increases immunogenicity and protective efficacy of malaria DNA vaccine, *Proc. Natl. Acad. Sci. U.S.A.* **95**, 7648–7653.

Smith, G.J. III, Helf, M., Nesbet, C., Betita, H.A., Meek, J., Ferre, F. (1999) Fast and accurate method for quantitating *E. coli* host-cell DNA contamination in plasmid DNA preparations, *BioTechniques* **26**, 518–522, 524–526.

Spellerberg, M.B., Zhu, D., Thompsett, A., King, C.A., Hamblin, T.J., Stevenson, F.K. (1997) DNA vaccines against lymphoma: promotion of anti-idiotypic antibody responses induced by single chain Fv genes by fusion to tetanus toxin fragment C, *J. Immunol.* **159**, 1885–1892.

Syrengelas, A.D., Levy, R. (1999) DNA vaccination against the idiotype of a murine

B cell lymphoma: mechanism of tumor protection, *J. Immunol.* **162**, 4790–4795.

Tedeschi, V., Akatsuka, T., Shih, J.W., Battegay, M., Feinstone, S.M. (1997) A specific antibody response to HCV E2 elicited in mice by intramuscular inoculation of plasmid DNA containing coding sequences for E2, *Hepatology* **25**, 459–462.

Walther, W., Stein, U., Voss, C., Schmidt, T., Schleef, M., Schlag, P.M. (2003) Stability analysis for long-term storage of naked DNA: impact on nonviral in vivo gene transfer, *Anal. Biochem.* **318**, 230–235.

Walther, W., Stein, U., Fichtner, I., Voss, C., Schmidt, T., Schleef, M., Nellessen, T., Schlag, P.M. (2002) Intratumoral low-volume jet-injection for efficient nonviral gene transfer, *Mol. Biotechnol.* **21**, 105–115.

Wang, R., Doolan, D.L., Le, T.P., Hedstrom, R.C., Coonan, K.M., Charoenvit, Y., Jones, T.R., Hobart, P., Margalith, M., Ng, J., Weiss, W.R., Sedegah, M., de Taisne, C., Norman, J.A., Hoffman, S.L. (1998) Induction of antigen-specific cytotoxic T lymphocytes in humans by a malaria DNA vaccine, *Science* **282**, 476–480.

Wild, J., Grüner, B., Metzger, K., Kuhröber, A., Pudollek, H.-P., Hauser, H., Schirmbeck, R., Reimann, J. (1998) Polyvalent vaccination against hepatitis B surface and core antigen using dicistronic expression plasmids, *Vaccine* **16**, 353–360.

Yasutomi, Y., Robinson, H.L., Lu, S., Mustafa, F., Lekutis, C., Arthos, J., Mullins, J.I., Voss, G., Manson, K., Wyand, M., Letvin, N.L. (1996) Simian immunodeficiency virus-specific cytotoxic T-lymphocyte induction through DNA vaccination of rhesus monkeys, *J. Virol.* **70**, 678–681.

Youssef, S., Maor, G., Wildbaum, G., Grabie, N., Gour, L.A., Karin, N. (2000) C-C chemokine-encoding DNA vaccines enhance breakdown of tolerance to their gene products and treat ongoing adjuvant arthritis, *J. Clin. Invest.* **106**, 361–371.

Zhang, J., Silvestri, N., Whitton, J.L., Hassett, D.E. (2002) Neonates mount robust and protective adult-like CD8$^+$ T-cell responses to DNA vaccines, *J. Virol.* **76**, 11911–11919.

28
Vectors and Gene Therapy

Edward A. Burton[1], David J. Fink[2], and Joseph C. Glorioso[2]
[1]*University of Pittsburgh, Pittsburgh, PA, USA*
[2]*University of Michigan, Ann Arbor, MI, USA*

1	**Introduction**	**882**
2	**The Science of Gene Transfer**	**882**
3	**Principles of Vector Engineering**	**885**
3.1	Retroviruses	885
3.2	Lentiviruses	886
3.3	Adenoviruses	887
3.4	Adeno-associated Viruses	892
3.5	Herpes Simplex Virus	894
3.6	Vector Targeting	898
3.7	Regulation of Gene Expression	900
3.8	Nonviral Vectors	901
4	**Clinical Applications and Genes**	**903**
4.1	Single Gene Disorders	903
4.1.1	Hematological Disease	903
4.1.2	Restoration of Circulating Proteins	904
4.1.3	Respiratory Disease	906
4.1.4	Neurological Disease	907
4.1.5	Muscle	908
4.2	Delivery of Proteins for a Pharmacological Action	909
4.2.1	Transplantation	909
4.2.2	Ischemic Heart Disease	910
4.2.3	Neurological Disease	911
4.2.4	Cancer Gene Therapy	912

Pharmacology. From Drug Development to Gene Therapy. Edited by Robert A. Meyers.
Copyright © 2008 Wiley-VCH Verlag GmbH & Co. KGaA, Weinheim
ISBN: 978-3-527-32343-2

5   **Adverse Events   913**
5.1   Multiple Organ Failure Secondary to Cytokine Storm   913
5.2   Leukemia Secondary to Insertional Mutagenesis   914

6   **From Bench to Clinic – HSV-mediated Gene Therapy of Pain as an Example   916**

7   **Future Prospects – What will Gene Therapy Likely be About in 10 Years?   918**

Bibliography   919
Books and reviews   919
Primary Literature   920

Keywords

Adeno-associated Virus
A nonenveloped single-stranded DNA virus that may be modified to produce a gene transfer vector.

Adenovirus
A nonenveloped double-stranded DNA virus that may be modified to produce a gene transfer vector.

***Ex vivo* Gene Transfer**
Transfer of genetic material to cells cultured outside the body of a living organism.

Gene Therapy
The introduction of genetic sequences into cells of a living organism, resulting in an alteration of cell or tissue function in a manner that corrects or treats a pathological process.

Gene Transfer Vector
Reagent used to deliver genetic material to the interior of cells.

Herpes Simplex Virus
An enveloped neurotropic double-stranded DNA virus that may be modified to produce a gene transfer vector.

***In vivo* Gene Transfer**
Transfer of genetic material to cells by introduction of a vector into the body of a living organism.

Lentivirus

An enveloped single-stranded RNA virus that may be modified to produce a gene transfer vector.

Nonviral Vector

Gene transfer vector that does not contain viral components.

Replication defective

A virus that has been modified to prevent its replication in target cells following gene transfer.

Tropism

The natural host cell range of a vector.

Viral Vector

Gene transfer vector made by genetic engineering of a virus.

■ Gene therapy may be defined as *the introduction of genetic sequences into cells of a living organism, resulting in an alteration of cell or tissue function in a manner that corrects or treats a pathological process.*

This might be accomplished in one of two broad ways: (1) The therapeutic genetic material is transported *ex vivo* into cells taken from a patient – the cells can be subsequently reintroduced, with or without expansion, as an homologous cell transplant. The reintroduced cells engraft and produce a therapeutic product that can alter the biology of the transduced cell to correct a genetic abnormality or deficiency, or may serve as a factory for production of a protein product used by other tissues exposed to the circulation. (2) The therapeutic genetic material is introduced into the cells of the body by direct *in vivo* gene transfer. Direct *in vivo* gene transfer may be used if procurement of appropriate cell explants requires unacceptably invasive procedures, or for gene transfer to essentially nonregenerating tissues (e.g. brain or heart).

The genetic material transferred ("transgene") may encode a complete therapeutic gene to replace a defective function, or coding sequences whose products interfere with an acquired or inherited pathologic cellular function. Gene transfer may also be used to enhance normal function to achieve a therapeutic effect, such as the induction of an immune response or the reversal of autoimmune activity. Finally, a large effort in gene therapy has been directed toward the use of gene transfer to destroy unwanted tissue, such as malignant cells, or fight infectious agents, such as human immune deficiency virus (HIV).

The diverse potential gene therapy applications suggest that genes as molecular medicines hold great promise for the future. In part this promise is beginning to be realized, but much more research (and testing in patients) is required before gene therapy becomes standard medical practice.

1
Introduction

In this article, we discuss the science and the current status of gene therapy. This includes a review of methods used for gene transfer, current attempts to apply gene therapy to treat disease, and a discussion of serious adverse reactions to gene therapy. One example of gene therapy will be described in more detail in order to better acquaint the reader with the steps needed to develop this type of therapy. Finally, an attempt will be made to make some projections regarding the future of gene therapy research and practice by describing where the field may be headed in the next 10 years.

2
The Science of Gene Transfer

A major effort in gene therapy research has concerned the development of efficient, safe methods to introduce genetic information into cells either outside or within the body. These gene delivery tools are referred to as *gene vectors* and can be constructed from modified viruses ("viral vectors") or directly from chemical constructs ("nonviral vectors").

The advent of gene cloning and the ability to make recombinant viruses in the early 1980s portended an era in which viral gene vectors would become the working tools for gene therapists (Table 1). All that was needed was the removal of a critical gene from the virus that allowed it to grow or cause disease (Table 2) and replace that gene with one that is useful to the cell. Gene therapy researchers soon found that reporter genes like the *Escherichia coli lacZ* gene encoding β-galactosidase could be introduced into

almost any tissue by various recombinant viruses, and β-gal activity detected using a colorigenic agent. Depending on the target cell, a nonintegrating or integrating vector could be used to introduce the reporter gene. Curing a disease using this technology should have been a simple matter of replacing the reporter transgene with a therapeutic gene. So why did this clear path to success fail to rapidly yield new therapeutic products? To answer this question, it is important to understand the technology of virus-mediated gene transfer and the nature of clinical studies targeted by this approach to treatment.

Why choose viruses? It has been known for many years that viruses can deliver their genes to cells by the process of virus infection. Depending on the class of virus, a variety of highly evolved mechanisms for redirecting cellular processes for making new virus particles come into play. Viruses are essentially inert particles outside the body and are vulnerable to the outside world, making their expectant viability short-lived, in the absence of available hosts. The life cycle of viruses, in the simplest terms, involve virus attachment to a susceptible cell, entry into the cell, capsid removal in a process referred to as *uncoating* to expose the virus genome in an active form, either in the cytoplasm or nucleus. The virus genes are transcribed and expressed as proteins or active RNA molecules, requiring at least partial use of the cellular transcriptional and translational machinery. The most sophisticated viruses have hundreds of genes (e.g. vaccinia), whereas the most simple have as few as four to six genes (e.g. polyoma virus and adeno-associated virus). The viral genome, single- or double-stranded DNA or RNA, is replicated and encapsidated into new virus particles that are released by cell lysis or by a

Tab. 1 Major viruses used to construct viral vectors.

	Genome	Genomic integration?	Envelope?	Latent infection?	Helper virus?	Cellular receptor	Route of cellular entry	Disease caused by wild-type virus
Lentivirus	ssRNA; 9.5 kb	Yes	Yes	Yes	No	CD4, CXCR5 ([a]phosphatidyl serine)	Plasmalemma ([a]endosome)	AIDS
Adenovirus	dsDNA; 35 kb	No	No	No	No	CAR, integrin $\alpha v \beta 5$	Endosome	Respiratory infection; conjunctivitis; gastroenteritis
Adeno-associated virus	ssDNA; 5 kb	Yes	No	Yes	Yes	Integrin $\alpha v \beta 5$, FGF-1R	Endosome	None known
Herpes simplex virus	dsDNA; 150 kb	No	Yes	Yes	No	Glycosaminoglycan, nectin1α and HVEM	Plasmalemma	Cold sore; rarely encephalitis

[a]Although wild-type HIV enters cells through the plasmalemma, vectors pseudotyped with the vesicular stomatitis virus G-spike glycoprotein enter through the endocytotic pathway.

Tab. 2 Properties of some viral vectors.

Vector		Transgene insert capacity [kb]	Genes removed from vector genome to prevent replication/toxicity	Complementation of essential functions	Easy preparation of high titers and pure stock?	Easy insertion of transgene sequences?	Toxicity
Lentivirus	HIV-based	6	All except 5' portion of gag	Transient plasmid transfection	No	Yes	Insertional mutagenesis
Adenovirus	E1, E3 deleted Ad5	8	E1, E3	Complementing cell line	Yes	No	Inflammation
	'Gutless'	30	All	Complementing cell line and helper virus	No	No	Inflammation
Adeno-associated virus	AAV2-based	4.5	All	Helper virus or transient plasmid transfection	No	Yes	Insertional mutagenesis
Herpes simplex virus	Genomic HSV-1 vectors	30–40	ICP4, ICP27, ICP22, ICP47, ICP0, U_L41	Complementing cell line	Yes	No	Minimal
	Amplicon	120	All	Transient BAC transfection	No	No	Minimal

process called *budding* in which the virus capsid is enclosed in a membrane or envelope. These nascent particles are then competent to invade other cells. For details of viral replication and life cycles, see excellent and exhaustive chapters in Field's Virology. Summary figures of the life cycles of major viruses used as vectors are shown below.

Viruses have evolved sophisticated mechanisms for either rapid spread or the ability to remain relatively quiescent in cells of the body until an opportunity presents itself for transmission to a naïve host. Many viruses (e.g. adenovirus) do not persist in the host but rather rapidly replicate and produce large numbers of infectious particles that can be spread to other susceptible hosts. Vectors based on such viruses are less useful for long-term gene delivery but can be used for applications that require transient transgene expression, such as the induction of immunity or destruction of tumors. The life cycle of other viruses (e.g. retroviruses and lentiviruses) involves a persistent phase in which the virus genome may become integrated into a host chromosome and can thus be passed on to daughter cells following cell division. Vectors created from these viruses can be useful for applications in which persistent transgene expression is required. Herpes viruses persist in the host as nonintegrated forms that either remain associated with nondividing cells or can replicate their genetic information in synchrony with cell division. Most viruses that persist in the host have evolved sophisticated means for transiently avoiding host detection by the immune system, often reaching a stalemate between their elimination by the immune system and their disease-causing activity. Most human infecting viruses that persist do so by a system referred to

as *latency* where few, if any, viral genes are expressed in cells where latency is established and virus persistence generally lasts for the life of the host.

Early studies of viral vector-mediated gene transfer for therapeutic purposes have been focused on a few viruses (Tables 1 and 2). The choice of viral vector for a specific application depends on the biology of the wild-type virus and the degree to which the virus life cycle and genes have been characterized. As more insight is gained into virus biology, it is likely that additional viral gene transfer vectors will be developed.

3
Principles of Vector Engineering

3.1
Retroviruses

It has been known for some time that retroviruses can integrate their genomes into the host cell by a process of reverse transcription, using reverse transcriptase to allow the RNA tumor virus genome to become integrated into the DNA genome of a cell. Virus entry into the nucleus is largely dependent on cell division and thus these viruses most efficiently infect dividing cells.

One of the best-studied retroviruses is the mouse Moloney leukemia virus. It was discovered in the 1980s that "packaging" cell lines could be engineered to express the virus coat protein and envelope protein constitutively. On transfection of these packaging cells with a DNA copy of the virus, infectious packaged particles were produced, even though the vector genome contained only terminal repeat elements and the packaging signal from the original virus – the internal sequences having been replaced by nonviral genes. These infectious packaged particles could be used to transduce other cells, and by virtue of their terminal repeat elements, the nonviral genes were incorporated into cellular DNA. Following successful transfer of the adenosine deaminase (*ADA*) gene in preclinical studies, this first virus gene transfer vector was used in the first gene transfer clinical trials in the early 1990s in an attempt to treat the ADA-deficiency form of severe combined immunodeficiency (SCID). Gene transfer with these first-generation vectors was not efficient enough to produce a therapeutic outcome, and indeed the study design almost ensured failure. An initially unrecognized shortcoming of retroviruses and lentiviruses is the propensity for the vector genome to integrate into the cell genome, preferentially near sites of active transcription. This process can lead to rare insertional mutagenesis events and activation of cellular genes that have oncogenic potential. In a more recent clinical trial using a retroviral vector to treat X-lined SCID, two of the patients cured of the disease by gene transfer developed leukemic transformation as a result of insertional mutagenesis (see Sect. 5.2). Investigators are now attempting to engineer retroviral vectors, which are either directed in their integration activity or lack the ability to activate cellular genes.

3.2
Lentiviruses

Vectors constructed from modified lentiviruses, a group of RNA viruses closely related to the oncogenic retroviruses (Figs. 1 and 2), have come to the forefront in the last five years because of their efficiency of gene transduction, their larger capacity for foreign DNA, and their ability to infect nondividing cells. Engineering human lentiviruses to create a vector requires retention of the natural integrase function part of the nucleocapsid and the viral polymerase (Fig. 3). Methods have been developed in which elements of lentiviruses, the Moloney virus, and the envelope components of vesicular stomatitis virus (VSV-G) have been incorporated into three expression plasmids, which can be transfected into cells for vector production (Fig. 4). Transfection methods are not as efficient as using packaging cell lines for retroviral vectors, but lentiviral vectors can be concentrated by centrifugation since the VSV-G envelope component is stable. Another advantage of VSV-G is that it utilizes a common cell surface proteoglycan, which is ubiquitously expressed

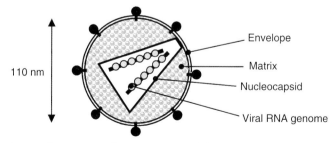

Fig. 1 The structure of Human Immunodeficiency Virus – A schematic depiction of a mature HIV-1 virion is shown, to illustrate key structural components of this prototypical lentivirus.

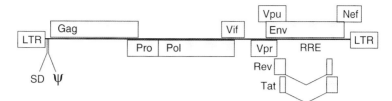

Fig. 2 The HIV-1 genome – The HIV-1 RNA genome is illustrated diagrammatically (not to scale) to demonstrate overlapping genomic locations and splicing of viral genes. Abbreviations: LTR, long terminal repeat (containing promoter for viral transcripts); SD, major splice donor; Ψ, packaging signal; RRE, rev-response element. The names of viral genes are shown within the boxes. *gag* encodes the core antigens, *pol/pro* encodes the reverse transcriptase and protease enzymes necessary for genomic integration and posttranslational processing of viral proteins respectively, and *env* encodes the viral envelope proteins necessary for cell entry. *tat* encodes a transactivator of viral transcription and *rev* encodes a splicing/export regulator – see Fig. 3.

on many cells as a receptor, and thus the host range for the lentiviral vector is greatly broadened. It should be noted that despite the use of human immune deficiency virus (HIV) components for many applications, this vector does not cause AIDS or other diseases. Other lentiviruses may also be suitable for the construction of lentiviral-based vectors. Nevertheless, lentiviral vectors have the same propensity for random integration that has been observed with retroviral vectors, although chromosomal breaks are less targeted by lentivirus than by oncogenic retrovirus since the lentivirus has the ability to cut and religate double-stranded DNA as part of the enzyme systems that are contained within the particle. Lentiviral vectors have proven especially useful in transduction of brain and bone marrow stem cells. They have yet to be tested clinically, but this is likely to occur within the next few years.

3.3
Adenoviruses

After retroviruses, adenoviruses have been used most often for gene transfer (Fig. 5).

Replication-defective viruses lacking the tumor-causing gene of adenovirus, *E1a*, had been made in the early 1980s and propagated in cell lines that contained the *E1a* gene integrated into the cell chromosome (see Figs. 6, 7). Such cell lines were designated as complementing cells since the missing viral function was supplied *in trans* on infection. The deletion of E1a prevented the virus from replicating in most wild-type cells (Fig. 7), although there was leaky expression of the other viral functions, including structural proteins and the viral polymerase. Transduction of a number of target tissues in experimental models was demonstrated using early adenoviral (AdV) vectors. Deletion and complementation of further adenoviral genes enabled generation of more efficient and less toxic vectors. One attractive property of AdV vectors is their remarkable ability to express transgenes at very high levels. Because the wild-type virus causes a respiratory infection, it was initially thought that Ad vectors would prove to be ideal for gene transfer to lung, for example, in the common inherited respiratory disease, cystic fibrosis. Unfortunately,

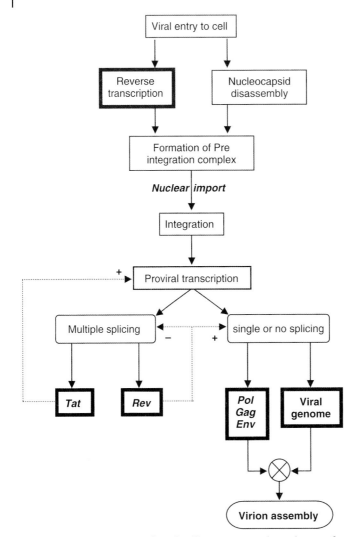

Fig. 3 Major events in the life cycle of lentiviruses – The early part of the life cycle is depicted in the upper portion of the diagram; entry, reverse transcription, formation of the preintegration complex (PIC) and nuclear import of the PIC culminate in the integration of proviral DNA into the host cell genome. The late part of the cycle is characterized by transcription of viral genes. All of the viral genes are encoded by a single primary transcript, and the expression of different proteins is controlled by regulation of RNA splicing and posttranslational protein processing. Initially, multiply spliced RNA isoforms encode regulatory proteins (*tat* and *rev*) that *trans*activate proviral transcription, and drive a shift toward the production of unspliced or singly spliced RNA. The latter encodes the virion structural proteins and forms the viral genome, enabling assembly of virions. Vectors are constructed by deleting all viral genes from the genome contained in the particle, thereby disrupting replication at multiple levels – see Fig. 4.

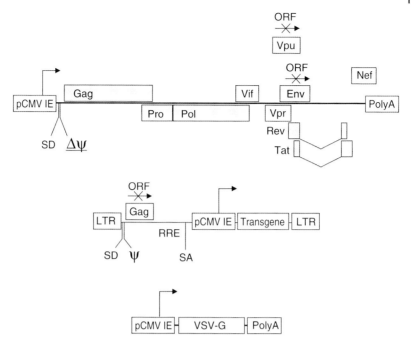

Fig. 4 Construction of replication-defective lentivirus vectors – The system described by Naldini et al. is illustrated. Replication-defective lentiviral vectors may be generated by cotransfection of mammalian cells with the three plasmids shown. A. The ***packaging construct*** provides all of the genes that encode viral structural proteins. Thus, gag-pol, rev, and tat are expressed from this construct. The genes encoding these essential proteins are not incorporated into the virion, however, as the viral LTRs and packaging signal (ψ) are deleted from this vector. In addition, the accessory gene *Vpu* and envelope gene contain frame-shift mutations, abolishing expression of the relevant proteins. B. The ***transfer vector*** contains an expression cassette for the therapeutic or experimental transgene, in addition to the viral LTRs and packaging signals. This vector sequence is transcribed, and the resulting RNA is packaged into lentiviral particles generated from the structural proteins encoded by plasmid A. As the transfer vector contains no sequences encoding functional viral genes (the *gag* gene is truncated and frame shifted), the resulting vectors are replication defective. C. The ***envelope plasmid*** contains an expression cassette encoding a viral envelope protein to replace that encoded by the lentiviral *env* gene, which is deleted from the packaging construct. The G-spike envelope glycoprotein from Vesicular Stomatitis Virus is commonly used to pseudotype lentiviral vectors.

AdV vectors have not proven useful for this application for two major reasons. First, adenoviral receptors are not present on the apical (airway) surface of airway cells, and so intrabronchial or aerosol application of the vector does not give rise to efficient infection of the appropriate target cell required for cystic fibrosis transmembrane conductance regulator (CFTR) expression in the lung. Second, innate and acquired immune response to vector enhanced by the leaky gene expression in the first-generation Ad vector constructs made them susceptible to immune elimination. The immune response to Ad vectors has proven to be a difficult problem for many

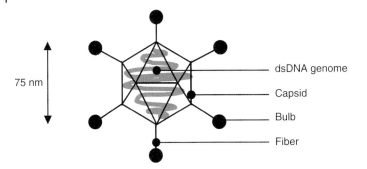

Fig. 5 The structure of Adenovirus – A schematic depiction of a mature adenovirus virion is shown to illustrate key structural components of the virus.

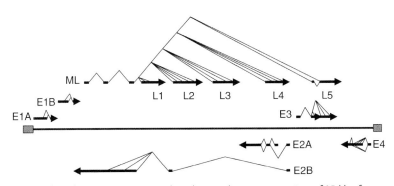

Fig. 6 The adenovirus genome – The adenoviral genome consists of 35 kb of dsDNA, in which the viral gene-encoding sequence is enclosed by two inverted terminal repeats (grey boxes). Although there are only eight basic transcriptional units, approximately 40 transcripts are produced by a bewildering array of alternative splicing events. In particular, the major late promoter gives rise to transcripts that share a tripartite leader sequence, culminating in a splice boundary with one of a possible 18 coding sequences. These are grouped, according to the polyA signal at which the transcripts terminate, into L1, L2, and so on. Viral transcription depends on the presence of the viral gene E1A (see Fig. 7); first-generation vectors were deleted for E1A and E1B and the genes supplied *in trans* using special cell lines. Later vectors are deleted for other genes, for example E3, in addition to E1. The so-called "gutless" vectors contain only the packaging signals and transgene DNA, the viral genome being supplied *in trans* by use of a helper virus to express structural proteins, and thus allow the generation of virion-like particles. These vectors can accommodate up to 30 kb of transgene sequence, but are difficult to prepare in high titer and purity.

proposed applications. Alterations to the vector, which eliminate all of the viral components from the vector genome, improve vector stability *in vivo*, but this is not sufficient to eliminate immune rejection of AdV-infected cells. This was most dramatically demonstrated by the finding that AdV inoculation of liver in immune-competent mice results in high levels of hepatocyte transduction, but expression is lost.

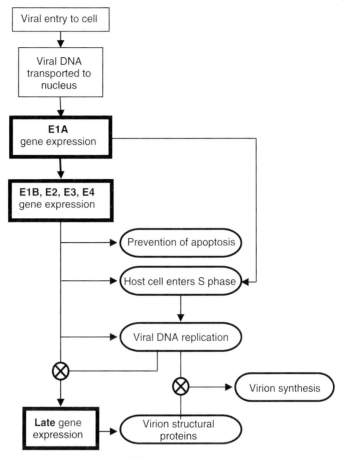

Fig. 7 Major events in the life cycle of adenovirus – The major events in regulation of viral gene expression are shown. Following entry to the nucleus, expression of the viral gene *E1A* is essential to allow expression of the remaining components of the viral genome. The gene expression program of adenovirus results in the subversion of a number of cellular processes, facilitating the production of progeny virions. There is no latent infection and the result of infection is cell lysis and release of adenoviral particles. Deletion of the E1 region halts the viral transcriptional program, and the resulting particles can be used as gene transfer vectors. Later versions of these vectors have multiple genes deleted to enhance the cloning capacity of the vectors and reduce cytotoxicity resulting from leaky expression of the remaining viral genes.

In contrast, the use of immunodeficient mice in the same experiments resulted in long-term gene expression. In addition to immune rejection, AdV vectors cannot be administered to patients with high levels of circulating antibody, and the vector cannot be readily repeat dosed in patients, even those without preexisting immunity, since vector inoculation results in high-titer antibody production. There have been attempts to protect AdV from immune recognition by coating the particle and AdVs of alternative serotypes or from other species or have been isolated with different coat protein structures in the hope that these particles will avoid immune recognition. The AdV particle itself, however, has the ability to induce cytokines (for example interleukin-6) that can result in elimination of the virus genome. A liver gene transfer clinical trial, using high-titer AdV, led to the death of one patient as a result of a vector-induced cytokine storm, leading to organ failure (see Sect. 5.1). There are two important uses of AdV vectors that are likely to be effective in the future. The first is the use of AdVs carrying immune-activating genes in the treatment of solid tumors, and the second is the use of recombinant AdVs for vaccination against newly arising infectious agents. Both applications take advantage of high-level transgene expression, efficient gene delivery, and immunogenicity of the vector substrate.

3.4
Adeno-associated Viruses

Adeno-associated virus (AAV) was initially discovered as a contaminant of adenoviral preparations (Figs. 8, 9 and 10). AAV-based vectors have enjoyed a broad appeal following their initial development. The reasons for this include the following: (1) AAV causes no known disease; (2) the AAV genome can be manipulated as a simple plasmid; (3) the small size of AAV allows the particle to infiltrate many different tissues; (4) certain tissues (e.g. muscle) are transduced very efficiently. Although its small size (22 nm) does not allow packaging of more than 5 kb of foreign sequence, this is sufficient to accommodate most gene coding sequences as cDNAs (i.e. the coding sequence of a gene with the introns and flanking regions deleted). *In vitro*, wild-type AAV integrates into a specific location on chromosome 19q, but this specific integration event is dependent on *replicase*, a viral gene that must be eliminated from vectors because of its considerable toxicity to cells. AAV replication requires several helper functions that can be provided by either adenovirus or herpes simplex virus. Like adenovirus, AAV is highly susceptible to neutralization and cannot be easily repeat dosed, but AAV vector-mediated transgene expression in some tissues provides for long-term expression; the lack of induction of immunity to the transgene product may reflect low infectivity in antigen-producing cells, such as the dendritic cells located in the skin. The optimal method for producing AAV is still

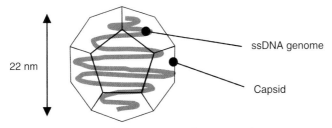

Fig. 8 The structure of adeno-associated virus – A schematic depiction of a mature adeno-associated virus virion is shown, to illustrate key structural components of the virus.

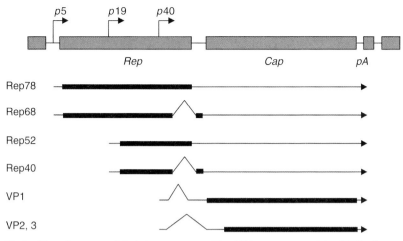

Fig. 9 The adeno-associated virus genome – The AAV genome consists of 5 kb of ssDNA. The coding sequences are flanked by inverted terminal repeats (grey boxes). There are two major genes, *rep* (encoding proteins necessary for gene expression, genomic integration, and replication) and *cap* (encoding the structural components of the virion). There are three viral promoters giving rise to six transcripts by alternative splicing. All of the transcripts terminate at a single polyA signal. Seven proteins are encoded by the six transcripts because the VP2,3 transcript can be translated using one of two different translational start codons. Gene transfer vectors are generated by deletion of *rep* and *cap*, supplying these genes *in trans* by cotransfection of a plasmid, to allow generation of particles. Unfortunately, the products of the *rep* gene are toxic to host cells, and so packaging cell lines have not been possible to generate.

under development, but the most common approach is a triple-plasmid transfection method in which one plasmid is the vector, another expresses the replicase and capsid functions, and the final plasmid provides the adenovirus helper functions. This method produces AAV vector particles without contamination from helper virus since the adenovirus packaging signals have been removed, but is not very efficient. The scale-up manufacture of AAV is also complicated by the remarkably low transduction efficiency of AAV, compared with other vectors. Transduction with AAV *in vivo* thus requires very high doses of virus per cell. Although AAV may integrate into the host genome during its normal life cycle, this is inefficient and cell division is usually required. In contrast to other vectors, AAV appears to require concatemerization in the nucleus for expression, a process that can take weeks for maximum transgene expression. Unless the efficiency of AAV transduction can be improved, its utility as a vector for the treatment of patients will be limited; manufacturing considerations will preclude treatment of more than a few patients at the required doses of $>10^{12}$ per patient. High vector dosing also risks provoking toxic immune responses. Despite these concerns, AAV remains promising. For certain applications, such as gene transfer to the heart, it may prove to be the vector of choice. In addition, new serotypes are proving to be more efficient in some tissues such as liver where previous vectors based on AAV type 2, for

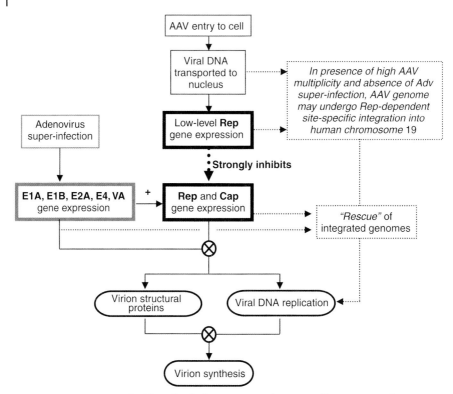

Fig. 10 Major events in the life cycle of adeno-associated virus – Following entry of AAV into the cell, one of two chains of events may ensue the following: 1. In the absence of super infection with a helper virus (AdV is shown, but HSV can also provide helper functions), concatemerized AAV genomes may undergo *rep*-dependent site-specific integration into human chromosome 19, giving rise to a latent infection. Alternatively, the viral genome may persist in the cell nucleus. Low-level expression of rep proteins is strongly inhibitory to expression of viral transcripts. 2. Infection of an AAV-harboring cell with adenovirus, or transfection with a plasmid containing the minimal essential AdV helper functions (E1A, E1B, E2A, E4, and VA) allows high-level expression of *rep* and *cap*, and also forces the cell to enter the S-phase of the cell cycle. This allows replication of AAV viral DNA, synthesis of virion components and assembly of AAV virions. High-level expression of *rep* and *cap*, in association with AdV helper functions can rescue integrated genomes from the chromosome of a latently infected cell. Replication-defective vectors are generated by deletion of *rep* and *cap* from the AAV genome. The vector particles are prepared by cotransfection of packaging cells with a *rep/cap* plasmid, an AdV helper function plasmid, and a gene transfer plasmid containing the transgene of interest and the AAV packaging signals. As the resulting particles are deficient in the *rep* gene, integration into the host chromosome is very inefficient and occurs randomly, but with a predilection for transcriptionally active genes.

example, were considerably less effective. Perhaps, when increased manufacturing and transduction efficiency is achieved, opportunities for engineering better vectors may arise.

3.5
Herpes Simplex Virus

The last vector under serious consideration for human studies is Herpes simplex virus

(HSV) type 1 (Figs. 11, 12, 13 and 14). The wild-type virus causes the common cold sore, and is transmitted through the skin by direct contact with a lesion from an infected individual. The wild-type virus can replicate in skin and mucous membranes but does not persist in the epithelium, instead entering sensory nerve terminals in the skin from which they are transported in a retrograde manner to the nerve cell body in sensory ganglia (Fig. 13). In the sensory ganglia, the lytic viral life cycle is curtailed within days, after which the wild-type virus enters a latent state,

with concomitant silencing of lytic genes. During latency, only the latency locus is transcriptionally active, and latently infected nuclei accumulate a stable intron called the *latency-associated transcript* or LAT RNA. The ability to persist in neurons for life suggests that HSV may be engineered for gene transfer to nerves and that vector delivery can result from simple skin inoculation. The general strategy for engineering HSV vectors from the wild-type virus is to eliminate genes that contribute to virus replication and reactivation from latency while taking advantage

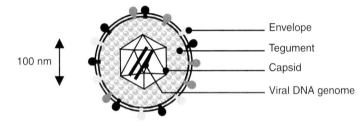

Fig. 11 The structure of herpes simplex virus – A schematic depiction of a mature HSV-1 virion is shown to illustrate the key structural components of the viral particle.

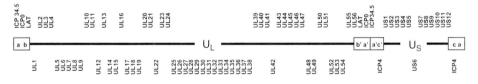

Fig. 12 The HSV-1 genome – The HSV-1 genome is illustrated diagrammatically. The genome is 154 kb and encodes 84 genes. The genome is divided into unique long and short segments flanked by repeat sequences. Genes that are essential and nonessential for viral replication *in vitro* are indicated. Nonessential genes (which encode a variety of functions that optimize the interaction of HSV with the host organism) can be removed from the virus

without compromising replication *in vitro*, allowing their replacement with transgenes of interest. The capacity for the insertion of foreign DNA sequences into the HSV genome is large; genomic vectors can accommodate around 40 kb of transgenic material and amplicons (particles that have all viral genes removed and supplied in trans) can accommodate 120 kb of foreign sequence.

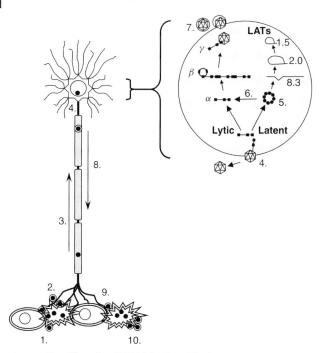

Fig. 13 The life cycle of HSV-1 *in vivo* – The key events occurring during infection of a human host are depicted schematically as follows: 1 – Lytic cycle of replication at epithelial port of entry; 2 – Virions released from epithelia enter sensory nerve terminals; 3 – Nucleocapsid and tegument undergoes retrograde axonal transport to soma; 4 – Viral DNA enters neuronal nucleus and either initiates lytic cascade of gene expression or becomes latent; 5 – During latency, viral genome remains episomal and nuclear. Only the LAT genes are expressed; 6 – Immunosuppression, intercurrent illness, or other stimulus "reactivates" lytic infection; 7 – Virions formed by budding from nuclear membrane; 8 – Nucleocapsid and glycoproteins transported separately by anterograde axonal transport; 9 – Virion assembly and egress from nerve terminal; 10 – Recurrent epithelial infection at or near the site of primary lesion.

of the latent genome as a platform for transgene expression (Fig. 14). The virus depends on expression of four genes, activated upon entry into the nucleus and referred to as *immediate early functions* for replication to occur. In the absence of these genes, other viral functions fail to be expressed or are expressed at exceedingly low levels. Thus, despite the fact that the virus contains approximately 84 genes (Fig. 12),

engineering HSV vectors is not as complex as it may seem. Two of the immediate early genes are essential functions, but complementation of all four genes is required for high virus vector yield on production in complementing cells. The latency promoter elements have been partially characterized and can be used to drive the transgene expression for considerable time periods in sensory nerves. While

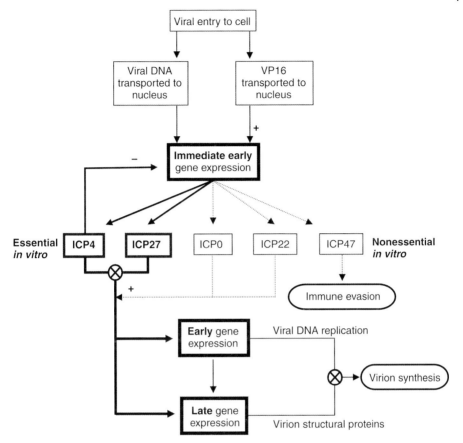

Fig. 14 Regulation of HSV-1 gene expression during lytic infection – This flow chart illustrates the important regulatory events in gene expression occurring during lytic HSV-1 infection. In order to proceed to the later stages of infection, during which the viral genome is replicated and new virions assembled, both of the essential immediate-early genes *ICP4* and *ICP27* must be expressed. Deletion of one or other essential *IE* gene results in a replication-defective virus by eliminating early and late gene expression; these vectors are easily propagated and prepared to high titer and purity in cell lines expressing ICP4 and ICP27. Later vectors have multiple *IE* genes deleted to reduce cytotoxicity. In addition, many of the large number of genes that are nonessential for replication *in vitro* can be deleted to allow insertion of multiple or large transgene sequences. Herpes amplicon genomes contain the HSV origin of replication and packaging signals, in addition too the transgene of interest, but do not contain any viral coding sequences. A BAC containing the HSV genome expresses all viral structural genes in a cotransfection preparation, to allow generation of particles. Although the amplicon system may be thought advantageous owing to the absence of viral genes and large capacity for insertion of transgenic material, (120 kb), amplicons are very difficult to prepare in useful amounts and current technology strongly favors the use of replication-defective genomic vectors.

multiple essential viral genes have been complemented in cell lines engineered for this purpose, a packaging cell line has not yet been produced that takes full advantage of the large genome for delivering foreign DNA. This may be difficult since a number of the virus functions are toxic to cells and their expression requires coordinated regulation, a feat difficult to accomplish using virus genes embedded in cellular chromosomes. Nevertheless, efforts are ongoing to eliminate more virus functions, creating additional room for foreign sequences. The large genome of HSV of 152 kb in length suggests its potential utility for transferring multiple genes and perhaps even genomic sequences. Current vectors can accommodate up to 50 kb.

Another class of HSV-based vectors is referred to as *amplicons*. These are plasmids that mimic defective interfering particles that arise spontaneously during high multiplicity passage of the virus in cell culture. Amplicons can be generated with wild-type or conditional mutant virus as a helper, provided the amplicon contains a packaging signal and an origin of replication. As the viral genes are supplied *in trans*, the capacity of insertion of cloned DNA is large. Unfortunately, the *Ori* signal increases the recombination frequency, and it is therefore difficult to avoid recombination between the amplicon and helper virus, so that completely pure vector stocks are difficult to obtain. This problem can be ameliorated to a substantial degree by using helper plasmids for amplicon packaging, but virus reconstitution may occur. Manufacture of amplicons is a difficult task for use in patients, since consistent preparations are difficult to achieve. Thus, vectors that are produced by complementation are more likely to be developed as gene therapy products, at least with current

technology. As is the case with AdV and AAV-based vectors, a substantial proportion of the population has been infected with HSV and has antibodies against the virus. However, antiviral immunity is not effective in preventing HSV infection, rather it is the extent of virus replication and frequency of reactivation that is controlled by the immune response. Immune competent individuals can have HSV reactivation events, but this frequency is considerably greater in immune-compromised individuals. Reactivation, of course, does not occur with replication-defective vectors.

3.6
Vector Targeting

Over the past decade, substantial emphasis has been placed on manipulating the host range of viral vectors. Targeting could be used (1) to transduce cells that are not naturally infected by the wild-type virus or (2) to increase the uptake of vector into a limited subset of cells. In the best-case scenario, a vector could be engineered to be defective in its natural targeting function, but redirected to recognize an epitope on a desired target cell, allowing systemic vector inoculation, to achieve distributed, yet targeted, transduction. Enveloped viruses have been retargeted by using different envelope glycoproteins from other enveloped viruses. In addition, novel ligands have been inserted into the coding sequence of specific virus envelope genes. However, virus binding to target cells has not always led to infection, since a second fusion step is required either at the cell surface or within the endosome compartment (Figs. 15, 16). Recent studies with AAV have discovered sequences that can be modified without disrupting virus uncoating. Although efficient retargeting has

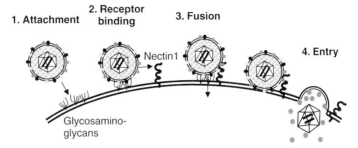

Fig. 15 Cell entry of an enveloped virus – HSV-1 is shown for illustration. Following an initial attachment event (involving interaction of HSV glycoproteins gC and gB with cell surface glycosaminoglycans), a specific receptor interaction occurs between viral glycoprotein gD and cell surface nectin-1 (also called HveC). This results in fusion of viral envelope with the cell membrane, a process dependent on viral glycoproteins gB and gH/L. The nucleocapsid and tegument proteins then enter the cytoplasm, leaving the viral glycoproteins on the cell surface. Subsequently, the nucleocapsid and some of the tegument proteins are transported to the cell nucleus. The viral DNA is uncoated and enters the nucleus with some of the tegument proteins, initiating viral gene transcription (see Fig. 14).

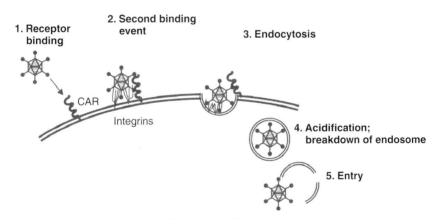

Fig. 16 Adenovirus is shown for illustration. Following an initial receptor binding event, involving interaction of the terminal bulb of the virus fibre protein with the coxsackie-adenovirus receptor (CAR), a second receptor interaction occurs between the AdV penton base protein and cell surface integrins. This results in the endocytosis of the receptor and virus. As the endosome matures, and its environment acidifies, viral components cause the endosome to break down, releasing the partially degraded viral particle into the cell. The nucleocapsid is then transported to the nucleus, where uncoating and nuclear entry of the viral genome are followed by viral gene expression.

not yet been achieved with AAV vectors, enhancement of entry into cells that express low levels of AAV receptor has been achieved by modification of the capsid to display a cell-specific receptor on the AAV virion. The most effective retargeting of viral vectors has involved the modification of coat protein components of adenovirus. Adenovirus infects cells by binding to the coxsackie/adenovirus receptor (CAR) using the extended knob structure of the hexon capsid protein at the particle surface. The virus penton base binds to a specific integrin, $\alpha V\beta 5$, using a specific motif arginine-glutamate-aspartate (RGD). This dual receptor binding recognition is typical of many viruses and ensures specificity. The adenovirus is endocytosed and is released from endosome as it acidifies. A number of strategies have been used to retarget adenoviruses. These include extension of the hexon, using an antibody ligand or a receptor ligand, or engineering the knob function directly by genetic engineering. In addition, the RGD amino acid motif has been altered, so that different integrins can be recognized. This combination has specifically altered receptor interactions that lead to adenovirus infection, in a quantitatively significant manner. Such retargeting holds promise for safe, directed *in vivo* use, especially for targeting cancer cells involved in metastasis.

3.7
Regulation of Gene Expression

If gene delivery cannot be restricted to the cell of interest, targeting of gene expression can be attempted using promoters with tissue specificity. It should be noted that promoter function in the background of a virus genome may be unpredictable. In addition, some tissue-specific promoters are complex, requiring large amounts of sequence (including elements located within introns) to be active, and most vector systems cannot accommodate such large sequences. Considerable effort has gone into determining the critical motifs for promoter specificity and a variety of interesting sequences have been characterized, including locus control regions, matrix attachment functions, transcription factor recognition sequences, and insulator elements. Transcriptional control has proven to be a complex problem to unravel; native promoters in their minimum state have not proven satisfactory. Moreover, as indicated earlier, the context of the gene is important, such that some promoters are quite active until the virus genome becomes integrated or is subject to chromatin formation. Engineering vectors that respond to chromatin remodeling for gene expression has not been satisfactorily worked out, so that gene control in vectors often relies on empirical rather than rational methods. There are exceptions; "housekeeping" gene promoters tend to be functional most often (if not most vigorously), although targeted gene expression involves another level of complexity in design. For some vectors, the virus contains naturally occurring strong constitutive promoters, such as the retrovirus LTRs, or tissue-specific promoters such as the nerve-specific latency promoter of HSV. While this is a promising area of investigation for further gene vector development, the use of enhancer elements out of context can lead to an expression that is not appropriately controlled.

A related issue concerns control of when and how long the gene product should be expressed. Some vector-expressed hormones, for example, are highly active in small doses – long-term expression could be harmful or could lead to malignant transformation. It would be highly useful if a gene switch were available for use in vectors, in which a safe and bioavailable drug could be used to turn gene expression on and off. Several systems have been developed (Table 3). The common theme shared by these systems is that a chimeric transcription factor both (1) recognizes a specific target promoter driving the therapeutic transgene, and (2) is activated by a drug. These systems require the constitutive expression of one or more transcriptional activator gene products. There are several problems associated with all of the available systems: the promoters are usually "leaky" (low-level transcription persists even in the absence of the activating drug or presence of the repressor); the constitutively expressed chimeric transcription factors are frequently immunogenic; maintenance of activator gene transcription is as difficult as effecting long-term expression of any transgene; and the targeted promoter may become unresponsive due to methylation, chromatin structure, and so on. Despite these difficulties, evidence for gene switch function in animal models appears promising; perhaps these systems will be improved in various ways, including humanization of the activator gene products to reduce immunogenicity. Another strategy for achieving the same end result might be engineered gene products that are constitutively expressed, but functionally inert in the absence of an "activator" drug. Such a system might be simpler to apply, but more difficult to design or apply broadly and may only work in special cases. This remains a fertile area of investigation for the field.

3.8
Nonviral Vectors

A compelling argument for the gene therapy field has been that if nonviral vectors could be developed with similar efficiency and maintenance of transgene expression could be done as viral vectors, several difficult problems in the field would be addressed. These include scalable and more controlled manufacturing processes, since DNA can be readily produced in bioreactors to very high concentrations. The products would be more consistent and better characterized, and delivery could be simple, involving direct injection into tissue. Theoretically, the immune response to nonviral vectors should be attenuated because there are no protein components in the particles – if true, repeat dosing might also be possible. These arguments have been especially attractive to the pharmaceutical industry and thus a considerable amount of resources has been invested in the field of nonviral gene delivery.

Despite these efforts, several problems have arisen that have been very difficult to address. The first is that DNA alone has proven to be highly immunogenic, particularly when CpG repeat sequences are present, and when used with various delivery agents such as cationic liposomes. The second is that targeting is generally not possible, even when specific ligands are attached to the DNA or the delivery vehicle, and gene delivery by nonviral vectors is relatively inefficient compared to viral vector-mediated gene transfer. Third, transgene expression is highly variable and generally very short lived. There have been some exceptions to these general observations. DNA delivery to some tissues such as skeletal muscle is reasonably efficient, and nonviral vector-mediated DNA delivery has proven to be useful for immune priming as part of vaccine strategies.

Tab. 3 Examples of inducible promoter systems.

Type	Inducer/ repressor	DNA response element	Chimeric Transcription factor(s)				Mechanism of regulation
			Name	DNA binding domain	Ligand Binding domain	Transactivation domain	
Tet-off	Tetracyclines	Bacterial tet operon sequences (tetO)	tTA (tet transactivator)	Bacterial tet repressor		HSV VP-16	tTA binds to tetO in absence of tetracycline
Tet-on	Tetracyclines	Bacterial tet operon sequences (tetO)	rtTA (reverse tet transactivator)	Mutated bacterial tet repressor		HSV-VP-16	rtTA binds to tetO in presence of tetracycline
Progesterone regulated	Mifepristone (RU486)	Yeast Gal4 upstream activating sequence (UASG)	GL-VP	Yeast Gal4 transcription factor	Mutated human progesterone receptor	HSV VP-16 or human NFκB p65	GL-VP binds to UASG in presence of RU486
Ecdysone regulated	Ecdysone, muristerone	Drosophila ecdysone response element	1.VgEcR	Drosophila ecdysone receptor		HSV VP-16	VgEcR forms active complex with hRXRα or drosophila USP in presence of ecdysone
			2. Human retinoic acid receptor X or drosophila ultraspiracle (USP)				
Rapamycin regulated	Rapamycin	ZFHD1 response element	1. ZFHD1-FKBP 2. FRAP-p65	Human ZFHD1 none	Human FKBP Truncated human FRAP	None Truncated human NFκB p65	Rapamycin binding brings together functional units of bipartite transcription factor

4
Clinical Applications and Genes

4.1
Single Gene Disorders

Gene delivery to treat Mendelian single gene disorders would allow the fundamental genetic abnormalities to be addressed, rather than the current best practice of intermittently delivering gene products or devising some other compensatory strategy for the genetic lesion. The list of potential gene therapy targets in this category is very large – theoretically, any genetic disease could be treated this way. There are, however, a few examples that have been instructive in terms of understanding the factors likely to determine a successful outcome, and some disease targets are attractive, because the factors governing successful development of therapy are likely to be less stringent than in other diseases. The following paragraphs present a selection of applications, including some where clinical efficacy has already been demonstrated and others where practical gene therapy seems a remote prospect at present.

4.1.1 Hematological Disease
These disorders provide an attractive target for the gene therapist. The diseases are often very severe or fatal and have limited effective therapy at present. Many of the diseases are well characterized at a molecular level, so that the genes that should be delivered are well known. Finally, many of these conditions result from defects in genes necessary for the function of cells during or after differentiation from bone marrow multipotent precursors. Consequently, the transduction event may be carried out *ex vivo* in autologous harvested bone marrow stem cells, so that the vector

only enters the target cells, and a degree of selection or expansion is possible before the cells are returned to the host. A list of possible disease targets in this category is shown in Table 4.

Gene therapy for SCID has been ongoing for more than a decade, beginning in 1990. While there are some 60 genetic defects that lead to the SCID phenotype, the availability of patients and a clear understanding of the disease process has focused attention on two genes, ADA deficiency and the gamma c chain of the cytokine receptor (γc). ADA deficiency leads to toxicity to developing immune cells (T and B lymphocytes) and γc deficiency results in a defective growth factor receptor on T and B cells that is needed for responsiveness to cytokine induction of proliferation and maturation of immune lymphocytes. Current management of ADA deficiency is carried out by infusing the ADA protein into the blood, which is taken up by immune cells primarily macrophage. This results in partial restoration of the immune system. The enzyme is PEGalated to enhance stability in the serum and to increase uptake. The first landmark SCID-ADA clinical trial was carried out by French Anderson and Michael Blease, who were then members of the National Institutes of Health (NIH). The patients were given autologous bone marrow cells derived from the circulation that had been infected with a Moloney-based retroviral vector carrying the ADA gene. Infusion of these cells did prove to be safe, but patients continued to receive PEG-ADA for safety reasons. Other trials have continued along these lines until a recent study in Italy carried out by Claudio Bordignon has attempted this treatment in the absence of PEG-ADA therapy. Patients appear to be responding without toxicity and it is likely that the potential success of this trial

Tab. 4 Possible disease targets for gene transfer to hematopoietic stem cells.

Disease	Gene
Red Cell Defects	
β-Thalassaemia	β-Globin
Sickle-cell disease	β-like globin
G6PD deficiency	G6PD
Porphyria	Ferrochelatase, others
Cytoskeletal defects	Spectrin
Leukocyte defects	
Chronic granulomatous disease	gp91phox, p47phox
Leukocyte adhesion defect	CD18
Stem-cell defects	
Fanconi anemia	FANC A–E
Immune deficiency syndromes	
Severe combined immunodeficiency (SCID)	γc, ADA, JAK3 kinase
Wiskott–Aldrich syndrome	WASP
CD40 ligand deficiency	CD154
Agammaglobulinemia	BTK
Lysosomal storage disease	
Gaucher disease	Glucocerebrosidase
Hurler's syndrome	α-Iduronidase
Leukodystrophies	X-adrenoleukodystrophy ALDP
Metachromatic leukodystrophy	Arylsulphatase A

can be attributed to the removal of PEG-ADA therapy. ADA expression should lead to selection of the gene-repaired cells *in vivo*, whereas continued use of PEG-ADA prevents this selection. This brings up an important point for gene therapy, which is that the most efficient outcomes may occur in circumstances where transduction occurs in a tissue where there is cellular turnover, and the transduced cells acquire a selective growth advantage. This seems to have contributed to the unprecedented clinical success of the SCIDX gene therapy trial described in the section below.

A number of other targets for HSC gene therapy are contemplated, including hemoglobinopathies, leukodystrophies, lysosomal storage diseases, porphyrias, and leukocyte defects.

4.1.2 Restoration of Circulating Proteins

Some hereditary diseases are caused by genetic defects that abolish the expression of circulating proteins. Hemophilias are the commonest of these disorders. Absence of circulating clotting factor VIII (hemophilia A) or IX (hemophilia B) results in defective blood coagulation, with a tendency to bleed spontaneously into joints (hemarthrosis), following dental extractions or surgical procedures, or following even minor trauma causing life-threatening hemorrhage. Both diseases are transmitted as Mendelian X-linked traits and are therefore usually manifested only in boys. Current treatment involves infusion of purified protein factors, providing temporary resolution of the clotting defect at large expense, inconvenience, and at a finite risk of transmitting infection, where factors are obtained from pooled blood donations.

These diseases are attractive targets for gene therapists for several reasons. First, they are relatively common and disabling. Second, the blood levels of the clotting factors necessary to restore physiological clotting function are low; levels of >1% normal are rarely associated with spontaneous hemorrhage; levels above 5% normal are associated with posttraumatic bleeding only; and levels above 20% normal are associated with a normal phenotype. This means that complete restoration of the blood levels produced physiologically (by the liver and endothelium) is not necessary to have a clinical impact, and also that the regulation of expression levels might not be as critical as in some diseases, where, for example, stoichiometry with other components of a multiprotein complex is important, or the levels of a potently bioactive protein controlled closely to prevent toxicity. Finally, the requirements for restoration of function are that the protein should be present in the bloodstream, and so the site or tissue of transduction might not be critical, as long as the "depot" tissue has access to the circulation. This means that transduction of more accessible sites than the site of physiological production (the liver) might be possible, or that engineered cells created by *ex vivo* transduction might be able to correct the underlying defect.

Using animal models of hemophilia (there are both mouse and dog models), transient restoration of hemostatic levels of factors VIII and IX was demonstrated using first- and second-generation adenoviruses. However, the inflammatory response that occurs in response to adenovirus was responsible for limiting the time span of gene expression, an effect that was partially mitigated using a gutless AdV vector. Similar studies using lentiviruses in mouse models have shown a sustained increase in levels of factor IX, but not of factor VIII owing to an immune response to the human protein used in the mouse model. More recently, adeno-associated viral vectors have been shown to allow sustained expression of clotting factors at therapeutic levels, following transduction of either liver or muscle in animal models. In one clinical trial, hemophilia B patients have been treated with hepatic arterial infusions of an AAV2 vector carrying the factor IX gene. At low dosage (2×10^{11} particles), no toxicity or elevation of factor IX above background was detectable. One patient received an intermediate dosage (1×10^{12} particles). Circulating factor IX levels of 10 to 12% were detectable within 2 to 3 weeks after transduction. Unfortunately, the levels of factor IX then dropped back to the baseline as the levels of circulating transaminases increased, indicative of hepatocellular injury. A similar dose of vector produced a therapeutic level of factor IX lasting 1 to 2 years in the canine model. It is unclear at present whether the pattern seen in the single reported patient will be reiterated, or whether there will clinical benefit, in other patients. Another study using AAV2 injected into muscle reported a transient increase in factor IX levels at a lower vector dose, but no measurable increase at a higher vector dose. Finally, a phase I trial used endogenous fibroblasts transduced with the factor VIII gene *ex vivo* to investigate cell-based delivery systems. Following expansion, $1–4 \times 10^8$ cells were reimplanted into the omentum of six patients. Four of these had detectable elevations in serum factor VIII levels, but these were transient and all had returned to baseline by one year. It seems that better understanding of the processes regulating antibody responses to factors VIII and

IX, the immune response to viral vector components, and the regulatory events involved in long-term gene expression and implanted cell senescence, may be necessary to take this work forward.

α1-antitrypsin (α1AT) deficiency is another example of a genetic disease associated with loss of a circulating protein. This serine protease inhibitor is normally produced in the liver and secreted into the circulation. Patients with loss of the circulating enzyme inhibitor develop abnormal lung proteolysis and a severe form of emphysema. As one primary site of pathology is the lung, it has been suggested that therapy directed at local extracellular expression in the lung might be easier to accomplish than systemic delivery, and equally therapeutically efficacious for the lung disease. However, to prevent the liver disease that accompanies α1AT deficiency in the circulation, it will be necessary to express normal α1AT in the liver. This is because the liver pathology is caused by misfolding of a mutant protein rather than loss of its function, and so local synthesis of wild-type protein will be necessary to suppress production of the mutant. Animal studies have been carried out using adeno-associated virus and adenovirus vectors expressing α1AT. By hepatic or muscular delivery of the vectors, it is possible to produce detectable levels of circulating protein for sustained periods. One reported clinical trial used a liposome complex to deliver the AAT gene to the nasal epithelium of subjects with α1AT deficiency. Other clinical trials have yet to commence, including one aiming to express circulating α1-AT in skeletal muscle using an AAV vector.

4.1.3 Respiratory Disease

Cystic fibrosis (CF) is the commonest autosomal recessive genetic disorder in the western world, with an estimated gene carrier frequency of $1:20$, resulting in $1:1600$ livebirths being affected by the condition. CF is a multiorgan disease affecting the respiratory system, pancreas, digestive system, skin, and reproductive organs. The product of the *CF* gene, the CFTR is an integral membrane protein involved in ionic flux in exocrine glands. Its loss results in extremely thickened secretions causing bacterial colonization, repeated infection, and bronchiectasis in the lungs, and exocrine dysfunction in the pancreas. The latter is amenable to enzyme replacement therapy; however, despite optimal antibiotic therapy, CF patients generally die in their teens or in their 20s from the respiratory complications of the disease.

Gene therapy has focused on the introduction of the normal *CFTR* gene into bronchial airway epithelial cells to restore normal CFTR function and thereby alleviate the respiratory problems that cause fatality. In principle, the airway epithelium should be easily accessible to viral and nonviral vectors applied topically, through aerosols or bronchoscopic instillation. As the nasal epithelium is histologically similar to that found in the bronchioles and exhibits similar functional deficits in cystic fibrosis, some studies have focused on gene transfer to nasal epithelium to show proof of principle. Early studies showed proof of principle that a number of different vector platforms could introduce the *CFTR* gene into airway epithelium, resulting in expression of CFTR. Despite early optimism, however, clinical gene transfer to correct the abnormal pulmonary phenotype of CF has proved very difficult and therapeutic results have yet to be achieved. Latest clinical gene transfer trials show that adenovirus and adeno-associated virus vectors are extremely inefficient in transducing the bronchial epithelium, and there are major problems with repeat dosing each of these vectors (as would be necessary because of short-lived gene expression) owing to immunity. Although nonviral techniques, including liposomes and cationic lipid formulations, can be repeatedly administered, they appear even less efficient than the viral techniques, and are not entirely devoid of toxicity – one study reporting fever, muscle and joint pain in half of the subjects after aerosol delivery. Recent advances have included identification of factors such as mucus and glycocalyx that contribute to the poor efficiency of transduction *in vivo*. Although measures designed to mitigate these effects may enhance gene transfer, unfortunately, the location of receptors for adenovirus and AAV on the basal (nonairway) surface of the bronchiolar epithelium may prove an insurmountable obstacle to the use of these vectors for topical gene transfer in CF, unless their tropism can be redirected to apical receptors. Recently, other viral vectors have been developed that may transduce airway cells via the apical (airway) surface, including lentivirus pseudotyped with envelope glycoproteins from viruses that naturally infect the airway epithelia via the apical surface. Finally, inefficient transduction of epithelia has been demonstrated using nonviral vectors and oligonucleotides via the bronchial circulation, raising the possibility that gene delivery to the basal surface of the cells may be achievable. It remains to be seen whether these modified vectors or other approaches can solve the problems of efficiency, gene expression longevity, and toxicity inherent in techniques used hitherto.

4.1.4 Neurological Disease

Gene transfer to the brain presents a number of formidable challenges. Brain tissue is inaccessible to vectors from the circulation, enclosed in dense bone, extremely sensitive to functional disruption by mechanical manipulation, nonregenerating and physiologically vital. This means that *ex vivo* transduction cannot be carried out, except in rare circumstances where there is good reason to think that bone marrow stem cell transduction will allow correction of a neurological phenotype. For example, in the severe childhood cerebral inflammatory type of adrenoleukodystrophy, bone marrow transplantation early in the course of the illness appears to arrest the progressive cerebral disease, and it is reasonable to suppose that genetic modification of endogenous bone marrow stem cells might also be efficacious. For most neurogenetic diseases, however, *in vivo* gene transfer will be necessary to correct the genetic abnormality present in the brain or spine. This might be achieved through direct inoculation of vector into the area of the brain in which the pathological process is manifest. For example, replacement of the *Parkin* gene in juvenile onset Parkinson's disease might be targeted to the substantia nigra as the bulk of the initial pathology appears here. Alternatively, some viruses are transported into the CNS from peripheral sites, or within the CNS from one location to another, by axonal transport. This may allow vector inoculation at a remote and more accessible site, for example, muscle inoculation in gene therapy targeted at diseases of the motor neuron.

The pathology in many types of hereditary neurological diseases is widely distributed, and there is no good method at present for widespread *in vivo* gene delivery in the brain, as would be needed to correct the phenotype of recessive diseases like Friedreich's ataxia, fragile X mental retardation, or Hallervorden-Spatz disease. Consequently, clinical optimism at present is limited to diseases in which the pathology is localized, or rare conditions in which the missing gene product is normally located extracellularly or can be taken up by cells adjacent and remote to those transduced. Examples of the latter groups of diseases include the rare mucopolysaccharidoses with CNS involvement, where successful phenotypic outcomes have been seen following gene transfer in animal models.

Two further barriers present obstacles for gene therapy of single-gene diseases of the CNS. First, most of the adult-onset and many of the childhood-onset conditions are inherited in an autosomal dominant pattern and are caused by pathological gain of function or dominant negative effects. Examples of these diseases include the spinocerebellar ataxias, Huntington's disease, inherited prion diseases, and familial Alzheimer's diseases, the commonest forms of dystonia and some developmental diseases. Gene therapy in these cases would depend on gene targeting, possibly with gene replacement, rather than gene delivery on its own. There has been progress in this field, including development of RNA interference technology, but there have been no clinical gene therapy trials in these diseases. Second, the majority of these disease run their course over years and decades, and, as the brain is not an accessible site for repeated vector inoculation, long-term expression of transgenes would be highly desirable before gene therapy for these disease could be contemplated. It is likely that, for these type of applications, success will be achieved by exploiting the properties of viruses that persist long-term in the nervous system as part of their natural life cycle.

4.1.5 Muscle

Duchenne muscular dystrophy (DMD) is a common (1 : 3500 male births) genetic disease of muscle that results in progressive muscle wasting and death by the age of 15 to 20 from respiratory impairment or cardiac disease. It is caused by the loss of a muscle protein, dystrophin, which forms part of a large complex of proteins that localize to the sarcolemma of muscle fibers and function to maintain the integrity of the muscle cell membrane during contraction. The dystrophin gene is very large (the cDNA is >10 kb) and therefore can only be accommodated within gutless adenovirus or herpes simplex virus vectors – both of which are inefficient vehicles for transduction of muscle. Much work has been carried out in trying to develop truncated functional versions of the dystrophin gene that may be accommodated in adeno-associated virus vectors, which appear more promising as vectors in muscle tissue. A group of conditions, the sarcoglycanopathies, are closely related to DMD. They are caused by mutations in genes encoding other components of the protein complex of which dystrophin is part. These genes are smaller and can be readily accommodated within adeno-associated virus vectors. Successful correction of either the dystrophin- or sarcoglycan-deficient phenotypes presents a number of significant challenges, however, even if a useful vector system can be developed. First, the tissue compartment requiring transduction by the vector is vast and is distributed throughout the body, necessitating many multiple points of inoculation or systemic delivery. Second, functional recovery of an individual muscle is likely to depend on the transduction of a threshold proportion of muscle fibers, by introduction of a transgene at a number of sites along the syncitial muscle fiber, so inefficient or incomplete transduction would likely be ineffective even if distributed over the large tissue compartment. Although a number of preclinical and clinical studies have shown proof of concept that dystrophin and other missing proteins can be expressed transiently in dystrophic muscle, no clinical studies have yet demonstrated any phenotypic benefit.

4.2
Delivery of Proteins for a Pharmacological Action

Gene therapy has much broader potential application than the delivery of genes that are missing in inherited Mendelian recessive diseases. There are many examples of potently active biological proteins whose delivery to specific sites might be useful to correct the abnormalities in certain diseases. Delivery of these proteins might be best accomplished by gene transfer, either because of convenience or costs issues (it is very expensive to manufacture purified recombinant proteins, and difficult to continuously administer them to sites such as the brain or joints), or because of biological necessity (for example, proteins that act intracellularly, or proteins intended to act at the cell surface of targeted cells only, would have to be expressed within the target cell unless some form of highly efficient protein transduction could be developed). The following paragraphs describe some potential applications of gene therapy to allow protein pharmacology rather than gene function replacement.

4.2.1 Transplantation
Rejection is a serious and common consequence of organ transplantation, necessitating the use of potent and toxic immunosuppressant drugs, often with incomplete suppression of rejection. Rejection of transplanted tissue depends on host CD4 and CD8 T-cells becoming activated in response to the transplantation of foreign antigens. There has been much work focusing on molecular definition of the events that follow stimulation of the T-cell receptor by antigen bound to the surface of antigen presenting cells (APC). It appears that interaction of T-cell CD28 with antigens CD80 and CD86 present on the antigen presenting cells favors immune activation, whereas signaling through another T-cell receptor, CTLA-4, results in downregulation of the immune response. Systemic blockade of the CD28 – CD80/86 interaction in animal models, using a chimeric antibody, results in systemic immune suppression. Recent work has examined the possibility of expressing the blocking antibody locally in the allograft by gene transfer; although this improved graft survival, it also resulted in systemic immune suppression. A similar approach to blocking the interaction between T-cell ligand CD154 with the APC receptor CD40 resulted in suppression of acute rejection, but not chronic rejection. Following costimulation, T helper cells secrete cytokines, with particular profiles that correlate with either rejection (Th1 response) or lack of rejection (Th2 response). Consequently, it has been suggested that creating a Th2 response in the transplanted tissue may prevent rejection. As most cytokines are associated with severe adverse side effects on systemic administration, the local production of Th2 cytokines, for example IL-10, in the graft has been suggested, using gene transfer. This approach enabled modest prolongation of graft survival in animal models. Other parallel approaches have focused on genetic modification of antigen presenting cells, causing them to synthesize immune

tolerance–inducing factors like TGF-β, or factors that specifically cause elimination of activated T cells, for example, *Fas* ligand. Finally, another approach to the induction of immune tolerance using gene transfer relies on the observation that hosts carrying allogeneic bone marrow transplants exist in a state of mixed host-donor hematopoietic cell chimerism, in which specific tolerance to donor antigens develops. On the basis of this observation, gene transfer strategies have been devised in which donor MHC molecules are expressed in host hematopoietic cells using *ex vivo* gene transfer. In several animal models, this seems to induce hyporesponsiveness to the transplanted antigens, allowing prolonged graft survival without compromising systemic immunity. None of these approaches has yet proven sufficiently successful in preclinical studies to warrant testing in a clinical trial, although the field is moving rapidly and the potential applications for gene transfer expanding in parallel with understanding the processes involved in transplant rejection.

4.2.2 Ischemic Heart Disease

Ischemic heart disease is the leading cause of death in the western world, and is most commonly caused by atheromatous occlusion of the coronary vessels. The blood supply to the myocardium becomes compromised and there may be a supply/demand mismatch resulting in cardiac ischemia or infarction. Conventional therapy includes addressing factors that may contribute to the development of atheroma, drugs that improve cardiac perfusion or reduce cardiac oxygen and energy demand, or various re-vascularization procedures. The success rate of these procedures is less than perfect, and restenosis is common after revascularization procedures like angioplasty or bypass grafting.

Consequently, there has been considerable interest in gene therapy approaches that might help to encourage endogenous neovascularization in areas of ischemic myocardium through the local expression of potent peptide factors that encourage growth of new blood vessels (for example vascular endothelial growth factors, VEGF1 and VEGF2, and fibroblast growth factors FGF1 and FGF4), or the introduction of genes encoding transcription factors that are instrumental in executing the coordinated neovascularization response (for example hypoxia-inducible factor-1α, HIF1α). Transfer of these genes to ischemic myocardium or limb tissues has been demonstrated in preclinical studies using adenovirus and adeno-associated virus vectors in addition to nonviral vectors. First- and second-generation AdV gene transfer, as elsewhere in the body, gives rise to nonsustained gene expression and a local inflammatory response. In many of the preclinical studies, expression of the growth factor or transcription factor resulted in significant angiogenesis. Clinical studies have demonstrated the feasibility of intracardiac or intracoronary administration of the gene transfer reagents encoding angiogenic growth factors. Most of the studies have been small and primarily aimed at assessing safety rather than efficacy. Even so, markers of cardiac ischemia that would not be expected to be susceptible to placebo artifact, such as SPECT scanning or angiography, were improved in two of the trials examining VEGF2 expression in the myocardium or endocardium. A single double-blind placebo-controlled trial examined intracoronary gene transfer using an adenovirus vector encoding FGF-4. This trial did not demonstrate any statistically significant benefit from the treatment. Understanding the factors, for example, the longevity of gene expression, that underlie successful revascularization is still incomplete and it is expected that further advances in gene delivery technology and vascular biology will pave the way for success in this field.

4.2.3 Neurological Disease

The common sporadic form of Parkinson's disease does not have a known or defined genetic basis, yet many potential protein-based interventions have been identified through work in tissue culture and animal models. These include intracellular proteins (for example antiapoptotic factors to prevent cell loss or enzymes to enable functional rescue of the abnormal neurochemical phenotype following cell loss) or extracellular proteins (for example growth factors that might allow restoration of the damaged basal ganglia circuitry). One recent study described the intraputaminal infusion of recombinant glial cell-line derived neurotrophic factor (GDNF) in PD patients, with beneficial effects on functional imaging surrogates of cell integrity. The infusion of GDNF may prove to be clinically efficacious and was associated with few minor adverse effects. The route of administration is, however, cumbersome and expensive; therefore, *GDNF* gene delivery has many possible advantages over the local infusion of recombinant factor. These advantages might include the capacity for prolonged local synthesis and delivery of the factor *in situ*, in addition to convenience and cost issues. However, it will be essential to develop vectors that allow regulated gene expression and sustained transgene expression before *GDNF* gene delivery might be contemplated.

Using a different approach for *PD* gene therapy, a clinical trial is about to commence using an AAV vector to transfer a gene encoding the enzyme glutamic acid decarboxylase (GAD) to the brain. This strategy is based on a number of observations concerning the functional abnormalities present in the basal ganglia of patients with PD. Neurons of the subthalamic nucleus (STN) are generally overactive in PD and secrete an excitatory neurotransmitter, glutamate, which acts to increase the firing rate of postsynaptic neurons in the internal *globus pallidus* and *substantia nigra pars reticulata*. It is known that electrically evoked reduction in STN overactivity in PD can be therapeutically efficacious. GAD is involved in the synthesis of an inhibitory transmitter, γ-amino butyric acid (GABA). STN neurons expressing GAD produce mixed excitatory/inhibitory postsynaptic responses. This may functionally alleviate the effects of STN overactivity by partially antagonizing the postsynaptic responses to STN overactivity. The clinical trial has recently begun to recruit patients and will address toxicity and dosing issues rather than therapeutic effectiveness in the first instance.

Other examples of gene transfer–mediated protein pharmacology in neurology might include the targeting of neuroimmunological regulatory molecules in diseases with a prominent inflammatory or immune component, such as multiple sclerosis (MS). For example, it is known that the antiinflammatory cytokine β-interferon is weakly efficacious when administered systemically in relapsing-remitting MS. Various animal models of autoimmune myelin destruction have shown that pathological effects can be mitigated by expression of a range of antiinflammatory cytokines in the cerebrospinal fluid and extracellular fluid of the CNS parenchyma, following transduction of the meninges as depot sites for production. It is possible that this may be a viable way to deliver immunomodulatory molecules to the CNS.

4.2.4 Cancer Gene Therapy

Despite recent advances in clinical oncology and radiotherapy, many types of cancer are still associated with a poor prognosis, and many of the current best treatments are highly toxic. Gene therapy thus provides an attractive experimental approach to developing novel therapeutic reagents to tackle malignancy. Of human clinical gene therapy trials carried out so far, the majority have been in patients with various cancers, reflecting both the desperate need for better treatments and the perceived potential for this technology to yield favorable results.

The aims of cancer gene therapy are rather different to those of other gene therapy applications, in that the gene therapist seeks to selectively destroy target cells. This has been accomplished in a number of ways, including the following:

(a) *Suicide gene therapy.* The transgene product is toxic to expressing cells. An example is the HSV-thymidine kinase-ganciclovir (TK-GCV) system in which expression of viral TK allows activation of a prodrug (GCV) that interferes with DNA replication in rapidly dividing cells.

(b) *Radiosensitization.* The transgene product enhances the toxicity of gamma irradiation in the tumor. TNF-α is an example.

(c) *Immunotherapy.* The transgene product stimulates an immune response directed against tumor. Examples include CD80, TNFα, GM-CSF, IL-2, interferon-γ, and IL-12.

(d) *Restoration of cellular functions altered during oncogenesis.* Many tumors acquire means of avoiding apoptosis in

response to the mutations in cellular DNA that often occur during oncogenesis. A common example is the loss of p53 signaling that occurs in many types of solid tumors. Replacement of p53 function in this instance can cause the malignant cells to undergo apoptosis. Other examples might include delivery of other tumor suppressor genes that are mutated in the tumor, or targeting oncogene products or their related cellular pathways to suppress tumor growth.

(e) *Disruption of tumor blood supply.* Most tumors excite an angiogenic response that allows continuing, and adequate, metabolic support for the expanding the tumor mass. Gene therapy can be designed to interfere with this process, causing the tumor to outgrow its blood supply and undergo necrosis.

The mode of action of these reagents is to effect selective destruction of malignant cells. It follows that some means of targeting is essential to prevent destruction of normal tissue. This might be accomplished in several ways. Firstly, strategies might be designed that rely on limiting the expression of a universally toxic gene product to cancer cells. For example, targeted viral delivery, by engineering the tropism of the vector, or targeted transgene transcription in malignant cells, by using specific regulatory elements in the transgene expression cassette, might accomplish the limited spatial expression of a toxic suicide gene product. Secondly, strategies might be deigned that rely on the differential toxicity of a gene product expressed in both normal and malignant cells. Gene products that are directly and selectively toxic to cancer cells could be expressed by both normal and malignant cells, with a preferential effect on the latter. An example might include the HSV-TK system, where the rapid cell division characteristic of malignant cells renders them especially sensitive to disruption in cellular DNA synthesis. Alternatively, gene products could be expressed within a tissue, in order to induce an immune response, which is preferentially directed against the tumor, by virtue of its abnormal antigenic signature. The first of these general approaches is still in early stages of development, as the problems inherent in effecting targeted vector transduction and cell-specific vector-mediated transcription have yet to be fully overcome. In addition, these targeting strategies will depend upon better definition of tumor-specific features, such as tumor-restricted cell surface receptors and cis-acting regulatory elements that are preferentially active in cancer cells. This type of strategy is extremely attractive, however, because there is a theoretical possibility that avid and highly specific targeting would allow systemic administration of the vector, with resulting selective destruction of metastatic tumor deposits. This is rarely achievable in current practice, with few notable examples, such as the ablation of metastatic well-differentiated thyroid tumors through targeting a defined cellular phenotype, the uptake of iodine, allowing selective sequestration of radioactive iodine. It is hoped that similar molecular targeting through gene therapy will allow parallel approaches to be taken in targeting defined cellular processes unique to tumor tissue.

Various gene transfer vectors have been used in preclinical and clinical trials of cancer gene therapy, including replication-deficient lentiviruses, adenoviruses and herpes simplex viruses, and conditionally replicating HSV and adenoviruses. It is not yet known which vector is optimal, and it is likely that different vectors will show utility for specific applications.

For example, the high-level transient expression and immunogenicity of AdV may have application for suicide gene therapy and immunotherapy applications in rapidly dividing tumors, whereas the long-term gene expression and capacity for multiple transgenes seen with HSV vectors may make them good candidates for use in slower growing tumors where multiple simultaneous pathways must be targeted to achieve tumor eradication, for example, glioblastoma.

5
Adverse Events

Considering the number of patients treated with gene therapy in clinical trials, there have been relatively few serious adverse events that have threatened the lives of participants. Nevertheless, those that have occurred have been rather dramatic.

5.1
Multiple Organ Failure Secondary to Cytokine Storm

In the late 1990s, a dose-escalation phase I trial was carried out by the Human Gene Therapy Institute at the University of Pennsylvania. This trial involved the use of replication-defective adenovirus, carrying the gene encoding ornithine transcarbamylase (OTC), to treat inherited OTC deficiency. OTC normally functions as part of the urea cycle, to detoxify nitrogen produced during hepatic amino acid metabolism. The disease phenotype varies in severity; the most significant disease is associated with a completely defective gene. Failure to detoxify hepatic nitrogen leads to hyperammonemia and metabolic coma, which may be fatal if left untreated. It was hoped that successful safety testing of the AdV-OTC vector would eventually lead to the treatment of children suffering from this fatal disease, following successful gene transfer in preclinical studies. However, following review of the protocol, the study was redesigned to enroll adult patients with mild disease. One such patient, Jesse Gelsinger, received the highest dose of vector $(3.8 \times 10^{23}$ infectious particles) at the top end of the dose-escalation schedule. Within hours, he developed a fever, accompanied by biochemical evidence of hepatic damage. Inflammatory cytokines appeared in the blood, followed by signs of disseminated intravascular coagulation, and respiratory and multiorgan failure. He died within four days of receiving the vector. A second patient had received a similar dose of vector, but did not experience severe side effects.

It was concluded from this study that adenovirus introduced through the hepatic portal vein was not confined to the liver, and that the virus had a greater propensity to infect Kupffer cells than hepatocytes in humans. Kupffer cells are reticuloendothelial cells, which were probably responsible for the release of high levels of circulating cytokines following transduction with recombinant adenovirus. This result differed enormously from the experience in mouse models of OTC deficiency, in which the AdV vector largely infected hepatocytes by the same route of administration. Studies in primates showed toxicity similar to that observed in the patient who died.

This outcome demonstrated that the initial immune response to very high doses of vector can be potentially life threatening. Indeed, high doses of any virus will probably result in toxicity, due to the significant load of virus proteins, rather than the transgene. A fire storm of criticism directed at the field of gene therapy followed this unfortunate adverse event. The development of stricter control over gene therapy clinical research was an inevitable result. This outcome at Penn essentially eliminated the use of adenovirus-based vector for liver gene transfer and reduced the interest in using adenovirus *in vivo* for applications other than cancer gene therapy or vaccines, where the immunogenicity of the vector would be advantageous. This has, in turn, focused attention on other vector systems and accelerated progress in other areas.

5.2
Leukemia Secondary to Insertional Mutagenesis

The one true cure of an inherited disease by gene therapy was achieved in the treatment of severe combined immunodeficiency (SCID). There are 60 genetic defects that can lead to the SCID phenotype. Deficiency of the common γc chain of the cytokine receptor results in failure of maturing B and T cells to respond to cytokine induction for both proliferation and maturation. The γc gene is located on the X chromosome, and correspondingly, the disease is inherited as a Mendelian X-linked recessive trait. Death at an early age, secondary to recurrent infections is the usual outcome, unless the children can be treated by donor-matched bone marrow transplantation, which has approximately an 80% success rate. Children without matched donors are treated by transplant with a relatively low success rate and at considerable risk.

Replacement of the missing γc chain gene by *ex vivo* gene transfer to autologous CD34+ hematopoietic stem cells was carried out in patients after successful outcomes in preclinical studies, using a retroviral vector encoding the γc cDNA under transcriptional control of the retroviral

LTR promoter. The transduced cells were reintroduced into the patients, and initial results showed repopulation of bone marrow with differentiating cell lineages and appearance of the missing differentiated cell types in peripheral blood. Correspondingly, there was recovery of immune functions, with many of the 10 treated patients no longer experiencing recurrent infections and dependence on antibiotic therapy (see above).

Unfortunately, after an interval of three years, it became apparent that two of the patients had developed clonal expansion of a T-lymphocyte subpopulation, with peripheral lymphocytosis, bone marrow infiltration and splenomegaly – clinical signs of leukemia. In each case, the clone, which in retrospect was detectable in samples from the patients at earlier time points in the follow-up process, contained a single copy of the retrovirus integrated into the host cell chromosome 11, within or near the *LMO2* gene. The leukemia cells contained additional dyskaryotic abnormalities, including a t(6 : 13) translocation in one patient and clonal populations with various abnormalities including trisomy 11 in the other. Both patients are undergoing chemotherapy at the time of writing this review.

It is acknowledged that there was no reason to suspect that this outcome would occur – a decade of clinical trials using retroviruses to transduce hematopoietic stem cells preceded the SCIDX trial, without a single case of leukemia occurring. In all reports of mice receiving retrovirally transduced HSCs, there is one description of a single animal that developed myeloid leukemia secondary to integration of the vector within a protooncogene that was previously implicated in leukemogenesis. LMO2 is a leukemogenic oncoprotein, as determined by murine transgenic overexpression experiments, which is activated in human childhood acute leukemia. It is transcriptionally active in progenitor cells, which may explain the propensity of the vector to integrate within this gene. It is unclear how integration into this gene contributed to the formation of leukemia in the SCIDX trial patients. The prolonged latency between retroviral integration and malignant clonal emergence argues that additional factors must have been involved, other than insertional mutagenesis following the transduction event. For example, unregulated expression of the γc chain from the viral LTR promoter may have contributed to malignant transformation; there are reported precedents of leukemias that are dependent on γc cytokine signaling. Furthermore, the disease may have provided unique circumstances resulting in oncogenic interaction between multiple factors. The combination of LMO2 upregulation, unregulated γc expression, and the disease-related immune deficiency preventing detection and eradication of malignant clones may have allowed subclones with additional oncogenic mutations to emerge. These possibilities are currently being investigated further.

The implications for the development of gene therapy mediated by integrating vectors are significant. First, there will be more interest in the integration of vectors into protooncogenes, and preclinical trials and toxicity studies will have to address site of integration issues. Second, vector design may be modified to incorporate tissue-specific regulatory elements, self-inactivating viral LTR sequences and insulators to prevent the inadvertent activation of neighboring genes following integration. Third, it may be desirable to incorporate a suicide gene into the vectors so that transduced clones that become malignant can be eradicated pharmacologically. Finally, research in understanding the processes that determine the site of vector integration may be expanded, with the aim of learning how to manipulate the mechanisms involved and direct insertion into an inert part of the genome.

While there is still great skepticism regarding the future of gene therapy, the majority of workers remain optimistic that many of the problems encountered are not substantially more difficult than those seen in other fields where new technology is under development, including transplantation and cancer chemotherapy.

6
From Bench to Clinic – HSV-mediated Gene Therapy of Pain as an Example

One example of therapeutic gene transfer is the use of HSV vectors in the treatment of chronic pain. Chronic pain is defined as pain that persists beyond the course of the acute insult, or pain that accompanies a chronic primary process that cannot be cured. Although the majority of chronic pain can be effectively treated with existing remedies, a significant minority of patients cannot, resulting in substantial morbidity and cost. The neuroanatomic pathways involved in pain are identical to those involved in the perception of acute painful stimuli, but alterations in gene expression in neuronal and nonneuronal elements at many levels of the neuraxis produce an altered substrate that result in symptoms that are refractory to medical management. The traditional pharmacologic approach to chronic pain is epitomized by the search for small molecule agonists that would be selective for elements in the pain pathway, but most of those components are not unique to nociceptive neurotransmission.

Opioid receptors, for example, are present at all levels of the neuraxis, including the central and peripheral terminals of primary nociceptors, second-order neurons in dorsal horn of spinal cord, and nuclei in the brain and brain stem and are also found in nonneural tissues including bladder, gut, and inflammatory cells. Even though opiate drugs are highly effective, their continuous use for treatment of chronic pain is limited by side effects that occur because activation of receptors in nonnociceptive pathways results in sedation, constipation, urinary retention, and respiratory suppression. Continued use results in tolerance so that increasing doses of the drug are required to achieve maintain the therapeutic effect and abuse is a potential problem. The gene therapy approach to the treatment of chronic pain exploits gene transfer to achieve local release of neuroactive peptides to reduce pain. HSV-based vectors are uniquely suited to this purpose because subcutaneous inoculation of the vector can be used to transduce dorsal root ganglia (DRG) in an anatomically predictable manner to effect the release of analgesic peptides from axonal terminals of the DRG neurons in the dorsal horn of spinal cord.

Animal models have been developed that recapitulate the essential features of inflammatory pain, neuropathic pain, and pain caused by metastatic cancer, which can be used to predict the response of human patients to analgesic drugs. We tested HSV vectors in each of these models. We constructed an HSV vector containing the coding sequence for human proenkephalin under the control of a human cytomegalovirus immediate-early promoter (HCMV IEp) in a vector background deleted for a single essential immediate-early HSV gene (*ICP4*), termed *vector SHPE*. We demonstrated *in vitro* that neurons transduced with the vector produce human proenkephalin, and release enkephalin into the medium, and demonstrated *in vivo* that subcutaneous inoculation of the vector resulted in transduction of DRG neurons and production of proenkephalin *in vivo*. In the formalin test, a model of inflammatory pain created by injection of a dilute solution of formalin, inoculation with SHPE produced a substantial and statistically significant reduction pain that was reversed by intrathecal naltrexone, a relatively selective delta opiate receptor antagonist. The effect of vector inoculation was maximal in animals tested one week after vector administration, waned over the subsequent three weeks, but could be reestablished by reinoculation of the vector.

Pain resulting from nerve damage (neuropathic pain) can be modeled by selective ligation of a single spinal nerve. Subcutaneous inoculation of SHPE into the plantar surface of the foot one week after selective L5 spinal nerve ligation provided an antiallodynic effect that began one week after inoculation and persisted for five weeks. Like the analgesic effect of SHPE in the formalin model of inflammatory pain, the antiallodynic effect of SHPE inoculation in neuropathic pain was reversed by intraperitoneal naloxone, and reinoculation of the vector after the initial effect had waned promptly reestablished the allodynic effect. The antiallodynic effect of SHPE-mediated enkephalin expression was continuous throughout the day, was additive with morphine, shifting the ED_{50} for morphine from 1.8 mg kg^{-1} to 0.15 mg kg^{-1}, and the effect of SHPE-mediated enkephalin expression persisted in the face of tolerance to morphine. Animals treated with the maximum dose of morphine (10 mg kg^{-1} twice a day) developed tolerance by one week, so that

morphine no longer provided any antiallodynic effect. In contrast, animals that had been inoculated with SHPE continued to demonstrate an antiallodynic effect even after three weeks of morphine treatment.

An important consideration in moving from preclinical animal studies to human trials is the selection of an appropriate condition so that the potential risks of the novel therapy are justified, and even though chronic pain is a cause of significant suffering, the condition itself is not life threatening. Therefore, we examined the analgesic effect of the subcutaneous inoculation of SHPE in a murine model of pain resulting from cancer metastatic to bone. Tumor-bearing mice develop a spontaneous pain behavior that can be rated. Animals inoculated with a control vector manifested spontaneous pain-related behavior that increased over the subsequent two weeks, while mice inoculated with SHPE one week after establishment of the tumor showed a substantial and statistically significant reduction in pain-related behavior, and an effect that was synergistic with morphine and could be reversed by intrathecal naltrexone.

On the basis of the preclinical data in the several different rodent models of pain, we are moving forward with plans for a human trial. The plans for this phase I/II safety/dose-escalation trial of the proenkephalin-expressing vector was reviewed by the recombinant DNA Advisory Committee (RAC) of the NIH in June 2002, and the request for an investigational new drug (IND) waiver to the Food and Drug Administration has been submitted. The HSV vector for the human trial will be deleted for two IE HSV genes (*ICP4* and *ICP27*) and contains deletions in the promoters for two other IE genes (*ICP22* and *ICP47*). The proenkephalin transgene has been placed in both copies of ICP4, so that in the unlikely event of recombination with a latent wild-type virus, the recombinants would be replication defective. In the trial, we will enroll patients with cancer metastatic to a vertebral body, resulting in pain refractory to maximal medical management. The primary outcome of this phase I/II trial will involve standard measures of safety assessed by common criteria. Secondary measures will include an evaluation of the focal pain using an analog pain "thermometer", global measures of total pain using a similar tool, as well as assessment of pain-related phenomena such as sleep and depression and the concurrent use of analgesic medication, including opiate drugs.

In animal models, HSV-mediated gene transfer to DRG neurons achieved by subcutaneous inoculation is effective in expressing peptides to be released locally from sensory neurons to achieve focal therapeutic effects. The proposed human trial will allow us to determine whether the same approach may be used in the treatment of patients, and will be the first step in the use of this therapy for pain and polyneuropathy. Proenkephalin is not the only transgene that may be used in gene therapy for chronic pain. In other studies, we have found that HSV-mediated expression of glutamic acid decarboxylase, antiinflammatory peptides (interleukin 4 or the tumor necrosis factor alpha soluble receptor), or the glial cell derived neurotrophic factor, all have analgesic effects in different models of chronic pain. HSV-based vectors may ultimately serve as the platform to deliver a number of different genes whose products have analgesic properties in the treatment of specific types of chronic pain.

7
Future Prospects – What will Gene Therapy Likely be About in 10 Years?

Gene transfer as a method to alter the biology of cells has almost unlimited potential providing safe and effective methods for gene delivery and expression can be developed. It appears likely that this can be achieved and indeed certain human viruses have largely accomplished this task. Vectors that integrate have great potential for gene delivery to dividing cells where long-term expression is required. The retroviruses are currently the vector of choice and lentiviruses in particular may become the dominant vector type since cell division is not required for vector entry into the nucleus and integration can be mediated by the vector integrase. However, integration is essentially random with a propensity for integrating at sites of open chromatin and active genes. The problems associated with gene inactivation by insertional mutagenesis or the activation of potential oncogenes is not just theoretical, posing safety concerns with the use of these vectors. Future work on the development of these viruses will endeavor to target integration, remove promiscuous enhancers in the vector LTRs, and attempt to take advantage of tissue-specific enhancers that may limit expression to certain stages of development or cell type. Also, the possibility exists that certain phage integrases may be useful if expressed from the vector along with movable elements that might achieve targeting to specific loci or chromosomal sites. Another important development may result from a better understanding of mechanisms of vector uncoating and gene expression. For example, AAV transduces many cell types with poor efficiency, requiring large multiplicities to achieve transgene expression. Uncoating may be enhanced through use of different serotypes or through manipulation of the capsid. AAV may also be delivered in recombinant form within the genome of larger vectors such as HSV, where transient expression of rep, for example, may induce excision and subsequent integration of the AAV genome into a safe site within chromosome 19. HSV has a very large packaging potential, which can be fully realized if there were a packaging cell line available. The engineering of such cell lines is possible and may be achieved in the coming years. Other possibilities for improvement involve the establishment of precise methods of vector targeting and transgene expression. There are likely to be numerous viral or cellular genomic sequences that act in cis to influence transgene expression and these must be discovered, characterized, and applied in the context of the virus genome. The rules that govern gene expression in the virus genome are still unclear. Engineering the virus coat or envelope will continue until suitable methods are developed. Secondary targeting at the nuclear membrane may also be possible. The future will also include multigene therapies requiring the interaction of multiple gene functions to achieve a therapeutic outcome including genes, which trigger the differentiation and survival of stem cells that can rebuild damaged tissues. In general, gene transfer may become a very important tool for directed tissue development.

Diseases that are the most likely targets for gene therapy within the next 5 to 8 years will include the modification of responses in the host that either lead to improved immunity to infectious diseases or cancer, alter the host response to painful stimuli, reduce autoimmune reactions, and improve transplant tissue survival or improve the outcome for damaged tissue such as ischemia in the heart. Also, in the short term, it is likely that certain metabolic diseases such as hemophilia or inborn errors of metabolism that result in immunodeficiency or toxic metabolic states will show signs of success. Longer term, the use of gene transfer for tissue engineering, and stem cell applications for tissue repair will began to unfold. While these comments are only speculative, there is reason to believe that many of these applications are nearing the era of real benefit to patients and even if only a few of these applications are successful in the near term, gene therapy as a practical modality of medical therapy will have reached its early stages of promise.

See also Liposome Gene Transfection; Medicinal Chemistry; Somatic Gene Therapy.

Bibliography

Books and reviews

Bagley, J., Iacomini, J. (2003) Gene therapy progress and prospects: gene therapy in organ transplantation, *Gene Ther.* **10**, 605–611.

Burton, E.A., Glorioso, J.C., Fink, D.J. (2003) Gene therapy progress and prospects: Parkinson's disease, *Gene Ther.* **10**, 1721–1727.

Burton, E.A., Fink, D.J., Glorioso, J.C. (2002) Gene delivery using herpes simplex virus vectors, *DNA Cell Biol.* **21**, 915–936.

Burton, E.A., Wechuck, J.B., Wendell, S.K., Goins, W.F., Fink, D.J., Glorioso, J.C. (2001) Multiple applications for replication-defective Herpes Simplex virus vectors, *Stem Cells* **19**, 358–377.

Cheng, S.H., Smith, A.E. (2003) Gene therapy progress and prospects: gene therapy of lysosomal storage disorders, *Gene Ther.* **10**, 1275–1281.

Fields, B.N., Knipe, D.M., Howley, P.M. (1996) *Fields Virology*, 3rd Edition Lippincott- Raven, Philadelphia, PA.

Griesenbach, U., Ferrari, S., Geddes, D.M., Alton, E.W. (2002) Gene therapy progress and prospects: cystic fibrosis, *Gene Ther.* **9**, 1344–1350.

Khan, T.A., Sellke, F.W., Laham, R.J. (2003) Gene therapy progress and prospects: therapeutic angiogenesis for limb and myocardial ischemia, *Gene Ther.* **10**, 285–291.

Luciw, P.A. (1996) Chapter 60: Human Immunodeficiency Viruses and Their Replication, in: Field's, B.N., Knipe, D.M., Howley, P.M. (Eds.) *Fields Virology*, Lippincott-Raven, Philadelphia, PA pp. 1881–1952.

Niidome, T., Huang, L. (2002) Gene therapy progress and prospects: nonviral vectors, *Gene Ther.* **9**, 1647–1652.

Roizman, B., Sears, A.E. (1996) Chapter 72: Herpes Simplex Viruses and Their Replication, in: Fields, B.N., Knipe, D.M., Howley, P.M. (Eds.) *Fields Virology*, Lippincott-Raven, Philadelphia, PA pp. 2231–2295.

St George, J.A. (2003) Gene therapy progress and prospects: adenoviral vectors, *Gene Ther.* **10**, 1135–1141.

Stecenko, A.A., Brigham, K.L. (2003) Gene therapy progress and prospects: alpha-1 antitrypsin, *Gene Ther.* **10**, 95–99.

Walsh, C.E. (2003) Gene therapy progress and prospects: gene therapy for the hemophilias, *Gene Ther.* **10**, 999–1003.

Primary Literature

Aitken, M.L., Moss, R.B., Waltz, D.A., Dovey, M.E., Tonelli, M.R., McNamara, S.C., Gibson, R.L., Ramsey, B.W., Carter, B.J., Reynolds, T.C. (2001) A phase I study of aerosolized administration of tgAAVCF to cystic fibrosis subjects with mild lung disease, *Hum. Gene Ther.* **12**, 1907–1916.

Aiuti, A., Vai, S., Mortellaro, A., Casorati, G., Ficara, F., Andolfi, G., Ferrari, G., Tabucchi, A., Carlucci, F., Ochs, H.D., Notarangelo, L.D., Roncarolo, M.G., Bordignon, C. (2002) Immune reconstitution in ADA-SCID after PBL gene therapy and discontinuation of enzyme replacement, *Nat. Med.* **8**, 423–425.

Aiuti, A., Slavin, S., Aker, M., Ficara, F., Deola, S., Mortellaro, A., Morecki, S., Andolfi, G.,

Tabucchi, A., Carlucci, F., Marinello, E., Cattaneo, F., Vai, S., Servida, P., Miniero, R., Roncarolo, M.G., Bordignon, C. (2002) Correction of ADA-SCID by stem cell gene therapy combined with nonmyeloablative conditioning, *Science* **296**, 2410–2413.

Akkina, R.K., Walton, R.M., Chen, M.L., Li, Q.X., Planelles, V., Chen, I.S. (1996) High-efficiency gene transfer into CD34+ cells with a human immunodeficiency virus type 1-based retroviral vector pseudotyped with vesicular stomatitis virus envelope glycoprotein G, *J. Virol.* **70**, 2581–2585.

Amalfitano, A., Hauser, M.A., Hu, H., Serra, D., Begy, C.R., Chamberlain, J.S. (1998) Production and characterization of improved adenovirus vectors with the E1, E2b, and E3 genes deleted, *J. Virol.* **72**, 926–933.

Anderson, D.B., Laquerre, S., Goins, W.F., Cohen, J.B., Glorioso, J.C. (2000) Pseudotyping of glycoprotein D-deficient herpes simplex virus type 1 with vesicular stomatitis virus glycoprotein G enables mutant virus attachment and entry., *J. Virol.* **74**, 2481–2487.

Armentano, D., Thompson, A.R., Darlington, G., Woo, S.L. (1990) Expression of human factor IX in rabbit hepatocytes by retrovirus-mediated gene transfer: potential for gene therapy of hemophilia B, *Proc. Natl. Acad. Sci. U. S. A.* **87**, 6141–6145.

Babiss, L.E., Young, C.S., Fisher, P.B., Ginsberg, H.S. (1983) Expression of adenovirus E1a and E1b gene products and the Escherichia coli XGPRT gene in KB cells, *J. Virol.* **46**, 454–465.

Bagley, J., Iacomini, J. (2003) Gene therapy progress and prospects: gene therapy in organ transplantation, *Gene Ther.* **10**, 605–611.

Bai, Q., Burton, E.A., Goins, W.F., Glorioso, J.C. (2002) Modifying the tropism of HSV vectors for gene therapy applications, in: *Vector Targeting for Therapeutic Gene Delivery*, Douglas, J., Curiel, D. (Eds.) John Wiley & Sons, New York.

Barr, D., Tubb, J., Ferguson, D., Scaria, A., Lieber, A., Wilson, C., Perkins, J., Kay, M.A. (1995) Strain related variations in adenovirally mediated transgene expression from mouse hepatocytes in vivo: comparisons between immunocompetent and immunodeficient inbred strains, *Gene Ther.* **2**, 151–155.

Batshaw, M.L., Roan, Y., Jung, A.L., Rosenberg, L.A., Brusilow, S.W. (1980) Cerebral dysfunction in asymptomatic carriers of ornithine transcarbamylase deficiency, *N. Engl. J. Med.* **302**, 482–485.

Bellon, G., Michel-Calemard, L., Thouvenot, D., Jagneaux, V., Poitevin, F., Malcus, C., Accart, N., Layani, M.P., Aymard, M., Bernon, H., Bienvenu, J., Courtney, M., Doring, G., Gilly, B., Gilly, R., Lamy, D., Levrey, H., Morel, Y., Paulin, C., Perraud, F., Rodillon, L., Sene, C., So, S., Touraine-Moulin, F., Pavirani, A., et al. (1997) Aerosol administration of a recombinant adenovirus expressing CFTR to cystic fibrosis patients: a phase I clinical trial, *Hum. Gene Ther.* **8**, 15–25.

Ben-Gary, H., McKinney, R.L., Rosengart, T., Lesser, M.L., Crystal, R.G. (2002) Systemic interleukin-6 responses following administration of adenovirus gene transfer vectors to humans by different routes, *Mol. Ther.* **6**, 287–297.

Bensadoun, J.C., Pereira de Almeida, L., Fine, E.G., Tseng, J.L., Deglon, N., Aebischer, P. (2003) Comparative study of GDNF delivery systems for the CNS: polymer rods, encapsulated cells, and lentiviral vectors, *J. Controlled Release* **87**, 107–115.

Blaese, R.M., Culver, K.W., Miller, A.D., Carter, C.S., Fleisher, T., Clerici, M., Shearer, G., Chang, L., Chiang, Y., Tolstoshev, P., et al. (1995) T lymphocyte-directed gene therapy for ADA-SCID: initial trial results after 4 years, *Science* **270**, 475–480.

Bloom, D.C., Lokensgard, J.R., Maidment, N.T., Feldman, L.T., Stevens, J.G. (1994) Long-term expression of genes in vivo using non-replicating HSV vectors, *Gene Ther.* **1**, S36–S38.

Brigham, K.L., Lane, K.B., Meyrick, B., Stecenko, A.A., Strack, S., Cannon, D.R., Caudill, M., Canonico, A.E. (2000) Transfection of nasal mucosa with a normal alpha1-antitrypsin gene in alpha1-antitrypsin-deficient subjects: comparison with protein therapy, *Hum. Gene Ther.* **11**, 1023–1032.

Buning, H., Ried, M.U., Perabo, L., Gerner, F.M., Huttner, N.A., Enssle, J., Hallek, M. (2003) Receptor targeting of adeno-associated virus vectors, *Gene Ther.* **10**, 1142–1151.

Burton, E.A., Glorioso, J.C., Fink, D.J. (2003) Gene therapy progress and prospects: Parkinson's disease, *Gene Ther.* **10**, 1721–1727.

Burton, E.A., Bai, Q., Goins, W.F., Glorioso, J.C. (2001) Targeting gene expression using HSV vectors, *Adv. Drug Delivery Rev.* **53**, 155–170.

Burton, E.A., Wechuck, J.B., Wendell, S.K., Goins, W.F., Fink, D.J., Glorioso, J.C. (2001) Multiple Applications For Replication-Defective Herpes Simplex Virus Vectors, *Stem Cells* **19**, 358–377.

Caplen, N.J., Alton, E.W., Middleton, P.G., Dorin, J.R., Stevenson, B.J., Gao, X., Durham, S.R., Jeffery, P.K., Hodson, M.E., Coutelle, C., et al. (1995) Liposome-mediated CFTR gene transfer to the nasal epithelium of patients with cystic fibrosis, *Nat. Med.* **1**, 39–46.

Cavazzana-Calvo, M., Hacein-Bey, S., de Saint Basile, G., Gross, F., Yvon, E., Nusbaum, P., Selz, F., Hue, C., Certain, S., Casanova, J.L., Bousso, P., Deist, F.L., Fischer, A. (2000) Gene therapy of human severe combined immunodeficiency (SCID)-X1 disease, *Science* **288**, 669–672.

Chao, H., Monahan, P.E., Liu, Y., Samulski, R.J., Walsh, C.E. (2001) Sustained and complete phenotype correction of hemophilia B mice following intramuscular injection of AAV1 serotype vectors, *Mol. Ther.* **4**, 217–222.

Chao, H., Liu, Y., Rabinowitz, J., Li, C., Samulski, R.J., Walsh, C.E. (2000) Several log increase in therapeutic transgene delivery by distinct adeno-associated viral serotype vectors, *Mol. Ther.* **2**, 619–623.

Chen, X., Schmidt, M.C., Goins, W.F., Glorioso, J.C. (1995) Two herpes simplex virus type 1 latency-active promoters differ in their contributions to latency-associated transcript expression during lytic and latent infections, *J. Virol.* **69**, 7899–7908.

Chow, C.M., Athanassiadou, A., Raguz, S., Psiouri, L., Harland, L., Malik, M., Aitken, M.A., Grosveld, F., Antoniou, M. (2002) LCR-mediated, long-term tissue-specific gene expression within replicating episomal plasmid and cosmid vectors, *Gene Ther.* **9**, 327–336.

Colombo, F., Zanusso, M., Casentini, L., Cavaggioni, A., Franchin, E., Calvi, P., Palu, G. (1997) Gene stereotactic neurosurgery for recurrent malignant gliomas, *Stereotact. Funct. Neurosurg.* **68**, 245–251.

Corbeau, P., Kraus, G., Wong-Staal, F. (1996) Efficient gene transfer by a human immunodeficiency virus type 1 (HIV-1)-derived vector utilizing a stable HIV packaging cell line, *Proc. Natl. Acad. Sci. U. S. A.* **93**, 14070–14075.

Croyle, M.A., Chirmule, N., Zhang, Y., Wilson, J.M. (2002) PEGylation of E1-deleted adenovirus vectors allows significant gene expression on readministration to liver, *Hum. Gene Ther.* **13**, 1887–1900.

Crystal, R.G., McElvaney, N.G., Rosenfeld, M.A., Chu, C.S., Mastrangeli, A., Hay, J.G., Brody, S.L., Jaffe, H.A., Eissa, N.T., Danel, C. (1994) Administration of an adenovirus containing the human CFTR cDNA to the respiratory tract of individuals with cystic fibrosis, *Nat. Genet.* **8**, 42–51.

Curiel, D.T. (1999) Strategies to adapt adenoviral vectors for targeted delivery, *Ann. N. Y. Acad. Sci.* **886**, 158–171.

David, A., Chetritt, J., Guillot, C., Tesson, L., Heslan, J.M., Cuturi, M.C., Soulillou, J.P., Anegon, I. (2000) Interleukin-10 produced by recombinant adenovirus prolongs survival of cardiac allografts in rats, *Gene Ther.* **7**, 505–510.

Davidson, B.L., Allen, E.D., Kozarsky, K.F., Wilson, J.M., Roessler, B.J. (1993) A model system for in vivo gene transfer into the central nervous system using an adenoviral vector, *Nat. Genet.* **3**, 219–223.

DeLuca, N.A., McCarthy, A.M., Schaffer, P.A. (1985) Isolation and characterization of deletion mutants of herpes simplex virus type 1 in the gene encoding immediate-early regulatory protein ICP4, *J. Virol.* **56**, 558–570.

DeMatteo, R.P., Chu, G., Ahn, M., Chang, E., Burke, C., Raper, S.E., Barker, C.F., Markmann, J.F. (1997) Immunologic barriers to hepatic adenoviral gene therapy for transplantation, *Transplantation* **63**, 315–319.

Desmaris, N., Bosch, A., Salaun, C., Petit, C., Prevost, M.C., Tordo, N., Perrin, P., Schwartz, O., de Rocquigny, H., Heard, J.M. (2001) Production and neurotropism of lentivirus vectors pseudotyped with lyssavirus envelope glycoproteins, *Mol. Ther.* **4**, 149–156.

Dmitriev, I.P., Kashentseva, E.A., Curiel, D.T. (2002) Engineering of adenovirus vectors containing heterologous peptide sequences in the C terminus of capsid protein IX, *J. Virol.* **76**, 6893–6899.

Dobson, A.T., Margolis, T.P., Gomes, W.A., Feldman, L.T. (1995) In vivo deletion analysis

of the herpes simplex virus type 1 latency-associated transcript promoter, *J. Virol.* **69**, 2264–2270.

Dobson, A.T., Margolis, T.P., Sedarati, F., Stevens, J.G., Feldman, L.T. (1990) A latent, nonpathogenic HSV-1-derived vector stably expresses beta-galactosidase in mouse neurons, *Neuron* **5**, 353–360.

Dobson, A.T., Sederati, F., Devi Rao, G., Flanagan, W.M., Farrell, M.J., Stevens, J.G., Wagner, E.K., Feldman, L.T. (1989) Identification of the latency-associated transcript promoter by expression of rabbit beta-globin mRNA in mouse sensory nerve ganglia latently infected with a recombinant herpes simplex virus, *J. Virol.* **63**, 3844–3851.

Dolman, C.L., Clasen, R.A., Dorovini-Zis, K. (1988) Severe cerebral damage in ornithine transcarbamylase deficiency, *Clin. Neuropathol.* **7**, 10–15.

Dull, T., Zufferey, R., Kelly, M., Mandel, R.J., Nguyen, M., Trono, D., Naldini, L. (1998) A third-generation lentivirus vector with a conditional packaging system, *J. Virol.* **72**, 8463–8471.

During, M.J., Kaplitt, M.G., Stern, M.B., Eidelberg, D. (2001) Subthalamic GAD gene transfer in Parkinson disease patients who are candidates for deep brain stimulation, *Hum. Gene Ther.* **12**, 1589–1591.

Einfeld, D.A., Schroeder, R., Roelvink, P.W., Lizonova, A., King, C.R., Kovesdi, I., Wickham, T.J. (2001) Reducing the native tropism of adenovirus vectors requires removal of both CAR and integrin interactions, *J. Virol.* **75**, 11284–11291.

Emery, D.W., Yannaki, E., Tubb, J., Stamatoyannopoulos, G. (2000) A chromatin insulator protects retrovirus vectors from chromosomal position effects, *Proc. Natl. Acad. Sci. U. S. A.* **97**, 9150–9155.

Emi, N., Friedmann, T., Yee, J.K. (1991) Pseudotype formation of murine leukemia virus with the G protein of vesicular stomatitis virus, *J. Virol.* **65**, 1202–1207.

Ferrari, G., Rossini, S., Giavazzi, R., Maggioni, D., Nobili, N., Soldati, M., Ungers, G., Mavilio, F., Gilboa, E., Bordignon, C. (1991) An in vivo model of somatic cell gene therapy for human severe combined immunodeficiency, *Science* **251**, 1363–1366.

Fields, B.N., Knipe, D.M., Howley, P.M. (1996) *Fields Virology*, 3rd Edition, Lippincott-Raven, Philadelphia, PA.

Fink, J.K., Correll, P.H., Perry, L.K., Brady, R.O., Karlsson, S. (1990) Correction of glucocerebrosidase deficiency after retroviral-mediated gene transfer into hematopoietic progenitor cells from patients with Gaucher disease, *Proc. Natl. Acad. Sci. U. S. A.* **87**, 2334–2338.

Fink, D.J., Sternberg, L.R., Weber, P.C., Mata, M., Goins, W.F., Glorioso, J.C. (1992) In vivo expression of beta-galactosidase in hippocampal neurons by HSV-mediated gene transfer, *Hum. Gene Ther.* **3**, 11–19.

Frenkel, N., Singer, O., Kwong, A.D. (1994) Minireview: the herpes simplex virus amplicon–a versatile defective virus vector, *Gene. Ther.* **1**(Suppl 1), S40–S46.

Friedman, R.L. (1985) Expression of human adenosine deaminase using a transmissible murine retrovirus vector system, *Proc. Natl. Acad. Sci. U. S. A.* **82**, 703–707.

Furlan, R., Poliani, P.L., Marconi, P.C., Bergami, A., Ruffini, F., Adorini, L., Glorioso, J.C., Comi, G., Martino, G. (2001) Central nervous system gene therapy with interleukin-4 inhibits progression of ongoing relapsing-remitting autoimmune encephalomyelitis in Biozzi AB/H mice, *Gene Ther.* **8**, 13–19.

Gansbacher, B. (2003) Report of a second serious adverse event in a clinical trial of gene therapy for X-linked severe combined immune deficiency (X-SCID). Position of the European Society of Gene Therapy (ESGT), *J. Gene. Med.* **5**, 261–262.

Gill, S.S., Patel, N.K., Hotton, G.R., O'Sullivan, K., McCarter, R., Bunnage, M., Brooks, D.J., Svendsen, C.N., Heywood, P. (2003) Direct brain infusion of glial cell line-derived neurotrophic factor in Parkinson disease, *Nat. Med.* **9**, 589–595.

Giraud, C., Winocour, E., Berns, K.I. (1994) Site-specific integration by adeno-associated virus is directed by a cellular DNA sequence, *Proc. Natl. Acad. Sci. U. S. A.* **91**, 10039–10043.

Girod, A., Ried, M., Wobus, C., Lahm, H., Leike, K., Kleinschmidt, J., Deleage, G., Hallek, M. (1999) Genetic capsid modifications allow efficient re-targeting of adeno-associated virus type 2, *Nat. Med.* **5**, 1438.

Goins, W.F., Lee, K.A., Cavalcoli, J.D., O'Malley, M.E., DeKosky, S.T., Fink, D.J., Glorioso, J.C. (1999) Herpes simplex virus type 1 vector-mediated expression of nerve growth factor protects dorsal root ganglion neurons from peroxide toxicity, *J. Virol.* **73**, 519–532.

Goins, W.F., Sternberg, L.R., Croen, K.D., Krause, P.R., Hendricks, R.L., Fink, D.J., Straus, S.E., Levine, M., Glorioso, J.C. (1994) A novel latency-active promoter is contained within the herpes simplex virus type 1 UL flanking repeats, *J. Virol.* **68**, 2239–2252.

Goins, W.F., Yoshimura, N., Phelan, M.W., Yokoyama, T., Fraser, M.O., Ozawa, H., Bennett, N.J., de Groat, W.C., Glorioso, J.C., Chancellor, M.B. (2001) Herpes simplex virus mediated nerve growth factor expression in bladder and afferent neurons: potential treatment for diabetic bladder dysfunction, *J. Urol.* **165**, 1748–1754.

Gordon, Y.J., Johnson, B., Romanowski, E., Araullo Cruz, T. (1988) RNA complementary to herpes simplex virus type 1 ICP0 gene demonstrated in neurons of human trigeminal ganglia, *J. Virol.* **62**, 1832–1835.

Goss, J.R., Goins, W.F., Lacomis, D., Mata, M., Glorioso, J.C., Fink, D.J. (2002) Herpes simplex-mediated gene transfer of nerve growth factor protects against peripheral neuropathy in streptozotocin-induced diabetes in the mouse, *Diabetes* **51**, 2227–2232.

Goss, J.R., Mata, M., Goins, W.F., Wu, H.H., Glorioso, J.C., Fink, D.J. (2001) Antinociceptive effect of a genomic herpes simplex virus-based vector expressing human proenkephalin in rat dorsal root ganglion, *Gene Ther.* **8**, 551–556.

Grines, C.L., Watkins, M.W., Helmer, G., Penny, W., Brinker, J., Marmur, J.D., West, A., Rade, J.J., Marrott, P., Hammond, H.K., Engler, R.L. (2002) Angiogenic Gene Therapy (AGENT) trial in patients with stable angina pectoris, *Circulation* **105**, 1291–1297.

Guillot, C., Guillonneau, C., Mathieu, P., Gerdes, C.A., Menoret, S., Braudeau, C., Tesson, L., Renaudin, K., Castro, M.G., Lowenstein, P.R., Anegon, I. (2002) Prolonged blockade of CD40-CD40 ligand interactions by gene transfer of CD40Ig results in long-term heart allograft survival and donor-specific hyporesponsiveness, but does not prevent chronic rejection, *J. Immunol.* **168**, 1600–1609.

Guillot, C., Mathieu, P., Coathalem, H., Le Mauff, B., Castro, M.G., Tesson, L., Usal, C., Laumonier, T., Brouard, S., Soulillou, J.P., Lowenstein, P.R., Cuturi, M.C., Anegon, I. (2000) Tolerance to cardiac allografts via local and systemic mechanisms after adenovirus-mediated CTLA4Ig expression, *J. Immunol.* **164**, 5258–5268.

Hacein-Bey, S., Basile, G.D., Lemerle, J., Fischer, A., Cavazzana-Calvo, M. (1998) gammac gene transfer in the presence of stem cell factor, FLT-3L, interleukin-7 (IL-7), IL-1, and IL-15 cytokines restores T-cell differentiation from gammac(-) X-linked severe combined immunodeficiency hematopoietic progenitor cells in murine fetal thymic organ cultures, *Blood* **92**, 4090–4097.

Hacein-Bey, H., Cavazzana-Calvo, M., Le Deist, F., Dautry-Varsat, A., Hivroz, C., Riviere, I., Danos, O., Heard, J.M., Sugamura, K., Fischer, A., De Saint Basile, G. (1996) Gamma-c gene transfer into SCID X1 patients' B-cell lines restores normal high-affinity interleukin-2 receptor expression and function, *Blood* **87**, 3108–3116.

Hacein-Bey-Abina, S., von Kalle, C., Schmidt, M., Le Deist, F., Wulffraat, N., McIntyre, E., Radford, I., Villeval, J.L., Fraser, C.C., Cavazzana-Calvo, M., Fischer, A. (2003) A serious adverse event after successful gene therapy for X-linked severe combined immunodeficiency, *N. Engl. J. Med.* **348**, 255–256.

Hacein-Bey-Abina, S., Le Deist, F., Carlier, F., Bouneaud, C., Hue, C., De Villartay, J.P., Thrasher, A.J., Wulffraat, N., Sorensen, R., Dupuis-Girod, S., Fischer, A., Davies, E.G., Kuis, W., Leiva, L., Cavazzana-Calvo, M. (2002) Sustained correction of X-linked severe combined immunodeficiency by ex vivo gene therapy, *N. Engl. J. Med.* **346**, 1185–1193.

Haj-Ahmad, Y., Graham, F.L. (1986) Development of a helper-independent human adenovirus vector and its use in the transfer of the herpes simplex virus thymidine kinase gene, *J. Virol.* **57**, 267–274.

Hao, S., Mata, M., Goins, W., Glorioso, J.C., Fink, D.J. (2003) Transgene-mediated enkephalin release enhances the effect of morphine and evades tolerance to produce a sustained antiallodynic effect in neuropathic pain, *Pain* **102**, 135–142.

Harding, B.N., Leonard, J.V., Erdohazi, M. (1984) Ornithine carbamoyl transferase deficiency: a neuropathological study, *Eur. J. Pediatr.* **141**, 215–220.

Heim, D.A., Hanazono, Y., Giri, N., Wu, T., Childs, R., Sellers, S.E., Muul, L., Agricola, B.A., Metzger, M.E., Donahue, R.E., Tisdale, J.F., Dunbar, C.E. (2000) Introduction of a xenogeneic gene via hematopoietic stem cells leads to specific tolerance in a rhesus monkey model, *Mol. Ther.* **1**, 533–544.

Hermonat, P.L., Muzyczka, N. (1984) Use of adeno-associated virus as a mammalian DNA cloning vector: transduction of neomycin resistance into mammalian tissue culture cells, *Proc. Natl. Acad. Sci. U. S. A.* **81**, 6466–6470.

Hershfield, M.S. (1995) PEG-ADA: an alternative to haploidentical bone marrow transplantation and an adjunct to gene therapy for adenosine deaminase deficiency, *Hum. Mutat.* **5**, 107–112.

Hershfield, M.S., Chaffee, S., Sorensen, R.U. (1993) Enzyme replacement therapy with polyethylene glycol-adenosine deaminase in adenosine deaminase deficiency: overview and case reports of three patients, including two now receiving gene therapy, *Pediatr. Res.* **33**, S42–S47; discussion S47-8.

Hofmann, A., Nolan, G.P., Blau, H.M. (1996) Rapid retroviral delivery of tetracycline-inducible genes in a single autoregulatory cassette, *Proc. Natl. Acad. Sci. U. S. A.* **93**, 5185–5190.

Hoppe, U.C., Marban, E., Johns, D.C. (2000) Adenovirus-mediated inducible gene expression in vivo by a hybrid ecdysone receptor, *Mol. Ther.* **1**, 159–164.

Hyde, S.C., Southern, K.W., Gileadi, U., Fitzjohn, E.M., Mofford, K.A., Waddell, B.E., Gooi, H.C., Goddard, C.A., Hannavy, K., Smyth, S.E., Egan, J.J., Sorgi, F.L., Huang, L., Cuthbert, A.W., Evans, M.J., Colledge, W.H., Higgins, C.F., Webb, A.K., Gill, D.R. (2000) Repeat administration of DNA/liposomes to the nasal epithelium of patients with cystic fibrosis, *Gene Ther.* **7**, 1156–1165.

Iida, A., Chen, S.T., Friedmann, T., Yee, J.K. (1996) Inducible gene expression by retrovirus-mediated transfer of a modified tetracycline-regulated system, *J. Virol.* **70**, 6054–6059.

Im, S.A., Gomez Manzano, C., Fueyo, J., Liu, T.J., Ke, L.D., Kim, J.S., Lee, H.Y., Steck, P.A., Kyritsis, A.P., Yung, W.K. (1999) Antiangiogenesis treatment for gliomas: transfer of antisense-vascular endothelial growth factor inhibits tumor growth in vivo, *Cancer Res.* **59**, 895–900.

Kaiser, J. (2003) Gene therapy. Seeking the cause of induced leukemias in X-SCID trial, *Science* **299**, 495.

Kanno, H., Hattori, S., Sato, H., Murata, H., Huang, F.H., Hayashi, A., Suzuki, N., Yamamoto, I., Kawamoto, S., Minami, M., Miyatake, S., Shuin, T., Kaplitt, M.G. (1999) Experimental gene therapy against subcutaneously implanted glioma with a herpes simplex virus-defective vector expressing interferon-gamma, *Cancer Gene Ther.* **6**, 147–154.

Kantoff, P.W., Kohn, D.B., Mitsuya, H., Armentano, D., Sieberg, M., Zwiebel, J.A., Eglitis, M.A., McLachlin, J.R., Wiginton, D.A., Hutton, J.J., et al. (1986) Correction of adenosine deaminase deficiency in cultured human T and B cells by retrovirus-mediated gene transfer, *Proc. Natl. Acad. Sci. U. S. A.* **83**, 6563–6567.

Kashentseva, E.A., Seki, T., Curiel, D.T., Dmitriev, I.P. (2002) Adenovirus targeting to c-erbB-2 oncoprotein by single-chain antibody fused to trimeric form of adenovirus receptor ectodomain, *Cancer Res.* **62**, 609–616.

Kawada, T., Nakazawa, M., Nakauchi, S., Yamazaki, K., Shimamoto, R., Urabe, M., Nakata, J., Hemmi, C., Masui, F., Nakajima, T., Suzuki, J., Monahan, J., Sato, H., Masaki, T., Ozawa, K., Toyo-Oka, T. (2002) Rescue of hereditary form of dilated cardiomyopathy by rAAV-mediated somatic gene therapy: amelioration of morphological findings, sarcolemmal permeability, cardiac performances, and the prognosis of TO-2 hamsters, *Proc. Natl. Acad. Sci. U. S. A.* **99**, 901–906.

Kay, M.A., Manno, C.S., Ragni, M.V., Larson, P.J., Couto, L.B., McClelland, A., Glader, B., Chew, A.J., Tai, S.J., Herzog, R.W., Arruda, V., Johnson, F., Scallan, C., Skarsgard, E., Flake, A.W., High, K.A. (2000) Evidence for gene transfer and expression of factor IX in haemophilia B patients treated with an AAV vector, *Nat. Genet.* **24**, 257–261.

Keir, S.D., Mitchell, W.J., Feldman, L.T., Martin, J.R. (1995) Targeting and gene expression in spinal cord motor neurons following intramuscular inoculation of an HSV-1 vector, *J. Neurovirol.* **1**, 259–267.

Khan, T.A., Sellke, F.W., Laham, R.J. (2003) Gene therapy progress and prospects: therapeutic angiogenesis for limb and myocardial ischemia, *Gene Ther.* **10**, 285–291.

Kim, S.H., Chung, J.M. (1992) An experimental model for peripheral neuropathy produced by segmental spinal nerve ligation in the rat, *Pain* **50**, 355–363.

Kim, V.N., Mitrophanous, K., Kingsman, S.M., Kingsman, A.J. (1998) Minimal requirement for a lentivirus vector based on human immunodeficiency virus type 1, *J. Virol.* **72**, 811–816.

Kitada, T., Asakawa, S., Hattori, N., Matsumine, H., Yamamura, Y., Minoshima, S., Yokochi, M., Mizuno, Y., Shimizu, N. (1998) Mutations in the parkin gene cause autosomal recessive juvenile parkinsonism, *Nature* **392**, 605–608.

Knowles, M.R., Hohneker, K.W., Zhou, Z., Olsen, J.C., Noah, T.L., Hu, P.C., Leigh, M.W., Engelhardt, J.F., Edwards, L.J., Jones, K.R., et al. (1995) A controlled study of adenoviral-vector-mediated gene transfer in the nasal epithelium of patients with cystic fibrosis, *N. Engl. J. Med.* **333**, 823–831.

Kochanek, S., Schiedner, G., Volpers, C. (2001) High-capacity 'gutless' adenoviral vectors, *Curr. Opin. Mol. Ther.* **3**, 454–463.

Koeberl, D.D., Alexander, I.E., Halbert, C.L., Russell, D.W., Miller, A.D. (1997) Persistent expression of human clotting factor IX from mouse liver after intravenous injection of adeno-associated virus vectors, *Proc. Natl. Acad. Sci. U. S. A.* **94**, 1426–1431.

Kohn, D.B., Sadelain, M., Glorioso, J.C. (2003) Occurrence of leukaemia following gene therapy of X-linked SCID, *Nat. Rev. Cancer* **3**, 477–488.

Koponen, J.K., Kankkonen, H., Kannasto, J., Wirth, T., Hillen, W., Bujard, H., Yla-Herttuala, S. (2003) Doxycycline-regulated lentiviral vector system with a novel reverse transactivator rtTA2S-M2 shows a tight control of gene expression in vitro and in vivo, *Gene Ther.* **10**, 459–466.

Kordower, J.H., Emborg, M.E., Bloch, J., Ma, S.Y., Chu, Y., Leventhal, L., McBride, J., Chen, E.Y., Palfi, S., Roitberg, B.Z., Brown, W.D., Holden, J.E., Pyzalski, R., Taylor, M.D., Carvey, P., Ling, Z., Trono, D., Hantraye, P., Deglon, N., Aebischer, P. (2000) Neurodegeneration prevented by lentiviral vector delivery of GDNF in primate models of Parkinson's disease, *Science* **290**, 767–773.

Krisky, D.M., Marconi, P.C., Oligino, T., Rouse, R.J., Fink, D.J., Glorioso, J.C. (1997) Rapid method for construction of recombinant HSV gene transfer vectors, *Gene Ther.* **4**, 1120–1125.

Krisky, D.M., Marconi, P.C., Oligino, T.J., Rouse, R.J., Fink, D.J., Cohen, J.B., Watkins, S.C., Glorioso, J.C. (1998) Development of herpes simplex virus replication-defective multigene vectors for combination gene therapy applications, *Gene Ther.* **5**, 1517–1530.

Krisky, D.M., Wolfe, D., Goins, W.F., Marconi, P.C., Ramakrishnan, R., Mata, M., Rouse, R.J., Fink, D.J., Glorioso, J.C. (1998) Deletion of multiple immediate-early genes from herpes simplex virus reduces cytotoxicity and permits long-term gene expression in neurons, *Gene Ther.* **5**, 1593–1603.

Lachmann, R.H., Efstathiou, S. (1997) Utilization of the herpes simplex virus type 1 latency-associated regulatory region to drive stable reporter gene expression in the nervous system, *J. Virol.* **71**, 3197–3207.

Lamartina, S., Silvi, L., Roscilli, G., Casimiro, D., Simon, A.J., Davies, M.E., Shiver, J.W., Rinaudo, C.D., Zampaglione, I., Fattori, E., Colloca, S., Gonzalez Paz, O., Laufer, R., Bujard, H., Cortese, R., Ciliberto, G., Toniatti, C. (2003) Construction of an rtTA2(s)-m2/tts(kid)-based transcription regulatory switch that displays no basal activity, good inducibility, and high responsiveness to doxycycline in mice and non-human primates, *Mol. Ther.* **7**, 271–280.

Lang, F.F., Yung, W.K., Sawaya, R., Tofilon, P.J. (1999) Adenovirus-mediated p53 gene therapy for human gliomas, *Neurosurgery* **45**, 1093–1104.

Le Gal La Salle, G., Robert, J.J., Berrard, S., Ridoux, V., Stratford-Perricaudet, L.D., Perricaudet, M., Mallet, J. (1993) An adenovirus vector for gene transfer into neurons and glia in the brain, *Science* **259**, 988–990.

Ledley, F.D., Grenett, H.E., McGinnis-Shelnutt, M., Woo, S.L. (1986) Retroviral-mediated gene transfer of human phenylalanine hydroxylase into NIH 3T3 and hepatoma cells, *Proc. Natl. Acad. Sci. U. S. A.* **83**, 409–413.

Lee, L.Y., Patel, S.R., Hackett, N.R., Mack, C.A., Polce, D.R., El-Sawy, T., Hachamovitch, R., Zanzonico, P., Sanborn, T.A., Parikh, M., Isom, O.W., Crystal, R.G., Rosengart, T.K. (2000) Focal angiogen therapy using intramyocardial delivery of an adenovirus vector coding for vascular endothelial growth factor 121, *Ann. Thorac. Surg.* **69**, 14–23; discussion 23-4.

Li, X., Mukai, T., Young, D., Frankel, S., Law, P., Wong Staal, F. (1998) Transduction of CD34+ cells by a vesicular stomach virus protein G (VSV-G) pseudotyped HIV-1 vector. Stable gene expression in progeny cells, including dendritic cells, *J. Hum. Virol.* **1**, 346–352.

Lim, B., Apperley, J.F., Orkin, S.H., Williams, D.A. (1989) Long-term expression of human adenosine deaminase in mice transplanted with retrovirus-infected hematopoietic stem cells, *Proc. Natl. Acad. Sci. U. S. A.* **86**, 8892–8896.

Linden, R.M., Ward, P., Giraud, C., Winocour, E., Berns, K.I. (1996) Site-specific integration by adeno-associated virus, *Proc. Natl. Acad. Sci. U. S. A.* **93**, 11288–11294.

Loeser, J., Butler, S., Chapman, C., Turk, D. (2001) *Bonica's Management of Pain*, 3rd Edition, Lippincott Williams & Wilkins, Philadelphia, PA.

Loiler, S.A., Conlon, T.J., Song, S., Tang, Q., Warrington, K.H., Agarwal, A., Kapturczak, M., Li, C., Ricordi, C., Atkinson, M.A., Muzyczka, N., Flotte, T.R. (2003) Targeting recombinant adeno-associated virus vectors to enhance gene transfer to pancreatic islets and liver, *Gene Ther.* **10**, 1551–1558.

Losordo, D.W., Vale, P.R., Hendel, R.C., Milliken, C.E., Fortuin, F.D., Cummings, N., Schatz, R.A., Asahara, T., Isner, J.M., Kuntz, R.E. (2002) Phase 1/2 placebo-controlled, double-blind, dose-escalating trial of myocardial vascular endothelial growth factor 2 gene transfer by catheter delivery in patients with chronic myocardial ischemia, *Circulation* **105**, 2012–2018.

Luo, J., Kaplitt, M.G., Fitzsimons, H.L., Zuzga, D.S., Liu, Y., Oshinsky, M.L., During, M.J. (2002) Subthalamic GAD gene therapy in a Parkinson's disease rat model, *Science* **298**, 425–429.

Machein, M.R., Kullmer, J., Fiebich, B.L., Plate, K.H., Warnke, P.C. (1999) Vascular endothelial growth factor expression, vascular volume, and, capillary permeability in human brain tumors, *Neurosurgery* **44**, 732–740.

Mack, C.A., Song, W.R., Carpenter, H., Wickham, T.J., Kovesdi, I., Harvey, B.G., Magovern, C.J., Isom, O.W., Rosengart, T., Falck-Pedersen, E., Hackett, N.R., Crystal, R.G., Mastrangeli, A. (1997) Circumvention of anti-adenovirus neutralizing immunity by administration of an adenoviral vector of an alternate serotype, *Hum. Gene Ther.* **8**, 99–109.

Maestri, N.E., Clissold, D., Brusilow, S.W. (1999) Neonatal onset ornithine transcarbamylase deficiency: A retrospective analysis, *J. Pediatr.* **134**, 268–272.

Maestri, N.E., Brusilow, S.W., Clissold, D.B., Bassett, S.S. (1996) Long-term treatment of girls with ornithine transcarbamylase deficiency, *N. Engl. J. Med.* **335**, 855–859.

Manno, C.S., Chew, A.J., Hutchison, S., Larson, P.J., Herzog, R.W., Arruda, V.R., Tai, S.J., Ragni, M.V., Thompson, A., Ozelo, M., Couto, L.B., Leonard, D.G., Johnson, F.A., McClelland, A., Scallan, C., Skarsgard, E., Flake, A.W., Kay, M.A., High, K.A., Glader, B. (2003) AAV-mediated factor IX gene transfer to skeletal muscle in patients with severe hemophilia B, *Blood* **101**, 2963–2972.

Marconi, P., Tamura, M., Moriuchi, S., Krisky, D.M., Niranjan, A., Goins, W.F., Cohen, J.B., Glorioso, J.C. (2000) Connexin 43-enhanced suicide gene therapy using herpesviral vectors, *Mol. Ther.* **1**, 71–81.

Markowitz, D., Goff, S., Bank, A. (1988) Construction and use of a safe and efficient amphotropic packaging cell line, *Virology* **167**, 400–406.

Mastrangeli, A., Harvey, B.G., Yao, J., Wolff, G., Kovesdi, I., Crystal, R.G., Falck-Pedersen, E. (1996) "Sero-switch" adenovirus-mediated in vivo gene transfer: circumvention of anti-adenovirus humoral immune defenses against repeat adenovirus vector administration by changing the adenovirus serotype, *Hum. Gene Ther.* **7**, 79–87.

Mazarakis, N.D., Azzouz, M., Rohll, J.B., Ellard, F.M., Wilkes, F.J., Olsen, A.L., Carter, E.E., Barber, R.D., Baban, D.F., Kingsman, S.M., Kingsman, A.J., O'Malley, K., Mitrophanous, K.A. (2001) Rabies virus glycoprotein pseudotyping of lentiviral vectors enables retrograde axonal transport and access to the nervous system after peripheral delivery, *Hum. Mol. Genet.* **10**, 2109–2121.

McLaughlin, S.K., Collis, P., Hermonat, P.L., Muzyczka, N. (1988) Adeno-associated virus general transduction vectors: analysis of proviral structures, *J. Virol.* **62**, 1963–1973.

Mercier, S., Gahery-Segard, H., Monteil, M., Lengagne, R., Guillet, J.G., Eloit, M., Denesvre, C. (2002) Distinct roles of adenovirus vector-transduced dendritic cells, myoblasts, and endothelial cells in mediating an immune response against a transgene product, *J. Virol.* **76**, 2899–2911.

Miao, C.H., Ohashi, K., Patijn, G.A., Meuse, L., Ye, X., Thompson, A.R., Kay, M.A. (2000) Inclusion of the hepatic locus control region, an intron, and untranslated region increases and stabilizes hepatic factor IX gene expression in vivo but not in vitro, *Mol. Ther.* **1**, 522–532.

Min, W.P., Gorczynski, R., Huang, X.Y., Kushida, M., Kim, P., Obataki, M., Lei, J., Suri, R.M., Cattral, M.S. (2000) Dendritic cells genetically engineered to express Fas ligand induce donor-specific hyporesponsiveness and prolong allograft survival, *J. Immunol.* **164**, 161–167.

Miyanohara, A., Sharkey, M.F., Witztum, J.L., Steinberg, D., Friedmann, T. (1988) Efficient expression of retroviral vector-transduced human low density lipoprotein (LDL) receptor in LDL receptor-deficient rabbit fibroblasts in vitro, *Proc. Natl. Acad. Sci. U. S. A.* **85**, 6538–6542.

Miyoshi, H., Takahashi, M., Gage, F.H., Verma, I.M. (1997) Stable and efficient gene transfer into the retina using an HIV-based lentiviral vector, *Proc. Natl. Acad. Sci. U. S. A.* **94**, 10319–10323.

Miyoshi, H., Blomer, U., Takahashi, M., Gage, F.H., Verma, I.M. (1998) Development of a self-inactivating lentivirus vector, *J. Virol.* **72**, 8150–8157.

Miyoshi, H., Smith, K.A., Mosier, D.E., Verma, I.M., Torbett, B.E. (1999) Transduction of human CD34+ cells that mediate long-term engraftment of NOD/SCID mice by HIV vectors, *Science* **283**, 682–686.

Mizuguchi, H., Xu, Z.L., Sakurai, F., Mayumi, T., Hayakawa, T. (2003) Tight positive regulation of transgene expression by a single adenovirus vector containing the rtTA and tTS expression cassettes in separate genome regions, *Hum. Gene Ther.* **14**, 1265–1277.

Mizuguchi, H., Koizumi, N., Hosono, T., Utoguchi, N., Watanabe, Y., Kay, M.A., Hayakawa, T. (2001) A simplified system for constructing recombinant adenoviral vectors containing heterologous peptides in the HI loop of their fiber knob, *Gene Ther.* **8**, 730–735.

Molinier-Frenkel, V., Gahery-Segard, H., Mehtali, M., Le Boulaire, C., Ribault, S., Boulanger, P., Tursz, T., Guillet, J.G., Farace, F. (2000) Immune response to recombinant adenovirus in humans: capsid components from viral input are targets for vector-specific cytotoxic T lymphocytes, *J. Virol.* **74**, 7678–7682.

Moriuchi, S., Oligino, T., Krisky, D., Marconi, P., Fink, D., Cohen, J., Glorioso, J.C. (1998) Enhanced tumor cell killing in the presence of ganciclovir by herpes simplex virus type 1 vector-directed coexpression of human tumor necrosis factor-alpha and herpes simplex virus thymidine kinase, *Cancer Res.* **58**, 5731–5737.

Morral, N., O'Neal, W., Rice, K., Leland, M., Kaplan, J., Piedra, P.A., Zhou, H., Parks, R.J., Velji, R., Aguilar-Cordova, E., Wadsworth, S., Graham, F.L., Kochanek, S., Carey, K.D., Beaudet, A.L. (1999) Administration of helper-dependent adenoviral vectors and sequential delivery of different vector serotype for long-term liver-directed gene transfer in baboons, *Proc. Natl. Acad. Sci. U. S. A.* **96**, 12816–12821.

Mount, J.D., Herzog, R.W., Tillson, D.M., Goodman, S.A., Robinson, N., McCleland, M.L., Bellinger, D., Nichols, T.C., Arruda, V.R., Lothrop, C.D., Jr., High, K.A. (2002) Sustained phenotypic correction of hemophilia B dogs with a factor IX null mutation by liver-directed gene therapy, *Blood* **99**, 2670–2676.

Muller, O.J., Kaul, F., Weitzman, M.D., Pasqualini, R., Arap, W., Kleinschmidt, J.A., Trepel, M. (2003) Random peptide libraries displayed on adeno-associated virus to select for targeted gene therapy vectors, *Nat. Biotechnol.* **21**, 1040–1046.

Naldini, L., Blomer, U., Gallay, P., Ory, D., Mulligan, R., Gage, F.H., Verma, I.M., Trono, D. (1996) In vivo gene delivery and stable transduction of nondividing cells by a lentiviral vector, *Science* **272**, 263–267.

Nathwani, A.C., Davidoff, A.M., Hanawa, H., Hu, Y., Hoffer, F.A., Nikanorov, A., Slaughter, C., Ng, C.Y., Zhou, J., Lozier, J.N., Mandrell, T.D., Vanin, E.F., Nienhuis, A.W. (2002) Sustained high-level expression of human factor IX (hFIX) after liver-targeted delivery of recombinant adeno-associated virus encoding the hFIX gene in rhesus macaques, *Blood* **100**, 1662–1669.

Niranjan, A., Moriuchi, S., Lunsford, L.D., Kondziolka, D., Flickinger, J.C., Fellows, W., Rajendiran, S., Tamura, M., Cohen, J.B., Glorioso, J.C. (2000) Effective treatment of experimental glioblastoma by HSV vector-mediated TNFalpha and HSV-tk gene transfer in combination with radiosurgery and ganciclovir administration, *Mol. Ther.* **2**, 114–120.

No, D., Yao, T.P., Evans, R.M. (1996) Ecdysone-inducible gene expression in mammalian cells and transgenic mice, *Proc. Natl. Acad. Sci. U. S. A.* **93**, 3346–3351.

Noone, P.G., Hohneker, K.W., Zhou, Z., Johnson, L.G., Foy, C., Gipson, C., Jones, K., Noah, T.L., Leigh, M.W., Schwartzbach, C., Efthimiou, J., Pearlman, R., Boucher, R.C., Knowles, M.R. (2000) Safety and biological efficacy of a lipid-CFTR complex for gene transfer in the nasal epithelium of adult patients with cystic fibrosis, *Mol. Ther.* **1**, 105–114.

Oligino, T., Poliani, P.L., Wang, Y., Tsai, S.Y., O'Malley, B.W., Fink, D.J., Glorioso, J.C. (1998) Drug inducible transgene expression in brain using a herpes simplex virus vector, *Gene Ther.* **5**, 491–496.

Palmer, T.D., Hock, R.A., Osborne, W.R., Miller, A.D. (1987) Efficient retrovirus-mediated transfer and expression of a human adenosine deaminase gene in diploid skin fibroblasts from an adenosine deaminase-deficient human, *Proc. Natl. Acad. Sci. U. S. A.* **84**, 1055–1059.

Palmer, J.A., Branston, R.H., Lilley, C.E., Robinson, M.J., Groutsi, F., Smith, J., Latchman, D.S., Coffin, R.S. (2000) Development and optimization of herpes simplex virus vectors for multiple long-term gene delivery to the peripheral nervous system, *J. Virol.* **74**, 5604–5618.

Park, F., Ohashi, K., Kay, M.A. (2000) Therapeutic levels of human factor VIII and IX using HIV-1-based lentiviral vectors in mouse liver, *Blood* **96**, 1173–1176.

Parker, J.N., Gillespie, G.Y., Love, C.E., Randall, S., Whitley, R.J., Markert, J.M. (2000) From the cover: engineered herpes simplex virus expressing IL-12 in the treatment of experimental murine brain tumors, *Proc. Natl. Acad. Sci. U. S. A.* **97**, 2208–2213.

Paulus, W., Baur, I., Boyce, F.M., Breakefield, X.O., Reeves, S.A. (1996) Self-contained, tetracycline-regulated retroviral vector system for gene delivery to mammalian cells, *J. Virol.* **70**, 62–67.

Pawliuk, R., Westerman, K.A., Fabry, M.E., Payen, E., Tighe, R., Bouhassira, E.E., Acharya, S.A., Ellis, J., London, I.M., Eaves, C.J., Humphries, R.K., Beuzard, Y., Nagel, R.L., Leboulch, P. (2001) Correction of sickle cell disease in transgenic mouse models by gene therapy, *Science* **294**, 2368–2371.

Perricone, M.A., Morris, J.E., Pavelka, K., Plog, M.S., O'Sullivan, B.P., Joseph, P.M., Dorkin, H., Lapey, A., Balfour, R., Meeker, D.P., Smith, A.E., Wadsworth, S.C., St George, J.A. (2001) Aerosol and lobar administration of a recombinant adenovirus to individuals with cystic fibrosis. II. Transfection efficiency in airway epithelium, *Hum. Gene Ther.* **12**, 1383–1394.

Podsakoff, G.M. (2001) Lentiviral vectors approach the clinic but fall back: National Institutes of Health Recombinant DNA Advisory Committee review of a first clinical protocol for use of a lentiviral vector, *Mol. Ther.* **4**, 282–283.

Poliani, P.L., Brok, H., Furlan, R., Ruffini, F., Bergami, A., Desina, G., Marconi, P.C., Rovaris, M., Uccelli, A., Glorioso, J.C., Penna, G., Adorini, L., Comi, G., t Hart, B., Martino, G. (2001) Delivery to the central nervous system of a nonreplicative herpes simplex type 1 vector engineered with the interleukin 4 gene protects rhesus monkeys from hyperacute autoimmune encephalomyelitis, *Hum. Gene Ther.* **12**, 905–920.

Ponnazhagan, S., Erikson, D., Kearns, W.G., Zhou, S.Z., Nahreini, P., Wang, X.S., Srivastava, A. (1997) Lack of site-specific integration of the recombinant adeno-associated virus 2 genomes in human cells, *Hum. Gene Ther.* **8**, 275–284.

Puck, J.M., Deschenes, S.M., Porter, J.C., Dutra, A.S., Brown, C.J., Willard, H.F., Henthorn, P.S. (1993) The interleukin-2 receptor gamma chain maps to Xq13.1 and is mutated in X-linked severe combined immunodeficiency, SCIDX1, *Hum. Mol. Genet.* **2**, 1099–1104.

Qian, H.S., Channon, K., Neplioueva, V., Wang, Q., Finer, M., Tsui, L., George, S.E., McArthur, J. (2001) Improved adenoviral vector for vascular gene therapy: beneficial effects on vascular function and inflammation, *Circ. Res.* **88**, 911–917.

Ragot, T., Vincent, N., Chafey, P., Vigne, E., Gilgenkrantz, H., Couton, D., Cartaud, J., Briand, P., Kaplan, J.C., Perricaudet, M., et al. (1993) Efficient adenovirus-mediated transfer of a human minidystrophin gene to skeletal muscle of mdx mice, *Nature* **361**, 647–650.

Raper, S.E., Yudkoff, M., Chirmule, N., Gao, G.P., Nunes, F., Haskal, Z.J., Furth, E.E., Propert, K.J., Robinson, M.B., Magosin, S., Simoes, H., Speicher, L., Hughes, J., Tazelaar, J., Wivel, N.A., Wilson, J.M., Batshaw, M.L. (2002) A pilot study of in vivo liver-directed gene transfer with an adenoviral vector in partial ornithine transcarbamylase deficiency, *Hum. Gene Ther.* **13**, 163–175.

Reddy, P.S., Sakhuja, K., Ganesh, S., Yang, L., Kayda, D., Brann, T., Pattison, S., Golightly, D., Idamakanti, N., Pinkstaff, A., Kaloss, M., Barjot, C., Chamberlain, J.S., Kaleko, M., Connelly, S. (2002) Sustained human factor VIII expression in hemophilia A mice following systemic delivery of a gutless adenoviral vector, *Mol. Ther.* **5**, 63–73.

Reiser, J., Harmison, G., Kluepfel-Stahl, S., Brady, R.O., Karlsson, S., Schubert, M. (1996) Transduction of nondividing cells using pseudotyped defective high-titer HIV type 1 particles, *Proc. Natl. Acad. Sci. U. S. A.* **93**, 15266–15271.

Rivera, V.M., Clackson, T., Natesan, S., Pollock, R., Amara, J.F., Keenan, T., Magari, S.R., Phillips, T., Courage, N.L., Cerasoli, F., Jr., Holt, D.A., Gilman, M. (1996) A humanized system for pharmacologic control of gene expression, *Nat. Med.* **2**, 1028–1032.

Rock, D.L., Nesburn, A.B., Ghiasi, H., Ong, J., Lewis, T.L., Lokensgard, J.R., Wechsler, S.L. (1987) Detection of latency-related viral RNAs in trigeminal ganglia of rabbits latently infected with herpes simplex virus type 1, *J. Virol.* **61**, 3820–3826.

Rosen, C.A., Sodroski, J.G., Haseltine, W.A. (1985) The location of cis-acting regulatory sequences in the human T cell lymphotropic virus type III (HTLV-III/LAV) long terminal repeat, *Cell* **41**, 813–823.

Rosenfeld, M.A., Siegfried, W., Yoshimura, K., Yoneyama, K., Fukayama, M., Stier, L.E., Paakko, P.K., Gilardi, P., Stratford-Perricaudet, L.D., Perricaudet, M., et al. (1991) Adenovirus-mediated transfer of a recombinant alpha 1-antitrypsin gene to the lung epithelium in vivo, *Science* **252**, 431–434.

Rosenfeld, M.A., Yoshimura, K., Trapnell, B.C., Yoneyama, K., Rosenthal, E.R., Dalemans, W., Fukayama, M., Bargon, J., Stier, L.E., Stratford-Perricaudet, L., et al. (1992) In vivo transfer of the human cystic fibrosis transmembrane conductance regulator gene to the airway epithelium, *Cell* **68**, 143–155.

Rosengart, T.K., Lee, L.Y., Patel, S.R., Sanborn, T.A., Parikh, M., Bergman, G.W., Hachamovitch, R., Szulc, M., Kligfield, P.D., Okin, P.M., Hahn, R.T., Devereux, R.B., Post, M.R., Hackett, N.R., Foster, T., Grasso, T.M., Lesser, M.L., Isom, O.W., Crystal, R.G. (1999) Angiogenesis gene therapy: phase I assessment of direct intramyocardial administration of an adenovirus vector expressing VEGF121 cDNA to individuals with clinically significant severe coronary artery disease, *Circulation* **100**, 468–474.

Roth, D.A., Tawa, N.E., Jr., O'Brien, J.M., Treco, D.A., Selden, R.F. (2001) Nonviral transfer of the gene encoding coagulation factor VIII in patients with severe hemophilia A, *N. Engl. J. Med.* **344**, 1735–1742.

Ruffini, F., Furlan, R., Poliani, P.L., Brambilla, E., Marconi, P.C., Bergami, A., Desina, G., Glorioso, J.C., Comi, G., Martino, G. (2001) Fibroblast growth factor-II gene therapy reverts the clinical course and the pathological signs of chronic experimental autoimmune encephalomyelitis in C57BL/6 mice, *Gene Ther.* **8**, 1207–1213.

Ruiz, F.E., Clancy, J.P., Perricone, M.A., Bebok, Z., Hong, J.S., Cheng, S.H., Meeker, D.P., Young, K.R., Schoumacher, R.A., Weatherly, M.R., Wing, L., Morris, J.E., Sindel, L., Rosenberg, M., van Ginkel, F.W., McGhee, J.R., Kelly, D., Lyrene, R.K., Sorscher, E.J. (2001) A clinical inflammatory syndrome attributable to aerosolized lipid-DNA administration in cystic fibrosis, *Hum. Gene Ther.* **12**, 751–761.

Sacks, W.R., Greene, C.C., Aschman, D.P., Schaffer, P.A. (1985) Herpes simplex virus type 1 ICP27 is an essential regulatory protein, *J. Virol.* **55**, 796–805.

Sailaja, G., HogenEsch, H., North, A., Hays, J., Mittal, S.K. (2002) Encapsulation of recombinant adenovirus into alginate microspheres circumvents vector-specific immune response, *Gene Ther.* **9**, 1722–1729.

Sakhuja, K., Reddy, P.S., Ganesh, S., Cantaniag, F., Pattison, S., Limbach, P., Kayda, D.B., Kadan, M.J., Kaleko, M., Connelly, S. (2003) Optimization of the generation and propagation of gutless adenoviral vectors, *Hum. Gene Ther.* **14**, 243–254.

Samulski, R.J., Zhu, X., Xiao, X., Brook, J.D., Housman, D.E., Epstein, N., Hunter, L.A. (1991) Targeted integration of adeno-associated virus (AAV) into human chromosome 19, *EMBO J.* **10**, 3941–3950.

Sarkar, N., Ruck, A., Kallner, G.S.Y.H., Blomberg, P., Islam, K.B., van der Linden, J., Lindblom, D., Nygren, A.T., Lind, B., Brodin, L.A., Drvota, V., Sylven, C. (2001) Effects of intramyocardial injection of phVEGF-A165 as sole therapy in patients with refractory coronary artery disease–12-month follow-up: angiogenic gene therapy, *J. Intern. Med.* **250**, 373–381.

Scherr, M., Battmer, K., Blomer, U., Schiedlmeier, B., Ganser, A., Grez, M., Eder, M. (2002) Lentiviral gene transfer into peripheral blood-derived CD34+ NOD/SCID-repopulating cells, *Blood* **99**, 709–712.

Schlegel, R., Tralka, T.S., Willingham, M.C., Pastan, I. (1983) Inhibition of VSV binding and infectivity by phosphatidylserine: is phosphatidylserine a VSV-binding site? *Cell* **32**, 639–646.

Schmeisser, F., Donohue, M., Weir, J.P. (2002) Tetracycline-regulated gene expression in replication-incompetent herpes simplex virus vectors, *Hum. Gene Ther.* **13**, 2113–2124.

Schroder, A.R., Shinn, P., Chen, H., Berry, C., Ecker, J.R., Bushman, F. (2002) HIV-1 integration in the human genome favors active genes and local hotspots, *Cell* **110**, 521–529.

Schwei, M.J., Honore, P., Rogers, S.D., Salak-Johnson, J.L., Finke, M.P., Ramnaraine, M.L., Clohisy, D.R., Mantyh, P.W. (1999) Neurochemical and cellular reorganization of the spinal cord in a murine model of bone cancer pain, *J. Neurosci.* **19**, 10886–10897.

Seshidhar Reddy, P., Ganesh, S., Limbach, M.P., Brann, T., Pinkstaff, A., Kaloss, M., Kaleko, M., Connelly, S. (2003) Development of adenovirus serotype 35 as a gene transfer vector, *Virology* **311**, 384–393.

Shapiro, E., Krivit, W., Lockman, L., Jambaque, I., Peters, C., Cowan, M., Harris, R., Blanche, S., Bordigoni, P., Loes, D., Ziegler, R., Crittenden, M., Ris, D., Berg, B., Cox, C., Moser, H., Fischer, A., Aubourg, P. (2000) Long-term effect of bone-marrow transplantation for childhood-onset cerebral X-linked adrenoleukodystrophy, *Lancet* **356**, 713–718.

Shi, W., Bartlett, J.S. (2003) RGD inclusion in VP3 provides adeno-associated virus type 2 (AAV2)-based vectors with a heparan sulfate-independent cell entry mechanism, *Mol. Ther.* **7**, 515–525.

Smith, C., Lachmann, R.H., Efstathiou, S. (2000) Expression from the herpes simplex virus type 1 latency-associated promoter in the murine central nervous system, *J. Gen. Virol.* **3**, 649–662.

Snyder, R.O., Flotte, T.R. (2002) Production of clinical-grade recombinant adeno-associated virus vectors, *Curr. Opin. Biotechnol.* **13**, 418–423.

Snyder, R.O., Miao, C.H., Patijn, G.A., Spratt, S.K., Danos, O., Nagy, D., Gown, A.M., Winther, B., Meuse, L., Cohen, L.K., Thompson, A.R., Kay, M.A. (1997) Persistent and therapeutic concentrations of human factor IX in mice after hepatic gene transfer of recombinant AAV vectors, *Nat. Genet.* **16**, 270–276.

Sonntag, K.C., Emery, D.W., Yasumoto, A., Haller, G., Germana, S., Sablinski, T., Shimizu, A., Yamada, K., Shimada, H., Arn, S., Sachs, D.H., LeGuern, C. (2001) Tolerance to solid organ transplants through transfer of MHC class II genes, *J. Clin. Invest.* **107**, 65–71.

Spivack, J.G., Fraser, N.W. (1987) Detection of herpes simplex virus type 1 transcripts during latent infection in mice, *J. Virol.* **61**, 3841–3847.

Starcich, B., Ratner, L., Josephs, S.F., Okamoto, T., Gallo, R.C., Wong-Staal, F. (1985) Characterization of long terminal repeat sequences of HTLV-III, *Science* **227**, 538–540.

Stecenko, A.A., Brigham, K.L. (2003) Gene therapy progress and prospects: alpha-1 antitrypsin, *Gene Ther.* **10**, 95–99.

Stevens, J.G., Wagner, E.K., Devi Rao, G.B., Cook, M.L., Feldman, L.T. (1987) RNA complementary to a herpesvirus alpha gene mRNA is prominent in latently infected neurons, *Science* **235**, 1056–1059.

Su, H., Arakawa-Hoyt, J., Kan, Y.W. (2002) Adeno-associated viral vector-mediated hypoxia response element-regulated gene expression in mouse ischemic heart model, *Proc. Natl. Acad. Sci. U. S. A.* **99**, 9480–9485.

Su, H., Lu, R., Kan, Y.W. (2000) Adeno-associated viral vector-mediated vascular endothelial growth factor gene transfer induces neovascular formation in ischemic heart, *Proc. Natl. Acad. Sci. U. S. A.* **97**, 13801–13806.

Suzuki, M., Singh, R.N., Crystal, R.G. (1996) Regulatable promoters for use in gene therapy applications: modification of the 5'-flanking region of the CFTR gene with multiple cAMP response elements to support basal, low-level gene expression that can be upregulated by exogenous agents that raise intracellular levels of cAMP, *Hum. Gene Ther.* **7**, 1883–1893.

Suzuki, Y., Isogai, K., Teramoto, T., Tashita, H., Shimozawa, N., Nishimura, M., Asano, T., Oda, M., Kamei, A., Ishiguro, H., Kato, S., Ohashi, T., Kobayashi, H., Eto, Y., Kondo, N.

(2000) Bone marrow transplantation for the treatment of X-linked adrenoleukodystrophy, *J. Inherit. Metab. Dis.* **23**, 453–458.

Sykes, M. (2001) Mixed chimerism and transplant tolerance, *Immunity* **14**, 417–424.

Takanashi, J., Kurihara, A., Tomita, M., Kanazawa, M., Yamamoto, S., Morita, F., Ikehira, H., Tanada, S., Kohno, Y. (2002) Distinctly abnormal brain metabolism in late-onset ornithine transcarbamylase deficiency, *Neurology* **59**, 210–214.

Takayama, T., Kaneko, K., Morelli, A.E., Li, W., Tahara, H., Thomson, A.W. (2002) Retroviral delivery of transforming growth factor-beta1 to myeloid dendritic cells: inhibition of T-cell priming ability and influence on allograft survival, *Transplantation* **74**, 112–119.

Tao, N., Gao, G.P., Parr, M., Johnston, J., Baradet, T., Wilson, J.M., Barsoum, J., Fawell, S.E. (2001) Sequestration of adenoviral vector by Kupffer cells leads to a nonlinear dose response of transduction in liver, *Mol. Ther.* **3**, 28–35.

Tratschin, J.D., West, M.H., Sandbank, T., Carter, B.J. (1984) A human parvovirus, adeno-associated virus, as a eucaryotic vector: transient expression and encapsidation of the procaryotic gene for chloramphenicol acetyltransferase, *Mol. Cell. Biol.* **4**, 2072–2081.

Tuchman, M., McCullough, B.A., Yudkoff, M. (2000) The molecular basis of ornithine transcarbamylase deficiency, *Eur. J. Pediatr.* **159**(Suppl 3), S196–S198.

Vale, P.R., Losordo, D.W., Milliken, C.E., McDonald, M.C., Gravelin, L.M., Curry, C.M., Esakof, D.D., Maysky, M., Symes, J.F., Isner, J.M. (2001) Randomized, single-blind, placebo-controlled pilot study of catheter-based myocardial gene transfer for therapeutic angiogenesis using left ventricular electromechanical mapping in patients with chronic myocardial ischemia, *Circulation* **103**, 2138–2143.

Wade-Martins, R., Smith, E.R., Tyminski, E., Chiocca, E.A., Saeki, Y. (2001) An infectious transfer and expression system for genomic DNA loci in human and mouse cells, *Nat. Biotechnol.* **19**, 1067–1070.

Walsh, C.E. (2003) Gene therapy progress and prospects: gene therapy for the hemophilias, *Gene Ther.* **10**, 999–1003.

Wang, L., Muramatsu, S., Lu, Y., Ikeguchi, K., Fujimoto, K., Okada, T., Mizukami, H., Hanazono, Y., Kume, A., Urano, F., Ichinose, H.,

Nagatsu, T., Nakano, I., Ozawa, K. (2002) Delayed delivery of AAV-GDNF prevents nigral neurodegeneration and promotes functional recovery in a rat model of Parkinson's disease, *Gene Ther.* **9**, 381–389.

Wesseling, J.G., Bosma, P.J., Krasnykh, V., Kashentseva, E.A., Blackwell, J.L., Reynolds, P.N., Li, H., Parameshwar, M., Vickers, S.M., Jaffee, E.M., Huibregtse, K., Curiel, D.T., Dmitriev, I. (2001) Improved gene transfer efficiency to primary and established human pancreatic carcinoma target cells via epidermal growth factor receptor and integrin-targeted adenoviral vectors, *Gene Ther.* **8**, 969–976.

Woolf, C.J., Salter, M.W. (2000) Neuronal plasticity: increasing the gain in pain, *Science* **288**, 1765–1769.

Wu, H., Seki, T., Dmitriev, I., Uil, T., Kashentseva, E., Han, T., Curiel, D.T. (2002) Double modification of adenovirus fiber with RGD and polylysine motifs improves coxsackievirus-adenovirus receptor-independent gene transfer efficiency, *Hum. Gene Ther.* **13**, 1647–1653.

Xiao, X., Li, J., Samulski, R.J. (1998) Production of high-titer recombinant adeno-associated virus vectors in the absence of helper adenovirus, *J. Virol.* **72**, 2224–2232.

Xie, Q., Bu, W., Bhatia, S., Hare, J., Somasundaram, T., Azzi, A., Chapman, M.S. (2002) The atomic structure of adeno-associated virus (AAV-2), a vector for human gene therapy, *Proc. Natl. Acad. Sci. U. S. A.* **99**, 10405–10410.

Yaksh, T.L. (1999) Spinal systems and pain processing: development of novel analgesic drugs with mechanistically defined models, *Trends Pharmacol. Sci.* **20**, 329–337.

Ye, X., Rivera, V.M., Zoltick, P., Cerasoli, F., Jr., Schnell, M.A., Gao, G., Hughes, J.V., Gilman, M., Wilson, J.M. (1999) Regulated delivery of therapeutic proteins after in vivo somatic cell gene transfer, *Science* **283**, 88–91.

Zhang, X.Y., La Russa, V.F., Bao, L., Kolls, J., Schwarzenberger, P., Reiser, J. (2002) Lentiviral vectors for sustained transgene expression in human bone marrow-derived stromal cells, *Mol. Ther.* **5**, 555–565.

Zielske, S.P., Gerson, S.L. (2002) Lentiviral Transduction of P140K MGMT into Human CD34(+) Hematopoietic Progenitors at Low Multiplicity of Infection Confers Significant Resistance to BG/BCNU and Allows Selection in Vitro, *Mol. Ther.* **5**, 381–387.

Zou, L., Zhou, H., Pastore, L., Yang, K. (2000) Prolonged transgene expression mediated by a helper-dependent adenoviral vector (hdAd) in the central nervous system, *Mol. Ther.* **2**, 105–113.

Zufferey, R., Nagy, D., Mandel, R.J., Naldini, L., Trono, D. (1997) Multiply attenuated lentiviral vector achieves efficient gene delivery in vivo, *Nat. Biotechnol.* **15**, 871–875.

Zwaagstra, J., Ghiasi, H., Nesburn, A.B., Wechsler, S.L. (1989) In vitro promoter activity associated with the latency-associated transcript gene of herpes simplex virus type 1, *J. Gen. Virol.* **70**, 2163–2169.

Zwaagstra, J.C., Ghiasi, H., Nesburn, A.B., Wechsler, S.L. (1991) Identification of a major regulatory sequence in the latency associated transcript (LAT) promoter of herpes simplex virus type 1 (HSV-1), *Virology* **182**, 287–297.

Zwaagstra, J.C., Ghiasi, H., Slanina, S.M., Nesburn, A.B., Wheatley, S.C., Lillycrop, K., Wood, J., Latchman, D.S., Patel, K., Wechsler, S.L. (1990) Activity of herpes simplex virus type 1 latency-associated transcript (LAT) promoter in neuron-derived cells: evidence for neuron specificity and for a large LAT transcript, *J. Virol.* **64**, 5019–5028.

Zwiebel, J.A., Freeman, S.M., Kantoff, P.W., Cornetta, K., Ryan, U.S., Anderson, W.F. (1989) High-level recombinant gene expression in rabbit endothelial cells transduced by retroviral vectors, *Science* **243**, 220–222.

29
Somatic Gene Therapy

M. Schweizer, E. Flory, C. Münk, Uwe Gottschalk, and K. Cichutek
Paul-Ehrlich-Institut, Langen, Germany

1   Introduction   934

2   Gene Transfer Methods   936
2.1   Nonviral Vectors and Naked Nucleic Acid   938
2.2   Viral Vectors   939
2.2.1   Retroviral Vectors   939
2.2.2   Lentiviral Vectors   940
2.2.3   Adenoviral Vectors   940
2.2.4   AAV (Adeno-associated Viral) Vectors   941
2.2.5   Poxvirus Vectors   941

3   Clinical Use   941
3.1   Overview on Clinical Gene Therapy Trials   941
3.2   Gene Therapy of Monogeneic Congenital Diseases   941
3.3   Tumor Gene Therapy   943
3.4   Gene Therapy of Cardiovascular Diseases   944
3.5   Preventive Vaccination and Gene Therapy of Infectious Diseases   944
3.6   Clinical Gene Therapy for the Treatment of Other Diseases   945

4   Manufacture and Regulatory Aspects   945

5   First Experience with the Clinical Use of Gene Transfer
        Medicinal Products   949

        Bibliography   949
        Books and Reviews   949
        Primary Literature   950

Pharmacology. From Drug Development to Gene Therapy. Edited by Robert A. Meyers.
Copyright © 2008 Wiley-VCH Verlag GmbH & Co. KGaA, Weinheim
ISBN: 978-3-527-32343-2

1
Introduction

Innovative biotechnologicals of the future include gene transfer medicinal products. It can be assumed that by mid-2003, ~4000 patients or healthy individuals would have been treated within a clinical gene therapy trial, ~600 of those in Europe, and ~260 in Germany (The data originate from some statistics published in the Internet by Wiley Genetic Medicine Clinical Trials Online, http:///www.wiley.co.uk.genetherapy, and are reproduced by courtesy of the publisher.). Most of the clinical trials are currently in phase I or II due to a great diversity of ongoing developments, clinical experience must first be gained, before target-orientated product development and phase III clinical trials can be initiated. In this regard, investigator-driven gene therapy strategies developed by biomedical laboratories together with special clinic teams are very distinct from those developed by pharmaceutical industry. Investigator-driven gene therapy strategies are being invented by teams of biomedical researchers and physicians while developing a new approach for the treatment of a special disease in a defined stage. This is used, for the first time, on a selected group of patients in first clinical trials of phase I/II and aimed at proving the safety of the medicinal product. In clinical trials sponsored by pharmaceutical industry, this phase of orientation has often already been completed and further development in phase II or III is aimed at dose finding or proving efficacy. Concerning product development, there are no standard approaches because, at this stage of development, little experience has been gained and the types of gene transfer medicinal products are very diverse.

Therefore, in the following sections, the main current clinical developments will be described while a brief outline of a single example of a manufacturing process is given, also due to manifold diversity.

Gene transfer medicinal products for human use are medicinal products used for *in vivo* diagnosis, prophylaxis, or therapy (Fig. 1). They contain or consist of:

1. genetically modified cells,
2. viral vectors, nonviral vectors or so-called naked nucleic acids, or
3. recombinant replication-competent microorganisms used for purposes other than the prevention or therapy of the infectious diseases that they cause.

The aim of the nucleic acid or gene transfer is the genetic modification of human somatic cells, either in the human body, that is, *in vivo*, or outside the human body, that is, *ex vivo*, in the latter case followed by transfer of the modified cells to the human body. The simplest case of genetic modification of a cell results from addition of a therapeutic gene encompassed by an expression vector. At least in theory, nucleic acid transfer may also be aimed at exchange of individual point mutations or other minimal genetic aberrations. Scientifically, this process is termed *homologous recombination* with the aim of repairing a defective endogenous gene at its locus. In principle, this can be achieved by so-called homologous recombination achieved by transferring oligonucleotides, where – thanks to 5′ and 3′ flanking homology regions – the new correct DNA sequence is replacing the existing defective one. In practice, homologous recombination is technically not yet achievable with the efficiency that will be required for clinical use.

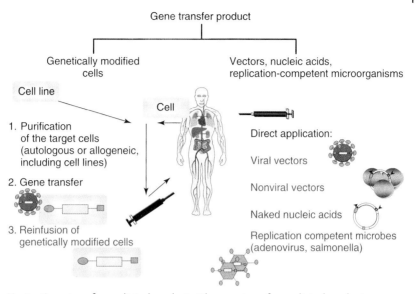

Fig. 1 Gene transfer medicinal products. The gene transfer medicinal products mentioned here are identical with those described in Table 1 of the European "Note for guidance on the quality, preclinical, and clinical aspects of gene transfer medicinal products (CPMP/BWP/3088/99)." The definition given is in compliance with the legally binding definition of gene therapeutics in Part IV, Annex I of Directive 2003/63/EC amending Directive 2001/83/EC.

Normally, genetic modification of cells is nowadays achieved by the transfer of an expression vector on which the therapeutic gene is located. The vector is transferred to cells via a delivery system (Fig. 2) such as a viral vector particle, a nonviral vector complex or a plasmid. In the latter case, the expression vector is inserted into and therefore part of a bacterial plasmid, which allows its manufacture and amplification in bacteria. Viral expression vectors contain the sequence signals (nucleic acid sequences) required for transfer by a particular viral vector particle. For retroviral vectors, for example, such signals are encompassed by the flanking "long terminal repeat" (LTR) sequences, the packaging signal psi (Ψ) required for incorporation of the expression vector by the retroviral vector particle, and other sequence signals. For nonviral vector complexes and naked nucleic acid, the expression vector is part of a bacterial carrier, the so-called plasmid DNA. Nonviral vectors are, for example, plasmid DNA mixed with a transfection reagent, whereas naked DNA does not contain a transfection reagent.

Another example of a gene transfer medicinal product is a recombinant microorganism such as conditionally replication-competent adenoviruses for tumor therapy. Here, neither is an endogenous cellular gene repaired by homologous recombination nor is a nonadenoviral therapeutic gene transferred. The transfer of conditional replicating adenoviruses to the malignant tumor cells induces cell lysis and local tumor ablation. The entire genome of the adenovirus is transferred without an additional therapeutic gene. The adenoviral genome may therefore be considered as the therapeutic gene.

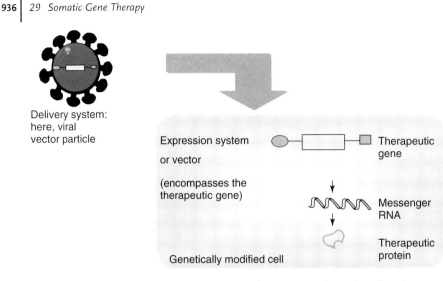

Delivery system:
here, viral
vector particle

Expression system
or vector

(encompasses the
therapeutic gene)

Therapeutic
gene

Messenger
RNA

Therapeutic
protein

Genetically modified cell

Fig. 2 Delivery system and expression vector used as gene transfer medicinal products. The terminology complies with the definition of gene therapeutics in Part IV, Annex I of Directive 2003/63/EC amending Directive 2001/83/EC.

Gene transfer efficiency plays a central role in gene transfer. It depends on a number of factors, for example, target cell, type of application (*ex vivo* or *in vivo* strategy), the tissue or organ containing the target cells, the physiological situation, and the disease and disease stage. Table 1 shows the most common viral vectors currently in clinical use. The vectors shown are replication incompetent and only transfer the expression vector void of any viral genes as much as possible. So-called integrating vectors mediate chromosomal integration of the expression vector (e.g. retroviral vectors), whereas nonintegrating vectors lead to an episomal status of the expression vector in the cell (e.g. adenoviral vectors), or to its cytoplasmatic replication (e.g. α-virus-derived vectors, vaccinia). Vectors derived from vaccinia, for example, used for tumor vaccination, may be replication incompetent such as modified vaccinia ancara (MVA) or ALVAC or replication competent, but attenuated like vaccinia.

After uptake by human somatic cells, the expression vector is transcribed like a normal cell gene. The resulting messenger RNA (mRNA) is translated and the therapeutic protein is synthesized by the cellular machinery. When so-called ribozyme genes are used, the mRNA acts like a catalytic enzyme and is itself the therapeutic gene product. As already mentioned, when a recombinant microorganism such as a conditionally replication-competent adenovirus (RCA) is used, the genome of the microorganism may be seen as the therapeutic gene.

2
Gene Transfer Methods

The objective of clinical gene transfer is the transfer of nucleic acids for the purpose of genetically modifying human cells (Fig. 3).

Whether a viral, a nonviral vector, or a naked plasmid DNA is used depends on

Tab. 1 Gene transfer methods (vectors/delivery systems).

Delivery system	Description	Chromosomal integration
Naked nucleic acid	Plasmid DNA, in absence of transfection reagents	No (after im inoculation)
Nonviral vector	Plasmid DNA/transfection reagent mixture	No (application dependent)
Viral vector		
Retroviral vector	Derived from murine leukemia virus (MLV)	Yes
Lentiviral vector	Derived from HIV-1	Yes
Adenoviral vector	Deletions in the virus genes E1, E3 or E4, E2ts, combinations thereof or "gutted" (gene-depleted)	No
Conditionally replication-competent adenovirus	No therapeutic gene except for the virus genome	No
Adeno-associated virus (AAV) vector	Wild-type AAV-derived	Yes /no (application dependent)
Smallpox virus vector	MVA ("Modified Vaccinia Ancara")	No
	ALVAC ("Avian Vaccinia")	No
	Vaccinia	No
Alphavirus vector	SFV	No
Herpes-viral vector	Herpes simplex virus	No

Note: SFV: Semliki Forest virus; MLV: murine leukemia virus.

the target cell of the genetic modification and whether an *in vivo* modification of the cell is at all possible. For a monogeneic disease affecting immune cells, it is for example, possible to purify CD34-positive cells or lymphocytes from the peripheral blood (e.g. by leukapharesis), to genetically modify the cells in culture, and to return the treated cells. Before reapplication, the treated cells may or may not be enriched. Currently, long-term correction of cells is only possible when integrating vectors such as retroviral or lentiviral vectors are used. Owing to chromosomal integration of the expression vector, the genetic modification is passed on to the daughter cells during cell division and persists. Only long-term expression may still be a problem. For therapy of a monogeneic disease such as cystic fibrosis, the target cells are primarily the endothelial cells of the bronchopulmonary tract, which can only be subjected to *in vivo* modification attempts. Although long-term correction would be desirable, *in vivo* modification using adenoviral vectors appeared to be more promising, because the target cells are largely in a resting state of the cell cycle amenable to adenoviral gene transfer due to expression of the cell surface receptors used by adenoviruses for cell entry. In addition, the amount and titers of adenoviral vectors seemed suitable. These examples illustrate that a number of factors contribute to the choice of the treatment strategy, the vector, and the route of administration. No single "ideal" vector is therefore suitable

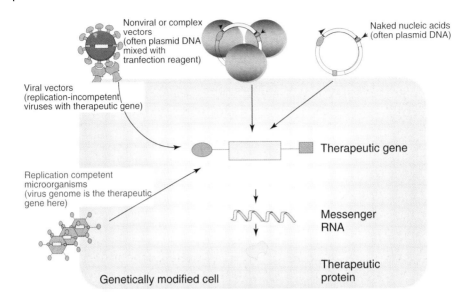

Fig. 3 Delivery systems used in clinical gene transfer. During gene therapy, an expression vector (therapeutic genes) is transferred to somatic cells via a delivery system, for example, a viral or nonviral vector (replication incompetent), a naked nucleic acid, or a recombinant, mostly conditionally replication-competent microorganism. The gene transfer, termed *transfection* when a viral vector is used or termed *transfection* when naked DNA or a nonviral vector is used, leads to genetic modification of the cell. The gene transfer can be carried out *in vivo*, that is, directly in or on the human body, or *ex vivo*, that is, in cell culture followed by the transfer of the modified cells to the human body.

for a large variety of gene therapies. In the past 15 years, many novel gene transfer techniques have been developed and used in clinical studies. In the following section and in Table 1, specific characteristics of the vectors most commonly used in the clinic are summarized.

2.1
Nonviral Vectors and Naked Nucleic Acid

The advantage of nonviral gene transfer systems compared with viral gene transfer systems is the smaller size limitations for the genes to be transferred. The expression vectors are nowadays usually part of a bacterial plasmid that can easily be amplified and grown in bacterial cultures. Plasmid DNA of up to 20 kb pairs encompassing an expression vector of up to 17 kb pairs can easily be manufactured. Promising methods for the *in vivo* administration of plasmid DNA include intradermal or intramuscular injection for the so-called naked nucleic acid transfer. Needle injection or application by medical devices such as gene guns can be used for this purpose. For so-called nonviral vectors, for example, synthetic liposomes or other transfection reagents mixed with plasmid DNA, the DNA-binding liposomes mediate contact with the cellular plasma membrane thus releasing the DNA into the cytoplasma of the cell where uptake by the nucleus has to occur subsequently. During receptor-mediated uptake of nonviral vectors, cell surface proteins (receptors), for example, asialoglycoprotein or the transferrin receptor, mediate cellular uptake of the DNA complex containing a specific receptor ligand.

2.2
Viral Vectors

During evolution, viruses have been optimized to efficiently enter mammalian cells and replicate. Infected mammalian cells transcribe the viral genes and synthesize the viral gene products with high efficiency, sometimes to the disadvantage of endogenous protein production. Viral vectors are replication-incompetent particles derived from viruses by genetic engineering, which no longer transfer to cells the complete set or any viral genes. Instead, an expression vector with one or more therapeutic genes is transferred to cells. Since no complete viral genome is transferred, virus replication is impossible or, in some cases, it is impaired like with first- or second-generation adenoviral vectors. The following section briefly describes the properties of the current frequently used viral vectors.

2.2.1   Retroviral Vectors
The retroviral vectors in clinical use have mainly been derived from murine leukemia virus (MLV). MLV causes leukemia in mice and replication-competent retrovirus (RCR) in a contaminated vector preparation was shown to cause leukemia in severely immunosuppressed monkeys. RCR absence has therefore to be verified before human use of retrovirally modified cells. MLV vector

use *in vivo* has been very rare. The genome of the retroviral vectors consists of two copies of single-stranded RNA, which contains one or more coding regions flanked by the viral control elements, the so-called "long-terminal repeat" regions. In the infected cells, the RNA is translated into double-stranded viral DNA and integrated into the cell. The integrated vector DNA is the expression vector. MLV vectors allow efficient genetic modification of proliferating cells by chromosomally integrating the expression vector.

Advantages of retroviral vectors include high gene transfer (transduction) efficiency, and long-term modification of cells due to stable integration of the expression vector into the chromosome of the cells. In addition, the MLV envelope proteins can be exchanged against those from other viruses (which is termed *vector pseudotyping*). This allows preparation of MLV vectors with improved transduction efficiency for certain cell types. Disadvantages of retroviral vectors include the small size of the coding region (~9 kb pairs or less), the restriction of transduction to proliferating cells only, insertional mutagenesis due to integration and the low titer of usually not more than 10^8 transducing units per milliliter of vector preparation. Although chromosomal integration occurs generally at random, it may lead to activation of cellular cancer genes, so-called proto-oncogenes, or, theoretically, to inactivation of tumor suppressor cells. In conjunction with additional genetic mutations, this may result in very low frequency in malignant cell transformation. Hundreds of patients that have been treated with retrovirally modified hematopoietic cells years ago have not shown any signs of cancer related to the gene transfer except for two patients treated during an SCID-X1 (severe combined immunodeficiency disease) gene therapy trial in France. In the latter two leukemia cases, the vector-mediated over-expression of the proto-oncogene LMO2, possibly in conjunction with the therapeutic γc chain gene (which may influence cell proliferation and signal transduction) and the SCID-X1 disease, are the probable cause of the leukemia (see the following sections).

2.2.2 Lentiviral Vectors

Lentiviral vectors have been derived from human immunodeficiency virus type 1 (HIV-1), simian immunodeficiency virus (SIV) isolated from various old-world monkeys, feline immunodeficiency virus (FIV) and equine infectious anemia virus (EIAV) isolated from horses. Lentiviruses cause an acquired immunodeficiency syndrome and a replication-competent virus has therefore to be excluded before human use by batch-to-batch analysis and verification of the absence of replication-competent lentivirus (RCL). Lentiviral vectors may transfer coding regions of up to 9 kb pairs and allow pseudotyping just like MLV vectors. Their advantage is the dual capacity to transfer therapeutic genes into nonproliferating cells in conjunction with persistent genetic modification due to chromosomal integration. This could be useful for *ex vivo* modification of stem cells and *in vivo* modification of neuronal cells. Most lentiviral vectors have been pseudotyped with the G-protein of vesicular stomatitis virus (VSV-G) or the envelope proteins of Gibbon ape leukemia virus. The first clinical study using lentiviral vectors was started in 2003 and involves the *ex vivo* modification of autologous lymphocytes of HIV-infected patients with a therapeutic ribozyme gene shown *in vitro* to inhibit HIV-1 replication.

2.2.3 Adenoviral Vectors

The adenoviral genome consists of double-stranded DNA that persists episomally, that is, inside the nucleus, but not integrated into the chromosome of the cell. Therefore, the genetic modification may be lost during cell proliferation. Adenoviral vectors are the currently preferred vectors for the *in vivo* transduction of a variety of human somatic cells including nonproliferating cells. In contrast to lentiviral vectors, they allow insertion of larger coding regions of therapeutic genes above 10 kb pairs and are not associated with a detectable risk of insertional oncogenesis. In addition, vector titers above 10^{11} transducing units per milliliter can usually be achieved. The lack of long-term expression is in part due to the fact that certain adenovirus genes have been kept on first or second-generation adenoviral expression vectors, and because of the frequent generation of RCA during production. So-called gutless vectors are void of any adenoviral genes, but have to be purified from RCA after production.

Some wild-type (replicating) adenovirus strains cause inflammations of the airways and the conjunctivae. Adenoviral vectors may therefore also be transferred by inhalation of aerosols and inflammations observed following vector applications are mainly local, transient, and associated with very high titer applications. High-titer adenoviral vectors are no longer systemically administrated, because one patient died during systemic administration of a maximum dose of $\sim 10^{13}$ vector particles during gene therapy of the monogeneic disease OTCOTC ("ornithine transcarbamylase") deficiency, a life-threatening metabolic disorder.

2.2.4 AAV (Adeno-associated Viral) Vectors

Adeno-associated viruses (AAVs) belong to the family of parvoviruses. Their genome consists of single-stranded DNA. Wild-type AVV can only replicate in the presence of helper viruses like adenovirus or herpesvirus and has not been associated with disease. AAV can infect hematopoietic cells including nonproliferating cells. Integration in infected human somatic cells is often confined to a distinct locus on human chromosome 19. AAV-derived vectors are usually classified as integrating vectors, although vector integration is unfortunately no longer confined to chromosome 19, but absence of integration may be observed, for example, following intramuscular administration The size of the coding region is very limited ($\sim$4 kb pairs).

2.2.5 Poxvirus Vectors

Poxvirus vectors encompass vaccinia derived from the smallpox vaccine and more attenuated variants like ALVAC or MVA. Their genome consists of single-stranded DNA of 130 to 300 kb pairs. Replication is restricted to the cytoplasm of cells and high amounts of protein are synthesized by the cell following transduction. Most applications, therefore, involve intramuscular vaccination.

3 Clinical Use

3.1 Overview on Clinical Gene Therapy Trials

A number of clinical trials show promising results (see Table 2). In the past few years, it has become increasingly clear that for each disease, the development of a particular and specific gene transfer method in connection with a particular treatment approach will probably be necessary. The first standard use of an approved gene transfer medicinal product is to be expected within the next seven years since $\sim$1% of the clinical gene therapy studies are in an advanced stage of phase II or phase III clinical trial.

Clinical gene therapy studies have been performed initially in North America and Europe. About 50 clinical gene transfer studies have been registered in Germany, with slightly more than 250 patients that have been treated (http://www.pei.de) (http://www.zks.uni-freiburg.de/dereg.html). A general overview on registered studies is listed on the following Web sites: (http://www.wiley.co.uk/genetherapy, or www.pei.de). In Germany, a public registry has been available since 2004.

Target diseases in most clinical gene therapy trials have been cancer, cardiovascular diseases, infectious diseases such as AIDS, or monogeneic congenital disorders. The vectors most frequently used *ex vivo* are MLV vectors derived from murine leukaemia virus (MLV), whereas vectors derived from adenovirus, pox viruses, and AAV are usually used *in vivo*. A growing number of studies involves the use of nonviral vectors or naked DNA.

3.2 Gene Therapy of Monogeneic Congenital Diseases

The idea underlying gene therapy is the replacement of a defective gene by its normal, functional counterpart; for example, a mutation of the gene encoding the γc chain of the interleukin-2 and other receptors is the cause of the congenital immune disorder SCID-X1.

Tab. 2 Promising clinical gene therapy trials.

Disease	Therapeutic gene	Pharmaceutical form/vector	Target cell	Remarks
Human severe combined immunodeficiency SCID-X1	γc Chain gene (e.g. interleukin-2-receptor part)	MLV vector	Bone marrow stem cells *ex vivo*	4 of 1 patient cured, 2 leukemias
PAOD	VEGFgene	Plasmid DNA	Muscle/ endothelial cells *in vivo* (im)	Improved blood flow
Head and neck tumor	Adenovirus genome (cell lysis/apoptosis)	Tumor cell specific replicating adenovirus	p53-Negative tumor cells *in vivo*	Local tumor remission in combination with chemotherapy
Graft versus host disease in donor lymphocyte transfer for leukemia treatment	Thymidin kinase gene of the herpes simplex virus, followed by treatment with Ganciclovir	T cells, MLV vectors	T-lymphocytes *ex vivo*	Successful treatment of host-versus-graft disease
Hemophilia B	Coagulation factor IX gene	AAV vector	Muscle cells *in vivo* (im)	Improved coagulation factor concentration

Note: PAOD: peripheral artery occlusive disease; VEGF: vascular endothelial growth factor; AAV: Adeno-associated virus; MLV: murine leukemia virus.

Owing to this defect, immunologically relevant receptors are unable to mediate the normal differentiation and immune function of lymphoid cells such as T cells and natural killer lymphocytes (NK). Therefore, newborn babies suffering from SCID-X1 have a very limited immune system and must live in a germ-free environment. Their life expectancy is strongly reduced. Conventional treatment, that is, bone marrow transplantation, can provide a cure to a certain extent, but involves a high risk if no HLA haploidentical donor is available. For the latter situation, gene therapy within the framework of a clinical study was considered in France.

In this study, autologous CD34-positive bone marrow stem cells were retrovirally modified to express the functional γc chain gene. T cells and other hemaotpoietic cells derived from corrected stem cells were shown to repopulate the hematopoietic cell compartment, and over a period of up to three years, 11 treated patients, mostly newborns, displayed a functional and nearly normal immune system. This represents the first reproducible cure of a disease by gene therapy.

A leukemia-like lymphoproliferative disease was diagnosed roughly three years after treatment of two obviously cured patients. Treatment had been started at the age of a few months. Subsequent analysis revealed that the leukemia-like disease was indeed caused by the MLV vector; the disease mechanism is termed *insertional oncogenesis* resulting from insertional mutagenesis of the proto-oncogene LMO2 (mentioned earlier). According to current knowledge, up to 50 cells with an integration in LMO2 may have been administered together with the $\sim 10^8$ genetically modified CD34-positive bone marrow cells.

Owing to the expression vector integration, the transcription of the LMO2 gene was deregulated and activated. Under normal circumstances, the body can cope with individual cells presenting preneoplastic changes like the one described. In the two treated children, however, further genetic changes must have accumulated to finally result in leukemia. Contributing factors discussed include the effect of the therapeutic γc chain gene, the product of which influences cell proliferation and differentiation, and other so far unknown genetic changes that may have occurred during the massive *in vivo* cell replication. In SCID-X1, the T-cell compartment is completely depleted, and is replenished after gene therapy by differentiation and replication of a few genetically corrected blood stem cells. During this process, genetic aberrations may occur with substantial frequency. However, further analysis will be required to understand the exact cause of leukemia development in SCID-X1 gene therapy. Since hundreds of patients treated with retrovirally modified cells in the past 10 years have not developed leukemia up to now, it is currently assumed that a practical risk of leukemia only exists in SCID-X1 gene therapy.

Gene therapy of hemophilia B also seems promising. Here, AAV vectors encoding a smaller, but functional version of the human coagulation factor IX gene were administered by intramuscular injection. A detectable increase in factor IX plasma concentration was observed. Even repeated AAV injections were well tolerated.

3.3
Tumor Gene Therapy

There are various gene therapy approaches that are being developed for the treatment of cancer. They are aimed at inhibiting molecular pathways underlying malignant cell transformation. In other cases, tumor cell ablation by directly applying cell-killing mechanisms or, more indirectly, by improving immunological defense mechanisms directed against tumor cells are attempted.

A number of gene therapy studies involving the adenoviral transfer of tumor suppressor genes like p53 have already been performed. This is aimed at reverting malignant cell transformation or at inducing apoptosis. However, transduction following, for example, needle inoculation into tumors has been shown to be limited to a few cells close to the needle tracks. Direct tumor cell ablation by local injection of conditional RCAs in head and neck tumors led to detectable local tumor regression by direct virus-mediated cell lysis, especially when chemotherapy was used in parallel. Here, virus replication improved transduction efficiency *in vivo*. For the treatment of malignant brain tumors, variant herpesviruses have been inoculated into the tumor in order to lyse the tumor cells *in vivo*, especially if prodrugs have been administered that are converted by the viral thymidin kinase gene to a toxic drug.

In addition, a number of clinical approaches have already been tested that led to an improvement of immune recognition of tumors. They involved intratumoral injection of vectors, which transfer foreign MHC genes, such as B7.1 or B7.2, or cytokine genes, for example, interleukin-2 or granulocyte-macrophage colony-stimulating factor (GM-CSF). Here, vaccinia derived vectors such as MVA or ALVAC have often been used. Autologous or allogeneic tumor cells were also modified *ex vivo* by transfer of immunostimulating genes. Promising results have been reported from a phase I-study in which autologous tumor cells were adenovirally modified with the GM-CSF gene and rapidly reinoculated to stimulate anti-tumor immunity.

3.4
Gene Therapy of Cardiovascular Diseases

Local intramuscular injection of plasmid DNA or adenoviral vectors encoding vascular epithelial growth factor or fibroblast growth factor, both able to induce the formation of new blood vessels, has been used to improve microcirculation in ischemic tissue. Needle injection of plasmid DNA has been used in leg muscle, catheter application, or needle injection was also tried in ischemic heart muscle. The formation of new blood vessels and an improvement in the microcirculation has been observed.

A narrowing of the blood vessels (restenosis) often occurs after coronary blood vessel dilatation by stent implantation. This is probably caused by the proliferation of smooth muscle cells following injuring of the blood vessel endothelium by the stent. Here, the role of adenoviral or plasmid DNA mediated transfer of the gene encoding inducible nitroxide synthase (iNOS) is thought to result in reduced cell proliferation.

3.5
Preventive Vaccination and Gene Therapy of Infectious Diseases

During the past five to ten years, effective medicines have been developed for the treatment of AIDS. Combinations of effective chemotherapeutics are able to inhibit various steps of the replication cycle of HIV-1. This often results in reduction of the viral load in the peripheral blood, sometimes down to a level barely detectable with modern techniques. Because of the requirement for long-term treatment and the massive adverse effects related to conventional treatment by chemotherapy, gene therapy of HIV infection could offer additional therapy options. *Ex vivo* retroviral transfer of HIV-inhibiting genes into peripheral blood lymphocytes or CD34-positive human cells has been attempted, so far with little success. The therapeutic molecules used include (1) decoy-RNA specifying multiple copies of the Rev- or the Tat-responsive element, so-called poly-TAR or poly-RRE sequences, (2) mini antibodies (single chain Fv; scFv), able to capture viral gene products within the cell, (3) trans-dominant negative mutants of viral proteins, for example, RevM10, or (4) ribozyme RNA, which enzymatically cleaves RNA. Other genes still under development are designed to prevent entry or chromosomal integration of HIV. It remains to be shown whether such gene therapy approaches present a suitable therapeutic option compared with existing chemotherapy.

The best prevention of infectious diseases is achieved by prophylactic vaccines. Clinical trials using vectored vaccines based on ALVAC or MVA have been initiated. Other clinical trials pursue the goal of developing vaccines against HIV-1, malaria, hepatitis B, tuberculosis, and influenza A virus infections. Vaccination regiments using poxvirus vectors such as ALVAC or MVA in combination with naked DNA as a prime vaccine, sometimes followed by further booster injections of recombinant viral antigens, are being tested in humans. Such regiments have been shown to prevent disease progression after lentivirus infection of monkeys. This illustrates the complexity of vaccination strategies that are currently pursued in vaccine research.

3.6
Clinical Gene Therapy for the Treatment of Other Diseases

Clinical gene therapy can also be used for the treatment of diseases not necessarily caused by single known gene defects, if promising therapeutic genes can be reasonably applied. Patients with chronic rheumatoid arthritis, for instance, should benefit from a reduction of the inflammations in joints. Such inflammations are caused or at least maintained by a cascade of events including the overexpression and increased release of a number of inflammatory cytokines. Monoclonal antibodies able to reduce the local concentration of the tumor necrosis factor (TNF) have already been successfully used to treat disease. Here, clinical gene transfer approaches involve the transfer of autologous synovial cells modified *ex vivo* by a therapeutic gene encoding interleukin-1 receptor antagonist. Alternatively, adenoviral vectors with the same gene have been directly injected into the affected joint.

4
Manufacture and Regulatory Aspects

The regulation of gene therapy is very complex and differs considerably in the European Union and the United States. In Part IV, Annex I of Directive 2003/63/EC (which replaces Annex I of Directive 2001/83/EC), a definition of so-called gene therapeutics is given. As gene therapy not only includes therapeutic but also preventive and diagnostic use of vectors, nucleic acids, certain microorganisms and genetically modified cells, the term "gene transfer medicinal products" as used in the relevant European guideline "Note for guidance on the quality, preclinical, and clinical aspects of gene transfer medicinal products (CPMP/BWP/3088/99)" seems more exact. An accurate listing of the medicinal products that belong to the group of gene transfer medicinal products can be found in the table contained in the guideline. The definition given in Sect. 1 of this article is in accordance with this guideline and is in agreement with the definition of gene therapeutic products of Directive 2003/63/EC. The annex of the latter Directive contains legally binding requirements for quality and safety specifications of gene transfer products. Although targeted at product licensing, these requirements may have a bearing on their characterization before clinical use. Active ingredients of gene transfer as defined medicinal products may include, for example, vectors, naked plasmid DNA, or certain microorganisms such as conditionally replicated adenovirus. For the *ex vivo* strategy, the active ingredients are the genetically modified cells.

Written approval by a competent authority in conjunction with positive appraisal by an ethics committee will in the future be necessary for the initiation of clinical gene therapy trials. Respective regulatory processes are currently established in all EU member states during transformation of Directive 2001/20/EC. The manufacture of clinical samples in compliance with good manufacturing practice (GMP) will become compulsory. Germline therapy is illegal in the EU. The law relevant for clinical gene therapy trials and manufacture of gene transfer medicinal products in Germany is the German Drug Law (AMG) and respective decrees and operation ordinances. The law governing the physicians' profession stipulates in the "Guidelines on gene transfer into human somatic cells" ("Richtlinien zum Gentransfer in menschlichen Körperzellen") that the competent ethics committee may seek advice from the central "Commission of Somatic Gene Therapy" of the Scientific Council of the German Medical Association before coming to its vote. The Paul-Ehrlich-Institut is the competent authority in Germany and offers information on current clinical trial regulations.

Gene transfer medicinal products will be licensed via the centralized procedure by the European Commission. The licensing process is coordinated by the EMEA ("European Agency for the Evaluation of Medicinal Products") following submission of a licensing application. The marketing authorization is governed by Council Regulation (EC) No. 2309/93. The recommendation in favor or against marketing authorization is made on the basis of Directives 75/319/EEC and 91/507/EEC by experts of the national competent authorities which are members of the "Committee for Proprietary Medicinal Products" (CPMP).

In the United States, the Center for Biologics Evaluation and Research "(CBER) of the "Food and Drug Administration" (FDA) is responsible for clinical trial approval and marketing authorization.

The assessment of the licensing application focuses on the quality, safety, efficacy, and environmental risk of a gene transfer medicinal product. The manufacturing process has to be designed and performed according to GMP regulations. Like other biologicals, gene therapy products have considerably larger size and complexity compared to chemicals, and analysis of the finished product is not sufficient to control their quality and safety. A suitable process management, in-process control of all critical parameters identified within process validation are decisive factors. Gene transfer medicinal products containing or consisting of genetically modified organisms are also subject to contained use regulations before licensing and until these organisms are applied to humans.

From the economic point of view, procedures for the manufacture of therapeutic DNA must be scalable and efficient, and at the same time simple and robust. Manufacturing processes are as manifold as the gene transfer methods used in gene therapy. As an example, manufacture of plasmid DNA for naked nucleic acid transfer can be briefly described as follows. The methods available for plasmid production today largely originate from lab procedures for the production of DNA for analytical purposes (mini preparations) and have been adapted to fit process scale. Toxic substances and those that present a hazard to the environment, expensive ingredients, and nonscalable methods must be avoided. In this context, the experience gained from industrial manufacture of raw materials with the aid of bacterial cultures and virus production for the purpose of vaccine production are useful for fermentation. Suitable methods for downstream processing above all include chromatographic methods with high

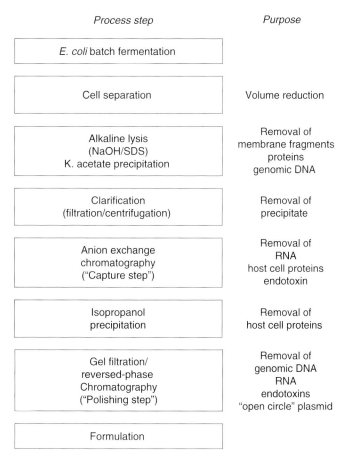

Fig. 4 Therapeutic plasmid DNA: typical manufacturing process.

Test	Specification (*method*)
Appearance	Clear colorless solution (visual inspection)
Size, restriction interfaces (identity)	Agreement with plasmid card (agarose gel electrophoresis, restriction enzyme assay)
Circular plasmid DNA (ccc)	>95% (Agarose gelelektrophorese, HPLC)
E. coli DNA	<0.02 µg/µg plasmid DNA (southern blot)
Protein	Not detectable (BCA protein assay)
RNA	Not (Agarose gel electrophoresis)
Endotoxin	<0.1 EU/µg plasmid DNA (LAL assay)
Sterility	No growth after 14 days (USP)
Specific activity	Conforms to reference standard (*in vitro* transfection)

Fig. 5 Therapeutic plasmid DNA: typical release specifications.

dynamic capacity and selectivity as well as high throughput.

In a typical procedure for the manufacture of therapeutic plasmid DNA (cf. Figs. 4 and 5), the first step is batch fermentation of *Escherichia coli* cells from a comprehensively characterized "Master Working Cell Bank" (MWCB). For this purpose, modern methods use high-density fermentation with optimized and safe *E. coli* K12 strains bearing a high number of copies of the required plasmid. The bacterial cells are harvested for further processing, resuspended in a small buffer volume, and lysed in an alkaline lysis procedure. By neutralization, the plasmid DNA is renatured while a large quantity of proteins, membrane components, and genomic DNA remain denatured. After separation of the precipitate by filtration, a chromatographic step can be performed as "capture step." Because of the anionic character of the nucleic acid, anion exchange chromatography (AEX) is the method of choice. In fractionated gradient elutions, differences in the charge enable the separation from contaminated RNA. Gel filtration (GF) or reversed phase (RP) steps can be used for fine purification. For final product analysis, evidence must be provided batch by batch that besides the correct identity and

homogeneity, critical impurities like microorganisms, host cell proteins, genomic DNA, RNA, or endotoxins have been reduced below the specified limits. Removal of endotoxins is critical for *in vivo* gene transfer efficiency achieved with naked DNA.

Some established methods from protein chemistry can be used for processing therapeutic DNA. In parallel with the processing of proteins, however, the fact cannot be concealed that nucleic acids have some very specific properties. These include the extremely high viscosity of DNA solutions, the high sensitivity of nucleic acids to gravity, the low static and dynamic capacity of their chromatographic adsorption, and the ability to penetrate filtration media with porosities well below their molecular weight ("spaghetti effect").

After first experience, plasmid concentrations of $\sim$200 mg L^{-1} fermentation broth can be obtained in high-density fermentation (optical density >50), corresponding to an yield of $\sim$800 mg plasmid DNA per kg of dry biomass. Thus, from a fermenter of 1000 L usable volume, $\sim$100 g plasmid DNA can be isolated per run in a batch fermentation at a purification yield of $\sim$50%. Consequently, capacities for production of kilogram amounts can be built up with existing technologies.

5
First Experience with the Clinical Use of Gene Transfer Medicinal Products

The development of somatic gene therapy is still in its infancy. A number of theoretical risks of gene therapy have been listed, and numerous approaches and gene transfer methods are being developed in the clinic, even more in preclinical experiments.

In spite of this, a few SCID patients have been apparently cured by gene therapy using retrovirally modified bone marrow stem cells. At the same time, the occurrence of leukemia in two of the $\sim$10 successfully treated children showed that theoretical risks cannot be clearly distinguished from clinically relevant risks due to the so far insufficient clinical experience. Trends, however, show that each pathological situation will require the development of a certain adapted gene therapy approach. Thus, in the long run, gene therapy will present real therapy or prevention options, especially for a number of up to now insufficiently treatable or untreatable diseases.

See also Gene Therapy and Cardiovascular Diseases; Liposome Gene Transfection; Medicinal Chemistry; Molecular Oncology; Genetic Vaccination; Vectors and Gene Therapy.

Bibliography

Books and Reviews

Anderson, F. (1995) Gene therapy, *Sci. Am.* **273**, 96B–98B.

Armentato, D., Sookdeo, C., White, G. (1994) Second generation adenovirus vectors for cystic fibrosis gene therapy, *J. Cell Biochem.* 18A, 102–107.

Birnboim, H.C. (1983) A rapid alkaline extraction method for the isolation of plasmid DNA, *Methods Enzymol.* **100**, 243–249.

Buchholz, C.J., Stitz, J., Cichutek, K. (1999) Retroviral cell targeting vectors, *Curr. Opin. Mol. Ther.* **5**, 613–621.

Cichutek, K. (2000) DNA vaccines: development, standardization and regulation, *Intervirology* **43**, 331–338.

Cohen-Haguenauer, O., Rosenthal, F., Gansbacher, B., Cichutek, K., et al. (2002) Euregenethy network. Opinion paper on the current status of the regulation of gene therapy in Europe, *Hum. Gene Ther.* **13**, 2085–2110.

Culver, K.W. (1994).*Gene Therapy*, Mary Ann Liebert, New York

Green, A.P., Prior, G.M., Helveston, N.M., Taittinger, B.E., et al. (1997) Preparative purification of supercoiled plasmid DNA for therapeutic applications, *Biopharmacology* **10**, 52–62.

Gottschalk, U.. (1997) The Industrial Perspective of Somatic Gene Therapy, in: Müller, S., Simon, J.W., Vesting J.W. (Eds) *Interdisciplinary Approaches to Gene Therapy*, Springer.

Gottschalk, U., Chan, S. (1998) Somatic gene therapy. Present situation and future perspective, *Arzneimittelforschung/Drug Res.* **48**, 1111–1120.

Hodgson, C.P. (1995) The vector void in gene therapy, *Biotechnology* **13**, 222–229.

Jain, K.K. (1996) *Vectors for Gene Therapy. Scrip Reports*, PJB Publications, Surrey.

Kotin, R.M. (1994) Prospects for the use of adeno-associated virus as a vector for human gene therapy, *Hum. Gene Ther.* **5**, 793–797.

Marquet, M., Horn, N.A., Meek, J.A. (1995) Process development for the manufacture of plasmid DNA vectors for the use in gene therapy, *Biopharmacology* **10**, 26–37.

Marquet, M., Horn, N.A., Meek, J.A. (1997) Characterization of plasmid DNA vectors for use in human gene therapy. Part 1. *Biopharmacology* **10**, 42–50; Part 2. (1997) *Biopharmacology* **10**, 40–45.

Morgan, R.A., Anderson, W.F. (1993) Human gene therapy, *Annu. Rev. Biochem.* **62**, 191–217.

Müller, M. (2003) Considerations for the Scale-up of Plasmid DNA Purification, in: Bowlen, B., Dürre, P. (Eds) *Nucleic Acid Isol. Meth.*, American Scientific Publishers, New York.

Mulligan, R.C. (1993) The basic science of somatic gene therapy, *Science* **260**, 926–932.

Nussenzweig, R.S., Long, C.A. (1994) Malaria vaccines: multiple targets, *Science* **265**, 1381–1384.

Prior, C., Bay, P., Ebert, B. (1995) Process development for the manufacture of inactivated HIV-1, *Pharm. Technol.* **19**, 30–52.

Randrianarison-Jewtoukoff, V., Perricaudet, M. (1995) Recombinant adenoviruses as vaccines, *Biologicals* **23**, 145–147.

Spooner, R.A., Deonarian, M.P., Epenetos, A.A. (1995) DNA vaccination for cancer treatment, *Gene Ther.* **2**, 1–11.

Tolstoshev, P., Anderson, W.F. (1993) Gene transfer techniques for use in human gene therapy, *Genome Res. Mol. Med. Virol.* **7**, 35–47.

Vile, R.G., Russell, S.J. (1995) Retroviruses as vectors, *Br. Med. Bull.* **51**, 12–15.

Primary Literature

Chandra, G., Patel, P., Kost, T.A., Gray, J.G. (1992) Large scale purification of plasmid DNA by fast protein liquid chromatography using a Hi-load Q sepharose column, *Anal. Biochem.* **203**, 169–177.

Gansbacher, B., Zier, K., Daniels, B. (1990) Interleukin-2 gene transfer into tumor cells abrogates tumorigenicity and induces protective immunity, *J. Exp. Med.* **172**, 1217–1222.

Horn, N.A., Meek, J.A., Budahazi, G., et al. (1995) Cancer gene therapy using plasmid DNA: purification of DNA for human clinical trials, *Hum. Gene Ther.* **6**, 565–573.

Mannino, R.J., Gould-Fogerite, S. (1988) Liposome-mediated gene transfer, *Biotechniques* **6**, 682–688.

Michael, S.I., Curiel, D.T. (1994) Strategies to achieve targeted gene delivery via the receptor-mediated endocytosis pathway, *Gene Ther.* **1**, 223–232.

Stitz, J., Buchholz, C.J., Cichutek, K., et al. (2000) Lentiviral vectors pseudotyped with envelope glycoproteins derived from gibbon ape leukemia virus and murine leukemia virus 10A1, *Virology* **273**, 16–20.

Stitz, J., Muhlebach, M.D., Cichutek, K., et al. (2001) A novel lentivirus vector derived from apathogenic simian immunodeficiency virus, *Virology* **291**, 191–197.

Wilson, J.W., Grossmann, M., Cabrera, J.A., et al. (1992) A novel mechanism for achieving transgene persistence in vivo after somatic gene transfer into hepatocytes, *J. Biol. Chem.* **267**, 11483–11489.

30

Virus-free Gene Transfer Systems in Somatic Gene Therapy

Oliver Kayser[1] and Albrecht F. Kiderlen[2]
[1] Pharmaceutical Biology, Rijksuniversiteit Groningen, Groningen, The Netherlands
[2] Robert Koch-Institut, Berlin, Germany

1   **What is Gene Therapy?   952**

2   **Strategies in Gene Therapy   953**

3   **Gene-transfection Systems   955**
3.1   Physical Gene-transfection Systems   956
3.1.1   Electroporation   956
3.1.2   Bioballistics   956
3.2   Chemical Gene-transfection Systems   956
3.2.1   Cationic Liposomes (Lipoplex)   957
3.2.2   Polymer Particles (Polyplex)   960
3.2.3   Poly-L-Lysine (PLL) and Poly-L-Arginine (PLA)   961
3.2.4   Polyethyleneimine (PEI)   962
3.2.5   Dendrimers   962
3.2.6   Chitosan   963
3.2.7   Poly(2-Dimethylamino)Ethylmethacrylate   963

4   **Perspectives   964**

         Bibliography   965
         Books and Reviews   965
         Primary Literature   965

Pharmacology. From Drug Development to Gene Therapy. Edited by Robert A. Meyers.
Copyright © 2008 Wiley-VCH Verlag GmbH & Co. KGaA, Weinheim
ISBN: 978-3-527-32343-2

Keywords

Liposomes
Microscopic spherical vesicles that form spontaneously when phospholipids are hydrated. The enclosed aqueous core may be used to transport hydrophilic, the uni- or multilamellar shell to transport lipophilic molecules.

Somatic
Referring to cells of the body, as opposed to sex cells or gametes of the germ line.

Transfection
Insertion of small pieces of DNA into a cell. If the DNA is expressed without integration into the host cell DNA, the transfection is transient. If the DNA integrates into the host cell DNA, it is replicated whenever the host cell divides, and the transfection is stable.

Vectors
Sensu strictu: DNA elements used to amplify and express foreign DNA in a host cell. *Sensu latu*: Also used synonymous with "gene-transfection systems," that is, biological, physical, and chemical carriers that augment the entry of pieces of DNA into a cell.

> In somatic gene therapy, nucleic acid is transferred into and subsequently expressed in somatic cells (i.e. not in stem cells) in order to alter or substitute gene functions as a means of prophylactic or therapeutic treatment of patients. The nucleic acid itself is the pharmaceutical drug. For transfer of genes, viral (retro, adeno, and adenovirus-associated viruses), physical (electroporation and bioballistics), and chemical systems are utilized. Chemical and physical systems are united as nonviral systems.

1
What is Gene Therapy?

Gene therapy may be defined as the expression of a gene that has been introduced into a target cell or a target tissue in order to alter an existing function or to introduce a new function with the aim of curing or protecting a patient from a specific disease. In many countries, this is restricted by law to somatic cells. In Germany, for example, genetic manipulation of germ cells is forbidden according to §5 Embryoschutz Gesetz (EschG) and is under penalty of up to 5-years imprisonment. German legislation on gene transfection as a form of therapy or medicine is still incomplete. An amendment specifically covering somatic gene therapy has not yet been passed. German Drug Regulation (§2 and §3 Deutsches Arzneimittelgesetz, AMG) defines DNA introduced for therapeutic purposes in a very general manner as a pharmaceutical product. German Gene Technology Regulation (§2 (3) Deutsches Gentechnikgesetz, GenTG) explicitly excludes the regulation of gene therapy. Interestingly, gene therapy might be indirectly affected: theoretically (*sensu strictu*), a patient undergoing gene therapy becomes a genetically modified organism. Consequently, his release from hospital should be subject to authorization. When discussing DNA as a pharmaceutical, a look at European legislation, for example, at the guidelines of the European Agency for the evaluation of medicinal products (EMEA) is helpful. According to Council Regulations (EEC) No. 2309/93–ANNEX (List A), DNA is considered a pharmaceutical product for gene therapy. The necessary vector is simply defined as an additive.

Most likely, gene therapy will only work for a limited number of "suitable" diseases in a restricted commercial environment. It is very costly and affords a highly complex technology as well as an individually tailored strategy for gene delivery, depending on the relevant circumstances and aims. Monogenetic diseases such as hemophilia, sickle cell anemia, adenosine-deaminase (ADA)-deficit, cystic fibrosis, or Duchenne muscular dystrophy are likely first candidates, as they require the replacement or substitution of only a single gene. Trisomy 21 (Down syndrome), on the other hand, which is also frequently mentioned in this context, is a poor candidate, as it is much more difficult to silence the additional chromosome 21 than to replace nonfunctional genes. Furthermore, the monogenetic origin of Down syndrome is under debate. In different forms of cancer and heart or circulatory failures or of acquired genetic dysfunctions such as hepatitis or AIDS, two or more genes must be substituted or otherwise manipulated. Here, successful gene therapy seems unlikely at the moment due to technical limitations in DNA transport into target cells and in tissue-specific forms of application.

Among the known innate diseases, gene therapy has been most intensively investigated in ADA deficiency and cystic fibrosis. Both reduce mean life expectancy to below 20 years, accompanied by severe symptoms that strongly affect the quality of life.

This review covers nonviral gene-transfection strategies of current interest with special reference to experimental results found *in vivo* and to clinical trials.

2
Strategies in Gene Therapy

Independent of the respective method of gene transfer, two basic strategies for gene therapy may be discriminated (Fig. 1). Following the *ex vivo* strategy, cells or tissue are first removed from the patient, then exposed *in vitro* to the therapeutic genetic construct. If the transfection has been successful, the material is reimplanted in the patient. In the alternative *in vivo* methods, the therapeutic gene or DNA-sequence is integrated into a vector and this construct is injected locally or systemically into the patient. Among other deficits, the latter method is characterized by poor tissue selectivity, rapid extracellular DNA degradation and the danger of inducing oncogenes when using viral vectors.

Further differentiation is possible at the molecular level (Fig. 2): An intact (therapeutic) gene may simply be added to the defect one (Fig. 2A), a missing gene may be substituted (Fig. 2B), or a malfunctioning gene product may be inhibited, for example, during gene translation by giving mRNA-complementary antisense oligonucleotides (Fig. 2C). The first antisense-oligonucleotide drug, Vitravene™ (with

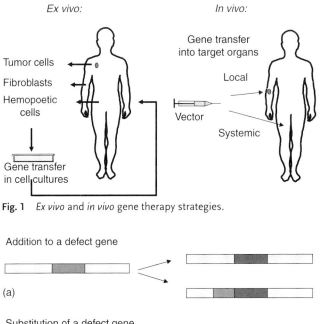

Fig. 1 *Ex vivo* and *in vivo* gene therapy strategies.

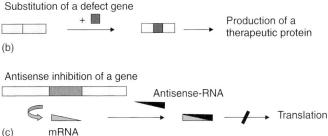

Fig. 2 Therapeutic gene functions.

formivirsen as the active ingredient), has been licensed for treating cytomegalovirus (CMV)-retinitis in AIDS patients.

The description of plasmid vectors, the biotechnology necessary for their production as pharmaceuticals and licensing specifications are not major subjects of this article. These can be studied in comprehensive overviews by Hutchins or Ferreira.

Intensive work is ongoing, both in designing new synthetic vectors and in improving DNA as a therapeutic agent. The transfection efficiency of "naked" DNA is low and it is rapidly degraded

in the cytosol. The expression of the therapeutic gene may be enhanced by eukaryotic promoters of viral origin such as CMV or simian virus. The influence of the 5′UTR-site on the translation efficiency of mRNA is also being studied. The insertion of at least one intron into the cDNA may lead to 100-fold enhancement of mRNA. The addition of a suitable terminal poly(A) signal (bovine growth factor) has similar effects. Special attention is given to the development of tissue-specific promoters, restricting transfected gene expression to the necessary therapeutic sites. A very elegant strategy for controlling the expression of the transfected gene is by turning it on or off with common oral drugs such as tetracycline or progesterone-antagonist. These interact with a mutated receptor acting as a transgene, thus initiating a signal transduction cascade, which finally induces the transcription (or its inhibition) of the respective gene for just as long as the drug is kept at a sufficient level.

3
Gene-transfection Systems

Owing to their rapid degradation in the cytosol, genes or DNA sequences are only rarely transfected as "naked" molecules. The commonly used gene transfer methods may be segregated into biological, physical, and chemical systems (Table 1). The biological systems involving viral vectors (retro, adeno, or pox viruses) make up 77% of all gene-transfection studies published to date. However, physical

and chemical methods have experienced a relative increase in recent years (12% from 1998 to 2003). This tendency reflects the often highly serious and hardly controllable side effects of viral systems. Despite recent modifications of wild-type vectors, the future of such systems for human application appears limited. One main problem of viral vectors is their strong immunogenicity. Already the first (high-dose) application may initiate an immune reaction against the given proteins, which may lead to all sorts of allergic reactions, even lethal anaphylactic shock, when repeated. Possible reversion of the virus to wild type is another danger. The potential induction of oncogenes by retroviruses must also be mentioned.

With this background, the development of chemical or physical gene transfer systems appears especially interesting, combining simple usage with maximum safety. Further requirements for an ideal gene transfer system are minimal infectivity and immunogenicity, defined

Tab. 1 Gene transfer methods in somatic gene therapy.

	Method	*Application*	*Tissue selectivity*	*Transfection efficiency*	*Expression duration*
Chemical	Liposomes, Ca-phosphate-precipitation	*Ex vivo*/(*in vivo*)	No	Low	Transient/stabile
Physical	Microinjection, electroporation, "particle-bombardment"	*Ex vivo*/(*in vivo*)	No	Moderate	Transient
Biological	Nonviral:ligand/ receptor	(*Ex vivo*)/*in vivo*	Yes	Low–moderate	Transient
	Viral: (e.g. retro-, adeno-, AAV)	*Ex vivo*/*in vivo*	Some	Moderate–high	Transient/stabile

From Gottschalk, U., Chan, S. (1998) Somatic gene therapy. Present situation and future perspective, *Arzneimittelforschung* **48**, 1111–1120.

chemical and physical characteristics, and the possibility of multiple dosing.

When looking for suitable alternatives to viral vectors, the pharmaceutical industry can offer a broad spectrum of thoroughly investigated and readily available medicinal carrier systems. As far as molecular transport and organ or cell specificity are concerned, the demands on modern drug delivery and gene transfer systems exhibit so much similarity that the latter may profit significantly in the fields of biotechnology and pharmacology. Among the chemical vectors, liposomes, polymer nanoparticles, and polylysine particles deserve special discussion. Physical transfection systems such as electroporation and bioballistics are further examples for an efficient transfer of existing know how in pharmaceutical technology to somatic gene therapy. It might be mentioned that gene transfer in a nonviral system must correctly be addressed as *transfection*, whereas, in biological systems, it should be referred to as *transduction*. Table 1 suggests a systematic arrangement of methods used in gene transfer technology. In the following sections, the most important contemporary nonviral gene transfer systems are described and assessed.

3.1
Physical Gene-transfection Systems

3.1.1 Electroporation
During electroporation, cells or tissues are exposed to an electric field of high voltage (up to 1 kV). Short, rapid pulses cause transient membrane instability and the formation of pores with a mean lifetime of up to minutes. Soluble DNA constructs that have been added to the culture medium or injected into the tissue may thereby enter the cell and ultimately reach the nucleus. The basic principle is also known to pharmacists as iontophoresis and is used for transdermal drug application. This gene-transfection method is so far well accepted by patients and is safe, especially due to the low risk of infection. To date, mainly liver, muscle, and skin cells have been transformed this way, mostly via the transdermal route.

3.1.2 Bioballistics
Bioballistical methods are already widely used in biotechnology, for example as "gene guns" for injecting DNA vaccines (Fig. 3). For this, linear or circular (plasmid-) DNA is adsorbed to nanometer-sized gold or tungsten particles. These are shot from a cylinder with compressed nitrogen or helium as propellant, thereby reaching speeds of up to 900 m s^{-1}. When applied to skin, the DNA/metal particles pass through dead tissue such as the *Stratum corneum* reaching living cells. Statistically, only one of 10 000 particles reaches the interior of viable cells, thereby loosing its DNA. For the DNA to then enter the nucleus, active transport mechanisms are probably necessary. Bioballistical gene transfer methods are obviously not suitable for systemic application. Further drawbacks are the need for very stable DNA and the high developing costs. Their greatest advantage, on the other hand, is the fact that related technologies are already approved and commercially available such as the Accell® (Powderject) (Fig. 3) or the Helios® (BioRad) systems, which are used for vaccination.

3.2
Chemical Gene-transfection Systems

A multitude of synthetic chemical vectors are being developed. Of these, cationic lipids and cationic polymers are probably

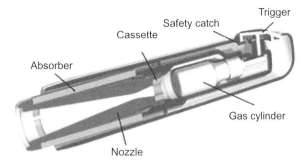

Fig. 3 Accela® gene gun (powderject). From: Burkoth, T.L., Bellhouse, B.J., Hewson, G., Longridge, D.J., Muddle, A.G., Sarphie, D.F. (1999) Transdermal and transmucosal powdered drug delivery, *Crit. Rev. Ther. Drug Carrier Syst.* **16**, 331–384.

the most thoroughly investigated. Already, in 1987, Felgner et al. could demonstrate *in vitro* gene transfection using cationic lipids. Transfer efficiency was systematically improved, leading to the first clinical studies on cystic fibrosis patients.

Irrespective of their highly variant molecular composition and 3D structure, chemical vectors such as liposomes and polymer particles have many biological and physical features in common. Positively charged amine functions are especially important, as these can be loaded with the negatively charged DNA molecules. Optimal interaction between plasmid DNA and cationic additives lead to the development of colloidal, positively charged particles, which may adhere to and be taken up by negatively charged cells a fact that is a cornerstone of chemical vector technology. Type and structure of the amine functions determine the stability of the complex, its cellular uptake in a phagosome, its release from the phagosome into the cytosol and dissociation of the DNA molecule, and even DNA transport to the nucleus.

Nucleic acids as drugs are still rather unusual in pharmaceutics. They are highly negatively charged and range in size from 10^3 kDa (oligonucleotides) to 10^6 kDa

(genes). Their targets are invariably intracellular. In contrast to most conventional pharmaceuticals, nucleic acids are too large and too strongly charged to pass cell membranes by simple passive means. Furthermore, free, that is, "naked" nucleic acids are rapidly degraded by cellular nucleases. Chemical vectors therefore have the additional job to protect the DNA they carry from enzymatic degradation. In the context of gene transfer, liposomes are also referred to as lipoplex, polymers as polyplex, and combinations as lipopolyplex particles.

3.2.1 Cationic Liposomes (Lipoplex)

Cationic liposomes were developed and already complexed with DNA over 20 years ago. However, it was in the Human Genome Project that their potential as gene transfer vehicles really became apparent to geneticists and pharmacists. Cationic liposomes consist of cationic phospholipids, which may be divided according to their number of tertiary amine functions into monovalent and multivalent cationic lipids. An overview of the most commonly used cationic lipids is given in Fig. 4.

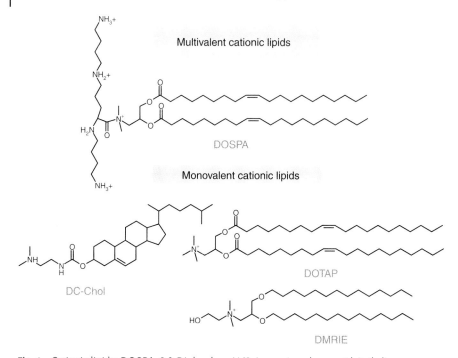

Fig. 4 Cationic lipids: DOSPA: 2,3-Dioleoyloxy-*N*-[2-(spermincarboxyamido)ethyl]-
N,*N*-dimethyl-1-propanamminiumchloride; DOTAP: 1,2-Dioleoyloxypropyl-3-*N*,*N*,*N*-
trimethyl-ammoniumchloride; DC-chol: 3β-[*N*-(*N'*,*N'*-dimethylaminoethane)
carbamoyl]-cholesterol; DMRIE: 1,2-Dimyristyloxypropyl-3-*N*,*N*-dimethylhydroxy-
ammoniumbromide. From Li, Z., Ma, Z. (2001) Nonviral gene therapy, *Curr. Gene Ther.* **1**,
201–226 and Simoes, S., Pires, P., Düzgünes, N., Pedroso de Lima, M.C. (1999) Cationic
liposomes as gene transfer vectors: barriers to successful application in gene therapy, *Curr.
Opin. Mol. Ther.* **1**, 147–157.

DOTAP (1,2-Dioleoyloxypropyl-3-*N*,*N*,*N*-trimethyl-ammoniumchloride) and DC-chol (3β-[*N'*,*N'*-dimethylaminoethane)-carbamoyl]-cholesterol are possibly the most important. However, owing to high toxicity, they must be mixed with helper lipids such as DOPE before processing to liposomes. A well-known transfection agent is Lipofectin®, which consists of equal parts DOTMA and DOPE.

The high general toxicity of the first cationic lipids initiated the synthesis of a variety of derivatives. The published *in vitro* data allows a first structure/activity analysis. The presence of a tertiary amine function and of 1 or 2 hydrophobic aliphatic chains are most important for producing stable liposomes and for binding negatively charged DNA. The tertiary amine functions can be combined with the hydrophobic lipid chains by either ester or ether bonds. Ester bonds are split more readily under physiological conditions than ether bonds and the lipoplex particles are consequentially metabolized more rapidly. These different metabolic characteristics are exemplified by DOTMA and DOTAP; the former is synthesized as ester, the latter as ether.

The aliphatic lipid chain may be saturated (DMRI) or contain double bonds (DOTAP, DOSPA). *In vivo*, dialkyl chains, with a length of 12 to 18 carbon atoms each, seem to promote the best gene transfection. A substitution of the alkyl chains with cholesterol, as in DC-chol, shows further advantages in the treatment of cystic fibrosis. Cholesterol structures have strong affinities to bronchoepithelial cells and interact less with plasma proteins.

Positively charged liposomes loaded with negatively charged DNA must maintain an overall positive charge in order to approach and contact target cells that are normally negatively charged. Liposomes that have been overloaded with DNA and have thus received a negative total charge exhibit low endocytosis rates and enhanced metabolic degradation. Proper selection of the cationic lipids and the lipid-to-DNA ratio are decisive for the rate of complexation and the colloidal structure of the product. Finally, conformations may change in time, a process also referred to as "aging" of the DNA/lipid complex.

Recent studies show that intracellular stability of the lipid/DNA complex and the necessary dissociation of the DNA molecule from its vector depend both on the pKs of the chosen lipids and on the pH of the product. Safinya et al. describe how not only the main cationic lipid but the helper lipids as well are influenced by the physical characteristics of the resulting lipid phase. For instance, when formulating DOTAP liposomes with DOPC, lamellar structures are achieved. However, when exchanging DOPC for DOPE as helper lipid, inverse hexagonal micelles are produced. One may speculate whether different lipid phase characteristics lead to defined biopharmaceutical variations.

Cationic liposomes have also been intensively investigated *in vivo*. In combination with neutral helper lipids, they appear to be well tolerated even at high concentrations; they are neither immunogenic nor do they induce toxic side effects. This applies to different routes of application such as intravenous, pulmonary, or nasal, none of which have been described as being significantly unpleasant by the recipient patients. Nevertheless, cationic liposomes also pose a number of problems such as high serum protein binding and extremely rapid metabolic degradation in the liver.

Liposomes are generally the most efficient at a diameter ranging from 400 to 500 nm. Larger particles are almost completely removed from the circulation by cells of the mononuclear phagocytes system of liver and lung and therefore do not reach other target areas. Pegylation is one means of improving pharmacokinetics. However, the useful extent of pegylation is restricted as further reduction of the zeta potential at the surface of the liposomes correlates with their reduced cellular uptake.

Low transfection rates are a further problem. Reasons are – among others – insufficient lysosomal release of the therapeutic DNA from its carrier and/or its rapid enzymatic degradation within the lysosome or in the cytosol. The DNA that was integrated in the liposomes must be released to become effective (see Fig. 5). Studies on microinjections of lipid/DNA complexes directly into the nucleus clearly show reduced transfection rates. As the nuclear pores have mean diameters of only 25 to 50 nm and passage for macromolecules is further controlled by the nuclear pore complex, passive diffusion into the karyosol is limited to particle sizes below 45 kDa. Conventional recombinant plasmids normally have a

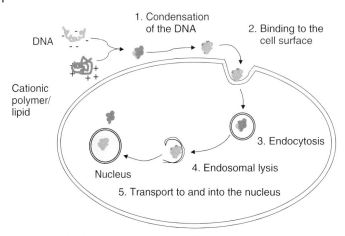

Fig. 5 Uptake, transport, and release of DNA in particulate gene transfer systems.

molecular weight ranging from 50 to 100 kDa and therefore require active transport into the nucleus.

Admission of plasmid DNA into the karyosol is steered by nuclear localization sequences, which are assisted by importin-beta, guanin-nucleotide-binding protein (Ran) and nuclear transport factor (NTF). In the karyosol, the therapeutic DNA is transcribed by RNA polymerases into mRNA, which is transported back into the cytosol where it attaches to ribosomes for translation into protein. In order to improve its transport into the nucleus, the therapeutic DNA may be coupled to such nucleus localizing sequences. The latter can be found naturally in certain viruses, which have developed this strategy for a most efficient nuclear invasion. For example, Rudolph et al. coupled DNA with short TAT sequences taken from the arginine-rich motif of the HIV-1-TAT protein and achieved significant enhancement of transfection. Of the 101 amino acid–long HIV-TAT sequence, they synthesized a 12 amino acid–long oligopeptide, bound it to polyarginine and thus achieved 390-fold enhanced transfection rates.

Unsatisfactory transfection rates and low cell or organ specificity also initiated the development of simple liposomes to virosomes or immunoliposomes. Virosomes are liposomes that contain viral proteins or fusiogenic peptides for enhanced DNA release from the endosome and for generally improved gene-transfection rates. Immunoliposomes are characterized by target-specific monoclonal antibodies bound to their surface. These were first developed in the 1980s for tumor-specific delivery of liposome-entrapped drugs and have since been modified for gene therapy.

3.2.2 Polymer Particles (Polyplex)

A further class of synthetic gene vectors that has received attention in past years is cationic polymers, which condense and package DNA with high efficiency. Polymerized or oligomerized branched or nonbranched amino acid chains composed of lysine or arginine are common. Polyethyleneimine, however, developed in 1995 by Boussif and already used for gene-transfection experiments *in vitro*

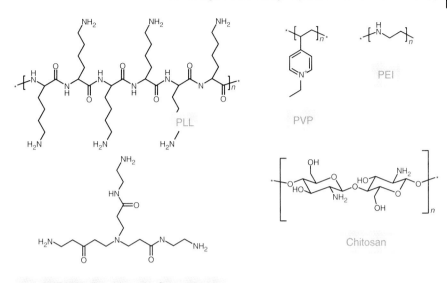

Fig. 6 Chemical structures of cationic polymers.

as well as *in vivo*, appears to be the most promising cationic polymer at the moment (see Fig. 6). Basically, cationic polymer gene transfer systems reveal the same pharmaceutical problems and intracellular barriers as described above for cationic liposomes.

3.2.3 Poly-L-Lysine (PLL) and Poly-L-Arginine (PLA)

Poly-L-lysine (PLL) has already been intensively used as polymeric gene transfer system. It is synthesized by polymerization of the *N*-carboxyanhydrid of lysine. Arginine is polymerized in a similar manner. PLL/DNA complexes are produced by dissolving both components in aqueous media and precipitating the particulate complexes. These particles, which normally range from 400 to 500 nm, are capable of transporting nucleic acids ranging from short molecules to large artificial yeast chromosomes. The first *in vivo* studies, however, revealed substantial toxicity combined with low DNA-transfection efficiency. Different chemical modifications and variations in particle size were then tested. Toxicity is substantially reduced by coating the particles with PEG derivatives, and the transfection rate is enhanced by attaching ligands such as transferrin, folate, or target-specific monoclonal antibodies. Interestingly, pegylation also achieved significant reduction in unwanted hepatic metabolization of the particles.

Apart from lysine, polymers of other cationic amino acids such as arginine and histidine were also investigated. Conjugation of histidine to ε-L-histidine enabled the development of highly interesting PLH/DNA complexes characterized by high transfection rates. One explanation for the elevated transfection efficiency may be that the highly protonated histidine structure that develops in the generally acidic (pH 6) endosomal environment may cause rapid destruction of the endosomal membrane and thus an enhanced release of the therapeutic DNA into the cytosol.

3.2.4 Polyethyleneimine (PEI)

Linear or branched polyethyleneimines generally range in size from 1.8 to 800 kDa. They are synthesized by cationic polymerization. Starting from 2-substituted-2-oxazoline-monomers, linear polyethyleneimine (PEI) with a mean molecular weight of 22 kDa A, also known as ExGEn 500, are produced by hydrolysis. PEI/DNA complexes have already been used in many *in vivo* studies in animals following iv injection; clinical studies, however, have not been reported to date. PEI/DNA complexes have repeatedly revealed very high transfection efficacy. One advantage of PEI/DNA complexes over lipoplex or PLL particles is their intrinsic buffer capacity at lysosomal pH, leading, as described above for PLL particles, to rapid destruction of the lysosomal membrane and DNA release. This effect, also termed *proton sponge*, is brought about by the chemical structure of PEI. Polymerization produces particles with primary amines at the surface and secondary as well as tertiary amines in the interior. This causes a shift in pKa from 6.9 to 3.9. The strong protonation at a pH below 6 induces an osmotic gradient across the endosomal membrane, resulting in an influx of water, swelling, and, finally, disruption of the endosome with release of the PEI/DNA particles into the cytosol.

Though the literature reveals some discrepancies, there seems to exist an inverse relationship between the molecular weight of the PEI particles and their transfection efficiency. The interesting physico-chemical characteristics of PEI-based gene transfer systems encouraged their further development, for example, to dendrimers (see below). In direct comparison, linear PEI complexes (e.g. PEI 22) seem to possess better transfection characteristics than branched ones (e.g. PEI 25). One explanation may be a premature dissociation and subsequent degradation of the DNA molecule.

Clinical trials with PEI complexes as gene transfer systems could so far not be undertaken because of their frequently intolerable general toxicity. Depending on the chemical structure, the lethal dose for mice ranges from 40 to 100 mg kg^{-1} body weight. The main problem lies in the strong interaction between PEI complexes and erythrocytes, leading to their aggregation and the danger of emboli. Pegylation of the PEI complexes may only partially help solve the problem, as a high degree of pegylation generally reduces particle uptake and thus transfection efficacy [77].

3.2.5 Dendrimers

The name ''dendrimer'' refers to the star- or tree-shaped, branched structures of this relatively new class of cationic gene transfer systems. They are frequently synthesized from polyamidoamines with special chemical or physical features. Probably best known are the ''starburst'' – dendrimers with particle sizes ranging from 5 to 100 nm. These particles reveal a highly regular branches ''dendritic'' symmetry. Starburst dendrimers are three-dimensional oligomeric or polymeric compounds, which, initiated from small molecules as nuclei, are built layer by layer (''generations'') by repeated chemical reaction cycles. This allows an exquisite steering of the final size, three-dimensional form, and surface chemistry of a starburst polymer by the individual selection of components and binding procedures for each generation.

The physical and chemical characteristics of dendrimers are mainly the result of number and type or amine functions on the particle surface, but the secondary and tertiary amines in the inside also affect their biological features. Despite their high molecular weights, dendrimers are soluble in water. They complex DNA with great efficiency, thus giving excellent vehicles for gene transfer. Their high transfer efficiency, however, is probably less due to high DNA adsorption rates and more to protonation of the amine functions after endosomal uptake. As described above for the PEI complexes, this induces an osmotic gradient, leading to osmotic lysis of the organelle and enhanced release of the complex into the cytosol. Dendrimer/DNA complexes have proven their gene transfer efficacy in *in vivo* studies. However, as already exhibited by the PEI complexes, they show strong, undesired interaction with erythrocytes, causing hemolysis. Again, the free primary amine functions on the particle surface are held responsible. Depending on the type of dendrimer and the target cell, cationic dendrimers also reveal general cytotoxicity at concentrations ranging from 50 to 300 µg mL^{-1}. On the other hand, no dendrimer has to date been reported to induce tumors or to substantially affect the immune system.

3.2.6 Chitosan

Chitosan is a fiber produced by hydrolyzing chitin, mostly from crustaceans. Owing to its free amine functions, chitosan may also be protonated (pKa = 5.6). In *in vitro* studies with Hela cells, chitosan/DNA complexes showed gene-transfection potency similar to that reported for PEI/DNA

complexes. Plain chitosan, however, is almost insoluble in water at neutral pH (but soluble at acidic pH). For this reason, tri-methylated, quaternary chitosan derivatives have been produced that are sufficiently soluble under physiological conditions and easily complex DNA molecules. In *in vitro* experiments with COS-1 and CaCo-2 cells, these innovative chitosan derivatives proved superior to nontreated chitosan polymer, particularly as they showed no unspecific cytotoxicity.

3.2.7 Poly(2-Dimethylamino) Ethylmethacrylate

Methacrylate polymers are used in pharmaceutical technology for microencapsulation. They are synthesized by polymerization of monomeric dimethylaminoacrylic acid to poly(2-dimethylamino)ethylmethacrylate (pDMAEMA), which is both simple and cheap. Their low general toxicity makes these polymers interesting also as gene transfer vehicles. In *in vitro* experiments with OVCAR-3 and COS-7 cells, some pDMAEMA/DNA particles showed high transfection rates. This proved to be highly dependent on their size and charge. In HEPES-buffer (pH 7.4), pDMAEMA particles exhibit a positive zeta potential of around 25 mV and an average size of 100 to 200 nm. Following endosomal uptake, again the outer primary amine functions are protonated, leading to osmotic lysis of the endosome and release of the pDMAEMA/DNA particles into the cytosol.

Studies on DNA absorption onto pDMAEMA particles show that linear DNA (e.g. antisense oligonucleotides) is adsorbed more strongly than circular plasmid DNA. However, this stronger adsorption has a negative influence on the gene transfer efficiency, as the DNA molecule is less likely to dissociate from the pDMAEMA particles in the cytosol. For this reason, circular DNA is preferred. As expected, DNA that is adsorbed to pDMAEMA is protected from degradation by DNAse I.

4
Perspectives

The nonviral gene-transfection systems introduced in this review bear significant advantages over the viral systems, but have serious drawbacks as well. One fact in favor is that many such systems are already well established in classical areas of pharmaceutical technology. Their production methods have already been optimized and safety aspect investigated in detail. Simple transfer of knowledge may substantially reduce developing costs. Nonviral systems are noninfectious. They allow significantly higher DNA-loading rates than viral systems, which reach their limits around 30 kb (Herpes virus). Nonviral systems are only weakly immunogenic and therefore allow – in stark contrast to viral systems – multiple application.

The main drawback of nonviral systems is that they normally only lead to transient expression of the therapeutic gene as it is not permanently integrated into the host genome. In consequence, the therapeutic gene transfer must be regularly repeated, possibly over a long period of time. Further disadvantages are insufficient cell or tissue specificity and low DNA transfer rates from the cytosol to the nucleus. Taken together, the gene-transfection performances of nonviral systems are even weaker than those of viral systems.

To date, it is still not possible to make a clear decision between viral and nonviral gene transfer systems. Mixed systems, hybrid vectors, which can be envisaged

as "de-nucleated" viruses, are in the pipeline. A combination of viral surface proteins and liposomes or the integration of therapeutic DNA into artificial cells or viruses are further innovative ideas for improving somatic gene therapy. Most important is rapid progress on three fields: In cell biology, unspecific and specific intracellular trafficking of macromolecules still raises questions. In biochemistry, further DNA carriers must be brought forward for testing, and pharmaceutical technology must supply improved and cell-/tissue-specific drug delivery systems. Brought together in a rational form, such progress should make somatic gene therapy possible for selected disease forms already in the near future.

Somatic gene therapy might develop into one of the most important therapeutic strategies of the near future. Innate or acquired genetic defects are held responsible for a number of diseases such as hemophilia, cystic fibrosis (mucoviscidosis), adenosine-deaminase deficit and AIDS. Substituting or supplementing malfunctioning or missing genetic information by transiently or permanently inserting the appropriate gene appears to be a plausible therapeutic strategy especially from the patients' point of view. Attempts in gene therapy began in the early 1990s with great expectations that have only partially been met. No disease with a defined genetic background has so far been causally cured by gene therapy. Viral gene transfer systems have caused severe problems that could not be brought under control to date. The death of the 18-year-old Jesse Gelsinger is a tragic evidence for the basic deficits of viral transfection systems. In consequence, attention is now focusing on chemical and physical gene transfer systems.

See also Liposome Gene Transfection; Somatic Gene Therapy; Genetic Vaccination; Vector System: Plasmid DNA.

Bibliography

Books and Reviews

Brooks, G. (2002) *Gene Therapy: The Use of DNA as a Drug*, Pharmaceutical Press, London.

EMEA Council Regulation 2309/93 as proclaimed 22nd July 1993 (OJ EC L 214).

Parker, A.L., Newman, C., Briggs, S., Seymour, L., Sheridan, P.J. (2003) Nonviral gene delivery: techniques and implications for molecular medicine, *Expert Rev. Mol. Med.* **22**, 113–142.

Pfeifer, A., Verma, I.M. (2001) Gene therapy: promises and problems, *Annu. Rev. Genomics Hum. Genet.* **2**, 177–211.

Rubanyi, G.M. (2001) The future of human gene therapy, *Mol. Aspects Med.* **22**, 113–142.

Primary Literature

Anwer, K., Shi, M., French, M.F., et al. (1998) Systemic effect of human growth hormone after intramuscular injection of a single dose of a muscle-specific gene medicine, *Hum. Gene Ther.* **9**, 659–670.

Arigita, C., Zuidam, N.J., Crommelin, D.J., Hennik, W.E. (1999) Association and dissociation characteristics of polymer/DNA complexes used for gene delivery, *Pharm. Res.* **16**, 1534–1541.

Barrett, A.D. (2002) Arilvax (Powderject), *Curr. Opin. Investig. Drugs* **3**, 992–995.

Behr, J. (1997) The proton sponge: a trick to enter cells the viruses did not exploit, *Chimia* **51**, 34–36.

Biggar, W.D., Klamut, H.J., Demacio, P.C., Stevens, D.J., Ray, P.N. (2002) Duchenne muscular dystrophy: current knowledge, treatment, and future prospects, *Clin. Orthop.* **401**, 88–106.

Blaese, R.M., Culver, K.W., Miller, A.D., et al. (1995) T lymphocyte-directed gene therapy for ADA-SCID: initial trial results after 4 years, *Science* **270**, 475–480.

Bordignon, C., Notarangelo, L.D., Nobili, N., et al. (1995) Gene therapy in peripheral blood lymphocytes and bone marrow for ADA-immunodeficient patients, *Science* **270**, 470–475.

Boussif, O., Lezoualch, F., Zanta, M.A., et al. (1995) A versatile vector for gene and oligonucleotide transfer into cells in culture and *in vivo*: polyethylenimine, *Proc. Natl. Acad. Sci. U.S.A.* **92**, 7297–7301.

Bragonzi, A., Dina, G., Villa, A., et al. (2000) Biodistribution and transgene expression with nonviral cationic vector/DNA complexes in the lungs, *Gene Ther.* **7**, 1753–1760.

Brissault, B., Kichler, A., Guis, C., Leborgne, C., Danos, O., Cheradame, H. (2003) Synthesis of linear polyethylenimine derivatives for DNA transfection, *Bioconjug. Chem.* **14**, 581–587.

Burkoth, T.L., Bellhouse, B.J., Hewson, G., Longridge, D.J., Muddle, A.G., Sarphie, D.F. (1999) Transdermal and transmucosal powdered drug delivery, *Crit. Rev. Ther. Drug Carrier Syst.* **16**, 331–384.

Chan, C.K., Jans, D.A. (2002) Using nuclear targeting signals to enhance non-viral gene transfer, *Immunol. Cell Biol.* **80**, 19–130.

Chemin, I., Moradpour, D., Wieland, S., et al. (1998) Liver-directed gene transfer: a linear polyethylenimine derivative mediates highly efficient DNA delivery to primary hepatocytes *in vitro* and *in vivo*, *J. Viral. Hepat.* **5**, 369–375.

Cloninger, M.J. (2002) Biological applications of dendrimers, *Curr. Opin. Chem. Biol.* **6**, 742–748.

Coleman, M.E., DeMayo, F., Yin, K.C., et al. (1995) Myogenic vector expression of insulin-like growth factor I stimulates muscle cell differentiation and myofiber hypertrophy in transgenic mice, *J. Biol. Chem.* **270**, 12109–12116.

De Jong, G., Telenius, A., Vanderbyl, S., Meitz, A., Drayer, J. (2001) Efficient *in vitro* transfer of a 60-Mb mammalian artificial chromosome into murine and hamster cells using cationic lipids and dendrimers, *Chromosome Res.* **9**, 475–485.

Dykes, G.M. (2001) Dendrimers: a review of their appeal and applications, *J. Chem. Technol. Biotechnol.* **76**, 903–918.

Felgner, P.L., Gadek, T.R., Holm, M., et al. (1987) Lipofection: a highly efficient, lipid-mediated DNA-transfection procedure, *Proc. Natl. Acad. Sci. U.S.A.* **84**, 7413–7417.

Felgner, P.L., Tsai, Y.J., Sukhu], L., et al. (1995) Improved cationic lipid formulations for *in vivo* gene therapy, *Ann. N. Y. Acad. Sci.* **772**, 126–139.

Feltquate, D.M. (1998) DNA vaccines: vector design, delivery, and antigen presentation, *J. Cell. Biochem.* **30–31**(Suppl.), 304–311.

Ferreira, G.N.M., Monteiro, G.A., Duarte, M.F., Cabral, P., Cabral, J.M.S. (2000) Downstream processing of plasmid DNA for gene therapy and DNA vaccine applications, *Trends Biotechnol.* **18**, 380–938.

Fischer, A. (2001) Gene therapy: some results, many problems to solve, *Cell Mol. Biol.* **47**, 1269–1275.

Flotte, T.R. (1999) Gene therapy for cystic fibrosis, *Curr. Opin. Mol. Ther.* **1**, 510–516.

Gebhart, C.L., Kabanov, A.V. (2001) Evaluation of polyplexes as gene transfer agents, *J. Control. Release* **73**, 401–416.

Gehl, J. (2003) Electroporation: theory and methods, perspectives for drug delivery, gene therapy and research, *Acta Physiol. Scand.* **177**, 437–447.

German Regulation for Gene Technology (Gentechnik Gesetz, GenTG) as proclaimed 16th December 1993. *BGBl* part I: 2066. Last altered Art. 1 G, 21st December 2004; 2005 I 186.

German Regulation for the Protection of Human Embryos (Embryoschutz Gesetz, EschG) as proclaimed 13th December 1990, *BGBl* part I (1990) pp. 2747.

Gossen, M., Freundlieb, S., Bender, G., Muller, G., Hillen, W., Bujard, H. (1995) Transcriptional activation by tetracyclines in mammalian cells, *Science* **268**, 1766–1769.

Gottschalk, U., Chan, S. (1998) Somatic gene therapy. Present situation and future perspective, *Arzneimittelforschung* **48**, 1111–1120.

Huang, M.T., Gorman, C.M. (1990) Intervening sequences increase efficiency of RNA 3′ processing and accumulation of cytoplasmic RNA, *Nucleic Acids Res.* **18**, 937–947.

Hutchins, B. (2000) Characterization of plasmids and formulations for non-viral gene therapy, *Curr. Opin. Mol. Ther.* **2**, 131–135.

Johnson-Saliba, M., Jans, D.A. (2001) Gene therapy: optimizing DNA delivery to the nucleus, *Curr. Drug Targets* **2**, 371–399.

Kanikkannan, N. (2002) Iontophoresis-based transdermal delivery systems, *BioDrugs* **16**, 339–347.

Kingdon, H.S., Lundblad, R.L. (2002) An adventure in biotechnology: the development of haemophilia A therapeutics – from whole-blood transfusion to recombinant DNA to gene therapy, *Biotechnol. Appl. Biochem.* **35**, 141–148.

Koltover, I., Wagner, K., Safinya, C.R. (2000) DNA condensation in two dimensions, *Proc. Natl. Acad. Sci. U.S.A.* **97**, 14046–14051.

Koltover, I., Salditt, T., Radler, J.O., Safinya, C.R. (1998) An inverted hexagonal phase of cationic liposome-DNA complexes related to DNA release and delivery, *Science* **281**, 78–81.

Kozak, M. (1991) Structural features in eukaryotic mRNAs that modulate the initiation of translation, *J. Biol. Chem.* **266**, 19867–19870.

Kozak, M. (1992) Regulation of translation in eukaryotic systems, *Ann. Rev. Cell. Biol.* **8**, 197–225.

Kukowska-Latallo, J.F., Bielinska, A.U., Johnson, J., Spindler, R., Tomalia, D.A., Baker, J.R. Jr. (1996) Efficient transfer of genetic material into mammalian cells using Starburst polyamidoamine dendrimers, *Proc. Natl. Acad. Sci. U.S.A.* **93**, 4897–4902.

Lee, E.R., Marshall, J., Siegel, C.S., et al. (1996) Detailed analysis of structures and formulations of cationic lipids for efficient gene transfer to the lung, *Hum. Gene Ther.* **7**, 1701–1717.

Li, Z., Ma, Z. (2001) Nonviral gene therapy, *Curr. Gene Ther.* **1**, 201–226.

Lin, A.J., Slack, N.L., Ahmad, A., et al. (2000) Structure and structure-function studies of lipid/plasmid DNA complexes, *J. Drug Target.* **8**, 13–27.

Lollo, C.P., Banaszczyk, M.G., Mullen, P.M., et al. (2002) Poly-L-lysine-based gene delivery systems. Synthesis, purification, and application, *Methods Mol. Med.* **69**, 1–13.

Ma, H., Diamond, S.L. (2001) Nonviral gene therapy and its delivery systems, *Curr. Pharm. Biotechnol.* **2**, 1–17.

Mahato, R.I., Smith, L.C., Rolland, A. (1999) Pharmaceutical perspectives of nonviral gene delivery, *Adv. Genet.* **41**, 95–156.

Malik, N., Wiwattanapatepee, R., Klopsch, R., et al. (2000) Dendrimers: relationship between structure and biocompatibility *in vitro* and preliminary studies on the biodistribution of 125J-labelled polyamidoamine dendrimers *in vivo*, *J. Control. Release* **65**, 133–148.

Mannisto, M., Vanderkerken, S., Toncheva, V., et al. (2002) Structure-activity relationships of poly(L-lysines): effects of pegylation and molecular shape on physicochemical and biological properties in gene delivery, *J. Control. Release* **83**, 169–182.

Marschall, P., Malik, N., Larin, Z. (1999) Transfer of YACs up to 2.3 Mb intact into human cells with polyethylenimine, *Gene Ther.* **6**, 1634–1637.

Merlin, J.L., N'Doye, A., Bouriez, T., Dolivet, G. (2002) Polyethylenimine derivatives as potent nonviral vectors for gene transfer, *Drug News Perspect.* **15**, 445–451.

Midoux, P., LeCam, E., Coulaud, D., Delain, E., Pichon, C. (2002) Histidine containing peptides and polypeptides as nucleic acid vectors, *Somat. Cell. Mol. Genet.* **27**, 27–47.

Newkome, G.R., Moorefield, C.N., Vogtle, F. (2001) *Dendrimers and Dendrons: Concepts, Syntheses, Applications*, Wiley-VCH, New York.

Niculescu-Duvaz, D., Heyes, J., Springer, C.J. (2003) Structure-activity relationship in cationic lipid mediated gene transfection, *Curr. Med. Chem.* **10**, 1233–1261.

Orr, R.M. (2001) Technology evaluation: fomivirsen, ISIS pharmaceuticals Inc/CIBA vision, *Curr. Opin. Mol. Ther.* **3**, 288–294.

Osaka, G., Carey, K., Cuthbertson, A., et al. (1996) Pharmacokinetics, tissue distribution, and expression efficiency of plasmid [33P]DNA following intravenous administration of DNA/cationic lipid complexes in mice: use of a novel radionuclide approach, *J. Pharm. Sci.* **6**, 612–618.

Petersen, H., Fechner, P.M., Marti, A.L., et al. (2002) Polyethylenimine-graft-poly(ethylene glycol) copolymers: influence of copolymer block structure on DNA complexation and biological activities as gene delivery system, *Bioconjug. Chem.* **13**, 845–854.

Plank, C., Tang, M.X., Wolfe, A.R., Szoka, F.C. Jr. (1999) Branched cationic peptides for gene delivery: role of type and number of cationic residues in formation and *in vitro* activity of DNA polyplexes, *Hum. Gene Ther.* **10**, 319–332.

Pouton, C.W., Lucas, P., Thomas, B.J., Uduehi, A.N., Milroy, D.A., Moss, S.H. (1998) Polycation-DNA complexes for gene delivery: a comparison of the biopharmaceutical properties of cationic polypeptides and cationic lipids, *J. Control. Release* **53**, 289–299.

Qin, L., Ding, Y., Pahud, D.R., Chang, E., Imperiale, M.J., Bromberg, J.S. (1997) Promoter attenuation in gene therapy: interferon-gamma and tumor necrosis factor-alpha inhibit transgene expression, *Hum. Gene Ther.* **8**, 2019–2029.

Rädler, J.O., Koltover, I., Salditt, T., Safinya, C.R. (1997) Structure of DNA-cationic liposome complexes: DNA intercalation in multilamellar membranes in distinct interhelical packing regimes, *Science* **275**, 810–814.

Romano, G., Claudio, P.P., Kaiser, H.E., Giordano, A. (1998) Recent advances, prospects and problems in designing new strategies for oligonucleotide and gene delivery in therapy, *In Vivo* **12**, 59–67.

Römpp, L. (1999) in Decjwer, W.D., Pühler, A., Schmid, E. (Eds.) *Biotechnologie und Gentechnik*, 2nd edition, Georg Thieme Verlag, Stuttgart, New York.

Rudolph, C., Plank, C., Lausier, J., Schillinger, U., Müller, R.H., Rosenecker, J. (2003) Oligomers of the arginine-rich motif of the HIV-1 TAT protein are capable of transferring plasmid DNA into cells, *J. Biol. Chem.* **278**, 11411–11418.

Safinya, C.R. (2001) Structures of lipid-DNA complexes: supramolecular assembly and gene delivery, *Curr. Opin. Struct. Biol.* **11**, 440–448.

Satkauskas, S., Bureau, M.F., Puc, M., et al. (2002) Mechanisms of *in vivo* DNA electrotransfer: respective contributions of cell electropermeabilization and DNA electrophoresis, *Mol. Ther.* **5**, 133–140.

Schaffer, D.V., Fidelman, N.A., Dan, N., Lauffenburger, D.A. (2000) Vector unpacking as a potential barrier for receptor-mediated polyplex gene delivery, *Biotechnol. Bioeng.* **67**, 598–606.

Schatzlein, A.G. (2001) Non-viral vectors in cancer gene therapy: principles and progress, *Anti-Cancer Drugs* **12**, 275–304.

Shi, N., Boado, R.J., Pardridge, W.M. (2001) Receptor-mediated gene targeting to tissues *in vivo* following intravenous administration of pegylated immunoliposomes, *Pharm. Res.* **18**, 1091–1095.

Simoes, S., Pires, P., Düzgünes, N., Pedroso de Lima, M.C. (1999) Cationic liposomes as gene transfer vectors: barriers to successful application in gene therapy, *Curr. Opin. Mol. Ther.* **1**, 147–157.

Stevenson, B.J., Carothers, A.D., Wallace, W.A., et al. (1997) Evidence for safety and efficacy of DOTAP cationic liposome-mediated CFTR gene transfer to the nasal epithelium of patients with cystic fibrosis, *Gene Ther.* **4**, 210–218.

Stiriba, S.E., Frey, H., Haag, R. (2002) Dendritic polymers in biomedical applications: from potential to clinical use in diagnostics and therapy, *Angew. Chem., Int. Ed. Engl.* **41**, 1329–1334.

Templeton, N.S. (2003) Myths concerning the use of cationic liposomes *in vivo*, *Expert Opin. Biol. Ther.* **3**, 57–69.

Thanou, M., Florea, B.I., Geldof, M., Junginger, H.E., Borchard, G. (2002) Quaternized chitosan oligomers as novel gene delivery vectors in epithelial cell lines, *Biomaterials* **23**, 153–159.

Tomalia, D.A., Killat, G.R. (1985) in: Kroschwitz, J.I. (Ed.) *Encyclopedia of Polymer Science and Engineering 1*, 2nd edition, Wiley, New York, pp. 680–739.

Tomlinson, E., Rolland, A.P. (1996) Controllable gene therapy: pharmaceutics of non viral gene delivery systems, *J. Control. Release* **39**, 357–372.

URL: http://www.wiley.co.uk/genmed/clinical/ (1st June 2003)

Vacik, J., Dean, B.S., Zimmer, W.E., Dean, D.A. (1998) Cell-specific nuclear import of plasmid DANN, *Gene Ther.* **6**, 1006–1014.

van Steenis, J.H., van Maarseveen, E.M., Verbaan, F.J. et al. (2003) Preparation and characterization of folate-targeted pEG-coated pDMAEMA-based polyplexes, *J. Control. Release* **87**, 167–176.

Verbaan, F. (2002) *Colloidal Gene Delivery Systems – In Vivo Fate of Poly(2-(Dimethyl Amino) Ethyl Methacrylate)-Based Transfection Complexes*, Ph.D.-thesis, Utrecht University, Holland, pp. 14–15.

Wagner, E., Ogris, M., Zauner, W. (1998) Polylysine-based transfection systems utilizing receptor-mediated delivery, *Adv. Drug Deliv. Rev.* **30**, 97–113.

Wang, Y., O'Malley, B.W., Tsai, S.Y. (1997) Inducible system designed for future gene therapy, *Methods Mol. Biol.* **63**, 401–413.

Wattiaux, R., Laurent, N., Wattiaux-De Coninck, S., Jadot, M. (2000) Endosomes, lysosomes: their implication in gene transfer, *Adv. Drug Deliv. Rev.* **41**, 201–208.

Wheeler, C., Felgner, P.L., Tsai, Y.J., et al. (1996) A novel cationic lipid greatly enhances plasmid DNA delivery and expression in mouse lung, *Proc. Natl. Acad. Sci. U.S.A.* **93**, 11454–11459.

Wightman, L., Kircheis, R., Rossler, V., et al. (2001) Different behavior of branched and linear polyethylenimine for gene delivery *in vitro* and *in vivo*, *J. Gene Med.* **3**, 362–372.

Wolff, J.A., Malone, R.W., Williams, P., et al. (1990) Direct gene transfer into mouse muscle *in vivo*, *Science* **247**, 1465–1468.

Yew, N.S., Wysokenski, D.M., Wang, K.X., et al. (1997) Optimization of plasmid vectors for high-level expression in lung epithelial cells, *Hum. Gene Ther.* **8**, 575–584.

Yu, R.Z., Geary, R.S., Leeds, J.M., et al. (1999) Pharmacokinetics and tissue disposition in monkeys of an antisense oligonucleotide inhibitor of Ha-ras encapsulated in stealth liposomes, *Pharm. Res.* **16**, 1309–1315.

Zauner, W., Ogris, M., Wagner, E. (1998) Polylysine-based transfection systems utilizing receptor mediated delivery, *Adv. Drug Deliv. Rev.* **30**, 115–131.

Zou, S.M., Erbacher, P., Remy, J.S., Behr, J.P. (2000) Systemic linear polyethylenimine (L-PEI)-mediated gene delivery in the mouse, *J. Gene Med.* **2**, 128–134.

Zuidam, N.J., Posthuma, G., de Vries, E.T.J., Crommelin, D.J.A., Hennink, W.E., Storm, G. (2000) Effects of physicochemical characteristics of poly(2-(dimethylamino) ethyl methacrylate)-based polyplexes on cellular association and internalization, *J. Drug Target.* **8**, 51–66.

31

Gene Therapy and Cardiovascular Diseases

Michael E. Rosenfeld[1] *and Alan D. Attie*[2]
[1] *Department of Pathobiology, University of Washington, Seattle, WA, USA*
[2] *Department of Biochemistry, University of Wisconsin-Madison, Madison, WI, USA*

1   Overview of Gene Therapy   975

2   Atherosclerosis: A Chronic Inflammatory Disease   976

3   Gene Therapy Targets for Cardiovascular Disease in the Lipoprotein
        Pathways   979
3.1   The Lipoprotein Pathways Provide Many Potential Gene
        Therapy Targets   979
3.2   Specific
        Genes are Critical for Dietary Lipid Absorption in the Intestine   980
3.3   The Intestine Exports Lipids on Chylomicron Particles   981
3.4   The Liver is a Major Producer of Plasma Lipoproteins   981
3.5   Lipoprotein Lipase as a Target for Gene Therapy   982
3.6   The LDL and VLDL Receptors are Attractive Targets
        for Gene Therapy   983
3.7   Increased Cholesterol and Phospholipid Efflux via ABCA1
        Can Prevent Atherosclerosis   984
3.8   Some Apolipoproteins Can Prevent Atherosclerosis   985
3.9   The Liver SR-B1 Receptor Protects against Atherosclerosis   986

4   Vascular and Inflammatory Targets for Gene Therapy   987
4.1   Adhesion Molecules and Leukocyte Counter Receptors   987
4.2   Cytokines   988
4.3   Chemokines and Chemokine Receptors   988
4.4   Interleukins, the TNF-α family, and Interferon-γ 989
4.5   Growth Factors and Receptors   990

5   Pro- and Antioxidant Enzymes   991

Pharmacology. From Drug Development to Gene Therapy. Edited by Robert A. Meyers.
Copyright © 2008 Wiley-VCH Verlag GmbH & Co. KGaA, Weinheim
ISBN: 978-3-527-32343-2

6   **Scavenger Receptors   992**

7   **Transcription Factors   993**

8   **Noninflammatory Gene Targets   994**
8.1   Cell Death   994
8.2   Proteases   994
8.3   Regulators of Vascular Tone and Blood Pressure   995
8.4   Coagulation Related Genes   995
8.5   Osteogenic Proteins   996

            Bibliography   996
            Books and Reviews   996
            Primary Literature   997

Keywords

ABCA1
A membrane lipid–transport protein involved in cholesterol and/or phospholipid efflux from cells. Its action is necessary for the extracellular assembly of lipoprotein particles.

Adhesion Molecules
These are proteins on the luminal surface of endothelial cells, bind to counter receptors on the membrane of leukocytes, and enable the leukocytes to attach tightly to the surface of the endothelial cells.

Angina Pectoris
Chest pain caused by reduced blood flow to the heart due to the blockage of coronary arteries by blood clots.

Angiogenesis
The process of formation of new blood vessels.

Angioplasty
An intervention to increase blood flow in a clogged artery. It involves insertion of a balloon catheter into the blocked artery and subsequent inflation of the balloon to break open or squash the atherosclerotic lesion and/or blood clot that is reducing blood flow.

Apical Membrane
In polarized cells (e.g. hepatocytes in the liver, enterocytes in the intestine), the membrane exposed to the outside world; in the hepatocytes, the bile canalicular membrane; in enterocytes, the membrane exposed to the intestinal lumen.

ApoA1
An apolipoprotein principally associated with HDL, an activator of lecithin cholesterol: acyltransferase. It interacts with the cells to mediate delivery of cholesterol ester from HDL particles.

ApoB100
An apolipoprotein associated with VLDL and LDL particles, synthesized in the liver, a ligand for the LDL receptor.

ApoB48
An apolipoprotein associated with chylomicrons, synthesized in the intestine; it is a truncated form of apoB100 and does not bind to the LDL receptor.

ApoE
An apolipoprotein principally associated with VLDL and chylomicrons, is responsible for the receptor-mediated clearance of IDL and chylomicron remnants, is a ligand for most members of the LDL-receptor superfamily. The apoE4 isoform is associated with increased risk of Alzheimer's Disease.

Apolipoproteins
The protein components of plasma lipoproteins.

Apoptosis
The programmed cell death of a cell or cellular suicide. It is a defined molecular pathway where proteolytic enzymes are activated to destroy key cellular proteins.

Atherosclerosis
An inflammatory disease in the arterial wall leading to the accumulation of cellular outgrowths that can become unstable, break off, and cause the formation of blood clots.

Basolateral Membrane
In polarized cells, the membrane exposed to the inside world; in hepatocytes, the sinusoidal membrane, which is exposed to venous circulation, in enterocytes, the basolateral membrane, which is exposed to the lymphatics and venous circulation.

Bile Acids
Detergent-like molecules formed from cholesterol. They are secreted by the liver and together with cholesterol and phospholipids, form bile. Bile forms micelles that emulsify lipids in the intestinal lumen aiding in their absorption.

Chemokines
A category of cytokines that function specifically to chemically attract leukocytes to sites of inflammation.

Chylomicron Remnants
Chylomicron particles that have been depleted of triacylglycerol after the lipoprotein lipase–mediated hydrolysis of their triacylglycerols.

Chylomicrons
Lipoprotein particles produced in the intestine to package and secrete dietary lipids. Chylomicrons are secreted into the mesenteric lymph.

Cytokines
Cell regulatory proteins secreted by many cell types that are key factors in the initiation and control of inflammation.

Familial Hypercholesterolemia
Elevation in LDL cholesterol due to mutations at the LDL-receptor locus.

Familial Hypoalphalipoproteinemia
Deficiency in HDL cholesterol due to mutations at the ABCA1 locus.

Fatty Streak
Earliest stage in the development of an atherosclerotic lesion. It consists of aggregates of macrophage-derived foam cells and lymphocytes that form underneath the endothelial lining of an artery.

Fibrous Cap
A thin layer of smooth muscle cells and connective tissue that encapsulates areas of dead cells and lipid in a developing atherosclerotic lesion. If the fibrous cap is too thin, it can break and enable formation of blood clots that can clog arteries.

Foam Cells
Primarily macrophages that have taken up large numbers of modified lipoprotein particles and have stored the excess lipid in non membrane bound cholesteryl-ester droplets and in increased numbers of secondary lysosomes.

Gallstones
Large crystals, usually composed of cholesterol, that form in the biliary tract and/or gall bladder when cholesterol levels in bile are too high relative to phospholipid and bile acids.

Growth Factors
Secreted by many cell types and by binding to specific receptors on the plasma membrane of adjacent cells, are potent regulators of cellular functions, including proliferation, migration, differentiation, and survival/apoptosis.

HDL
High-density lipoprotein, carries about 20% of plasma cholesterol. Its levels negatively correlate with risk of coronary heart disease. Is thought to mediate "reverse cholesterol transport."

Hemorrhage
Bleeding into a tissue. In atherosclerotic lesions, it occurs when the lesion forms fissures or ruptures and is an indication that the lesion is unstable.

IDL

An intermediate density lipoprotein, also called "VLDL remnant." It is the VLDL particle that has been depleted of triacylglycerol through the action of lipoprotein lipase.

Intima

The inner layer of a muscular artery. It is the space immediately behind the endothelium where atherosclerotic lesions develop. In normal, nondiseased human arteries, there is a diffuse thickening of the intima that contains connective tissue and sparse numbers of macrophages and smooth muscle cells.

Ischemia

The inadequate perfusion of a tissue with blood leading to the reduced availability of oxygen and nutrients in the tissue.

LDL

Low-density lipoprotein carries approximately two-thirds of plasma cholesterol. Its levels are positively correlated with the risk of coronary heart disease and is formed in the circulation from the catabolism of VLDL.

LDL Receptor

Expressed in most tissues and is mainly necessary for normal clearance of LDL from the bloodstream.

Lipoprotein Lipase

Catalyzes the hydrolysis of VLDL and LDL triacylglycerols to free fatty acids and glycerol, and is present on the luminal surface of the capillary endothelium.

Lipoproteins

Particles that transport lipids in the bloodstream.

Media

The middle layer of a muscular artery that contains concentric rings of smooth muscle cells oriented perpendicular to blood flow. The orientation allows the contraction of the smooth muscle cells to constrict the artery. Atherosclerotic lesions do not initially form in the media but can expand and replace the media in very advanced stages of the disease.

Myocardial Infarction

The necrotic death of heart tissue due to a sudden blockage of blood flow to the affected tissue. It most frequently occurs following the formation of a blood clot on top of an atherosclerotic lesion that has ruptured in a main coronary artery.

Necrotic Zones

Areas within an atherosclerotic lesion that contain dead cells and debris, and lipid droplets formed from dead foam cells and aggregated lipoproteins. The expansion of necrotic zones into a *necrotic core* can make the lesion unstable and at risk of rupture.

Neovascularization
The formation of new, small blood vessels within an advanced atherosclerotic lesion. Neovessels are often formed deep in the lesion where there is limited diffusion of oxygen and nutrients, and can be a conduit for bringing more leukocytes into the advanced lesions.

Restenosis
The process of reformation of an arterial lesion that reduces blood flow following an intervention procedure such as angioplasty. A restenotic lesion is not the same as an atherosclerotic lesion as it forms primarily because of the migration and proliferation of smooth muscle cells following injury to the artery caused by the intervention procedure. It occurs in up to 40% of people who have angioplasty to increase blood flow to the heart.

Scavenger Receptors
Bind to a wide range of molecules, including modified forms of LDL. Are involved in the accumulation of cholesterol in macrophages and smooth muscle cells in the arterial wall.

Statins
Drugs that inhibit the synthesis of cholesterol. They increase the abundance of the LDL receptor and thus reduce plasma LDL levels.

Tangier Disease
A severe HDL deficiency syndrome caused by homozygous mutations at the ABCA1 locus.

Thrombosis
The formation of blood clots. A thrombus consists of variable numbers of aggregated platelets, red blood cells, and fibrin. In the heart, brain, or peripheral blood vessels, it can be an *occlusive thrombus* that blocks blood flow, or a smaller *mural thrombus* that is attached to an atherosclerotic lesion and does not block blood flow.

Vasospasm
The transient constriction of a blood vessel. Depending on the extent of constriction, blood flow can be reduced leading to tissue ischemia.

VLDL
Very low-density lipoprotein, a triacylglycerol-rich lipoprotein assembled in the endoplasmic reticulum and Golgi of hepatocytes and then secreted into the bloodstream. While in the circulation, its triacylglycerol core is depleted through the action of lipoprotein lipase and it gives rise to low-density lipoprotein.

1
Overview of Gene Therapy

Gene therapy refers to the expression of a recombinant gene in a patient. The recombinant gene can be delivered to the patient directly or it can be incorporated into cells *in vitro*, followed by delivery of the genetically modified cells to the patient. DNA delivery can occur in the patient as naked DNA or within a biological or artificial delivery vehicle. The biological delivery vehicle is usually a virus. A wide variety of artificial delivery vehicles have been developed. They usually consist of lipid vesicles (liposomes) or positively charged polymers that complex with DNA and have a high affinity for cell surfaces that are negatively charged.

Genetic therapy for the treatment of cardiovascular disease (CVD) is in its infant stage despite the large number of potential target genes associated with the development of atherosclerosis. Cardiovascular disease lends itself to genetic therapy because of the focal nature of atherosclerotic lesions and the availability of techniques for direct delivery of the genes to the affected areas. The desire to conduct gene therapy for atherosclerosis is in large part motivated by the large number of transgenic mouse studies in which expression or deletion of a gene has a profound therapeutic effect on the animal. For example, overexpression of the apolipoprotein-A1 gene protects animals from atherosclerosis. A logical extension is to mimic these studies with gene therapy.

Although the gene therapy field is now more than 20 years old, it has not fulfilled its initial promise. From the beginning, it has been impossible to achieve sustained expression of foreign genes at high levels. There is still an incomplete understanding of the fundamental processes by which DNA enters the cells, is transported to the nucleus, integrates into chromosomal DNA, and interacts with transcriptional machinery.

Regardless of the vehicle, DNA must be administered into the circulatory system in order to gain access to a high proportion of cells in a solid tissue. However, most tissues are not in direct contact with blood. They are shielded from blood by a tight layer of endothelial cells that comprise the luminal surface of arteries and veins. Particles as large as viruses or DNA/polymer aggregates cannot cross the small gaps (fenestrae) between endothelial cells. An important exception is the vasculature that perfuses the liver. These vessels have large fenestrae, allowing large particles to gain access to the hepatocytes in the liver. For this reason, it is relatively easy to target the liver and quite difficult to target extrahepatic tissues.

There are three predominant types of viral vectors used in gene therapy; adenoviruses, adeno-associated viruses, and lentiviruses. *Adenoviruses* belong to a family of human DNA tumor viruses that can cause noncancerous respiratory tract infections in humans. Upon infection, the viral DNA remains episomal (outside the host genome), thus making expression transient. Adenoviruses can infect both dividing and nondividing cells. Adenoviral infection causes an inflammatory response, which curtails the infection and can produce severe reactions in some individuals.

Adeno-associated virus is a small nonpathogenic single-stranded DNA virus. On its own, it cannot replicate. It depends on simultaneous expression of genes provided by adenovirus. The virus infects a broad range of dividing and nondividing cells. It can maintain its DNA as an episome or can, at low frequency, integrate into the host cell's chromosomal DNA. Adeno-associated virus is potentially attractive because its expression tends to be long-lived and it does not elicit an inflammatory reaction the way adenoviruses do.

Lentiviruses are retroviruses, RNA viruses that replicate through a DNA intermediate. HIV is a lentivirus. Lentiviruses have been modified to infect a broad range of cells. They can infect nondividing cells. As is the case with adeno and adeno-associated virus, lentiviruses are produced that are replication-defective for gene therapy applications.

Injection of *naked DNA* into muscle results in transfection of the cells *in vivo*. Intravascular injection of naked DNA leads to uptake by hepatocytes in the liver. Some of the cells stably incorporate the foreign DNA and express its genes. Since animals are continually exposed to foreign DNA coming from the diet and from symbiotic and infectious microorganisms, they have evolved numerous mechanisms to protect their genomes from invasion by foreign DNA. These include degradation by nucleases, inefficient transport to the nucleus, cell death upon DNA uptake, and inactivation of promoters. Naked DNA is still very attractive because it avoids the complications of viral vectors. This justifies a continued effort to overcome the obstacles to efficient and prolonged expression of genes from the naked DNA.

Liposomes are vesicles formed from lipids, usually, phospholipids. Cationic lipids form stable complexes with DNA and can therefore be incorporated into liposomes. These complexes are routinely used by researchers to introduce DNA into cell lines *in vitro*. Their use *in vivo* is attractive because it does not raise the

safety issues associated with viral vectors. However, they are far less efficient than viruses so their utility is still limited.

An alternative to direct injection of DNA or a vehicle into a patient is to obtain cells from a patient and incorporate a foreign gene into the cells *in vitro*. Cells that have been selected for stably incorporating the foreign gene can then be given back to the patient. The benefits of this step cannot be overstated; instability of transfected DNA is a major unsolved problem with *in vivo* gene therapy. This approach has been used in atherosclerosis research with cells derived from bone marrow. Since the bone marrow contains precursors of red blood cells and cells of the immune system, this is a practical way to specifically target such cells. After reintroduction to the bone marrow, cells containing a foreign gene enter into the circulation and repopulate tissues. For example, the bone marrow is a source of circulating phagocytic cells ("monocytes" in the circulation, "macrophages" in most tissues, and "Kupffer cells" in the liver). Animal experiments have shown dramatic alterations in atherosclerosis susceptibility with the replacement of macrophages in the bone marrow. Partial hepatectomy stimulates a robust regenerative response in the liver. This makes possible the introduction of hepatocytes that have been genetically modified into a partially hepatectomized liver. The new cells respond to the proliferative signals and contribute to the new cell mass of the liver.

2
Atherosclerosis: A Chronic Inflammatory Disease

Atherosclerosis is thought to be the result of a chronic fibro-proliferative inflammatory response. Animal studies suggest that this inflammatory disease is initiated following the deposition, modification, and retention of lipoproteins within the artery wall. The initial inflammatory response involves the upregulation of expression of *adhesion molecules* and *chemokines* by endothelial cells and smooth muscle cells, leading to the recruitment of monocytes and lymphocytes into the arterial *intima*. The monocytes rapidly convert into tissue macrophages that have the capacity to scavenge modified

lipoproteins, secrete proinflammatory *cytokines* and *growth factors*, and further regulate immune functions via presentation of antigens. The *scavenger receptor* mediated uptake of modified lipoproteins transforms the macrophages into lipid-loaded *foam cells*, the accumulation of which is the hallmark of the fatty streak, the initial stage of atherosclerosis (Fig. 1).

The transition of the *fatty streak* into more advanced stages of the disease appears to involve the coalescence of deposited lipids coupled with the death of

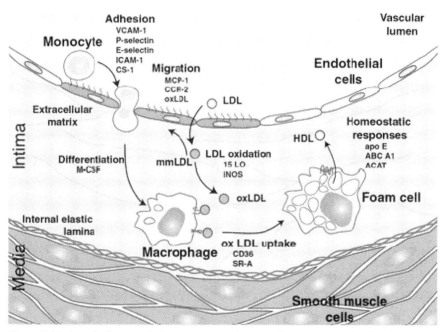

Fig. 1 Initiation of a fatty streak. Lipoproteins such as LDL become trapped within the extracellular matrix of the artery. The trapped lipoproteins are modified by processes such as oxidation or glycosylation (mmLDL, oxLDL) and become proinflammatory leading to the activation of endothelial cells to express adhesion molecules such as VCAM-1 and chemokines such as MCP-1. Monocytes are then recruited into the arterial intima and differentiate into macrophages most likely in response to increased expression of M-CSF. The modified lipoproteins are then taken up by scavenger receptors such as CD36 and the SRA1 expressed by the macrophages and this leads to foam cell formation. The excess cholesterol taken up by the foam cells is esterified by ACAT and stored in lipid droplets. It can be converted back to the more soluble free cholesterol and exported to extracellular HDL acceptors via cholesterol transporters, such as *ABC-A1*. (From Glass, C. K., Witztum, J. L. (2001) Atherosclerosis. The road ahead, *Cell* **104**(4), 503–516, included with permission of the Publisher.)

foam cells to form acellular *necrotic zones.* As in any classical inflammatory response, formation of the necrotic zones is accompanied by a wound-healing response where smooth muscle cells are recruited to encapsulate the necrotic zones by forming a *fibrous cap* around the lipid pools and necrotic debris (Fig. 2). With ongoing hyperlipidemia, however, there is a continuous influx, trapping, and modification of lipoproteins in the developing lesion that recruits additional inflammatory cells and leads to formation of new fatty streaks adjacent to or on top of the initial lesions. The combination of layering of new fatty streaks and erosion of the fibrous cap destabilizes the plaques allowing fissures, ruptures, and intraplaque *hemorrhage* to occur. While the exact mechanisms that cause plaques to rupture are currently unknown, the activation and/or death of macrophages with release of proteolytic enzymes such as *matrix metalloproteinases*, likely play a role. The resulting erosion and rupture exposes procoagulant proteins such as *tissue factor* to the blood and facilitates the formation of mural and *occlusive thrombi* (Fig. 3). The occlusion of the main coronary arteries causes the clinical outcomes of myocardial ischemia, *angina*, and ultimately *myocardial infarction*. Occlusion of cerebral vessels can lead to ischemic stroke while occlusion of peripheral blood vessels

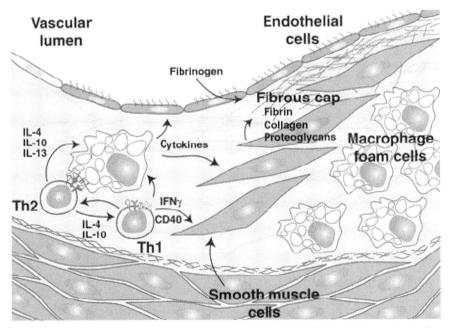

Fig. 2 Atherosclerotic lesion progression. Continued deposition of lipoproteins coupled with foam cell formation and interactions between foam cells, Th1 and Th2 T Helper cells and smooth muscle cells contribute to a chronic inflammatory response. Cytokines secreted by lymphocytes and macrophages exert both pro- and antiatherogenic effects. As part of a wound-healing response smooth muscle cells migrate from the medial portion of the arterial wall, proliferate, and secrete extracellular matrix proteins that form a fibrous cap. (From Glass, C.K., Witztum, J.L. (2001) Atherosclerosis. The road ahead, *Cell* **104**(4), 503–516, included with permission of the Publisher.)

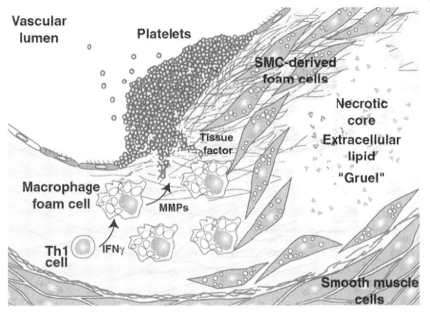

Fig. 3 Plaque rupture and thrombosis. The death of macrophage-derived foam cells and coalescence of trapped lipoproteins leads to the formation of an acellular necrotic zone and accumulation of extracellular cholesterol. Macrophage secretion of matrix metalloproteinases and neovascularization contribute to weakening of the fibrous cap. Plaque rupture exposes blood components to tissue factor, initiating coagulation, the recruitment of platelets, and the formation of a thrombus. (From Glass, CK and Witztum JL, Cell 2001; **104**(4): 503−516, included with permission of the Publisher.)

is associated with critical limb ischemia and gangrene.

3
Gene Therapy Targets for Cardiovascular Disease in the Lipoprotein Pathways

3.1
The Lipoprotein Pathways Provide Many Potential Gene Therapy Targets

A major risk factor for premature atherosclerosis is abnormalities in lipoprotein metabolism. In addition, people with diabetes mellitus frequently have lipoprotein abnormalities that elevate the risk of premature atherosclerosis that is already associated with diabetes.

Lipoprotein metabolism involves the interplay of the intestine, the liver, adipose tissue, and muscle. Endocrine organs also play a role, chiefly pancreatic islets, adrenals, the hypothalamus, and adipose tissue. However, the following discussion will emphasize the role of the liver because it is the most readily accessible target for gene therapy that is based upon the intravenous injection of DNA or DNA within a vector or carrier.

Animals transport large quantities of lipids through the bloodstream on carrier particles called lipoproteins. Lipoproteins consist of a shell of proteins called *apolipoproteins*, amphipathic lipids, primarily phospholipid and unesterified cholesterol, surrounding a core of

Tab. 1 Density, diameter, and composition of plasma lipoproteins.

Class	Density [g mL^{-1}]	Diameter [nm]	Chol	PL	Protein	TG	CE
Chylomicrons	0.93	75–1200	2	7	2	86	3
VLDL	0.93–1.006	30–80	7	18	8	55	12
IDL	1.006–1.019	25–35	9	19	19	23	29
LDL	1.019–1.063	18–25	8	22	22	6	42
HDL2	1.063–1.125	9–12	5	33	40	5	17
HDL3	1.125–1.210	5–9	4	35	55	3	13

Notes: Values represent percentage of dry mass. Chol = cholesterol; PL = phospholipids; TG = triacylglycerols; CE = cholesterol esters.

nonpolar lipid. The core composition consists of variable proportions of triacylglycerol and cholesterol ester.

When plasma is subjected to ultracentrifugation, most proteins sediment at the bottom of the centrifuge tube. Because they are associated with lipid and have a low buoyant density, lipoproteins float in the ultracentrifuge. The density at which they float is the basis for their classification (Table 1). In fasting plasma, most of the triacylglycerol is carried by very low-density lipoprotein (VLDL) particles. Cholesterol and cholesterol ester are carried by low-density lipoprotein (LDL) and high-density lipoprotein (HDL) particles, with LDL carrying about two-thirds of all cholesterol in human plasma.

3.2
Specific Genes are Critical for Dietary Lipid Absorption in the Intestine

It is important to remember that ordinarily, the major component of dietary fat is always triacylglycerol, not cholesterol. For example, milk and butter have very little cholesterol but are very high in triacylglycerol. Triacylglycerol (and other glycerolipids, such as phospholipids) is hydrolyzed in the intestinal lumen to yield monoglycerides and free fatty acids. These lipolysis products are then absorbed by the intestinal epithelial cells and resynthesized as triacylglycerols, phospholipids, and cholesterol esters. Thus, the intestine mediates both lipolysis (in the lumen) and reesterification (within the epithelial cells) of dietary lipids. The molecular mechanisms underlying intestinal absorption of fatty acids are still not understood. There is no consensus about whether a specific transporter is involved in fatty acid transport into the enterocytes.

Cholesterol absorption into the enterocyte is also not well understood. A specific inhibitor of cholesterol absorption, Ezetimibe, is in clinical use and is one line of evidence that there is a specific transporter for cholesterol at the membrane of the enterocyte that faces the intestinal lumen (the apical membrane).

The free fatty acids coming from intestinal lipolysis are solubilized into micelles within the intestinal lumen. These micelles consist of bile acids, cholesterol, and phosphatidylcholine. Bile acids are detergent-like molecules produced from cholesterol by the liver. Together with phospholipid and cholesterol, bile acids are secreted from the apical membrane of hepatocytes into the bile canaliculi, which drain into the bile duct and finally into the duodenum. As discussed below, conversion of cholesterol to bile acids and secretion of biliary cholesterol are the principal routes of cholesterol elimination.

Two membrane cholesterol transporters have been identified in the intestine. One consists of a heterodimer of two proteins, ABCG5, and ABCG8. This pair is located at the apical membrane and transports cholesterol out of the enterocyte into the lumen. In addition, the transporter transports plant sterols and thus protects animals from accumulation of these non-physiological sterol molecules. Mutations in ABCG5 or ABCG8 cause a rare disease called sitosterolemia, which involves elevated levels of cholesterol and plant sterols in the bloodstream. ABCA1 also transports cholesterol out of enterocytes. In contrast to ABCG5/ABCG8, this transporter appears to transport cholesterol across the basolateral membrane of the enterocyte, to the bloodstream and/or lymphatics. Overexpression of ABCG5/ABCG8 in transgenic mice reduces cholesterol absorption, making this an attractive target for therapeutic intervention.

3.3
The Intestine Exports Lipids on Chylomicron Particles

Since the intestine is primarily an absorptive organ, it must have the means of exporting newly absorbed lipids. The enterocyte reesterifies fatty acids and monoglycerides to form triacylglycerols and phospholipids. Absorbed cholesterol is esterified to form cholesterol esters. Triacylglycerols and cholesterol esters are then packaged into the core of lipoprotein particles unique to the intestine – *chylomicrons*. Rather than being secreted into the bloodstream, chylomicrons are secreted into the lymphatics. By secreting chylomicrons into the lymphatics, they gain entrance

into the general circulation via the thoracic duct. This guarantees that extrahepatic tissues, principally adipose tissue and muscle, are the first to be exposed to the newly secreted chylomicrons – if chylomicrons were secreted directly into the bloodstream, they would first be delivered to the liver, via the portal vein.

After entry into the bloodstream, chylomicrons interact with the luminal surface of the capillary beds of adipose tissue and muscle. Here resides the enzyme *lipoprotein lipase*, which hydrolyzes the triacylglycerols all the way to free fatty acids and glycerol. (Cholesterol esters are not substrates for lipoprotein lipase.) The free fatty acids are then absorbed where they are reesterified and stored in triacylglycerol droplets (in adipocytes) or oxidized for energy (in muscle). The chylomicron depleted of its triacylglycerol (a chylomicron remnant) is rapidly cleared from the circulation by the liver. There is significant variation in the abundance and activation state of lipoprotein lipase. This affects the efficiency of clearance of triacylglycerol-rich lipoproteins and is therefore an attractive target for gene therapy.

3.4
The Liver is a Major Producer of Plasma Lipoproteins

Adipose tissue and liver are quite active in the conversion of carbohydrate into fat. Adipose tissue stores the fat in the form of triacylglycerol droplets. However, these droplets are quite dynamic; they are continuously being formed and turned over. The turnover of adipocyte droplets occurs through the action of hormone-sensitive lipase. The free fatty acids that are released from adipocytes can go to the liver where they can be used to make ketone bodies and/or are reesterified to form triacylglycerol again. Whether derived from adipose tissue or from *de novo* synthesis, the liver does not generally store triacylglycerol. Triacylglycerol accumulation in the liver is generally regarded as a pathological state, termed *fatty liver* or *hepatic steatosis*.

3.5
Lipoprotein Lipase as a Target for Gene Therapy

In a healthy liver, triacylglycerol is packaged for secretion within the secretory pathway. This involves transfer of triacylglycerol to the endoplasmic reticulum lumen and interaction with apoB100 (Fig. 4). Within the secretory pathway, there are several steps in which triacylglycerol is incorporated into a growing VLDL particle. VLDL is then secreted into the bloodstream. Like chylomicrons, VLDL interacts with *lipoprotein lipase* while in the circulation. However, unlike chylomicrons, the depletion of triacylglycerol from VLDL yields a VLDL remnant, also termed *intermediate density lipoprotein* (IDL), which goes on to produce a stable lipoprotein,

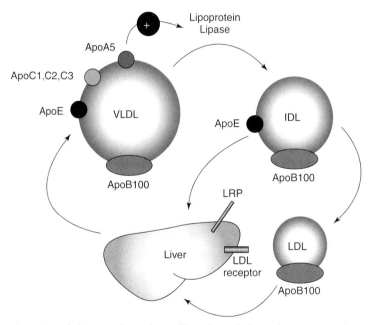

Fig. 4 Metabolic interrelationships of liver-derived plasma lipoproteins. The liver secretes VLDL, a particle enriched in triacylglycerol. It carries various apolipoproteins. ApoB100 is the only nonexchangeable protein on VLDL particles. ApoC2 and possibly, apoA5, are activators of lipoprotein lipase. This enzyme resides on the luminal surface of the capillary endothelium of adipose tissue and muscle and hydrolyzes the fatty acids from VLDL triacylglycerols. The resulting particle, IDL, can be cleared from the circulation by the liver or can become LDL. Clearance of IDL is mediated by apoE. Clearance of LDL is mediated by apoB100. The LDL receptor plays a critical role in the clearance of IDL and LDL; both apoE and apoB100 can bind to the LDL receptor. The LRP acts as a backup for IDL clearance; in the absence of the LDL receptor, it can clear IDL by binding to apoE.

LDL. Owing to the loss of most of the triacylglycerol, the predominant neutral lipids of LDL are cholesterol and cholesterol ester.

The catabolism of VLDL is dependent upon efficient hydrolysis of its triacylglycerol core by lipoprotein lipase. Lipoprotein lipase deficiency results in dramatic hypertriglyceridemia, liver enlargement (hepatomegaly), and inflammation of the pancreas (pancreatitis). However, elevated plasma VLDL can result from many other as-yet unidentified causes. It is very common in the human population and is associated with obesity, diabetes, and in some individuals, high-carbohydrate diets. Although these individuals have normal levels of lipoprotein lipase, increasing the level of this enzyme might still be a useful therapeutic strategy to lower plasma triacylglycerols. Since it is presently not feasible to target genes to the normal sites of expression of lipoprotein lipase (muscle and adipose tissue), expression in a nonphysiological site, the liver, has been tested in mice and in a naturally occurring feline model of lipoprotein lipase deficiency.

In addition to the expected role of lipoprotein lipase in catalyzing the hydrolysis of lipoprotein triacylglycerol, there is also a nonenzymatic property of potential therapeutic value. Lipoprotein lipase binds to lipoproteins and also binds to lipoprotein receptors in the LDL receptor family, most notably, the LDL receptor-related protein (LRP). In addition, lipoprotein lipase can bind to cell surface proteins that are enriched in acidic carbohydrate residues, the proteoglycans. The best evidence that these nonenzymatic functions are therapeutically relevant is the demonstration that a mutant form of lipoprotein lipase lacking enzymatic activity is still able to reduce plasma triacylglycerol by about 20 to 30%.

Lipoprotein lipase-mediated hydrolysis of triacylglycerol causes fatty acids to be taken up at the site of hydrolysis. In the liver, this leads to reesterification of the fatty acids and can result in an increase in cellular triacylglycerols. Through mechanisms not clearly understood, excessive triacylglycerol accumulation dampens the cell's responsiveness to insulin. In the liver, insulin normally suppresses glucose production. Thus, one potential side effect of expression of lipoprotein lipase in the liver is to reduce the ability of insulin to suppress glucose production, a potential problem for people who are already insulin-resistant or diabetic.

3.6
The LDL and VLDL Receptors are Attractive Targets for Gene Therapy

LDL is cleared from the circulation in large part through its interaction with the *LDL receptor*. Mutations affecting the expression or function of the LDL receptor are responsible for a common inherited disorder, *familial hypercholesterolemia*. Increased expression of the LDL receptor reduces LDL levels; thus, the LDL receptor has been used in gene therapy for hypercholesterolemia.

The VLDL receptor is a member of the LDL receptor family. It is expressed in a wide range of tissues, but not in the liver. However, adeno-associated virus was used to express this receptor in the livers of mice lacking the LDL receptor. These mice experienced a 40% reduction of cholesterol, due to enhanced clearance of both VLDL and LDL. Since patients who do not express the LDL receptor are immunologically naïve to this antigen, gene therapy with the VLDL receptor might be an effective treatment that would avoid the danger of immune rejection.

3.7
Increased Cholesterol and Phospholipid Efflux via ABCA1 Can Prevent Atherosclerosis

Epidemiological studies show an inverse relationship between HDL levels and risk of premature atherosclerosis. Unlike VLDL and chylomicrons, HDL is formed from its protein and lipid components in the bloodstream and interstitial fluids rather than within the secretory pathway of cells. The major apolipoproteins of HDL are apoA1 and apoA2. These proteins are secreted from hepatocytes and intestinal epithelial cells independently and also as minor components of VLDL and chylomicrons. ApoA1 and apoA2 bind to phospholipids. Phospholipids are available from the surface of VLDL after lipolysis. In addition, cells are able to efflux phospholipids and cholesterol through the action of ABCA1 (Fig. 5). Its crucial role in this process was established by the discovery that two types of severe inherited HDL deficiency syndromes are caused by mutations in ABCA1, Tangier Disease, and familial hypoalphalipoproteinemia (FHA).

Tangier Disease is a rare recessive disorder in which patients have almost no HDL. Cholesterol ester accumulates in macrophages and macrophage-rich tissues like spleen and liver. FHA is a very common dominant disorder in which people have low HDL (typically <30 mg dL^{-1}) and suffer from premature heart disease even without an elevation in LDL. Approximately 40% of patients with premature coronary heart disease have low HDL, making it the most common lipid disorder of heart disease patients.

Tangier Disease and FHA are caused by mutations in ABCA1. Tangier Disease patients are homozygous (or inherit two different mutant alleles). FHA patients are heterozygous for mutations at the ABCA1 locus. ABCA1 mutations lower HDL because they prevent phospholipid and/or cholesterol from effluxing and becoming associated with apoA1 and apoA2. In the absence of sufficient lipid, apoA1 is rapidly cleared by the kidneys.

Why do mutations in ABCA1 lead to premature heart disease? ABCA1 fulfills a rate-limiting step in the pathway by which cells get rid of cholesterol, and thus might be a critical protector against cholesterol overload. With the exception of hepatocytes, cells are unable to catabolize large quantities of cholesterol and must therefore protect themselves from cholesterol overload by expelling cholesterol to an appropriate extracellular carrier. It is interesting that ABCA1 is especially abundant in macrophages; macrophages can become engorged with cholesterol esters and form foam cells in the arterial wall. A mutation in ABCA1 might therefore predispose an individual to atherosclerosis by impeding cholesterol efflux (Fig. 1).

Proof-of-principle studies in mice nominate ABCA1 for the gene therapist's arsenal. Moderate overexpression of ABCA1 decreases atherosclerosis in mice, despite having a minimal effect on HDL levels. The most plausible explanation is that macrophage ABCA1 function is more important than HDL levels in protecting an animal from atherosclerosis. Indeed, if animals are transplanted with macrophages derived from mice lacking ABCA1, they show increased atherosclerosis. These animal studies suggest that increased expression of ABCA1 in macrophages might be a sensible gene therapy strategy for protection against or treatment of atherosclerosis.

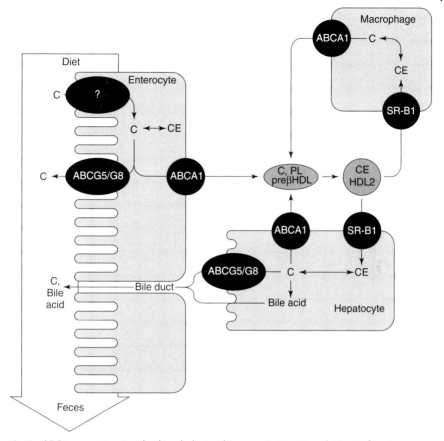

Fig. 5 ABC transporters involved in cholesterol transport. ABCG5 and ABCG8 function together as a heterodimer and mediate the transport of cholesterol from hepatocytes across the canalicular (apical) membrane into the bile. The ABCG5/G8 complex is also involved in cholesterol and plant sterol efflux from the enterocytes of the intestine to the intestinal lumen. This reduces the net absorption of cholesterol and prevents absorption of plant sterols. ABCA1 transports cholesterol and phospholipids on the sinusoidal (basolateral) surface of hepatocytes and enterocytes. In addition, ABCA1 is abundant in macrophages where it mediates cholesterol and phospholipid efflux. ApoA1 interacts with ABCA1 and mediates the formation of precursors to HDL (preβHDL). The esterification of the cholesterol in the preβHDL by the blood-borne enzyme, lecithin cholesterol acyl transferase (LCAT), produces mature HDL. Mature HDL can bind to the SR-B1 receptor and deliver cholesterol esters to hepatocytes. Much of the cholesterol ester is thus delivered and hydrolyzed by a cellular cholesterol esterase and secreted into bile as unesterified cholesterol.

3.8
Some Apolipoproteins Can Prevent Atherosclerosis

ApoA1 is a major protein constituent of HDL. It is an activator of an enzyme in the bloodstream, LCAT. This enzyme transfers a fatty acid from the *sn*-2 position of phosphatidylcholine to cholesterol to form a cholesterol ester. It enables HDL to "accept" cholesterol from cells or other lipoproteins and then to fill its core with the cholesterol by esterifying it. ApoA1 also interacts with ABCA1 to mediate cholesterol and phospholipid efflux from cells.

Overexpression of apoA1 in transgenic mice or injection of large quantities of the apoA1 protein produces dramatic effects on atherosclerosis – both prevention and regression of atherosclerotic lesions. ApoA1 overexpression is a very attractive prospect for gene therapy. The biggest difficulty is that apoA1 levels in human plasma are already quite high, ~ 1 mg mL^{-1}. Thus, with present technology, it would be quite difficult to achieve a significant increase in this steady state level.

ApoA5 is a newly discovered apolipoprotein that is associated with VLDL. Its deletion in mice results in elevated triacylglycerols and its overexpression in transgenic mice drives down triacylglycerol levels. It is likely that it plays a role in the ability of lipoprotein lipase to hydrolyze VLDL triacylglycerol. ApoA5 might be an attractive candidate for gene therapy of hypertriglyceridemia.

ApoE is a ligand for the LDL receptor and virtually all other members of the LDL receptor family. It is associated with VLDL and chylomicrons and to a varying extent, with HDL. Chylomicrons depend on apoE for their clearance from the circulation. In addition, although VLDL does have another competent LDL receptor ligand, apoB100, VLDL remnants are inefficiently cleared in the absence of apoE. There are three common allelic variants of apoE – apoE2, apoE3, and apoE4. ApoE2 has a greatly reduced affinity for its receptors and is therefore associated with impaired clearance of VLDL and chylomicron remnants. From these properties, one might predict that increasing apoE levels might be therapeutically desirable

by promoting efficient removal from the circulation of remnant lipoproteins. However, studies in transgenic mice and rabbits revealed two unexpected consequences of apoE overexpression. First, increased apoE synthesis in the liver leads to increased VLDL production. Second, increased apoE in the VLDL particle slows the hydrolysis of triacylglycerol by lipoprotein lipase.

3.9
The Liver SR-B1 Receptor Protects against Atherosclerosis

The scavenger receptor-B1 (SR-B1) is highly expressed in tissues that actively convert cholesterol into steroid hormones; for example, adrenals, ovaries, and testis. It is also highly expressed in hepatocytes. SR-B1 binds to HDL and mediates the selective uptake of cholesterol ester from the HDL particle into the cell. Unlike the uptake of LDL particles, the particle itself is spared and can then recycle back to pick up another cargo of cholesterol. The overexpression of SR-B1 in transgenic mice causes a drastic drop in HDL levels and protects the animals from atherosclerosis. Conversely, disruption of the gene raises HDL and increases the susceptibility of animals to atherosclerosis. Interestingly, increased SR-B1 expression increases the secretion of cholesterol into the bile, indicating that uptake of cholesterol from HDL effectively targets the HDL toward biliary secretion.

The foregoing might seem to contradict the known inverse relationship between HDL levels and atherosclerosis. However, increased HDL can be due to increased HDL production or decreased HDL turnover. Increased HDL production is thought to be beneficial because it promotes cholesterol flow back to the liver. However, increased HDL, if it is due to an impairment in its ability to deliver cholesterol to the liver, is not beneficial. The transgenic experiments in mice suggest that increased SR-B1 expression in the liver might be a viable approach to gene therapy for atherosclerosis.

4
Vascular and Inflammatory Targets for Gene Therapy

Small clinical trials of gene therapy for cardiovascular disease have been limited to induction of *angiogenesis* in the heart and legs for the treatment of *angina* and critical limb *ischemia* or to blocking of the proliferative response following injury induced by *angioplasty* and vascular grafting as a means of preventing *restenosis*. These trials have involved use of adenoviruses and DNA-containing liposomes for localized overexpression of angiogenic growth factors such as vascular endothelial growth factor (VEGF), fibroblast growth factor (FGF), hepatocyte growth factor (HGF) and antisense oligonucleotides or decoy oligonucleotides for inhibiting expression of cell cycle genes such as *c-Myc* or for preventing binding of transcription factors such as E2F to cis-acting response elements respectively. The localized overexpression of VEGF and other growth factors in the heart and limbs have had mixed results with some recorded successes in formation of collateral vessels, increased blood flow, and reduced pain. Large-scale clinical trials in the United States have been slowed because of the problems with virus-related inflammation and with VEGF-induced edema.

As discussed in the first section of this chapter, genes involved in lipid and lipoprotein metabolism are potential targets for reducing hyperlipidemia and the consequent deposition and retention of lipids and lipoproteins in the artery wall. However, there are still a considerable number of individuals who develop cardiovascular disease who do not have appreciably elevated lipids or are resistant to current therapies. Thus, other targets need to be considered. Genes involved in regulating leukocyte function and the inflammatory response within the artery wall are potential candidates.

4.1
Adhesion Molecules and Leukocyte Counter Receptors

The *adhesion molecules*, vascular cell adhesion molecule (VCAM-1) and intercellular adhesion molecule (ICAM-1), are members of the immunoglobulin superfamily of proteins. Together with their leukocyte counter receptors, the integrins VLA4 and MAC-1/CD11b:CD18, are potential targets for gene therapy. VCAM-1 and ICAM-1 are expressed by endothelial cells and support the tight binding of monocytes and lymphocytes to the endothelial cell plasma membrane. The selectins (E-, P-, and L-selectins) are also adhesion molecules that play a role in the initial tethering and rolling of leukocytes along the surface of the blood vessel. They are lectin-like molecules that recognize carbohydrate containing counterreceptors.

Knockouts of ICAM-1, E-, and P-selectins in mice all partially inhibit development of atherosclerosis. Thus, localized inhibition of expression of these genes might prevent initiation of lesions and limit progression of established lesions due to layering and the continuous influx of leukocytes. Adenovirus-mediated gene transfer to endothelial cells has been successful in both *in vitro* and *in vivo* studies and suggests that this approach could be used for inhibiting expression of the adhesion molecules.

The transient nature of adenoviral-mediated gene transfer is a cause for concern. Given that the atherosclerotic lesions develop over several decades, effective adenoviral therapy would require repeated injections. The use of retroviruses or adeno-associated viruses to incorporate the gene into the cellular genome might be a better alternative. However, this approach is also limited by the small percentage of endothelial cells that proliferate under normal circumstances. Blocking expression of the leukocyte integrins is even more problematic. Currently, this would require transfection of bone marrow stem cells and would likely compromise the capacity to mount an inflammatory response at other sites. Overexpression of secreted forms of the adhesion molecules may be an effective alternate approach.

4.2
Cytokines

Cytokines are cell regulatory proteins that are key factors in the initiation and control of inflammation. They are classified as members of several different families of proteins that include: the tumor necrosis factor (TNF) family, interleukins, interferons, colony-stimulating factors, growth factors, and chemokines. There are significant overlaps in the functions of many of the cytokines. This overlap is in part due to the convergence of signal transduction pathways from the different cytokine specific receptors leading to activation of the same transcription factors. However, in other cases cytokines can have opposite effects and are frequently designated as being either proinflammatory or anti-inflammatory. Serum cytokine levels are elevated in people with established cardiovascular disease. Virtually, every major pro- and anti-inflammatory cytokine is expressed by cells within atherosclerotic lesions and all vascular cell types are capable of responding to these proteins. Thus, there is significant potential for the inhibition and treatment of CVD by manipulating the production of or response to cytokines using gene transfer approaches.

4.3
Chemokines and Chemokine Receptors

Monocyte chemotactic protein (MCP-1) and IL-8 are two potent leukocyte chemoattractants (*chemokines*) that play a role in recruiting leukocytes into the sites of inflammation. MCP-1 is expressed by all of the cell types within atherosclerotic lesions. Recent data from studies on atherosclerosis-prone mice with targeted deletion of MCP-1 or the chemokine receptors CCR-2 or CXCR-2, and studies of bone marrow transplantation of cells overexpressing MCP-1 or devoid of IL-8, strongly suggest that these molecules play a critical role in the initiation of fatty streaks.

Recent gene therapy studies with an N-terminal deletion mutant of the human MCP-1 gene transfected into the skeletal muscle of the atherosclerosis-prone apoE knockout mice have demonstrated the potential for inhibiting atherosclerosis by blocking MCP-1 activity. However, as with the adhesion molecules, there are caveats with regard to targeting the MCP-1, IL-8, and/or CCR-2 and CXCR-2 genes for CVD gene therapy. Because MCP-1 is expressed by all of the cells within the lesions and IL-8 primarily by macrophages, it is unclear whether adenoviral or retroviral approaches would be successful in inhibiting MCP-1 or IL-8 expression by macrophages.

Primary macrophages are extremely difficult to transfect, therefore, blocking their capacity for expressing MCP-1, IL-8, or the receptors likely would require repeatedly knocking out the genes in bone marrow cells. This again raises the question, to what extent would this compromise the inflammatory response at other sites. Thus, localized overexpression of mutated forms of these proteins such as the N-terminal deletion mutant sited above is the most logical approach to targeting chemokines for prevention and treatment of cardiovascular disease.

4.4
Interleukins, the TNF-α family, and Interferon-γ

Currently, *in vitro* and limited *in vivo* data suggest that IL-1, IL-2, TNF-α, IL-3, IL-6, IL-12, IL-15, and IL-18 appear to have proatherogenic properties, while the IL-1 receptor antagonist (IL-1ra), IL-9, IL-10, IL-11 and possibly IL-4, and IL-13 are likely to be antiatherogenic. Thus, localized inhibition of proatherogenic cytokines and overexpression of antiatherogenic cytokines with gene therapy has significant potential for prevention and treatment of cardiovascular disease.

TNF-α and IL-1-β are the proinflammatory cytokines that have received the most attention. *In vitro* studies have clearly demonstrated that these two cytokines potently stimulate the expression of adhesion molecules and chemokines and suggest that they play an important role in the atherogenic process. Surprisingly, targeted deletion of TNF-α or the p55 TNF-α receptor is not protective of atherosclerosis in mouse models. Furthermore, the chronic administration of a TNF-α binding protein reduces fatty streak formation only in female apoE knockout mice. The effects

of deletion of IL-1 on atherosclerosis have not been reported. However, in knockouts of the IL-1ra, there was a trend toward increased foam-cell lesion area compared with the wild-type littermate controls. Successful gene therapy studies in animal models of cerebral, pancreatic, and articular inflammation with IL-1ra further support the potential for this approach to cardiovascular disease.

CD40 and CD40 ligand are members of the TNF receptor and protein families respectively. They are expressed by monocytes, macrophages, dendritic cells, lymphocytes, endothelial cells, and smooth muscle cells and play a role in many inflammatory processes including the expression of adhesion molecules, cytokines, chemokines, and matrix metalloproteinases. Recent data suggests that CD40/CD40 ligand play fundamental roles in the atherogenic process as CD40 ligand–apoE double knockout mice have significantly reduced atherosclerosis and lesions that contain reduced numbers of inflammatory cells, are connective tissue rich, and are likely resistant to plaque rupture. Thus, CD40 or CD40 ligand are both additional potential targets for localized CVD gene therapy.

Interferon gamma (IFN-γ) is an immuno-stimulatory cytokine that increases antigen presentation by macrophages and the activation of T lymphocytes. As macrophages and T lymphocytes are key cellular components of the atherosclerotic lesions at all stages of lesion development, gene therapy that targets IFN-γ expression could have a significant impact on the disease process. This is supported by several studies in mice that demonstrate a critical role for this cytokine. For example, atherosclerotic lesions are significantly reduced in IFN-γ-deficient mice crossed with either LDL-receptor knockout or apoE knockout mice and are increased with chronic administration of recombinant IFN-γ. Interleukin-18 (IL-18) in part promotes inflammatory responses through the release of IFN-γ. Administration of recombinant IL-18 to apoE knockout mice, like the administration of IFN-γ, significantly increases lesion size. Not surprisingly, in IFN-γ/apoE double knockout mice, there are no effects of IL-18 on lesion development.

IL-2 is another interleukin with probable proatherogenic properties. It also functions to alter T-lymphocytes by affecting a shift to a Th1 T helper cell phenotype. It is expressed within atherosclerotic lesions and serum levels are increased in people with ischemic heart disease and unstable angina pectoris. However, to date, IL-2 has not been shown to play a direct role in the development of lesions in animal models. In contrast to IL-2, IL-4 and IL-10 in part function to cause a shift toward an antiatherogenic Th2, T helper cell phenotype. There is reduced atherosclerosis in LDL-receptor knockout mice transplanted with bone marrow from IL-4 deficient mice but no increase in atherosclerosis in cholesterol-fed, IL-4 deficient mice. On the other hand, fatty streak formation in IL-4-deficient mice immunized with HSP65 or Mycobacterium tuberculosis is significantly reduced when compared with lesions in wild-type C57BL/6 mice.

In addition to causing a Th2 shift, IL-10 inhibits differentiation of monocytes to macrophages, macrophage presentation of antigens, generation of reactive oxygen and nitrogen species, and endothelial cell expression of ICAM-1. There is accelerated formation of atherosclerotic lesions in IL-10 knockout mice and reduced formation of lesions in IL-10 transgenic mice. Thus, localized overexpression of IL-4 and IL-10 could provide some protection against cardiovascular disease. There is also recent evidence that IL-6 may play a role in the development of atherosclerosis. Treatment of fat-fed C57BL/6 or apoE knockout mice with recombinant IL-6 significantly increases fatty streak formation.

4.5
Growth Factors and Receptors

Growth factors are potent regulators of cellular functions including proliferation, migration, differentiation, and survival/apoptosis. Many growth factors and growth factor receptors are expressed or deposited in atherosclerotic lesions. These include all forms of platelet-derived growth factor (PDGF), basic fibroblast growth factor (bFGF), vascular endothelial growth factor (VEGF), insulin-like growth factors (IGF-1 and IGF-2), thrombin, endothelin-1, angiotensin-II, heparin binding-epidermal growth factor (Hb-EGF), several forms of transforming growth factor-beta (TGF-β), and the hematopoietic growth factors: macrophage colony-stimulating factor (M-CSF), granulocyte colony–stimulating factor (G-CSF), and granulocyte-macrophage colony-stimulating factor (GM-CSF).

The original "Response to Injury" hypothesis of Glomset and Ross posited that denuding injury to the endothelium led to the activation and attachment of platelets with release of PDGF. This was thought to lead to increased smooth muscle cell migration and proliferation and development of atherosclerotic lesions. Over the past three decades, the paradigm has shifted to account for the crucial role of inflammatory cells and the potential protective role of smooth muscle migration and proliferation in the formation of the fibrous cap (Figs. 1–3). Thus, for gene therapy approaches to CVD, localized overexpression of growth factor genes could help stabilize lesions at risk of rupture and thrombosis. As proof of principle, transplant of fetal liver cells from mice deficient in PDGF-BB or chronic treatment with a PDGF-receptor antagonist or anti-PDGF receptor antibodies in apoE knockout mice leads to the formation of lesions that contain mostly macrophages, appear less mature, and have a reduced frequency of fibrous cap formation as compared with control mice. In contrast to primary atherosclerotic lesions, smooth muscle migration and proliferation contributes to *restenosis* following angioplasty and other interventions. Gene therapy approaches to inhibiting growth factor expression postinjury have been in development for several years.

Stimulating or inhibiting the expression of individual growth factors alone may not be sufficient to control vascular smooth muscle cell migration and proliferation. This is because both smooth muscle cell migration and proliferation are exceedingly complex processes and involve dissociation from the extracellular matrix through the activation and secretion of proteases, engagement of multiple growth factor receptors with activation of a variety of receptor associated and cytoplasmic kinases, activation of transcription factors, and production and activation of proteins involved in cell cycle traverse and DNA synthesis such as cyclins and cyclin-dependent kinases. Thus, there are potentially many targets other than growth factors or their specific receptors for gene therapy. This has been demonstrated by the ongoing clinical trials previously cited where antisense oligonucleotides or decoy oligonucleotides for inhibiting expression of cell cycle genes such as *c-Myc* or for preventing binding of transcription factors such as E2F are being tested as the means of preventing restenosis following angioplasty.

The hematopoietic growth factors M-CSF and GM-CSF play a role in the differentiation of monocytes and possibly in regulating macrophage proliferation and death within atherosclerotic lesions. Thus, these factors may also be good targets for gene therapy for both early and unstable lesions. This has been supported by data showing that M-CSF deficient mice crossed with apoE knockout mice have significantly reduced atherosclerosis. Furthermore, chronic administration of an antibody that blocks the M-CSF receptor (c-fms) also reduces early lesions in apoE knockout mice.

Angiogenic growth factors such as the VEGFs, HGF, and the angiopoietins have already been mentioned with regard to ongoing clinical trials for the induction of collateral circulation in people with occluded coronary and peripheral arteries. However, small *neovessels* also form in advanced atherosclerotic lesions and are additional conduits for recruitment of leukocytes into the established lesions. Blocking *neovascularization* could help reduce inflammation and stabilize the lesions. Thus, localized inhibition of expression of these factors or their respective receptors (FLT and FLK for VEGFs and Tie receptors for angiopoietins) are potential additional CVD targets.

5
Pro- and Antioxidant Enzymes

There is now ample evidence that polyunsaturated fatty acids, phospholipids, and cholesteryl-esters within lipoproteins that become trapped within the extracellular matrix of the artery wall can become oxidized. *In vitro* studies have demonstrated that macrophage scavenger receptors

(MSR) recognize oxidized lipoproteins and that foam cell formation is due in part to the accumulation of oxidized lipoproteins. The uptake of oxidized lipids can lead to intense oxidative stress within the foam cells and likely contributes to cell death.

It is currently unclear exactly how lipoproteins are oxidized within the artery wall. Several lines of evidence indicate that proinflammatory enzymes such as myeloperoxidase and the lipoxygenases can oxidize lipoproteins. Macrophages also express the bacteriocidal enzymes NADPH oxidase and the inducible form of nitric oxide synthase that generate the superoxide anion and nitric oxide respectively. These reactive oxygen and nitrogen species can also contribute to lipoprotein modification and oxidative stress within foam cells. Thus, it is possible that gene therapy could be used to inhibit expression of these enzymes within atherosclerotic lesions and thus reduce formation of the necrotic zones and help stabilize lesions that are susceptible to plaque rupture and thrombosis. This is supported by studies showing that mice deficient in 5-lipoxygenase or 12/15 lipoxygenase are protected from atherosclerosis and that mice transgenic for 12/15 lipoxygenase have accelerated formation of lesions.

In contrast to the lipoxygenases, knockout of myeloperoxidase and the NADPH oxidase subunits do not protect mice from atherosclerosis. As with other essential proinflammatory factors, a deficiency of these enzymes can have a significant effect on the capacity to mount an inflammatory response as is seen in people with a deficiency of NADPH oxidase and the resulting chronic granulomatous disease. Thus, future gene therapy to inhibit the expression or activity of these enzymes will require viral targeting to leukocytes only within the artery wall.

All cell types have protective mechanisms against the buildup of pro-oxidants that could disrupt cellular functions by oxidizing lipids, proteins, and DNA. These protective mechanisms include formation of the primary endogenous antioxidant glutathione by the enzyme complex glutamate cysteine ligase. Glutathione acts by enzymatically and chemically converting electrophilic centers to thioether bonds and as a substrate in the glutathione peroxidase mediated destruction of hydroperoxides. Complete glutathione redox systems are located in both the mitochondria and cytoplasm. Reduction of oxidized glutathione by glutathione reductase utilizes reducing equivalents supplied by NADPH and consumes NADPH at a higher rate than most other NADPH-dependent enzymes. Under conditions of oxidative stress with active glutathione redox cycling (as would occur in foam cells containing increased lipid peroxides), the cell's supply of glutathione and NADPH can be depleted, thus limiting many important redox sensitive and biosynthetic reactions and can lead to cell injury and death. Cells also contain superoxide dismutases that convert the superoxide anion to hydrogen peroxide and the enzyme catalase that converts hydrogen peroxide to water. Thus, targeted overexpression of the enzymes involved in glutathione metabolism – the superoxide dismutases and/or catalase could help reduce oxidative stress and foam cell death.

6
Scavenger Receptors

There are now known to be at least three families of broad specificity *scavenger receptors* that are expressed primarily by macrophages within human atherosclerotic lesions. These include the type A family (subtypes I–III and the *ma*crophage *receptor with collagenous structure or MARCO*), type B receptors that include CD36, SR-B1/CLA-1 and the splice variant SR-B2, and an additional group of receptors such as the mucin-like receptor macrosalin/CD68 and LOX-1. All of these receptors bind oxidized LDL, but CD36 now appears to be the major receptor on macrophages responsible for accumulation of oxidized LDL.

Recent studies of hyperlipidemic mice with targeted deletions of SRA I/II or CD36 have clearly established that both types of receptors play a fundamental role in foam cell formation and lesion development *in vivo*. Macrophages within human lesions also express a specific receptor that recognizes advanced glycosylation endproduct (AGE) proteins, the LDL receptor, VLDL receptor, and the LDL-receptor related protein/α_2-macroglobulin receptor (LRP). Because all of these receptors are expressed primarily by macrophages, this again brings up the problem that primary macrophages are extremely difficult to transfect and blocking their capacity for expressing scavenger receptors would likely require repeatedly knocking out the genes in bone marrow cells. Like adhesion molecules, an alternate approach that should be effective is the overexpression of soluble decoy scavenger receptors that would bind and clear modified lipoproteins and reduce lipoprotein trapping in the artery wall and the subsequent formation of foam cells. This is supported by a recent study showing that there is reduced atherosclerosis in LDL-receptor deficient mice treated with an adenoviral construct containing the human MSR AI extracellular domains.

7
Transcription Factors

Decoy oligonucleotides have been used to block binding of activated transcription factors to their consensus DNA response elements in the promoters of many genes. This may be a viable approach to reducing expression of many cytokines and other proinflammatory factors *in vivo* because activation of transcription factors such NF-κB, AP-1, and the STAT proteins are end points common to signal transduction pathways activated by various proinflammatory stimuli. Blocking the activation or expression of NF-κB could be a particularly effective therapy as there is activated NF-κB in all of the cell types within atherosclerotic lesions. In addition to blocking activation of NF-κB with decoy oligonucleotides, stimulating the activity of the natural inhibitors of NF-κB, the I-κB proteins, or inhibiting the expression or activity of the I-κB kinases that phosphorylate the I-κB proteins leading to the proteosomal degradation of the NF-κB inhibitors, may also be viable approaches. Targeting the expression of the NF-κB subunits p65 and p50 is another possible approach. Other transcription factors such as Egr-1, Nrf-1, and Nrf-2 may also be potential targets for cardiovascular disease. Egr-1 is an essential factor for regulating the expression of tissue factor, a key procoagulant protein expressed by cells in atherosclerotic lesions. Nrf-1 and Nrf-2 are important factors for regulating the expression of pro- and antioxidant enzymes and bind to consensus antioxidant response elements of these genes.

8
Noninflammatory Gene Targets

There are a large number of proteins that are not directly part of the inflammatory response that are potential targets for CVD gene therapy. These include proteins that regulate cell death, cellular proteases that may play a role in breaking down the arterial extracellular matrix, proteins that play a role in regulating blood pressure and vascular tone, pro- and anticoagulant proteins, and osteogenic proteins that may contribute to vascular calcification.

8.1
Cell Death

As noted, the death of macrophages likely plays a fundamental role in the formation of the necrotic zones of advanced lesions. There is ample evidence showing the presence of macrophages with fragmented DNA (a marker of cell death) located within or adjacent to these necrotic zones. The death of smooth muscle cells also plays a role in the thinning of the fibrous cap, and like the macrophages, smooth muscle cells with fragmented DNA have been documented within atherosclerotic lesions from both humans and experimental animals. Thus, strategies designed to reduce cell death within atherosclerotic lesions could help stabilize the plaques and prevent plaque rupture and formation of occlusive thrombi.

Although it is currently unclear what induces the death of either cell type *in vivo*, there is *in vitro* evidence that apoptosis (programmed cell death or cellular suicide) can be induced in both macrophages and smooth muscle cells by oxidized lipids and other proinflammatory factors. Thus, proteins known to play a role in apoptotic death are potential targets for gene therapy.

These include death-promoting proteins such as Fas (a death receptor that is a member of the TNF-α receptor family) and the Fas ligand, the cysteine proteases (caspases 3, 8, 9), and other death pathway effector proteins such as Fas-associated death domain (FADD) (Fas-associated protein with death domain), TNF receptor associated death domain (TRADD) (TNF receptor associated death domain protein), TRAF (TNF receptor associated factor), and receptor interacting protein (RID). There are also a number of antiapoptotic proteins such as c-FLIP (Fas-associated death domain (FADD) protein (FADD)-like interleukin-1 beta-converting enzyme [FLICE (caspase-8)]-inhibitory protein), BCL-2 and BCL-X that could provide protection against cell death if locally overexpressed.

8.2
Proteases

Secretion of proteolytic enzymes such as the matrix metalloproteinases (MMPs) by cells within the blood vessel plays an essential role in enabling the cells to migrate and proliferate. However, excess secretion of these enzymes by activated leukocytes or release of lysosomal enzymes such as cathepsins following the death of cells likely contributes to the breakdown of the extracellular matrix and to the fissure and rupture of the plaques. This is supported by data showing the presence of activated MMPs in unstable human atherosclerotic plaques. Thus, strategies designed to inhibit the expression of these proteolytic enzymes or the activation of the zymogen forms by membrane-associated enzymes such as the ADAM family of proteases could help prevent plaque destabilization and formation of occlusive thrombi. Cells within atherosclerotic lesions also express specific tissue inhibitors of metal-loproteinases (TIMPs) and thus localized overexpression of these inhibitors could also be an effective gene therapy approach for cardiovascular disease.

8.3
Regulators of Vascular Tone and Blood Pressure

Elevated blood pressure is a known risk factor for cardiovascular disease. It is well established that as atherosclerotic lesions progress, the affected blood vessel loses its capacity to adequately vasodilate. Controlling acute changes in vascular tone that cause *vasospasm* may be even more fundamental to CVD as evidence suggests that vasospasm may precipitate plaque rupture and the formation of occlusive thrombi. There are currently many drugs available for chronically controlling high blood pressure but very few for managing vasospasm. Thus, localized gene therapy that targets the production of vasoactive substances by arterial wall cells or the response of smooth muscle cells to these vasoactive substances leading to increased vasodilation and reduced vasospasm may be effective approaches for the treatment of cardiovascular disease.

Nitric oxide is an extremely potent vasodilator and most endothelial cells express an endothelium specific form of nitric oxide synthase (e-NOS). However, e-NOS expression and NO production are reduced in atherosclerotic arteries. Thus, a localized increase in the expression of e-NOS could help alleviate the impaired vasodilatory properties of atherosclerotic arteries. Endothelial cells also produce the vasodilatory prostaglandin, prostacyclin (PGI$_2$). PGI$_2$ is produced from arachidonic acid by the action of the cyclooxygenases followed by PGI$_2$ synthase. Thus,

increased expression of PGI$_2$ synthase could be an effective approach for increasing PGI$_2$ synthesis. Endothelial cells also produce a variety of vasoconstrictors such as endothelin-1 and endothelial cell hyperpolarizing factors. Thus, inhibiting expression of the proform of endothelin or the endothelin-converting enzyme that activates endothelin could help control vasoconstriction. There are also endogenous inhibitors of endothelin activation such as the endothelin-converting enzyme inhibitor that could also be locally overexpressed and play a beneficial role in regulating blood pressure. Similarly, endothelial cells express a form of the angiotensin-converting enzyme (ACE). Angiotensin-II is a potent vasoconstrictor. It is produced following the conversion of angiotensinogen to angiotensin-I by renin and from angiotensin-I to angiotensin-II by ACE. Thus, inhibition of endothelial expression of ACE could also be an effective therapy. Finally, blocking the response of smooth muscle cells to these various vasoconstrictors or increasing the response to the vasodilators by targeting expression of the specific smooth muscle cell receptors or the down stream signal transduction pathways may also be effective gene therapy targets.

8.4
Coagulation Related Genes

There are a variety of pharmacological agents that effectively inhibit *thrombosis*, and chronic administration of these drugs is associated with reduced frequencies of angina and myocardial infarction in people with established cardiovascular disease. However, because we still do not know what causes atherosclerotic plaques to rupture and because plaque rupture is unpredictable, administration of anticoagulants throughout the three to four decades that lesions develop may not be practical for most people due to the accompanying bleeding disorders. Thus, specifically blocking the expression of procoagulant proteins such as tissue factor by cells within atherosclerotic lesions, may be an effective approach to preventing localized formation of occlusive thrombi following plaque rupture. Tissue factor participates in the extrinsic pathway of coagulation and binds to and activates factor VIIa, which in turn activates factor X enabling it to convert prothrombin to thrombin and thrombin to convert fibrinogen to fibrin, the primary protein component of blood clots. Cells within atherosclerotic lesions also express a specific tissue factor inhibitor; thus an additional possibility would be to stimulate expression of this inhibitor. Another potential approach for reducing formation of occlusive thrombi is to increase the production of thrombolytic factors such as plasmin by increasing the localized expression of tissue plasminogen activator or reducing the expression of the plasminogen activator inhibitors.

8.5
Osteogenic Proteins

Bone mineral (calcium-phosphate) is deposited in most advanced atherosclerotic plaques and in heart valves. However, it is still controversial as to whether calcification of the plaques is a good prognostic indicator of subsequent CVD events. Nevertheless, preventing vascular calcification is beneficial for interventions such as angioplasty and for reducing the need for heart valve replacement. Vascular calcification is now known to be an active cellular mediated process that is analogous to the process by which cartilage is converted to

bone. It thus involves a balance between bone forming osteoblast type cells and bone removing osteoclast type cells and the expression of proteins that are both pro-osteogenic and antiosteogenic. These include the matrix gla proteins, osteopontin, osteoprotegrin, osteonectin, and the bone morphogenic proteins. Thus, localized gene therapy designed to either increase or inhibit expression of these proteins could have dramatic effects on reducing plaque calcification and complications resulting from "stiffening" of the blood vessels.

Bibliography

Books and Reviews

Freedman, S.B. (2002) Clinical trials of gene therapy for atherosclerotic cardiovascular disease, *Curr. Opin. Lipidol.* **13**, 653–661.

Glass, C.K., Witztum, J.L. (2001) Atherosclerosis. the road ahead, *Cell* **104**, 503–516.

Herweijer, H., Wolff, J.A. (2003) Progress and prospects: naked DNA gene transfer and therapy, *Gene Ther.* **10**, 453–458.

Khurana, R., Martin, J.F., Zachary, I. (2001) Gene therapy for cardiovascular disease: a case for cautious optimism, *Hypertension* **38**, 1210–1216.

Morishita, R. (2002) Recent progress in gene therapy for cardiovascular disease, *Circ. J.* **66**, 1077–1086.

Newby, A.C., Zaltsman, A.B. (2000) Molecular mechanisms in intimal hyperplasia, *J. Pathol.* **190**, 300–309.

Ross, R. (1999) Atherosclerosis – an inflammatory disease, *N. Engl. J. Med.* **340**, 115–126.

Springer, T.A., Cybulsky, M.I. (1996) Traffic signals on endothelium for leukocytes in health, inflammation, and atherosclerosis, in: Fuster, V., Ross, R., Topol, E.J. (Eds.) *Atherosclerosis and Coronary Artery Disease*, Lippincott-Raven, Philadelphia.

Tangirala, R.K., Tsukamoto, K., Chun, S.H., Usher, D., Pure, E., Rader, D.J. (1999) Regression of atherosclerosis induced by liver-directed gene transfer of apolipoprotein A-I in mice, *Circulation* **100**, 1816–1822.

Thomas, C.E., Ehrhardt, A., Kay, M.A. (2003) Progress and problems with the use of viral vectors for gene therapy, *Nat. Rev. Genet.* **4**, 346–358.

Von Der Thusen, J.H., Kuiper, J., Van Berkel, T.J., Biessen, E.A. (2003) Interleukins in atherosclerosis: molecular pathways and therapeutic potential, *Pharmacol. Rev.* **55**, 133–166.

Primary Literature

Aiello, R.J., Bourassa, P.A., Lindsey, S., Weng, W., Natoli, E., Rollins, B.J., Milos, P.M. (1999) Monocyte chemoattractant protein-1 accelerates atherosclerosis in apolipoprotein E-deficient mice, *Arterioscler. Thromb. Vasc. Biol.* **19**, 1518–1525.

Aiello, R.J., Brees, D., Bourassa, P.A., Royer, L., Lindsey, S., Coskran, T., Haghpassand, M., Francone, O.L. (2002) Increased atherosclerosis in hyperlipidemic mice with inactivation of ABCA1 in macrophages, *Arterioscler. Thromb. Vasc. Biol.* **22**, 630–637.

Babaev, V.R., Gleaves, L.A., Carter, K.J., Suzuki, H., Kodama, T., Fazio, S., Linton, M.F. (2000) Reduced atherosclerotic lesions in mice deficient for total or macrophage-specific expression of scavenger receptor-A, *Arterioscler. Thromb. Vasc. Biol.* **20**, 2593–2599.

Boisvert, W.A., Black, A.S., Curtiss, L.K. (1999) ApoA1 reduces free cholesterol accumulation in atherosclerotic lesions of ApoE-deficient mice transplanted with ApoE-expressing macrophages, *Arterioscler. Thromb. Vasc. Biol.* **19**, 525–530.

Boisvert, W.A., Curtiss, L.K. (1999) Elimination of macrophage-specific apolipoprotein E reduces diet-induced atherosclerosis in C57BL/6J male mice, *J. Lipid Res.* **40**, 806–813.

Boisvert, W.A., Santiago, R., Curtiss, L.K., Terkeltaub, R.A. (1998) A leukocyte homologue of the IL-8 receptor CXCR2 mediates the accumulation of macrophages in atherosclerotic lesions of LDL receptor-deficient mice, *J. Clin. Invest.* **101**, 353–363.

Boring, L., Gosling, J., Cleary, M., Charo, I. (1998) Decreased lesion formation in CCR2-/- mice reveals a role for chemokines in the initiation of atherosclerosis, *Nature* **394**, 894–897.

Brennan, M.L., Anderson, M.M., Shih, D.M., Qu, X.D., Wang, X., Mehta, A.C., Lim, L.L., Shi, W., Hazen, S.L., Jacob, J.S., Crowley, J.R., Heinecke, J.W., Lusis, A.J. (2001) Increased atherosclerosis in myeloperoxidase-deficient mice, *J. Clin. Invest.* **107**, 419–430.

Brown, D.L., Hibbs, M.S., Kearney, M., Isner, J.M. (1997) Differential expression of 92-kDa gelatinase in primary atherosclerotic versus restenotic coronary lesions, *Am. J. Cardiol.* **79**, 878–882.

Buono, C., Come, C.E., Stavrakis, G., Maguire, G.F., Connelly, P.W., Lichtman, A.H. (2003) Influence of interferon-gamma on the extent and phenotype of diet-induced atherosclerosis in the LDLR-deficient mouse, *Arterioscler. Thromb. Vasc. Biol.* **23**, 454–460.

Caligiuri, G., Rudling, M., Ollivier, V., Jacob, M.P., Michel, J.B., Hansson, G.K., Nicoletti, A. (2003) Interleukin-10 deficiency increases atherosclerosis, thrombosis, and low-density lipoproteins in apolipoprotein E knockout mice, *Mol. Med.* **9**, 10–17.

Chen, S.J., Rader, D.J., Tazelaar, J., Kawashiri, M., Gao, G., and Wilson, J.M. (2000) Prolonged correction of hyperlipidemia in mice with familial hypercholesterolemia using an adeno-associated viral vector expressing very-low-density lipoprotein receptor, *Mol. Ther.* **2**, 256–261.

Collins, R.G., Velji, R., Guevara, N.V., Hicks, M.J., Chan, L., Beaudet, A.L. (2000) P-Selectin or intercellular adhesion molecule (ICAM)-1 deficiency substantially protects against atherosclerosis in apolipoprotein E-deficient mice, *J. Exp. Med.* **191**, 189–194.

Cyrus, T., Pratico, D., Zhao, L., Witztum, J.L., Rader, D.J., Rokach, J., FitzGerald, G.A., Funk, C.D. (2001) Absence of 12/15-lipoxygenase expression decreases lipid peroxidation and atherogenesis in apolipoprotein e-deficient mice, *Circulation* **103**, 2277–2282.

Dawson, T.C., Kuziel, W.C., Osahar, T.A., Madea, N. (1999) Absence of CC chemokine receptor-2 reduces atherosclerosis in apolipoprotein E-deficient mice, *Atherosclerosis* **143**, 205–211.

Devlin, C.M., Kuriakose, G., Hirsch, E., Tabas, I. (2002) Genetic alterations of IL-1 receptor antagonist in mice affect plasma cholesterol level and foam cell lesion size, *Proc. Natl. Acad. Sci. U.S.A.* **99**, 6280–6285.

Elhage, R., Maret, A., Pieraggi, M.T., Thiers, J.C., Arnal, J.F., Bayard, F. (1998) Differential effects of interleukin-1 receptor antagonist and tumor necrosis factor binding protein on fatty-streak formation in apolipoprotein E-deficient mice, *Circulation* **97**, 242–244.

Fabunmi, R.P., Sukhova, G.K., Sugiyama, S., Libby, P. (1998) Expression of tissue inhibitor of metalloproteinases-3 in human atheroma and regulation in lesion-associated cells: a potential protective mechanism in plaque stability, *Circ. Res.* **83**, 270–278.

Fazio, S., Babaev, V.R., Burleigh, M.E., Major, A.S., Hasty, A.H., Linton, M.F. (2002) Physiological expression of macrophage apoE in the artery wall reduces atherosclerosis in severely hyperlipidemic mice, *J. Lipid Res.* **43**, 1602–1609.

Febbraio, M., Podrez, E.A. (2000) Targeted disruption of the class B scavenger receptor CD36 protects against atherosclerotic lesion development in mice, *J. Clin. Invest.* **105**, 1049–1056.

Forlow, S.B., Ley, K. (2001) Selectin-independent leukocyte rolling and adhesion in mice deficient in E-, P-, and L-selectin and ICAM-1, *Am. J. Physiol. Heart Circ. Physiol.* **280**, H634–H641.

Frenette, P.S., Wagner, D.D. (1997) Insights into selectin function from knockout mice, *Thromb. Haemost.* **78**, 60–64.

Galis, Z.S., Johnson, C., Godin, D., Magid, R., Shipley, J.M., Senior, R.M., Ivan, E. (2002) Targeted disruption of the matrix metalloproteinase-9 gene impairs smooth muscle cell migration and geometrical arterial remodeling, *Circ. Res.* **91**, 852–859.

George, J., Afek, A., Shaish, A., Levkovitz, H., Bloom, N., Cyrus, T., Zhao, L., Funk, C.D., Sigal, E., Harats, D. (2001) 12/15-Lipoxygenase gene disruption attenuates atherogenesis in LDL receptor-deficient mice, *Circulation* **104**, 1646–1650.

George, J., Mulkins, M., Shaish, A., Casey, S., Schatzman, R., Sigal, E., Harats, D. (2000) Interleukin (IL)-4 deficiency does not influence fatty streak formation in C57BL/6 mice, *Atherosclerosis* **153**, 403–411.

George, J., Shoenfeld, Y., Gilburd, B., Afek, A., Shaish, A., Harats, D. (2000) Requisite role for interleukin-4 in the acceleration of fatty streaks induced by heat shock protein 65 or mycobacterium tuberculosis, *Circ. Res.* **86**, 1203–1210.

Gupta, S., Pablo, A.M., Jiang, X., Wang, N., Tall, A.R., Schindler, C. (1997) IFN-gamma

potentiates atherosclerosis in ApoE knock-out mice, *J. Clin. Invest.* **99**, 2752–2761.

Harats, D., Shaish, A., George, J., Mulkins, M., Kurihara, H., Levkovitz, H., Sigal, E. (2000) Overexpression of 15-lipoxygenase in vascular endothelium accelerates early atherosclerosis in LDL receptor-deficient mice, *Arterioscler. Thromb. Vasc. Biol.* **20**, 2100–2105.

Huber, S.A., Sakkinen, P., Conze, D., Hardin, N., Tracy, R. (1999) Interleukin-6 exacerbates early atherosclerosis in mice, *Arterioscler. Thromb. Vasc. Biol.* **19**, 2364–2367.

Inoue, S., Egashira, K., Ni, W., Kitamoto, S., Usui, M., Otani, K., Ishibashi, M., Hiasa, K., Nishida, K., Takeshita, A. (2002) Anti-monocyte chemoattractant protein-1 gene therapy limits progression and destabilization of established atherosclerosis in apolipoprotein E-knockout mice, *Circulation* **106**, 2700–2706.

Jalkanen, J., Leppanen, P., Narvanen, O., Greaves, D.R., Yla-Herttuala, S. (2003) Adenovirus-mediated gene transfer of a secreted decoy human macrophage scavenger receptor (SR-AI) in LDL receptor knock-out mice, *Atherosclerosis* **169**, 95–103.

Jong, M.C., van Dijk, K.W., Dahlmans, V.E., Van der Boom, H., Kobayashi, K., Oka, K., Siest, G., Chan, L., Hofker, M.H., Havekes, L.M. (1999) Reversal of hyperlipidaemia in apolipoprotein C1 transgenic mice by adenovirus-mediated gene delivery of the low-density-lipoprotein receptor, but not by the very-low-density-lipoprotein receptor, *Biochem. J.* **338**Pt 2, 281–287.

Joyce, C.W., Amar, M.J., Lambert, G., Vaisman, B.L., Paigen, B., Najib-Fruchart, J., Hoyt, R.F., Jr., Neufeld, E.D., Remaley, A.T., Fredrickson, D.S., Brewer, H.B., Jr., Santamarina-Fojo, S. (2002) The ATP binding cassette transporter A1 (ABCA1) modulates the development of aortic atherosclerosis in C57BL/6 and apoE-knockout mice, *Proc. Natl. Acad. Sci. U.S.A.* **99**, 407–412.

Kawashiri, M., Zhang, Y., Usher, D., Reilly, M., Pure, E., Rader, D.J. (2001) Effects of coexpression of the LDL receptor and apoE on cholesterol metabolism and atherosclerosis in LDL receptor-deficient mice, *J. Lipid Res.* **42**, 943–950.

Kim, I.H., Jozkowicz, A., Piedra, P.A., Oka, K., Chan, L. (2001) Lifetime correction of genetic deficiency in mice with a single injection of helper-dependent adenoviral vector, *Proc. Natl. Acad. Sci. U.S.A.* **98**, 13282–13287.

King, V.L., Szilvassy, S.J., Daugherty, A. (2002) Interleukin-4 deficiency decreases atherosclerotic lesion formation in a site-specific manner in female LDL receptor−/− mice, *Arterioscler. Thromb. Vasc. Biol.* **22**, 456–461.

Kirk, E.A., Dinauer, M.C., Rosen, H., Chait, A., Heinecke, J.W., LeBoeuf, R.C. (2000) Impaired superoxide production due to a deficiency in phagocyte NADPH oxidase fails to inhibit atherosclerosis in mice, *Arterioscler. Thromb. Vasc. Biol.* **20**, 1529–1535.

Kozaki, K., Kaminski, W.E., Tang, J., Hollenbach, S., Lindahl, P., Sullivan, C., Yu, J.C., Abe, K., Martin, P.J., Ross, R., Betsholtz, C., Giese, N.A., Raines, E.W. (2002) Blockade of platelet-derived growth factor or its receptors transiently delays but does not prevent fibrous cap formation in ApoE null mice, *Am. J. Pathol.* **161**, 1395–1407.

Kozarsky, K.F., Donahee, M.H., Glick, J.M., Krieger, M., Rader, D.J. (2000) Gene transfer and hepatic overexpression of the HDL receptor SR-BI reduces atherosclerosis in the cholesterol-fed LDL receptor-deficient mouse, *Arterioscler. Thromb. Vasc. Biol.* **20**, 721–727.

Lemaitre, V., O'Byrne, T.K., Borczuk, A.C., Okada, Y., Tall, A.R., D'Armiento, J. (2001) ApoE knockout mice expressing human matrix metalloproteinase-1 in macrophages have less advanced atherosclerosis, *J. Clin. Invest.* **107**, 1227–1234.

Linton, M.F., Atkinson, J.B., Fazio, S. (1995) Prevention of atherosclerosis in apolipoprotein E-deficient mice by bone marrow transplantation, *Science* **267**, 1034–1037.

Luoma, J., Hiltunen, T. (1994) Expression of alpha 2-macroglobulin receptor/low density lipoprotein receptor-related protein and scavenger receptor in human atherosclerotic lesions, *J. Clin. Invest.* **93**, 2014–2021.

Lutgens, E., Daemen, M.J. (2002) CD40-CD40L interactions in atherosclerosis, *Trends Cardiovasc. Med.* **12**, 27–32.

Mallat, Z., Gojova, A., Marchiol-Fournigault, C., Esposito, B., Kamate, C., Merval, R., Fradelizi, D., Tedgui, A. (2001) Inhibition of transforming growth factor-beta signaling accelerates atherosclerosis and induces an unstable plaque phenotype in mice, *Circ. Res.* **89**, 930–934.

Mehrabian, M., Allayee, H., Wong, J., Shi, W., Wang, X.P., Shaposhnik, Z., Funk, C.D., Lusis, A.J., Shih, W. (2002) Identification of 5-lipoxygenase as a major gene contributing to atherosclerosis susceptibility in mice, *Circ. Res.* **91**, 120–126.

Murayama, T., Yokode, M., Kataoka, H., Imabayashi, T., Yoshida, H., Sano, H., Nishikawa, S., Nishikawa, S., Kita, T. (1999) Intraperitoneal administration of anti-c-fms monoclonal antibody prevents initial events of atherogenesis but does not reduce the size of advanced lesions in apolipoprotein E-deficient mice, *Circulation* **99**, 1740–1746.

Ni, W., Egashira, K., Kitamoto, S., Kataoka, C., Koyanagi, M., Inoue, S., Imaizumi, K., Akiyama, C., Nishida, K.I., Takeshita, A. (2001) New anti-monocyte chemoattractant protein-1 gene therapy attenuates atherosclerosis in apolipoprotein E-knockout mice, *Circulation* **103**, 2096–2101.

Pennacchio, L.A., Olivier, M., Hubacek, J.A., Cohen, J.C., Cox, D.R., Fruchart, J.C., Krauss, R.M., Rubin, E.M. (2001) An apolipoprotein influencing triglycerides in humans and mice revealed by comparative sequencing, *Science* **294**, 169–173.

Pinderski, L.J., Fischbein, M.P., Subbanagounder, G., Fishbein, M.C., Kubo, N., Cheroutre, H., Curtiss, L.K., Berliner, J.A., Boisvert, W.A. (2002) Overexpression of interleukin-10 by activated T lymphocytes inhibits atherosclerosis in LDL receptor-deficient mice by altering lymphocyte and macrophage phenotypes, *Circ. Res.* **90**, 1064–1071.

Ross, R., Glomset, J.A. (1973) Atherosclerosis and the arterial smooth muscle cell: proliferation of smooth muscle is a key event in the genesis of the lesions of atherosclerosis, *Science* **180**, 1332–1339.

Sano, H., Sudo, T., Yokode, M., Murayama, T., Kataoka, H., Takakura, N., Nishikawa, S., Nishikawa, S.I., Kita, T. (2001) Functional blockade of platelet-derived growth factor receptor-beta but not of receptor-alpha prevents vascular smooth muscle cell accumulation in fibrous cap lesions in apolipoprotein E-deficient mice, *Circulation* **103**, 2955–2960.

Savontaus, M.J., Sauter, B.V., Huang, T.G., Woo, S.L. (2002) Transcriptional targeting of conditionally replicating adenovirus to dividing endothelial cells, *Gene Ther.* **9**, 972–979.

Schreyer, S.A., Peschon, J.J., LeBoeuf, R.C. (1996) Accelerated atherosclerosis in mice lacking tumor necrosis factor receptor p55, *J. Biol. Chem.* **271**, 26174–26178.

Shichiri, M., Tanaka, A., Hirata, Y. (2003) Intravenous gene therapy for familial hypercholesterolemia using ligand-facilitated transfer of a liposome: LDL receptor gene complex, *Gene Ther.* **10**, 827–831.

Simons, M., Edelman, E.R. (1997) Antisense oligonucleotide inhibition of PDGFR-ß receptor subunit expression directs suppression of intimal thickening, *Circulation* **95**, 669–676.

Singaraja, R.R., Bocher, V., James, E.R., Clee, S.M., Zhang, L.H., Leavitt, B.R., Tan, B., Brooks-Wilson, A., Kwok, A., Bissada, N., Yang, Y.Z., Liu, G., Tafuri, S.R., Fievet, C., Wellington, C.L., Staels, B., Hayden, M.R. (2001) Human ABCA1 BAC transgenic mice show increased high density lipoprotein cholesterol and ApoAI-dependent efflux stimulated by an internal promoter containing liver X receptor response elements in intron 1, *J. Biol. Chem.* **276**, 33969–33979.

Smith, J.D., Trogan, E., Ginsberg, M., Grigaux, C., Tian, J., Miyata, M. (1995) Decreased atherosclerosis in mice deficient in both macrophage colony-stimulating factor (op) and apolipoprotein E, *Proc. Natl. Acad. Sci. U.S.A.* **92**, 8264–8268.

Sukhova, G.K., Schonbeck, U., Rabkin, E., Schoen, F.J., Poole, A.R., Billinghurst, R.C., Libby, P. (1999) Evidence for increased collagenolysis by interstitial collagenases-1 and -3 in vulnerable human atheromatous plaques, *Circulation* **99**, 2503–2509.

Suzuki, H., Kurihara, Y., Takeya, M., Kamada, N., Kataoka, M., Jishage, K., Sakaguchi, H., Kruijt, J.K., Higashi, T., Suzuki, T., van Berkel, T.J., Horiuchi, S., Takahashi, K., Yazaki, Y., Kodama, T. (1997) The multiple roles of macrophage scavenger receptors (MSR) in vivo: resistance to atherosclerosis and susceptibility to infection in MSR knockout mice, *J. Atheroscler. Thromb.* **4**, 1–11.

Thorngate, F.E., Rudel, L.L., Walzem, R.L., Williams, D.L. (2000) Low levels of extrahepatic nonmacrophage ApoE inhibit atherosclerosis without correcting hypercholesterolemia in ApoE-deficient mice, *Arterioscler. Thromb. Vasc. Biol.* **20**, 1939–1945.

Tsukamoto, K., Tangirala, R.K., Chun, S., Usher, D., Pure, E., Rader, D.J. (2000) Hepatic expression of apolipoprotein E inhibits progression of atherosclerosis without reducing cholesterol levels in LDL receptor-deficient mice, *Mol. Ther.* **1**, 189–194.

Whitman, S.C., Ravisankar, P., Daugherty, A. (2002) IFN-gamma deficiency exerts gender-specific effects on atherogenesis in apolipoprotein E−/− mice, *J. Interferon Cytokine Res.* **22**, 661–670.

Whitman, S.C., Ravisankar, P., Daugherty, A. (2002) Interleukin-18 enhances atherosclerosis in apolipoprotein E(−/−) mice through release of interferon-gamma, *Circ. Res.* **90**, E34–E38.

Whitman, S.C., Ravisankar, P., Elam, H., Daugherty, A. (2000) Exogenous interferon-gamma enhances atherosclerosis in apolipoprotein E−/− mice, *Am. J. Pathol.* **157**, 1819–1824.

Yoshimura, S., Morishita, R., Hayashi, K., Yamamoto, K., Nakagami, H., Kaneda, Y., Sakai, N., Ogihara, T. (2001) Inhibition of intimal hyperplasia after balloon injury in rat carotid artery model using cis-element 'decoy' of nuclear factor-kappaB binding site as a novel molecular strategy, *Gene Ther.* **8**, 1635–1642.

Yu, L., Li-Hawkins, J., Hammer, R.E., Berge, K.E., Horton, J.D., Cohen, J.C., Hobbs, H.H. (2002) Overexpression of ABCG5 and ABCG8 promotes biliary cholesterol secretion and reduces fractional absorption of dietary cholesterol, *J. Clin. Invest.* **110**, 671–680.

Zhao, L., Cuff, C.A., Moss, E., Wille, U., Cyrus, T., Klein, E.A., Pratico, D., Rader, D.J., Hunter, C.A., Pure, E., Funk, C.D. (2002) Selective interleukin-12 synthesis defect in 12/15-lipoxygenase-deficient macrophages associated with reduced atherosclerosis in a mouse model of familial hypercholesterolemia, *J. Biol. Chem.* **277**, 35350–35356.

32
Vector System: Plasmid DNA

Rajkumar Banerjee[1] and Leaf Huang[2]
[1]*Indian Institute of Chemical Technology, Hyderabad, India*
[2]*University of Pittsburgh, Pittsburgh, PA, USA*

1	Overview of Plasmid-mediated Gene Therapy	1004
2	Direct Delivery with Naked Plasmid DNA	1006
2.1	History and Recent Efforts Toward Attaining Long-term Expression	1006
2.2	Recent Therapeutic Uses: Treating Cancer	1007
2.3	Understanding Physiological Role of Protein-transduction Pathways	1008
2.4	Gene Transfer to Skeletal Muscle	1008
2.5	Gene Delivery for Myocardial Diseases	1009
2.6	Gene Therapy for Angiogenesis	1010
2.7	Gene Therapy for Autoimmune Diseases	1011
3	Improving Plasmid DNA-mediated Gene Transfer by Electroporation	1011
4	Improving Plasmid DNA Transfer Mediated by Gene Gun	1012
5	Lipid-based Vectors	1013
5.1	Idea Behind Lipid-based Vectors: Recent and Classical Uses	1013
5.1.1	Structures of First Generation Cationic Lipids	1014
5.2	Cellular Barriers for Transfection	1016
5.2.1	Structure of Lipid/DNA Complex	1016
5.2.2	Entry of DNA into Cells	1016
5.2.3	Fate of Complex Inside the Cell: Escape into Cytosol	1018
5.2.4	Entry of DNA in Nucleus	1019
6	Second Generation of Lipidic Delivery System (Lipopolyplex)	1019
6.1	Polycation-condensed DNA Entrapped in Cationic Liposome: LPD-I Formulation	1019
6.2	Polycation-condensed DNA in Anionic Liposomes: LPD-II Formulation	1021

Pharmacology. From Drug Development to Gene Therapy. Edited by Robert A. Meyers.
Copyright © 2008 Wiley-VCH Verlag GmbH & Co. KGaA, Weinheim
ISBN: 978-3-527-32343-2

7   **Emulsion-mediated Gene Transfer**   **1022**
7.1   General Development   1022
7.2   Reconstituted Chylomicron Remnants for Gene Transfer   1022

8   **Use of Cationic Liposome/DNA Complex (Lipoplex)**   **1023**
8.1   *In Vivo* Biodistribution Through Intravenous Injection: Therapeutic
          Implications   1023
8.2   Directly Injected Lipoplexes Used Against Cancer and Other
          Diseases   1024
8.3   Intraperitoneal Injection of Lipoplex for Treating Cancer   1026

9   **Gene Delivery by Polymeric Systems (Polyplex)**   **1026**
9.1   General Development and Uses   1026
9.2   Targeted Gene Delivery by Antibodies Conjugated with Polycations   1028

10   **Nonviral Vector Related Cytotoxicity**   **1028**

11   **Conclusion**   **1029**

          Acknowledgment   **1030**

          Bibliography   **1030**
          Books and Reviews   1030
          Primary Literature   1031

Keywords

Gene Therapy
A therapeutic technique to eradicate genetic malfunctions by introducing new gene or repairing defective gene in the host cell. The therapy, initially aimed toward treating inheritable disorders, is also used in treating acquired disorders such as AIDS, cancer and so on.

Lipoplex
A charged complex made of DNA and cationic lipid. The complex is formed by electrostatic combination of negatively charged DNA with positively charged cationic lipids. Preformed cationic liposomes made of cationic lipids and/or colipids interact and condense DNA by cooperative interaction of positively charged head group of aggregated surface of lipids with negatively charged DNA.

Lipopolyplex
An entity formed by mixing the preformed liposomes made of cationic, anionic or neutral lipids, and/or colipids with cationic polymer induced precondensed DNA. Electron microscopic studies revealed a lipid-based envelope, carrying the polyplex-containing core.

Nonviral Gene Delivery
A special gene delivery technique, which does not use viral mechanism to deliver genes to cells. It involves various physical techniques, chemical methods, and biomimetic synthetic agents to introduce genes to cells.

Polyplex
Another charged complex as lipoplex, but here the cationic entities are polymers. Cationic polymers associated with net positive charges also condense negatively charged DNA by electrostatic combination to form polyplex.

Abbreviations

CHEMS:	cholesteryl hemisuccinate
DC-Chol:	$3\tilde{\beta}$-[N-(N',N'-dimethylaminoethane)-carbamoyl] cholesterol
DDAB:	dimethyldioctadecylammonium bromide
14Dea2:	O,O'-ditetradecanolyl-N-(trimethylammonio acetyl) diethanolamine chloride
DHDEAB:	(N,N-di-n-hexadecyl-N,N-dihydroxyethylammonium bromide)
DMDHP:	N,N-(2-hydroxyethyl)-N-methyl-2,3-bis(myristoyloxy)-1-propanaminium iodide
DMRIE:	N-(2-hydroxyethyl)-N,N-dimethyl-2,3-bis(tetradecyloxy)-1-propanaminium chloride
DOPE:	1,2-dioeoyl-sn-glycero-3-phosphatidylethanolamine
DORIE:	N-[1-(2,3-dioleyloxy)propyl]-N-hydroxyethyl-N,N-dimethylammonium chloride
DOSPA:	2,3-dioleyloxy-N-[2(sperminecar-boxamido)ethyl]-N,N-dimethyl-1-propanaminium trifluoroacetate
DOTAP:	N-[1-(2,3-dioleyloxy)propyl]-N',N',N'-trimethylammonium chloride
DOTIM:	1-[2-[9-(Z)-octadecenoyloxy]ethyl]]-2-[8](Z)-heptadecenyl]-3-[hydroxyethyl]imidazolinium chloride
DOTMA:	N-[1-(2,3-dioleyloxy)propyl]-N,N,N-trimethylammonium chloride
GAP-DLRIE:	N-(3-aminopropyl)-N,N-dimethyl-2,3-bis(dodecyloxy)-1-propaniminium bromide
LPLL:	lipopoly(L-lysine)
MP:	monomethylphosphonate
PAMAM:	polyamidoamine
PEG:	polyethyleneglycol
PEI:	polyethyleneimines
PLL:	poly-L-lysine
PO:	phosphodiester
PS:	phosphorothioate
TC-Chol:	3β-[N-(N',N',N'-trimethylaminoethane)carbamoyl] cholesterol

■ In gene therapy, nonviral gene delivery has earned a special position on its own right. This delivery system enjoys several favorable properties, such as, the delivery efficiency is not limited by the size of the genetic cargo, and it is less immunogenic and less toxic than their viral counterpart. One of the methods of delivery is direct injection of naked DNA to the organs of interest. Plasmid DNAs (pDNA), which carry recombinant genes of interest, are used for introducing genes to cells and organs. Various physical methods, for example, gene gun and electroporation, increase the efficiency of the naked DNA incorporation. Lipid-based vectors have the advantage of protecting the DNA against degradation by endogenous DNase *in vivo*, and can be targeted to a specific cellular site in some special cases. Varieties of lipid-based systems have been designed, mostly containing cationic lipids of different structures. Second-generation vectors containing polymers are more stable and more targetable than the first generation vectors. Although significant progress has been made, nonviral vectors are still limited in their efficiency and by some cytotoxicity inherited in the bacterial pDNA, which hosts the gene of interest. Understanding mechanisms and means to overcome the cellular barriers for the DNA delivery will undoubtedly promote further development of pDNA mediated gene delivery.

1
Overview of Plasmid-mediated Gene Therapy

Postgenomic era has thrust new responsibilities on humankind. Many defective genes responsible for various disease phenotypes have already been discovered. It now becomes a daunting challenge for multidisciplinary field experts to think of strategies to introduce normal genes efficiently into the target cells and/or tissues to complement the defective genes. Hence, gene therapy faces new tasks. This methodology originally designed to correct inheritable disorders, is now being considered for treating acquired disorders, such as cancer and AIDS.

Gene therapy is largely classified into two modes of gene delivery, it either utilizes viruses or it does not. Replication defective viruses such as retrovirus, adenovirus, adeno-associated virus, herpes simplex virus, papilloma virus, Sendai

virus, and so on with part of the genes replaced by a therapeutic gene are used to transduce cells with very high efficiency. They are in use for various gene therapy approaches either clinically or experimentally. There are several drawbacks, which have partially eclipsed or limited the widespread use of viral vectors albeit their excellent transducing efficacy in cells and tissues. For example, induction of strong host-immune response followed by toxicity is common in adenoviral vector–based treatment, which limits the duration of the transgene expression. Additionally, the imposing immunogenicity makes repeated dosing impossible. Retroviral vector requires dividing cells for gene expression, but it poses the risk of random integration into the host genome, leading to mutation and neoplastic transformation. A large, industrial scale production of viral vectors is difficult. There is limitation for the size of the gene cassette to be included in viral vectors. These concerns have prompted the development of nonviral vectors as a less toxic and more scalable alternative for gene therapy. However, nonviral vectors still need improvement, both in efficiency as well as in the duration of the transgene expression. These aspects are the central concerns of the current nonviral vector development.

Nonviral vectors often use recombinant plasmid DNA (pDNA) as the carrier of the therapeutic gene. Recombinant DNA is an artificial, synthetic DNA-based recombinant molecule, made by addition of several DNA fragments obtained from different sources, whereas pDNA is an extrachromosomal, circular, predominantly supercoiled bacterial DNA, which can be produced on a large scale by fermentation in bacterial cultures. Through simple recombination techniques, any therapeutic or marker gene of any size can be introduced into pDNA. Nowadays with the help of existing advanced technologies, a single lot can produce multigram quantities of pDNA, which can be finally purified using simple physical and chemical methods. Generally, standard pDNA is 4–10 kbp in size (molecular weight: 1×10^6 to 3×10^6). Other than the usual bacterial sequences, pDNA for gene therapy contains an expressible sequence of

genomic DNA, popularly known as *complementary DNA* (cDNA) that codes for a specific protein. This genetic sequence, also called *transgene,* remains under the controlling influence of another gene sequence called *promoter,* located upstream of the coding sequence of transgene. This promoter sequence controls transcription, that is, transgene to messenger RNA conversion. A transcription termination gene is often inserted downstream of coding sequence to ensure proper termination of transgene transcription. A polyadenylation sequence and sometimes an intron, that is, a nonexpressible gene sequence, is also added to ensure proper processing of the m-RNA product of the transgene (see Fig. 1). The major advantage of plasmid expression vectors is that the cells upon transfection produce homogeneous, correctly folded, posttranslationally modified proteins within itself. This thwarts the attempt to purify and isolate proteins, which often leads to partial degradation or inactivation of the protein.

This chapter is, however, intended to summarily emphasize the role of pDNA as a gene-carrying cask, which finds its role in gene therapy using nonviral-based delivery techniques toward deciphering various biological functions, and use

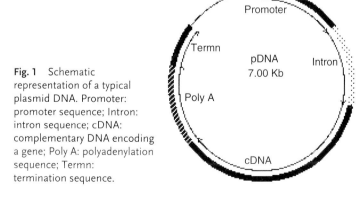

Fig. 1 Schematic representation of a typical plasmid DNA. Promoter: promoter sequence; Intron: intron sequence; cDNA: complementary DNA encoding a gene; Poly A: polyadenylation sequence; Termn: termination sequence.

those facts in finding gene therapy–based therapeutically useful tools against various disease pathologies.

2
Direct Delivery with Naked Plasmid DNA

2.1
History and Recent Efforts Toward Attaining Long-term Expression

The simplest of all DNA delivery systems is the injection of naked pDNA to the organ or tissue of interest. Skeletal muscle was first transfected by intramuscular (IM) injection of naked pDNA. Since then, a plethora of tissues such as, the interstitial space of liver, thyroid, heart muscles, brain, urological organs, and so on have been transfected with direct gene transfer. The delivery by direct injection of naked DNAs containing one or more anticancer genes was also tested against various tumors with mixed efficacies.

This technique of direct injection of pDNA was thoroughly used in several other experimentations as well. This technique of direct injection has become a useful tool to analyze the gene expression and promoter function in the respective organ. Utilizing viral promoter, such as that from cytomegalovirus (CMV), a high level of initial expression was attained, which, however, declined sharply to near background within two to three weeks. Although within two days of pDNA injection the maximum decrease in the expression level was observed, but the pDNA continued to be scantily detected till the end of 12 weeks (0.2 copies per genome). The major cause of this early decline was believed to be because of viral promoter activated immune responses, and this fact was later corroborated by experimentations in immunosuppressed mice that showed extended levels of transgene expressions.

Sustained therapeutic benefit needs assurance for long-lasting gene expression of pDNA associated therapeutic genes without eliciting any expression related cytotoxicity. Classically, several experimentations were performed, with fewer cases showing chances of extended expression time. For example, high-expressing human factor IX (hFIX) pDNA upon transfection in mouse liver yielded therapeutic-level gene expression over $1\frac{1}{2}$ years, eliciting no transgene expression–related cytotoxicity or long-term therapy related toxicity. However, with liver regeneration, there was a decline in transgene expression, which suggested the possibility of decline in maintenance of plasmid, rather than the possibility of transgene integration into the host genome. Hence, sustained gene expressions required a transcriptionally active vector DNA that could persist for a long time in the organ. Let us also not forget that a random genomic integration in host genome is contrary to health benefit. Therefore, with the help of this transcriptionally active vector, pDNA nonviral gene transfer could lead to extended life of transgene-expression level without leaving scope for genomic integration.

For extended transgene expressions of conventional plasmid vectors, a new technique was involved. The plasmid vector was modified to contain Eppstein–Barr virus (EBV) episomal vectors that consisted of *EBNA1* (EBV nuclear antigen-1) gene, and oriP element. Interestingly, nuclear localization and transcriptional upregulation of the oriP-bearing plasmid was assisted with the help of EBNA-1. This enabled efficacious transgene expression and long-term maintenance of the expression in cells transfected with the EBV/lipoplex. EBV plasmid vector played an important role in various disorders such as congenital, malignant, chronic, and infectious diseases. This plasmid was used in gene therapy against tumor malignancies, such as in reducing tumor size by intratumoral injection of EBV plasmid vector encoding *HSV1-TK* anticancer gene. *EBV* plasmid-based interleukin genes, *IL-12* and *IL-18* gene transfer to tumors elicited natural killer (NK) cell activities and cytotoxic T-cell (CTL) responses, which lead to tumor retardation. Cardiomyopathic animals experienced extended cardiac output upon intracardiomuscular transfer of EBV-based β-adrenergic receptor gene. EBV-based plasmid gene transfer was also used for genetic vaccination against acute viral infections.

Another school of thought sprouted while developing and fine-tuning the conditions for long-term transgene expression. We know that virus-mediated gene transfer lead to random integration into the host chromosome. This often leads to abnormality in gene expression. However, site-specific genetic integration into inconspicuous genomic sequence might be one of the most-sought-after preconditions for stable, long-lasting, and powerful transgene expressions mediated through recombinant plasmids. This became possible with phage integrases. These enzymes mediate unidirectional site-specific recombination between two specific DNA sequences, one containing phage attachment site (attP) and the other bacterial attachment site (attB). These DNA sequences are short, yet specific on a genetic scale. A plasmid containing the bacterial attachment site flanking the gene of interest in both the ends was transfected into cells. The integrases of the serine family showed efficient recombination in mammalian cells. They mediated efficient integration at introduced att sites or native sequences

with partial att sites (pseudo-attP). Human α_1-antitrypsin and hFIX gene associated with attB cassette, coadministered with integrase plasmid, upon liver delivery to mice showed elevated long-term expression (therapeutic level of protein obtained for about 8 months). Upon partial hepatectomy, the expression did not decline, indicating that the DNA was integrated to the mouse genome. Similar results were obtained during the functional restoration of human type VII collagen protein in skin cells obtained from recessive dystrophic epidermolysis bullosa (RDEB) patients. Additionally, this technique could be useful in developing big transgenic animals dedicated to the preparation of therapeutic proteins on large scales.

2.2
Recent Therapeutic Uses: Treating Cancer

Nonviral gene therapy had become a useful tool in generating various therapeutic effects in diverse animal models. One of these effects is to induce anticancer response in tumor models by introducing anticancer genes. NO synthase II (*NOS II*) gene that catalyzes nitric oxide (NO) production was incorporated in plasmid under CMV promoter control. This plasmid, upon injecting in medullary thyroid cancer (MTC), elicited anticancer effect in tumorigenic cells. The gene triggered a suicidal effect (apoptosis) on the tumor cells by the production of NO, which specifically activated the macrophages against the fast dividing tumor cells, leaving normal cells untouched. NO was also observed to mediate bystander antitumor effect: The activated *NOS* gene in a tumor cell induced the cytotoxicity in the neighboring tumor cells. The fact that NO mediated tumorigenic effect does not require transfection of all neoplastic cells promised a capable suicide gene therapy approach to human cancer.

Fas ligand is another apoptotic inducing molecule that showed similar bystander effect. The membrane protein receptor Fas and its ligand FasL mutual interaction initiate an apoptotic signal in Fas-bearing cells. pDNA could be used to deliver these apoptosis-inducing genes to initiate killing of transfected and nontransfected surrounding cells. On direct injection of FasL encoding pDNA vector into the inflamed thyroid, pathogenic lymphocytes were inhibited to enter into thyroid, leaving the already infiltrated T cells dead. Thus, FasL expressing in thyroicytes might lead to potential remedial therapy for the experimental autoimmune thyroiditis (EAT).

2.3
Understanding Physiological Role of Protein-transduction Pathways

Direct pDNA transfer technique could find its use in examining the role of a physiologically related protein-transduction signal pathway toward certain endogenous disease phenotype, such as investigating the functional role of the tissue kallikrein-kinin system (KKS) in the central control of blood pressure homeostasis. Kallikrein is a proteinase enzyme that converts kininogen to vasodialative kinin peptides. To understand the role of vasodialative KKS on the pathogenesis of hypertension, the human tissue kallikrein gene *CMV-cHK*, was intracerebroventricularly injected into hypertensive rats. Cortex, cerebellum, brain stem, hippocampus, and hypothalamus identifiably expressed human tissue kallikrein protein. The expression level and its effect could lead to verify the role of the KKS system.

Similarly, the method of Direct injection of pDNA to rat fibroblast had been used to study the consequences of over-expressing dominant negative forms of the ubiquitous mitogen-activated protein kinase (MAP-kinase) toward inhibition of cell proliferation. Direct pDNA microinjection technique was also used to demonstrate the absolute requirement of the protein Cyclin A in DNA synthesis, as opposed to the popular belief that the Cyclin A was uniquely involved in the mitotic activation only. An SV40 expression vector encoding the full-length, antisense Cyclin A RNA, upon direct microinjection into synchronized mammalian cells, completely suppressed Cyclin A expression at S phase, resulting in inhibition of DNA synthesis.

2.4
Gene Transfer to Skeletal Muscle

A variety of diseases such as muscular dystrophies, chronic ischemic limb syndromes and so on, were treated by the technique of direct gene transfer to skeletal muscle. Specifically engineered pDNAs and the vector systems were developed that enabled regulated and tissue-specific transgene expression in skeletal muscle *in vivo*. Naked pDNA–based gene transfer had been used in different animal models, for example, in correcting Duchenne Muscular Dystrophy, to supply sources of therapeutic protein systemically, for genetic vaccination against pathogens and tumor cells. However, larger animals showed limited clinical utility owing to inefficient gene expression in them.

On quantifying the gene-uptake in the muscles, the IM injection showed less than 1% uptake of injected dose and was limited to cells adjacent to the needle track. Using hypertonic sucrose, or muscle revitalizers, the efficiency and reproducibility of gene expression could be increased. In-traarterial injection of naked pDNA into the femoral arteries of rats showed 2 orders of magnitude higher transgene-expression level throughout the muscles of hind limb compared to that obtained in direct muscular injection. Myofibers were 10% more transfected through intravascular delivery than with the direct IM injection. This intraarterial injection technique was extended to the nonhuman primates also. Hypothetically, the pDNA upon intravascular injection extravasates out by the intravascular pressure following the convective flow across the endothelium, and was soon picked up by the *in situ* muscle cells with the help of membrane receptors. This was evidenced by the fact that the naked pDNA was taken up by hepatocytes *in vivo* by a receptor-mediated process. Several DNA receptors had been discovered in human leukocytes, peritoneal macrophages, and in wide variety of tissues and tumor cells. For the enhancement of IM gene expression, a fresh look is needed toward the poorly understood mechanism of molecular recognition and characterization of the cell surface receptor(s) involved in the binding and internalization of DNA. It is reported that rapid injection of pDNA in a large volume (e.g. 5 μg of DNA/20 g mouse in 1.5 to 2.0 mL of saline solution) through the tail vein left the injected DNA in the inferior vena cava. The DNA flowed back to the tissues linked to this vascular system, primarily the liver. The hydrodynamic pressure forced DNA into the liver cells before it was mixed with blood. By this process, the liver showed the highest expression of gene; internal organs such as lung, spleen, heart, and kidney were also efficiently transfected. It was also shown that briefly clamping the vena cava following tail vein injection of pDNA in a small volume efficiently transfected both liver and diaphragm. The result is potentially important because diaphragm is barely transfected by hydrodynamics-based method. The full-length dystrophin cDNA can be delivered to the diaphragm for the treatment of Duchenne Muscular Dystrophy. It is well known that patients with Duchenne Muscular Dystrophy often suffer from fatal respiratory failure due to the dystrophic diaphragm muscle collapse.

2.5
Gene Delivery for Myocardial Diseases

Myocardial gene delivery via direct injection or through coronary vasculature with naked pDNA usually showed low levels of gene transfection. However, the results so obtained had invaluable impact in characterizing the role of promoters in cardiac tissue and further helped in examining the effect on transferred foreign gene expression by the influences of naturally occurring mechanical and hormonal stimuli of the myocardium.

It was demonstrated that the tissue-specific promoter chimeras injected into the heart could respond accurately to shift in thyroid hormone levels *in vivo*. Injection of pDNA with gene constructs driven by cellular promoters resulted in detectable levels of reporter gene activities. The cellular promoter was derived from the rat α-myosin heavy chain (α-MHC) gene. The expression of this gene *in vivo* is restricted to cardiac muscle and is positively regulated by thyroid hormone. The regulatory portion of genes expressing specifically in cardiac muscles could be identified using this method. Direct DNA injection had been extended to evaluate and characterize the activation properties of a cardiac-specific promoter/enhancer of the slow/cardiac troponin C (cTnC) gene that express in cardiac striated muscles.

Myocardial direct DNA injection was also utilized to analyze the transcriptional regulation of brain creatine kinase (BCK) gene in the developing heart. pDNA constructs containing BCK promoter and *CAT* or luciferase reporter gene was delivered into the left lateral wall and apex of the ventricle on the heart. The study might provide insight into the embryonic gene expressing mechanism during cardiogenesis. Because the *BCK* gene, the major gene for cytoplasmic creatine kinase expressed in the embryonic heart, is downregulated during cardiogenesis, it is reinstated in response to stimuli such as ischemia, hypertrophy, or heart failure in the adult.

The method of direct pDNA injection was used to explore the effect of specific pathophysiological state on cardiac gene expression, such as ischemia, myocardial infarction, reperfusion injury, hypertension and so on. Ischemia is a disease state that is formed when tissues are starved of blood supply and nutrients because of deficient supply of blood through possibly narrowed or blocked arteries. Sporadic myocardial ischemia is prevalently associated with coronary arterial diseases. Ischemia related disease phenotype needs a therapeutic gene, which could be selectively upregulated by the elevated signals for ischemic activity and consequently downregulated when the activity represses. In this context, Prentice et al. introduced expression plasmids containing muscle-specific α-MHC promoters and hypoxia-responsive enhancer (HRE) elements linked to a reporter gene in cultured cells or into the rabbit myocardium, and measured the regulation of these constructs by hypoxia or experimental ischemia. It was shown that the expression of reporter gene was induced by both hypoxia *in vitro* and by a short interval of ischemia *in vivo*.

There were different reports concerning the stability of plasmid-based transgenes in both skeletal and cardiac muscles. It was shown that the rat cardiac myocytes could express *β-galactosidase* gene under the control of the Rous sarcoma virus promoter, by the injection of pDNA encoding the reporter gene directly into the left ventricular wall. *β*-galactosidase expressed in cardiac myocytes was detected in rat hearts for at least four weeks after injection of the *β-galactosidase* gene. In postmitotic cardiac and skeletal muscle cells, the transgene expression of the pDNA declines with time, probably due to the episomal localization of the DNA. The reason that the striated muscles showed higher capacity for uptake and expressing of pDNA following direct injection was not clear; the efficient gene transfer might be induced by cellular membrane rupturing and destabilization, followed by inflammation caused by the injection needle.

2.6
Gene Therapy for Angiogenesis

Because ischemia is formed as a result of deficient supply of blood to tissues, formation of new blood vessels is a remedy against this disease. One of the mechanisms that involves the formation of new blood vessels is angiogenesis. Angiogenesis is the process of new blood vessel development for the vascularization of various organs, for wound healing, and to allow cancer development and proliferation.

Therapeutic angiogenesis involves replenishing angiogenic growth factors by administering recombinant proteins or endothelial growth-factor gene. The recombinant proteins have severe limitation on its usage, as they are expensive and difficult to produce on a large scale.

On the other hand, gene therapy provides a systemic and long-term effect with modification in the effective dosage of the therapeutic agent. To evade potential problems of pathological angiogenesis, transient gene expression is usually preferred for this kind of treatment. Tsurumi et al. introduced naked pDNA encoding vascular endothelial growth factor (VEGF) by (IM injection into ischemic hind limb muscles of a rabbit model and observed that the vessels and blood-capillaries were increased in rabbit muscles injected with VEGF compared to controls. An enhanced vascularity-induced perfusion followed by increased blood flow in the ischemic limbs was also observed. In clinical trial, Simovic et al. introduced naked pDNA encoding human *VEGF* gene by direct IM injection to chronic ischemic limbs of patients, to treat peripheral neuropathy caused by critical limb ischemia. The patients showed decreased neuropathic disability in the treated limbs, indicating that long-term therapy might improve the integrity in tissues of ischemic limb and consequent retrieval of limb.

2.7
Gene Therapy for Autoimmune Diseases

Autoimmune disease is a pathogenic condition in which ones immune system erroneously targets and aggresses a person's own cells, tissues, and organs. The most prevalent symptom of this disease is inflammation, which is caused by the abundant presence of a large number of immune cells and molecules in the target site of the body. Autoimmune diseases or other inflammatory conditions were primarily and successfully confronted by gene therapy through the delivery of cytokines or cytokine inhibitors. Interferon γ. (IFN-γ), interleukin-1 (IL-1, α or β),

IL-12, and tumor necrosis factor α (TNFα) are recurrently addressed inflammatory cytokines in illnesses related to autoimmune/inflammatory diseases. Other than these cytokines, transforming growth factor β (TGF-β) is also a key regulatory cytokine, because TGF-β inhibits T and B cell responses, irregularity of which leads to elevation of autoimmunity invoked disease conditions.

In animal models, pDNA constructs with the encoding anti-inflammatory cytokine genes for IL-10, IL-4, and TGF-β1 were injected into either tibialis anterior or rectus femoris muscles in nonobese diabetic (NOD) mouse against autoimmune diabetic disease. Although there was no marked decrease in severity of insulitis, the diabetes was reduced in NOD mice injected with IL10 as compared to untreated NOD mice. In another experiment, treatment of autoimmunity prone NOD mice with pCMV-TGF-β1 resulted in considerable elevation of TGF-β1 level in the plasma. The increased levels of TGF-β1 exerted various immunosuppressive effects such as suppression of delayed-type hypersensitivity (DTH), and prevention of insulitic and diabetic incidence in this kind of mice. TGF-β1, IL-4, and IFN-γ gene coding plasmid vectors were also injected intramuscularly into rodent models for treating experimental allergic encephalomyelitis (EAE), systemic lupus erythematosus (SLE), colitis, and Streptococcal cell wall-induced arthritis (SCW arthritis).

3
Improving Plasmid DNA-mediated Gene Transfer by Electroporation

Electroporation is a process of exposing cells to controlled electric field for the purpose of cellular membrane permeability. The electric pulses, intensely localized to destabilize the membrane, allow molecules to enter cells. A variety of genetic materials were inserted into the cells *in vitro* by electroporation. Electrochemotherapy facilitates the cellular entry of hydrophilic anticancer agents such as bleomycin to obtain drastically improved antitumor effect in malignant melanoma.

Recently, *in vivo* electroporation has emerged as a leading technology for developing nonviral gene therapies and nucleic acid vaccines (NAV). Naked pDNA injections accompanied by electroporation showed 10 to 1000-fold increases in gene expressions as compared to the nonelectroporated direct injections. However, the duration of a gene expression following *in vivo* electroporation was dependent on target tissue and plasmid constructs. Despite this fact, a broader variety of cells showed reporter gene expressions.

The major advantage of electroporation is that a treatment-area specific *in vivo* gene expression is possible wherein specific tissue could be directed by using specifically designed electrodes. A high level of controlled expression of specific gene was obtained by using tissue-specific promoter directed against specific tissue with a different pulsing parameter.

Various disease pathologies underwent electroporation-mediated *in vivo* gene transfer. The successful utilization of this technique was done in targeting hepatic parenchyma, hepatocellular carcinoma (HCC), skin, skeletal muscle, mouse testes, melanoma, human primary myoblast, glomeruli, brain, human primary hematopoietic stem cells, human esophageal tumor, and rat skeletal muscle for correcting anemia of renal failure. Furthermore, electroporation of TGF-β1 gene to the wound models in diabetic mice

resulted in higher cell proliferation, denser yet organized extracellular matrix formation, collagen synthesis, and angiogenesis in the treated wound site.

Electroporation utilizing high electric field strength induces tissue damage. This restricts its usage. Efficient and safe electrotransfer for delivering exogenous material into tissues must be developed before the clinical potential of gene therapy can be realized. Recently, a novel syringe electrode was developed. With this electrode, electric field was directly delivered to the cells in which pDNA had been injected, the injected DNA could be confined to the high field region without affecting the adjacent areas. High transfection efficiency was observed with comparatively lower field strength that caused minimal tissue damage.

A technique called *microelectroporation* was utilized locally to introduce a transgene into chick embryo and for expressing the gene in a spatial and temporal manner. By the microelectroporation technique, DNA molecules were efficiently introduced into the optic vesicle, sensory placodes, surface ectoderm, neuroepithelium of the central nervous system (CNS), and into the somites and limb mesenchyme.

4
Improving Plasmid DNA Transfer Mediated by Gene Gun

Gene gun is a physical way of administering gene *in vitro* or *in vivo*. pDNA makes electrostatic complex with gold or tungsten microparticles. The DNA-metal particle upon targeting to specific tissue is forcibly expelled by a flow of regulated, highly compressed helium gas. The delivery is highly localized to the tissue part. The delivery to different tissue depths and areas is regulated by adjusting the speed and hence impact-pressure of the projectile. The process involves easy and speedy preparation of the delivery vehicle while keeping DNA intact. This technique sometimes allows DNA to gain direct access to nucleus bypassing the endosome/lysosome. These cellular compartments may induce possible enzymatic degradation. Because of the benefit of accessibility, this technique is especially suitable for gene transfer to skin and for superficial wounds. There are several examples in various animal models, which have shown a high level of transgene expression in the epidermis and dermis of the skin.

By the gene gun technique, mouse skin was transfected with IL-6 and hemagglutinin encoded DNA to elicit protective immune responses against equine influenza virus. Several different large animals such as rhesus monkeys, pigs, and horses were also immunized against virus by transfecting gene encoding the viral antigen.

Detectable transgene activities were also noticed in various nonsuperficial organs, such as lungs, pancreas, kidney, muscle, and cornea. Gene gun was also used to treat against tumor growth. Intradermal tumor upon *IL-12* gene delivery by gene gun gave detectable levels of the gene product at the treatment site. This eventually led to complete tumor regression within seven days. TGF-β1 encoded plasmid bombardment to rat tissue enhanced the tensile strength of the tissue by almost twofold, as compared to the control constituting nongene gun mediated direct injection. Porcine partial-thickness wounds, when transfected with a vector expressing epidermal growth factor (EGF) showed an increased rate of epithelial cell formation. This increased epithelialization shortened the wound healing time by 20%.

5
Lipid-based Vectors

5.1
Idea Behind Lipid-based Vectors: Recent and Classical Uses

The lipid-based DNA delivery system was first utilized on the premise that naked DNA upon injection *in vivo* might be degraded by endogenous DNase. The DNA would remain protected inside the lipid-based delivery vehicle during its run through the circulating blood stream. With necessary chemical modification, this vehicle would target the DNA toward specific cellular sites.

These lipids are a class of molecule that self-assemble in aqueous or organic media. Depending on its molecular architecture and in the presence or absence of cosolute, they assume structures such as micelle, emulsion, or liposome in aqueous media, and reverse micelle in organic media. However, among all the systems, liposomal systems found most biological usage, probably owing to its close resemblance with the cellular membrane. They constitute a bilayered structure, which can encapsulate water-soluble molecules in its aqueous hydrophilic core or water-insoluble molecules in its hydrophobic bilayer. Liposome-based drug delivery systems have shown promise in clinical use and several products have already been approved by the FDA. Fraley et al. had shown for the first time that encapsulating DNA in liposomal aqueous core could also deliver DNA to cellular targets. They used a composite liposomal system containing anionic and nonionic lipids. The DNA encapsulation efficiency for this system was low. Toward enhancing gene delivery and targeting ability of the liposome to specific tissue site, anionic liposomes encapsulating DNA were coated with target-specific antibody to make pH-sensitive immunoliposomes. These liposomes upon intraperitoneal (IP) injection, showed specific transfection to tumor cells in an ascites tumor model in nude mice. Very recently, the immunoliposomes were revisited for targeting brain. An exogenous gene was targeted to brain through the blood brain barrier by intravenous (i.v.) injection of pegylated immunoliposomes conjugated with antibody to rat transferrin receptor. The whole entity was targeted to brain via the transcytosis of transferrin receptor.

Felgner et al. for the first time used cationic liposomes for gene transfection. The primary idea was to electrostatically condense DNA with more than one equivalent of cationic lipid and the negatively charged cells would take up the net positively charged entity when fed to the cell. Overall gene delivery to the cells was very high compared to any contemporary nonviral gene delivery techniques. This opened up a new vista in the field of gene therapy. Soon a plethora of literature developed, which chronicled the painstaking fine-tuning of the chemical structure of lipids by systematic structure-activity studies. These studies were done to dig out the structure of the potentially most potent cationic lipid for gene transfection.

pDNA played a significant role in this context. pDNA reconstructed with recombinant marker/reporter gene and suitable promoter is primarily used as a tool to screen the efficient transfection lipid from a library of cationic lipidic molecules. The electrostatic lipid–DNA complex that is formed by the recombination of these first generation cationic lipids with DNA is termed *lipoplex*. Cationic polymers also condense DNA and, with or without the presence of lipid, these polymers can deliver DNA to cells. This makes the basis of the second-generation gene delivery systems. Cationic polymers, cationic dendrimers, and so on condense DNA to make a complex called "polyplex". If liposomes, cationic or anionic are used to encapsulate the precondensed cationic polymer–DNA complex, and are used to deliver DNA to cells, then the whole entity is termed *lipopolyplex*. We will talk about these second-generation gene delivery systems later in this chapter.

5.1.1 Structures of First Generation Cationic Lipids

In the process of finding out the best cationic transfection lipid, several groups throughout the world, over the last 15 to 17 years, explored different chemistries to evolve different chemical structures, which made quite a big library of molecules. It is very interesting to know that several architectural differences in the molecular infrastructure of cationic lipids evolved, which lead to the formation of cationic lipids of varied transfection ability. Here, we will briefly yet broadly classify the categories of cationic lipids with varied degrees of chemical moieties (Fig. 2).

1. *Lipids with glycerol backbone containing aliphatic carbon chain(s)*: DOTMA, DMRIE, DORIE, DOSPA, GAP-DLRIE, DOTAP, DMDHP and so on. These lipids are linked to glycerol moiety through ether or ester bond and have either a single cationic charge with none, single, or multiple hydroxyl groups, or have multiple cationic charges by possessing spermidine derivatives.

2. *Lipids with long-chain alkylamine/alkylamide moiety*: DDAB, DOGS, LPLL, GS2888, 14DEA2, diC14amidine,

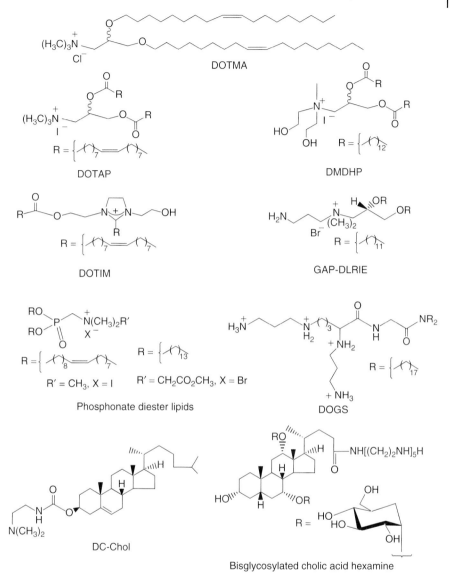

Fig. 2 Structures of some representative cationic lipids.

DHDEAB, TFX™ and so on. These are basically nonglycerol-based lipids with single or multiple charges. The charges arise because of the presence of ammonium or multiple amines or spermidines. Some of these lipids also possess multiple hydroxyl groups.

3. *Lipids with cholesterol moiety*: DC-Chol and other cholesterol derivatives, biglycosylated cholic acid derivative and cholesterol with polyamines, spermidines and so on.

4. *Lipids with L-α-phosphatidylethanolamine derivatives with spermidines*:

1,2-dipalmitoylphosphatidylethanol-amidospermine (DPPES) or L-α-phosphatidylcholine with phosphonate diester.

5. *Lipids with imidazole derivative*: DOTIM or nonglycerol-based lipids with long-chain alkyl acyl carnitine ester.

There were many other lipids that were synthesized and tested for gene transfection. Only a few of these lipids had shown consistent and relatively high level of transfection in various cell lines and in animal models *in vivo*. Most of these first generation formulations were not long circulating in the blood, owing to the fact that the DNA/cationic lipid complex disintegrates in the presence of negatively charged blood proteins. Additionally, they showed no specific targeting of cells. Finally, in spite of such a big library of molecules, no consensus thumb-rule could be predicted or ascertained regarding the magic structure of lipid, which might show best transfection in all kinds of cells consistently. This is because there were so many parameters involved in the whole process of transfection. In order to develop the potentially best nonviral gene delivery system, we have to understand various barriers confronting transfection. Here, we will briefly discuss these barriers.

5.2
Cellular Barriers for Transfection

To develop an efficient gene delivery system, it seems necessary to understand the extra- and intracellular processes involved in the overall transfection mechanism. This will lead to comprehending the challenge before the task of developing efficient lipid-based nonviral vectors for gene therapy applications. For this purpose, cationic liposomes and pDNA are used widely to understand the cellular mechanism involved in the transfection (see Fig. 3).

5.2.1 Structure of Lipid/DNA Complex
Positively charged cationic liposomes electrostatically interact with negatively charged nucleic acid sequences to form fused, aggregated complexes, which are capable of entering a cell. These aggregates have a very heterogeneous size distribution with respect to particle size and net charge. The lipid-to-DNA mass and charge ratio, which defines the size and net surface charge of the complex, is an important factor to determine transfection efficiency. Hence, the structural features associated with this kind of complex need complete interpretation. Structural features revealed by electron microscopy include lipid-coated DNA strands, aggregates of liposome intercalating DNA, DNA entrapped between the lamellae of aggregated multilamellar structure, and tubular structure consisting of fused liposome around DNA. Polycations such as polylysine or multivalent cationic lipid condense DNA into small compact particles. Cells can take these compacted DNA much more efficiently than the lipid/DNA condensed particles obtained by the interaction of DNA by monovalent cationic lipids.

5.2.2 Entry of DNA into Cells
The presence of glycophospholipids and negatively charged proteins such as proteoglycans, glycosaminoglycans and so on imparts negative charges on the cell surfaces. It was hypothesized that membrane fusion between cationic liposome and negatively charged cell membrane is the primary means of cell entry. The hypothesis was based on the supposition that cationic and anionic liposomes readily

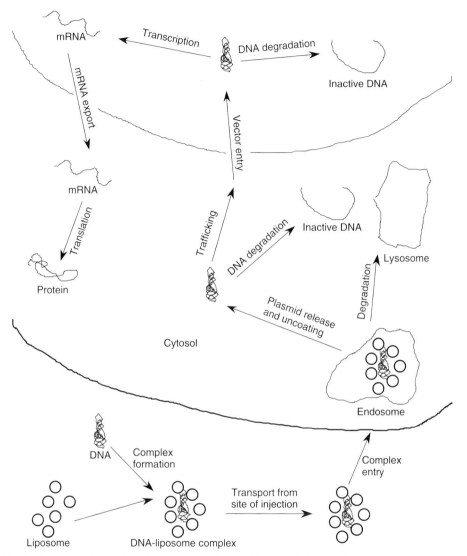

Fig. 3 Schematic illustration of the processes involved in gene delivery and expression.

fuse. It was conceptualized that the inter-action of the cationic complex with the cell is primarily electrostatic, and does not involve any specific receptor for the cationic moiety. Other experiments also suggested that the mechanism of DNA transfer to animal cells from cationic liposomes might not entail a simple fusion of liposomal and cellular membrane. However, it was shown that heparin sulfates, the highly anionic polysaccharides, serve as an important cell surface receptor for cationic lipid–DNA complexes. The nondifferentiated edged airway epithelial cells endocytose liposome–DNA complexes consequent to their relatively high negative charge and phagocytic activity compared to relatively more differentiated cells. Evidences now strongly suggest that slow endocytosis of intact lipid/DNA complex could be the primary method for cellular entry.

5.2.3 Fate of Complex Inside the Cell: Escape into Cytosol

After cellular entry, the lipoplex is engulfed into the lower pH compartment called *early endosomes* in the perimembranous region. The intracellular trafficking was ascertained by an experiment wherein a liposome composed of lipopolylysine (LPLL) and DOPE (1,2-dioleoyl-sn-glycero-3-phosphatidylethylamine) was first used to condense DNA to form electron-dense particles recognized by thin-section transmission EM and upon treatment to the cells a majority of them were found to reside in vesicular compartments. The endosomal contents usually pass into lysosome, the cell organelle in the perinuclear region that houses a host of degradative enzymes. The hydrolytic enzymes degrade most if not all of the lysosomal contents. So, it becomes necessary that the endosomal content must free itself at the early endosome stage to keep the DNA intact. Disruption of endosomal vesicle is visualized in the liposomal system containing DOPE as a helper colipid. DOPE, with its tendency to promote significant polymorphic changes in the lipid phase, stimulates membrane fusion or destabilization. This is followed by leakage of endosomal content into the cytoplasm. DOPE, in aqueous media, assumes inverted hexagonal phase II structure, which is frequently obtained in regions of membrane where it fuses with another membrane. Thus, one may assume that DOPE, or liposome formulation containing DOPE, might fuse with endosomal membrane and destabilize it to leak out the content from the endosome.

If the early endosomal release is not possible, then another way to keep DNA intact in lysosome is to protect the DNA from lysosomal degradation. Cationic liposomes formulated with cholesterol are believed to offer a useful role in keeping DNA intact. It was demonstrated that the lysosomal enzymes work at lower pH, that is, pH < 6. It was also shown that cholesterol-containing liposomes, which possess greater stability and lower ion-permeability compared to DOPE-containing liposomes, provide an improved stability to the lipid–DNA complex in the cytosol. It is easily conceivable that if the endosomal content passes onto lysosome before being released from endosomes, the lipoplex could remain secured in the lysosome.

Cationic lipids can destabilize a cellular membrane because of its intrinsic detergent property. Therefore, destabilization of endosomal and/or lysosomal membrane may be a contribution from the cationic lipids itself. In the same context, it was shown that the cationic lipid/DOPE or cationic lipid/cholesterol liposome formulation, exhibit surface anisotropies in terms of increased liposomal surface pH. The surface pH of the liposomal formulations exhibits at least two pH units higher than the pH of the solution at which they are made. Therefore, a liposomal solution made at physiological pH may in reality exhibit a surface pH > 9, which is detrimental for both the stability of endosome and activity of lysosomal enzymes. Endosomal disruptions were also done with fusogenic peptides, which promote pH-dependent fusion of small liposomes when associated with lipid bilayer. When these peptides were codelivered with lipid/DNA complex, they imparted formidable endosomal disruption by changing its usual random coil conformation into amphipathic α-helix conformation at lower pH, resulting in consequent cytoplasmic delivery of DNA.

5.2.4 Entry of DNA in Nucleus

The success of lipid-mediated gene transfer is severely limited by the inefficient transport of transfected DNA from the cytoplasm into the nucleus. In general, macromolecules enter the nucleus through nuclear pores. Molecular aggregates with size more than 55 Å in diameter or molecular weight greater than 40 KD utilize the nuclear pore complex (NPC) to access the nucleus. NPC bind with molecular aggregates associated with nuclear localization signal (NLS) peptide and help it to translocate across the nuclear membrane. One of the typical signals is the NLS from SV40 large T antigen (PKRRRKV), which had been conjugated to many different molecules to gain nuclear access. NLS peptide-conjugated pDNA was delivered efficiently inside the nucleus with an enhanced gene expression. Similarly, SV40 T antigen NLS codelivered with DOTAP cationic liposome mediated efficient gene transfer and expression in the cell. The genes delivered inside the nucleus require uncoating from the lipidic shell before the transcription starts. It is generally assumed that pDNA is displaced from the complex by anionic macromolecules in the nucleus. In this regard, an alternative hypothesis for cytosolic release of DNA from lipid/DNA complex had been proposed. Demonstration through model studies showed that the pDNA was released from cationic liposome/DNA complexes by anionic liposomes exhibiting compositions

mimicking the cytoplasmic face of the lipid monolayer of the cellular membrane. Membrane destabilization followed by flip-flop of the liposome/DNA complex by the anionic lipids by electrostatic interaction resulted in charge neutralized lipidic ion pairs followed by release of pDNA.

To evade the nuclear transport, an alternative approach was developed, which utilizes T7-based cytoplasmic expression vectors. Here, the inefficiently nuclear-transported DNA could be expressed in the cytoplasm itself.

6
Second Generation of Lipidic Delivery System (Lipopolyplex)

6.1
Polycation-condensed DNA Entrapped in Cationic Liposome: LPD-I Formulation

One of the prerequisites for a bioentity entering the cell and the nucleus is to possess a small size. The delivery of DNA was efficient through cationic lipidic formulation mediated gene delivery, but the nuclear transport from cytoplasm was quite an inefficient process. Generally, lipoplexes formed by multiple charged cationic lipids made small ($\sim$20 nm), highly condensed DNA/lipidic complex. These complexes were found to be more transfecting than the lipoplex formed by monocationic lipids and DNA. Synthetic cationic polymers like poly-L-lysine (PLL) could also condense DNA into very small compacted particles. This compact complex was allowed to freely mix with cationic liposomal solution. The overall complex so formed was termed lipid-protamine-DNA (LPD-I). A sucrose gradient ultracentrifugation of the heterogeneous mixture showed the existence of various populations associated with varied amounts of lipid. Negative-stain EM studies of purified complexes showed electron-dense structures ranging from elongated rod-shaped to ball-shaped particles. The purified fractions were several fold more transfection efficient than unpurified ones. The fractions that contained more lipids were more efficient in gene transfection than those containing fewer lipids. The transfection efficiency of LPD-I was many folds higher than the corresponding cationic liposome–DNA complex. It is hypothesized that (1) the small compacted structure of DNA resulted in high cellular and nuclear uptake, (2) the DNA is protected efficiently against enzymatic degradation, and (3) PLL may have mimicked the NLS for nuclear delivery of DNA. An alternative cationic polymer, protamine sulfate, from salmon sperm was used as a substitution for PLL. Protamine sulfate is a small (MW ~4000 vs ~18 500 for PLL), highly positively charged peptide and very basic due to the presence of 21 arginine residues, which contains an NLS. It is naturally occurring (whereas PLL is synthetic), a USP grade compound, FDA approved and finds use as an antidote to heparin-induced anticoagulation. With a routine history of human administration, the issues of toxicity and immunogenicity were minimal for protamine sulfate.

Both protamine sulfate and PLL were compared for their transfection efficiencies. With the same amount of DNA and cationic lipid, PLL reached its efficiency plateau at an amount that was half the amount of protamine sulfate, but the overall efficiency of protamine sulfate was 2 to 7-fold higher than PLL in different cell lines. The extent of transfection efficiency for LPD-I was 7 to 45-fold higher than the levels shown by DNA/cationic lipid complex. Phosphate and free-base forms of protamine showed lower levels of transfection and the activity was comparable to lipoplex. It is noteworthy that arginine, which exists as a salt of sulfate, and the lysine, which exists as a free base or as a phosphated salt, showed a variance in the relative transfection efficiencies even though the percentage of basic (arginine + lysine) residues remained relatively constant.

Upon i.v. injection, LPD-I made with DOTAP had shown very high gene expression in heart, lung, liver, spleen, and kidney, with the highest expression found in the lung. The *in vivo* gene expression had steadily increased with increase in cationic lipid and/or protamine, but the protamine–DNA charge ratio was kept below 2:1 to avoid the formation of large aggregates. After LPD injection, transgene expression was detected as early as 1 h, peaked at 6 h, and declined thereafter. Lung had consistently shown the highest gene expression, which lasted for 2 days. Even after 4 days of LPD injection, gene expression could still be detected in lung, spleen, and liver.

In a biodistribution study with labeled DNA and liposome, it was revealed that DNA was rapidly removed from circulation by the liver after injection of protamine–DNA complexes, and uptake by the lung was always less than 10% of injected dose at all time points. But DNA when formulated in LPD was trapped in lung to an extent of 40% within 5 min of LPD injection. In Southern blot analysis, it was revealed that the pDNA injected with LPD was detectable in the lung in a much higher quantity than the control, even after 6 h of i.v. injection. Intraportal injection gave significantly lower gene expression than with i.v. injection.

6.2
Polycation-condensed DNA in Anionic Liposomes: LPD-II Formulation

Some disadvantages always accompany the cationic lipid-mediated gene transfection. Cytotoxic effect in cells/tissues is the primary concern that requires early attention. The cationic lipids exhibit relatively large sizes, while complexation with DNA provide suboptimal DNA condensation and have limited efficiency and lack of tissue specificity, whereas anionic liposomes used in gene therapy have shown poor encapsulation efficiencies due to the large size and excessive negative charge of uncondensed pDNA. The utilization of anionic liposome was revisited during a recent approach, which also utilized the concept of condensing DNA by cationic polymers. A delivery vector was developed wherein polylysine-condensed pDNA was entrapped into folate-targeted anionic liposomes via charge interaction. It had structural similarity as LPD-I and it was named *LPD-II*. It differed from LPD-I in that anionic lipids instead of cationic lipids were used. This novel vector was more efficient and less cytotoxic compared to conventional cationic liposomal vectors.

Folate-targeted LPD-II particles were generated by mixing anionic liposomes composed of DOPE/CHEMS/folate-PEG-DOPE and the cationic DNA–polylysine (1 : 0.75, w/w) complexes. Structural analysis of LPD-II by negative-stain EM showed that the DNA–polylysine (which appears as rod shaped individually) and lipid complex appeared as a highly electron dense, spherical core with a low-density coating. The mean diameter of these particles was 74 ± 14 nm, that is, smaller than the empty liposomes.

KB cells expressing folate receptors were transfected with LPD-II particles containing luciferase reporter gene and high transfection efficiency was observed. The activity could be inhibited by the presence of excess free folate. Control LPD-II particles generated with nontargeted liposomes was only active at low lipid/DNA ratios, suggesting that the transfection by LPD-II particles was only receptor dependent when the overall charge was negative. Compared with DC-Chol/DOPE/DNA-liposome complexes, LPD-II showed ∼20 to 30-fold more transfection activity. On replacing DOPE with DOPC in the original formulation, the transfection was severely reduced. This indicated that the fusogenic activity of DOPE was essential for the transfection activity of LPD-II particles.

Their low physiological stability, inefficient cellular uptake, and the lack of tissue specificity currently limit the therapeutic applications of antisense oligonucleotides (ODN). The use of various vectors renders phosphodiester (PO) ODN resistant to enzymatic digestion. KB cells, which overexpress folate binding protein, were also transfected with LPD-II containing targeting ligand folate to deliver ODN against epidermal growth-factor receptor (EGFR). This resulted in downregulation of EGFR and growth inhibition of KB cells. The modified backbone-ODN, namely, phosphorothioate (PS) and monomethylphosphonate (MP) are more stable to enzymatic degradation compared to PO ODN, but they suffer from increased toxicity and decreased specificity. In a study, PO ODN against EGFR had shown growth inhibitory effect to KB cells compared to that of PS/PO ODN when delivered with LPD-II, indicating that LPD-II could also protect PO ODN from attack by enzymes inside cells.

7
Emulsion-mediated Gene Transfer

7.1
General Development

Emulsions are one of the most widely studied colloidal dispersion systems for the delivery of drugs. The oil-in-water emulsion is made of oil dispersed in an aqueous phase with a suitable emulsifier such as phospholipids, nonionic or ionic surfactants. Castor oil or soybean oil is predominantly used as the core oil phase. Nonionic surfactants such as Tween, Span, Brij, and pluronic copolymers are used as coemulsifiers. The ionic coemulsifiers are phospholipids or cationic lipids. A number of structure/activity studies had been done with different emulsion formulations, which were subsequently used for gene delivery *in vitro* and *in vivo*. The nonionic surfactants such as Tween, Span, Brij, and pluronic copolymers were found to be excellent coemulsifiers when used along with castor oil, DC-Chol, and DOPE. The *in vitro* transfection study on BL-6 cells showed that the Tween surfactant containing formulations had more serum resistivity and exhibited higher transfection in serum-containing media than in the absence of serum. One of the Brij containing formulations, that is, one with 2-oxyethylene chains, showed the highest transfection efficiency in the presence of serum. The toxicity of each formulation is minimal. In a DOTAP, soybean oil, and pDNA emulsion complex, it was observed that in spite of the change of zeta potential with varying amounts of DNA, the structure and the size of the emulsion complex remained mostly unchanged. The stability of this emulsion complex was shown to be high, and inhibited DNase-I digestion of pDNA. In serum-containing

media, the emulsion showed much higher transfection efficiency compared to lipofectamine/DNA transfection complex. On inclusion of polyethyleneglycol-PE in the emulsion complex, a high level transfection was observed even in the media containing 90% of serum. This result suggested that *in vivo* transfection could be done with this emulsion complex. Another soybean oil-DOTAP emulsion was used to transfer genes to the epithelial cells of the mouse nasal cavity via intranasal instillation. The emulsion showed enhanced stability against heparin exchange and exhibited higher level of transfection compared to commercially available liposome/DNA complex in nasal cavity mucosa.

7.2
Reconstituted Chylomicron Remnants for Gene Transfer

Chylomicrons are triglyceride rich lipoproteins that are slowly modified during circulation in blood. The core glyceride structure is hydrolyzed by the lipoprotein lipase. It is by the apolipoprotein-specific receptors that the hepatocytes in the liver consume these remnants. It had been shown that even reconstituted chylomicron remnants (RCR) formed by purified lipids could also be taken up by the hepatocytes following i.v. injections. In our lab, we modified the system and used it for delivery of DNA into liver cells. DNA being predominantly hydrophilic in nature cannot be included in the hydrophobic interior of the RCR. TC-Chol, a quaternary ammonium analog of DC-Chol, was used in various amounts to make complexes with DNA. The resultant hydrophobic complexes upon extraction from aqueous solution were emulsified with commercially available lipids (olive oil: L-α-phosphatidyl choline: L-α-lysophosphatidyl choline: cholesteryl oleate) by homogenization. DNA/TC-Chol complex was incorporated into the internal oil space of RCR and remained protected against Dnase-I digestion. The RCR containing DNA/TC-Chol complex, injected intraportally, gave the transgene luciferase expression in the liver 100-fold higher than with naked DNA injection. The expression was also obtained in the spleen, lung, and heart, but was 25 to 800-fold lower than that in the liver. The gene expressions obtained through tail vein injection was 100-fold lower than that of the mice injected intraportally. This was likely because the RCR did not contain any apolipoproteins on its surface, which could have otherwise facilitated the receptor-mediated uptake. Moreover, the colloidal stability might not have been as good as the ones containing apolipoproteins. RCR did not employ any protein or peptide that acts as an antigen. So, it could be injected repetitively by using a catheter method that had been established for multiple portal vein infusion. We have recently improved the formulation by adding pegylated lipid to the surface of RCR and showed that the circulation time of the particle was prolonged significantly.

8
Use of Cationic Liposome/DNA Complex (Lipoplex)

Lipoplexes are widely used for transferring genes to various *in vivo* targets with comparative ease and least toxic effect to the host. Use of lipoplexes in gene therapy clinical trials comprises almost one-fourth of the total gene therapy clinical trials. pDNA containing various therapeutic genes were used to treat a variety of disease pathologies. A vast amount of literature is available on the *in vitro*, preclinical, and clinical evaluations. Lipoplexes enjoy the property of easy administration in body without eliciting any extradiscomfort to the patient or the animal. Intravenous, intradermal, intraperitoneal, and direct injections are the common ways through which lipoplexes are injected in to the body. In the targeting front, several ligand associated cationic liposomes were developed to target genes to specific cell targets such as cancer. Recently, a cationic liposomal stealth gene delivery system was developed utilizing a sigma ligand associated polyethylene glycol–based lipid. The system could target and deliver genes specifically to sigma receptor overexpressing breast adenocarcinoma cells without showing any targeting ability to sigma receptor non-overexpressing cancer cells. Additionally, the stealth lipoplex was serum stable. The PEG lipid was chemically modified with a neuroleptic drug, haloperidol (used for over three decades to treat psychotic patients), to target cancer cells that overexpress sigma receptors. No conclusive links were ascertained between cancer pathogenicity and overexpressing sigma receptors in certain cancer cells. But, this versatile sigma receptor targeting stealth cationic liposomal system could be potentially used to target therapeutic anticancer genes to breast cancer or other cancer models that were implicated with overexpressing sigma receptors.

8.1
In Vivo Biodistribution Through Intravenous Injection: Therapeutic Implications

Intravenous injection is a widely used mode of gene delivery in animals. On i.v. lipoplex injection *in vivo*, the residence of DNA primarily in heart and lungs even after nine days with minimal toxicity was observed. Intravenous injected lipoplex expressed transgene in almost all organs including lung, kidney, heart, spleen, liver, brain and so on, and the expression stayed for nine weeks with apparently no treatment related toxicity. Toxicity and antitumor response was evaluated on mice and pigs with high doses of lipoplex containing *MHC* gene incorporated pDNA.

Recently, more work has been done to increase the overall transfection efficiency with much higher targeting capability and reproducibility of the liposomal delivery system. Intravenously administered lipoplex avidly reacts with blood components. So, it is necessary to keep the complex intact in the blood till it reaches the organ of interest. It was shown that in the presence of erythrocytes, cationic lipid/cholesterol formulation did not induce fusion between erythrocytes, whereas the cationic lipid/DOPE formulation possessing high fluidity in its structure induced fusion between the erythrocytes after a short incubation period. This offered an explanation as to why cholesterol makes a superior formulation with cationic lipids for *in vivo* purpose.

A repeated systemic i.v. injection of cytokine gene (*IFNβ*1) by lipoplexes gave a systemic expression of human interferon-β in mice, thereby increasing the possibility of cytokines used for therapeutic purposes in a systemic manner. An enhanced and highly selective liver targeting by i.v. injection of cationic lipoplex containing β-sitosterol beta-D-glucoside (*Sit-G*) gene was also observed. Intravenous injections showed gene expression in all major organs including heart, lung, liver, spleen, and kidney, with lung being most efficiently transfected. For efficient targeting and gene expression in the lung, i.v. injection was favored over intratracheal instillation. Uyechi et al. had shown by injecting fluorescently tagged lipoplexes through the vein that the entire lung lobe was homogeneously fluorescent, whereas intratracheal administration resulted in regional distribution of lipoplex, concentrated around bronchioles and distal airways.

LPD-I lipopolyplex particles upon i.v. injection were also distributed to spleen along with the major organs, where they were endocytosed and released to the cytoplasm. Administrations of these particles containing unmethylated CpG motif in pDNA elicit immunostimulation that subsequently showed tumorostatic effect. The effect of CpG will be discussed in detail in the later part of this chapter. However, the spleen delivery idea was utilized to deliver antigenic peptides entrapped in LPD particles to the cytoplasm of splenic antigen presenting cells. It is known that *E6* and *E7* are two oncogenes responsible for the maintenance of the malignant state of HPV-positive tumors. Therefore, an arginine containing small peptide epitope derived from tumor antigen, HPV-E7 protein was electrostatically attached to pDNA. The preattached peptide-DNA was condensed by protamine and finally the whole entity was enclosed in LPD using cationic lipid. The particle upon i.v. injection was delivered to the splenic APCs and thereby induced E7 mediated immune response against syngeneic HPV-induced tumor in mice.

8.2
Directly Injected Lipoplexes Used Against Cancer and Other Diseases

Direct injection to tissue is a common approach for cationic lipid-mediated gene therapy. Intratumoral injection of DNA-liposome complexes containing either E6 or E7 antisense plasmid resulted in significant growth inhibition of C3 tumors grown in a syngeneic mouse model. A direct injection of recombinant pDNA containing murine class I major histocompatibility complex (*MHC*) gene into localized arterial segment of various major organs showed that the direct gene transfer by liposomal transfection did not lead to treatment related toxicity, autoimmunity, or gonadal localization of the transgene in mice. The toxicity of gene delivery by DNA liposomes was also analyzed in pigs and rabbits *in vivo*. There were no clinically significant immunopathology in major organs such as, brain, heart, lung, liver, kidney, spleen, and skeletal muscles. To stimulate local tumor immunity in patients with stage IV melanoma, Nabel et al. injected pDNA encoding MHC class I protein complexed with cationic lipid directly into the cutaneous tumor nodules. Treated lesions exhibited the presence of T cell, followed by an enhanced reactivity of tumor infiltrating lymphocytes. As a result, local inhibition of tumor followed by complete diminution of tumor was observed in some of the treated patients. Mohr et al. had shown that direct lipolex injection to intrahepatic hepatocellular carcinoma produced by human HCC cells appeared far superior to systemic administration for gene therapy for localized intrahepatic tumors, because the direct administration to tumors left the surrounding normal hepatic cells untouched. In another typical example, *in vivo* direct intratumor injection of plasmid containing the coding sequence for the human *IL-2* gene complexed with cationic lipid formulation resulted in retention of intact pDNA in the tumor tissue and IL-2 secretion by cell cultures derived from the injected tumors.

Formulation of this lipid with the cationic lipid inhibited DNA degradation and enhanced *in vivo* transfection efficiency over pDNA alone.

Airway administration of liposome complexes was used for the treatment of pulmonary diseases including cystic fibrosis (CF). Cationic liposome/DNA complex showed no adverse effect toward airway epithelial integrity; hence, the cationic lipid-based delivery system proved to be appropriate for use in human trials for CF. A series of preclinical trials were done in CF patients with intranasal instillation to evaluate the risk factors associated with the treatment. Since there was no apparent toxicity associated with lipoplexes as was seen from these trials, progress has been made in delivering the complexes to the entire lung by aerosol in CF patients. By nebulization, lipoplex was delivered into the airways of mutant mice to obtain human cystic fibrosis transmembrane conductance regulator (CFTR) cDNA expression in the respiratory tract. A study conducted on CF patients revealed that pCMV-CFTR/cationic liposome complex on administration to the nasal epithelium gave no evidence of excess nasal inflammation, or any adverse events related to active treatment. Gene transfer and expression assayed by PCR revealed the presence of transgene DNA in seven of the eight treated patients up to 28 days after treatment. Intranasal instillation technique was also used in the mouse model, to incorporate cationic lipid/DNA complexes. The CFTR dysfunctional gene gives rise to several multiple defects in airway epithelia, one of them being altered $Cl-$ and $Na+$ permeability. Zhang et al. had shown that the goblet cells were more efficiently targeted with lipoplexes than any other cells in the entire spectrum of lung airway epithelia. This was ascertained by the fact that an efficiently reduced mucous sulfation to levels seen in non-CF airways was observed with lipoplex/DNA in spite of low levels of *CFTR* gene expression in lung epithelial cells in human bronchial xenograft model of mice as compared to non-CF airways of control mice. These kinds of apparent complexities in CFTR function presented challenges in the design of different lipoplex formulations that were capable of generating the endogenous patterns of *CFTR* gene expression in specific lung epithelial cells.

8.3
Intraperitoneal Injection of Lipoplex for Treating Cancer

IP injection of lipoplex was done to transfect cells in the peritoneum region. Nude mice bearing disseminated human ovarian tumors derived from the p185-overexpressing SKOV-3 ovarian cancer cells were injected with *E1A* gene/lipoplex intraperitoneally. These tumors resemble stage III of human ovarian cancer. The expression of E1A protein decreased the expression of p185 oncoprotein, and hence increased the survival rate of mice. Seventy percent of the treated group survived for 1.5 years from the last injection, but the untreated group barely survived more than 16 weeks. The treatment of complex containing 1/13 of the original lipid dose also worked as efficiently as the normal dose. There was no apparent toxicity or major organ pathologic change. There was no trace of E1A DNA in the liver, lung, heart, spleen, brain, uterus, and ovaries of the treated mice even after $1\frac{1}{2}$ years.

9
Gene Delivery by Polymeric Systems (Polyplex)

9.1
General Development and Uses

An alternative nonviral gene delivery system has been developed, which utilizes polymers, cationic or neutral. Cationic polymers are predominantly used since they efficiently condense DNA to very small particles. These complexes are called *polyplexes*. Wu et al. for the first time utilized polylysine-asialo-orosomucoid conjugate to condense pDNA and targeted the pDNA to liver. pDNA condensed with protamine/polylysine conjugate of iron transport protein, transferrin, was efficiently delivered to eukaryotic cells. pDNA was delivered to primary peripheral blood lymphocytes utilizing CD3 T-cell receptors. pDNA condensed by CD3 antibody–polylysine conjugate showed receptor-mediated endocytosis to efficiently internalize pDNA into T lymphocytes. Depending on the cell-binding ligand, specific targeting was obtained in different cell lines.

Several of the most effective polymeric delivery systems were polyamidoamine (PAMAM) dendrimers and polyethylenei-mines (PEI). Being nonbiodegradable, these synthetic polymers posed a potential toxicity to cell, and hence biodegradable polypeptides like PLL and protamine were used for condensation and delivery of gene but with limited efficacy in transfection. They were usually used with cationic lipids to obtain enhanced transfection activity. Among the biodegradable polymers, chitosan and β-cyclodextrin–based polymers were also used for gene transfection.

Although the cationic polymers shared the same mechanism of DNA condensation, the transfection efficiency greatly varied between polymers. Even different molecular weight and isomeric forms of the same polymer showed different physicochemical characteristics, transfection efficiency, and toxicity.

Ligand conjugated polymers were used for *in vivo* targeting and expression of gene. Kircheis et al. reported an enhanced level of transfection in subcutaneous Neuro2a tumors on intratumoral injection of transferrin-PEI/pDNA compared with naked pDNA injection. On pegylation, Tf-PEI/pDNA complex became serum resistant without losing its targetability, and the complex could be efficiently targeted to neuro2a tumors in mouse tumor model after i.v. injection. Neurotensin cross-linked PLL polyplexed with pDNA upon injection into the substantia nigra of rat, showed a high level of transfection in nigrostriatal dopamine neurons that was detectable up to 15 days.

EBV-based plasmid vector containing thymidine kinase (*TK*) gene coupled with PAMAM dendrimer (EBV/polyplex) was used in suicide gene therapy of cancer. Intratumoral injection of *TK* gene containing EBV/dendrimer polyplex into Huh7 HCC tumors in severely compromised immuno-deficient (SCID) mice showed remarkable suppression of tumor growth leading to prolongation of survival time. Gene transfer to the lung was obtained by i.v. injection of G9 PAMAM dendrimer-complexed pDNA into mice. This resulted in high levels of transgene expression in the alveoli at 12 and 24 h, followed by a second peak of expression three to five days after administration. But bronchial epithelium was primarily targeted with the direct endobronchial administration of this polyplex. Topical *in vivo* delivery of pDNA to the hairless mice skin was done with PAMAM dendrimer polyplex. The polyplex was incorporated in or coated on the surface of poly (DL-lactide-co-glycolide) (PLGA) or collagen-based biodegradable membranes.

In an effort to transfer gene to rabbit carotid artery, Turunen et al. used DNA/fractured dendrimer (generation 6) polyplex to obtain a high level of gene transfer (4.4%) compared with what was obtained by lipoplex. The arterial gene transfer was particularly useful because it could be used as a tool for treating various vascular diseases. *In vivo* gene transfer method, in this study, employed a gene delivery reservoir (collar) around the carotid artery, which served as a reservoir for the gene delivery solution. This type of local gene transfer with cationic polyplex provided a technically efficient way of treating arterial diseases during vascular surgeries, such as by-pass and other surgeries. These dendrimer-based polyplexes showed a clear advantage over polylysine in that polyplexes largely buffer the drop of endosomal pH inside the endosome leading to increase in *in vitro* transfection efficiencies.

Qin et al. used starburst PAMAM dendrimers to transfer genes into a murine cardiac transplantation model. These starburst dendrimers are a special class of its kind, which are highly branched spherical polymers with large numbers of amino groups on the surface. At the time of transplantation of whole heart in the recipient mice, the dendrimer/β-gal pDNA was directly injected into the graft tissue. X-gal staining revealed a highly efficient and widespread transgene expression in both myocytes and the graft infiltrating cells with the peak lasting up to 14 days. For organ transplantation, severe tissue-rejection is a common immune response. Viral IL-10, a cytokine synthesis inhibitory factor is able to regulate a variety of negative immune responses by suppressing the synthesis of IFN-γ, or inhibiting IL-1, IL-6, IL-8, IL-12, and TNF-α. Direct injection of this dendrimer/viral *IL-10* gene with α-MHC promoter polyplex to the cardiac tissue showed an increased survival of the cardiac allograft. As little as 0.31 µg of the injected pDNA led to an increased mean survival from 13.9 to 38.6 days.

9.2
Targeted Gene Delivery by Antibodies Conjugated with Polycations

Polyamines had shown efficient transfection to lung endothelium. An efficient targeted transfection vector to lungs could be achieved by conjugating a targeting ligand against platelet endothelial cell adhesion molecule-1 (PECAM-1) to polyamines. This ligand–polyamine complex was targeted efficiently to the pulmonary endothelial cells. A chemical vector was synthesized by covalent conjugation of polyethylenimine and anti-PECAM antibody (Ab). The cationic complex was shown to deliver DNA specifically to mouse lung endothelial cells. The highest gene expression was obtained at relatively low plus-to-minus charge ratios. The PEI, conjugated with a control IgG, did not enhance transfection of mouse lung endothelial cells. Intravenous injection of this anti-PECAM Ab-PEI /DNA showed an increased lung expression in mice compared to other modes of injection.

Immunostimulatory cytokine, TNF-α in blood was found to be about fivefold less in the mice injected with PEI-anti-PECAM Ab/DNA than in the mice injected with PEI/DNA. The decrease in TNF-α was partially reversible by pretreating mice with Ab to PECAM. Immunosuppressant dexamethasone, when injected along with anti-PECAM Ab/DNA, not only improved the persistence and level of gene expression in the lung but also shortened the refractory period for repeated dosing. This supported a potential therapeutic role of dexamethasone in lung gene transfer with Ab-polymer conjugates.

Similarly, Ferkol et al. targeted the polymeric immunoglobulin receptor (pIgR), which are expressed in lung and liver tissues and transferred pDNA to these tissues. The targeting ligand, anti-secretory component (SC) Fab antibody was covalently linked to PLL. The polycation upon condensing pDNA was delivered successfully to airway epithelium *in vivo*. Tissues that do not express the pIgR, spleen, and heart, were not transfected. In addition, conjugate prepared with irrelevant Fab fragments did not produce detectable transgene activity. This complex specifically targeted pIgR-bearing tissues, but after repeated dosing increased humoral immune response against anti-SC Fab antibody was observed.

10
Nonviral Vector Related Cytotoxicity

It is known from the 1980s that the bacterial DNA stimulates the formation of cytotoxic IFN-α, β, and IL-12 when the DNA is taken up by macrophages. It in turn leads to NK cell activation and production of proinflammatory cytokine IFN-γ. This is accompanied by the proliferation of B cell and hence reduction of apoptosis and release of IL-6 and IL-12. These proinflammatory effects were found to be due to some immunostimulatory sequences in prokaryotic DNA that contained unmethylated CpG dinucleotide motif flanked by two 5' purines and two 3' pyrimidines. pDNA, which is derived from bacterial DNA, induces these immune responses. The unmethylated CpG motif–containing sequence occurs four times more frequently in prokaryote DNA than in eukaryotic DNA. Moreover, the CpG motifs are usually 75% more methylated in mammalian DNA than in prokaryotic DNA. On methylation of the cytosine bases in plasmid, the immunostimulatory effect is decreased considerably. Immature dendritic cells tend to produce proinflammatory IFN-α, β, IL-6, IL-12, and TNF-α on exposure to CpG containing oligonucleotide or bacterial plasmid.

These immune-stimulatory effects leading to inflammatory cytokine productions had negative impact on the systemic gene delivery of cationic lipid/DNA complexes. On recognition of pDNA by splenic macrophages during circulation, there was every chance that the pDNA would elicit an immune response, which might lead to phagocytosis of the complex and hence to decreased transgene expression. A high level of proinflammatory cytokine also led to inactivation of several promoters, resulting in a decrease in transgene expression. The death of animals by high dose lipoplex injection for obtaining high transgene expression could be attributed both to the high concentration of lipid and to pDNA mediated toxicity. In the case of local lipoplex administration in animals, minimal toxicity was observed. However, on i.v. injection or intratracheal instillation, high levels of IFN-γ and TNF-α were observed. Pretreating cytokine-neutralizing antibodies during i.v. injection of lipoplex, CpG triggered inflammation and immune responses were minimized and prolonged gene expression was obtained. Repeated dosing without any antibody treatment led to silenced transgene expression after one or two weeks.

It is not clear though how cytokine production decreases the transgene expression, but various ongoing efforts to minimize CpG related immune responses and toxicity, and to enhance transgene expression is worth mentioning. Hofmann et al. had used PCR-amplified fragments containing encoded therapeutic gene and regulatory elements for preparing LPD. On delivering, a similar level of gene expression comparable to pDNA lipoplex was obtained. However, a much lower level of cytokine response was observed, which sustained the gene expression for a longer period than pDNA. PCR fragment contains fewer CpG motifs than the full-length pDNA, which led to reduced CpG triggered adverse effects. Yew et al. had shown that on mutating CpG or its flanking motifs in the plasmid, a decreased level of cytokine and increased transgene expression could be obtained. A limited interaction of plasmid with immune cells could also lead to decreased cytokine response. It could be achieved by sequentially injecting cationic liposomes and free pDNA. Song et al. used this process for the purpose of efficiently transfecting the lung by prolonging the residency time and interaction of DNA with pulmonary endothelium. Tan et al. used the same concept to show that sequential injection led to the formation of a lower level of cytokines as compared to lipoplex injection. It is evident from the above efforts that understanding the detailed mechanism of CpG induced immune response is required for increasing the efficacy of pDNA mediated gene delivery.

11
Conclusion

Since the first attempt of utilizing pDNA for gene delivery to cells, the two decades have seen many attempts to enhance the efficacy of genetic vectors, to test various therapeutically important genes, to understand the mechanism of gene delivery, associated toxicity, and factors inhibiting gene expression. A number of gene therapy clinical trials were also performed. Although no single vector is superior to other vectors, each *in vivo* gene transfer application will find its vector system for optimal performance. Understanding cellular barriers and possible means to overcome them will undoubtedly further improve the performance of a nonviral vector.

Acknowledgment

The original work from Leaf Huang's lab described in this review has been supported by NIH grants CA 74918, AR 45925, DK 44935, AI 48851. "Fast Track Research Grant for Young Scientists" from Department of Science & Technology, Govt. of India supported the work done in Rajkumar Banerjee's lab as described in this chapter.

See also Molecular Oncology; Somatic Gene Therapy; Therapeutic Angiogenesis; Vectors and Gene Therapy.

Bibliography

Books and Reviews

Bird, A.P. (1986) CpG-rich islands and the function of DNA methylation, *Nature* **321**, 209–213.

Budker, V., Budker, T., Zhang, G., Subbotin, V., Loomis, A., Wolff, J.A. (2000) Hypothesis: naked plasmid DNA is taken up by cells in vivo by a receptor-mediated process, *J. Gene Med.* **2**, 76–88.

Chonn, A., Cullis, P.R. (1995) Recent advances in liposomal drug-delivery systems, *Curr. Opin. Biotechnol.* **6**, 698–708.

Davidson, J.M., Krieg, T., Eming, S.A. (2000) Particle-mediated gene therapy of wounds, *Wound Repair. Regen.* **8**, 452–459.

Davis, L.I. (1995) The nuclear pore complex, *Annu. Rev. Biochem.* **64**, 865–896.

Demeneix, B., Behr, J.-P., Boussif, O., Zanta, M.A., Abdallah, P., Remy, J.-S. (1998) Gene transfer with lipospermines and polyethylenimines, *Adv. Drug Delivery Rev.* **30**, 85–95.

Groth, A.C., Calos, M.P. (2004) Phage integrases: biology and applications, *J. Mol. Biol.* **335**, 667–668.

Huang, L., Li, S. (1997) Liposomal gene delivery: a complex package, *Nat. Biotechnol.* **15**, 620–621.

Jaroszeski, M.J., Gilbert, R., Nicolau, C., Heller, R. (1999) In vivo gene delivery by electroporation, *Adv. Drug. Delivery Rev.* **35**, 131–137.

Kamps, J.A., Scherphof, G.L. (1998) Receptor versus non-receptor mediated clearance of liposomes, *Adv. Drug Delivery Rev.* **32**, 81–97.

Korzarsky, K.F., Wilson, J.M. (1993) Gene therapy: adenovirus vectors, *Curr. Opin. Genet. Dev.* **3**, 499–503.

Ledley, F.D. (1995) Nonviral gene therapy: the promise of genes as pharmaceutical products, *Hum. Gene Ther.* **6**, 1129–1144.

Marshall, D.J., Leiden, J.M. (1998) Recent advances in skeletal-muscle-based gene therapy, *Curr. Opin. Genet. Dev.* **8**, 360–365.

Mazda, O. (2002) Improvement of nonviral gene therapy by Epstein-Barr virus (EBV)-based plasmid vectors, *Curr. Gene Ther.* **2**, 379–392.

Mir, L.M., Bureau, M.F., Rangara, R., Schwartz, B., Scherman, D. (1998) Long-term, high level in vivo gene expression after electric pulse-mediated gene transfer into skeletal muscle, *Crit. Rev. Acad. Sci. III* **321**, 893–899.

Pante, N., Aebi, U. (1996) Molecular dissection of the nuclear pore complex, *Crit. Rev. Biochem. Mol. Biol.* **31**, 153–199.

Singh, M., Ravin, L.J. (1986) Parenteral emulsions as drug carrier systems, *J. Parenter. Sci. Technol.* **40**, 34–41.

Somiari, S., Malone, J.G., Drabick, J.J., Gilbert, R., Heller, R., Jaroszeski, M.J., Malone, R.W. (2000) Theory and in vivo application of electroporative gene delivery, *Mol. Ther.* **2**, 178–187.

Spooner, R.A., Deonarain, M.P., Epenetos, A.A. (1995) DNA vaccination for cancer treatment, *Gene Ther.* **2**, 173–180.

Webster, K.A., Prentice, H., Discher, D.J., Hicks, M.C., Bisphoric, N.H. (1998) in: Wheelan, W.J. (Ed.) *Molecular Biology in the Conquest of Disease*, Oxford University Press, Oxford, UK, p. 37.

Wolff, J.A. (1999) in: Friedmann, T. (Ed.) *Development of Human Gene Therapy*, Cold Spring Harbor Laboratory, Cold Spring Harbor, New York, p. 279.

Yang, N.S., Hogge, G.H., MacEwen, E.G. (1999) in: Huang, L. Hung, M.C. Wagner, E. (Eds.) *Nonviral Vectors for Gene Therapy*, Academic Press, San Diego, CA, p. 171.

Primary Literature

Acsadi, G., Dickson, D.R., Love, A., Jani, A., Walsh, F.S., Gurusinghe, A., Wolff, J.A., Davies, K.E. 1991. Human dystrophin expression in mdx mice after intramuscular injection of DNA constructs. *Nature* **352**, 815–818.

Aihara, H., Miyazaki, J. (1998) Gene transfer into muscle by electroporation in vivo, *Nat. Biotechnol.* **16**, 867–870.

Akao, T., Nakayama, T., Takeshia, K., Ito, A. (1994) Design of a new cationic amphiphile with efficient DNA-transfection ability, *Biochem. Mol. Biol. Int.* **34**, 915–920.

Alton, E.W., Middleton, P.G., Caplen, N.J., Smith, S.N., Steel, D.M., Munkonge, F.M., Jeffery, P.K., Geddes, D.M., Hart, S.L., Williamson, R., et al. (1993) Non-invasive liposome-mediated gene delivery can correct the ion transport defect in cystic fibrosis mutant mice, *Nat. Genet.* **5**, 135–142.

Alvarez-Maya, I., Navarro-Quiroga, I., Meraz-Rios, M.A., Aceves, J., Martinez-Fong, D. (2001) In vivo gene transfer to dopamine neurons of rat substantia nigra via the high-affinity neurotensin receptor, *Mol. Med.* **7**, 186–192.

Andree, C., Swain, W.F., Page, C.P., Macklin, M.D., Slama, J., Hatzis, D., Eriksson, E. (1994) In vivo transfer and expression of a human epidermal growth factor gene accelerates wound repair, *Proc. Natl. Acad. Sci. U.S.A.* **91**, 12188–12192.

Anwer, K., Shi, M., French, M.F., Muller, S.R., Chen, W., Liu, Q., Proctor, B.L., Wang, J., Mumper, R.J., Singhal, A., Rolland, A.P., Alila, H.W. (1998) Systemic effect of human growth hormone after intramuscular injection of a single dose of a muscle-specific gene medicine, *Hum. Gene Ther.* **9**, 659–670.

Ardehali, A., Fyfe, A., Laks, H., Drinkwater, D.C., Jr., Qiao, J.H., Lusis, A.J. (1995) Direct gene transfer into donor hearts at the time of harvest, *J. Thorac. Cardiovasc. Surg.* **109**, 716–719.

Aronsohn, A.I., Hughes, J.A. (1998) Nuclear localization signal peptides enhance cationic liposome-mediated gene therapy, *J. Drug Target.* **5**, 163–169.

Bailey, A.L., Cullis, P.R. (1997) Membrane fusion with cationic liposomes: effects of target membrane lipid composition, *Biochemistry* **36**, 1628–1634.

Banerjee, R., Das, P.K., Chaudhuri, A. (1998) Interfacial indazolization: novel chemical evidence for remarkably high exo-surface pH of cationic liposomes used in gene transfection, *Biochim. Biophys. Acta* **1373**, 299–308.

Banerjee, R., Das, P.K., Srilakshmi, G.V., Chaudhuri, A., Rao, N.M. (1999) Novel series of non-glycerol-based cationic transfection lipids for use in liposomal gene delivery, *J. Med. Chem.* **42**, 4292–4299.

Batteux, F., Tourneur, L., Trebeden, H., Charreire, J., Chiocchia, G. (1999) Gene therapy of experimental autoimmune thyroiditis by in vivo administration of plasmid DNA coding for Fas ligand, *J. Immunol.* **162**, 603–608.

Behr, J.P.-., Demeneix, B., Loeffler, J.-P., Perez-Mutul, J. (1989) Efficient gene transfer into mammalian primary endocrine cells with lipopolyamine-coated DNA, *Proc. Natl. Acad. Sci.* **86**, 6982–6986.

Belperron, A.A., Feltquate, D., Fox, B.A., Horii, T., Bzik, D.J. (1999) Immune responses induced by gene gun or intramuscular injection of DNA vaccines that express immunogenic regions of the serine repeat antigen from Plasmodium falciparum, *Infect. Immun.* **67**, 5163–5169.

Benita, S., Levy, M.Y. (1993) Submicron emulsions as colloidal drug carriers for intravenous administration: comprehensive physicochemical characterization, *J. Pharm. Sci.* **82**, 1069–1079.

Benn, S.I., Whitsitt, J.S., Broadley, K.N., Nanney, L.B., Perkins, D., He, L., Patel, M., Morgan, J.R., Swain, W.F., Davidson, J.M. (1996) Particle-mediated gene transfer with transforming growth factor-beta1 cDNAs enhances wound repair in rat skin, *J. Clin. Invest.* **98**, 2894–2902.

Bennett, R.M., Gabor, G.T., Merritt, M.M. (1985) DNA binding to human leukocytes. Evidence for a receptor-mediated association, internalization, and degradation of DNA, *J. Clin. Invest.* **76**, 2182–2190.

Bennett, M.J., Aberle, A.M., Balasubramaniam, R.P., Malone, J.G., Malone, R.W., Nantz, M.H. (1997) Cationic lipid-mediated gene delivery to murine lung: correlation of lipid hydration with in vivo transfection activity, *J. Med. Chem.* **269**, 4069–4078.

Bettan, M., Emmanuel, F., Darteil, R., Caillaud, J.M., Soubrier, F., Delaere, P., Macfoudi, D.B, Duverger, N., Scherman, D. (2000) High-level protein secretion into blood circulation after electric pulse-mediated gene transfer into skeletal muscle, *Mol. Ther.* **2**, 204–210.

Bielinska, A.U., Yen, A., Wu, H.L., Zahos, K.M., Sun, R., Weiner, N.D., Baker, J.R., Jr., Roessler, B.J. (2000) Application of membrane-based dendrimer/DNA complexes for solid phase transfection in vitro and in vivo, *Biomaterials* **21**, 877–887.

Bottega, R., Epand, R.M. (1992) Inhibition of protein kinase C by cationic amphiphiles, *Biochemistry* **31**, 9025–9030.

Boulton, T.G., Nye, S.H., Robbins, D.J., Ip, N.Y., Radziejewska, S.D., Morgenbesser, R.A., DePinho, R.A., Panayotatos, N., Cobbs, M.H., Yancopoulos, G.D. (1991) ERKs: a family of protein-serine/threonine kinases that are activated and tyrosine phosphorylated in response to insulin and NGF, *Cell* **65**, 663–675.

Brisson, M., He, Y., Li, S., Yang, J.-P., Huang, L. (1999) A novel T7 RNA polymerase autogene for efficient cytoplasmic expression of target genes, *Gene Ther.* **6**, 263–270.

Bryant, M., Drew, G.M., Houston, P., Hissey, P., Campbell, C.J., Braddock, M. (2000) Tissue repair with a therapeutic transcription factor, *Hum Gene Ther* **11**, 2143–2158.

Buschle, M., Cotten, M., Kirlappos, H., Mechtler, K., Schaffner, G., Zauner, W., Birnstiel, M.L., Wagner, E. (1995) Receptor-mediated gene transfer into human T

lymphocytes via binding of DNA/CD3 antibody particles to the CD3 T cell receptor complex, *Hum. Gene Ther.* **6**, 753–761.

Caplen, N.J., Alton, E.W., Middleton, P.G., Dorin, J.R., Stevenson, B.J., Gao, X., Durham, S.R., Jeffery, P.K., Hodson, M.E., Coutelle, C., Huang, L., Porteous, D.J., Williamson, R., Geddes, D.M. (1995) Liposome-mediated CFTR gene transfer to the nasal epithelium of patients with cystic fibrosis, *Nat. Med.* **1**, 39–46.

Chadwick, S.L., Kingston, H.D., Stern, M., Cook, R.M., O'Connor, B.J., Lukasson, M., Balfour, R.P., Rosenberg, M., Cheng, S.H., Smith, A.E., Meeker, D.P., Geddes, D.M., Alton, E.W. (1998) Safety of a single aerosol administration of escalating doses of the cationic lipid GL-67/DOPE/DMPE-PEG5000 formulation to the lungs of normal volunteers, *Gene Ther.* **5**, 937–942.

Chang, Y., Prud'homme, G.J. (1999) Intramuscular administration of expression plasmids encoding interferon-gamma receptor/IgG1 or IL-4/IgG1 chimeric proteins protects from autoimmunity, *J. Gene Med.* **1**, 415–423.

Chen, C.H., Ji, H., Suh, K.W., Choti, M.A., Pardoll, D.M., Wu, T.C. (1999) Gene gun-mediated DNA vaccination induces antitumor immunity against human papillomavirus type 16 E7-expressing murine tumor metastases in the liver and lungs, *Gene Ther.* **6**, 1972–1981.

Chesnoy, S., Lee, P.Y., Huang, L. (2003) Intradermal injection of transforming growth factor-beta1 gene enhances wound healing in genetically diabetic mice, *Pharm. Res.* **20**, 345–350.

Chesnoy, S., Durand, D., Doucet, J., Stolz, D.B., Huang, L. (2001) Improved DNA/emulsion complex stabilized by poly(ethylene glycol) conjugated phospholipid, *Pharm. Res.* **18**, 1480–1484.

Conry, R.M., LoBuglio, A.F., Loechel, F., Moore, S.E., Sumerel, L.A., Barlow, D.L., Curiel, D.T. (1995) A carcinoembryonic antigen polynucleotide vaccine has in vivo antitumor activity, *Gene Ther.* **2**, 59–65.

Coster, H.G. (1965) A quantitative analysis of the voltage-current relationships of fixed charge membranes and the associated property of "punch-through", *Biophys. J.* **5**, 669–686.

Cowdery, J.S., Chace, J.H., Yi, A.K., Krieg, A.M. (1996) Bacterial DNA induces NK cells to produce IFN-gamma in vivo and increases the toxicity of lipopolysaccharides, *J. Immunol.* **156**, 4570–4575.

Daleke, D.L., Hong, K.L., Papahadjopoulos, D. (1992) Endocytosis of liposomes by macrophages: binding, acidification and leakage of liposomes monitored by a new fluorescence assay, *Biochim. Biophys. Acta* **1024**, 352–366.

Danko, I., Fritz, J.D., Jiao, S., Hogan, K., Latendresse, J.S., Wolff, J.A. (1994) Pharmacological enhancement of in vivo foreign gene expression in muscle, *Gene Ther.* **1**, 114–121.

Davis, N.L., Brown, K.W., Johnston, R.E. (1996) A viral vaccine vector that expresses foreign genes in lymph nodes and protects against mucosal challenge, *J. Virol.* **70**, 3781–3787.

Davis, H.L., Whalen, R.G., Demeneix, B.A. (1993) Direct gene transfer into skeletal muscle in vivo: factors affecting efficiency of transfer and stability of expression, *Hum. Gene Ther.* **4**, 151–159.

Dileo, J., Banerjee, R., Whitmore, M., Nayak, J.V., Falo, L.D., Jr., Huang, L. (2003) Lipid-protamine-DNA-mediated antigen delivery to antigen-presenting cells results in enhanced anti-tumor immune responses, *Mol Ther.* **7**, 640–648.

Dowty, M.E., Williams, P., Zhang, G., Hagstrom, J.E., Wolff, J.A. (1995) Plasmid DNA entry into postmitotic nuclei of primary rat myotubes, *Proc. Natl. Acad. Sci. U.S.A.* **92**, 4572–4576.

Dubendorff, J.W., Studier, F.W. (1991) Creation of a T7 autogene. Cloning and expression of the gene for bacteriophage T7 RNA polymerase under control of its cognate promoter, *J. Mol. Biol.* **219**, 61–68.

Dujardin, N., Van Der Smissen, P., Preat, V. (2001) Topical gene transfer into rat skin using electroporation, *Pharm. Res.* **18**, 61–66.

Duzgunes, N., Goldstein, J.A., Friend, D.S., Felgner, P.L. (1989) Fusion of liposomes containing a novel cationic lipid, N-[2,3-(dioleyloxy)propyl]-N,N,N-trimethyl-ammonium: induction by multivalent anions and asymmetric fusion with acidic phospholipid vesicles, *Biochemistry* **28**, 9179–9184.

Dworetzky, S.I., Lanford, R.E., Feldherr, C.M. (1988) The effects of variations in the number and sequence of targeting signals on nuclear uptake, *J. Cell Biol.* **107**, 1279–1287.

Espinos, E., Liu, J.H., Bader, C.R., Bernheim, L. (2001) Efficient non-viral DNA-mediated gene transfer to human primary myoblasts using

electroporation, *Neuromuscl. Disord.* **11**, 341–349.

Farhood, H., Serbina, N., Huang, L. (1995) The role of dioleoyl phosphatidylethanolamine in cationic liposome mediated gene transfer, *Biochim. Biophys. Acta* **1235**, 289–295.

Fazio, V.M., Fazio, S., Rinaldi, M., Catani, M.V., Zotti, S., Ciafre, S.A., Seripa, D., Ricci, R., Farace, M.G. (1994) Accumulation of human apolipoprotein-E in rat plasma after in vivo intramuscular injection of naked DNA, *Biochem. Biophys. Res. Commun.* **200**, 298–305.

Feldherr, C.M., Akin, D. (1990) The permeability of the nuclear envelope in dividing and nondividing cell cultures, *J. Cell Biol.* **111**, 1–8.

Felgner, P.L., Gadek, T.R., Holm, M., Roman, R., Chan, H.W., Wenz, M., Northrop, J.P., Ringold, G.M., Danielsen, M. (1987) Lipofection: a highly efficient, lipid-mediated DNA-transfection procedure, *Proc. Natl. Acad. Sci. U.S.A.* **84**, 7413–7417.

Felgner, J.H., Kumar, R., Sridhar, C.N., Wheeler, C.J., Tsai, Y.J., Border, R., Ramsey, P., Martin, M., Felgner, P.L. (1994) Enhanced gene delivery and mechanism studies with a novel series of cationic lipid formulations, *J. Biol. Chem.* **269**(:) 2550–2561.

Ferkol, T., Perales, J.C., Eckman, E., Kaetzel, C.S., Hanson, R.W., Davis, P.B. (1995) Gene transfer into the airway epithelium of animals by targeting the polymeric immunoglobulin receptor, *J. Clin. Invest.* **95**, 493–502.

Ferkol, T., Palle, A.P., Eckman, E., Perales, J.C., Trzaska, T., Tosi, M., Redline, R., Davis, P.B. (1996) Immunologic responses to gene transfer into mice via the polymeric immunoglobulin receptor, *Gene Ther.* **3**, 669–678.

Fischer, D., Bieber, T., Li, Y., Elsasser, H., Kissel, T. (1999) A novel non-viral vector for DNA delivery based on low molecular weight, branched polyethylenimine: effect of molecular weight on transfection efficiency and cytotoxicity, *Pharm. Res.* **16**, 1273–1279.

Floch, V., Loisel, S., Guenin, E., Herve, A.C., Clement, J.C., Yaouanc, J.J., des Abbayes, H., Ferec, C. (2000) Cation substitution in cationic phosphonolipids: a new concept to improve transfection activity and decrease cellular toxicity, *J. Med. Chem.* **43**, 4617–4628.

Folkman, J., Merler, E., Abernathy, C., Williams, G. (1971) Isolation of a tumor factor responsible for angiogenesis, *J. Exp. Med.* **133**, 275–288.

Fraley, R., Subramani, S., Berg, P., Papahadjopoulos, D. (1980) Introduction of liposome-encapsulated SV40 DNA into cells, *J. Biol. Chem.* **255**, 10431–10435.

Friend, D.S., Papahadjopoulos, D., Debs, R.J. (1996) Endocytosis and intracellular processing accompanying transfection mediated by cationic liposomes, *Biochim. Biophys. Acta* **1278**, 41–50.

Fuller, D.H., Murphey-Corb, M., Clements, J., Barnett, S., Haynes, J.R. (1996) Induction of immunodeficiency virus-specific immune responses in rhesus monkeys following gene gun-mediated DNA vaccination, *J. Med. Primatol.* **25**, 236–241.

Gainer, A.L., Suarez-Pinzon, W.L., Min, W.P., Swiston, J.R., Hancock-Friesen, C., Korbutt, G.S., Rajotte, R.V., Warnock, G.L., Elliott, J.F. (1998) Improved survival of biolistically transfected mouse islet allografts expressing CTLA4-Ig or soluble Fas ligand, *Transplantation* **66**, 194–199.

Gao, X., Huang, L. (1991) A novel cationic liposome reagent for efficient transfection of mammalian cells, *Biochem. Biophys. Res. Commun.* **179**, 280–285.

Gao, X., Huang, L. (1993) Cytoplasmic expression of a reporter gene by co-delivery of T7 RNA polymerase and T7 promoter sequence with cationic liposomes, *Nucleic Acids Res.* **21**, 2867–2872.

Gao, X., Huang, L. (1996) Potentiation of cationic liposome-mediated gene delivery by polycations, *Biochemistry* **35**, 1027–1036.

Gao, X., Jaffurs, D., Robbins, P.D., Huang, L. (1994) A sustained, cytoplasmic transgene expression system delivered by cationic liposomes, *Biochem. Biophys. Res. Commun.* **200**, 1201–1206.

Gershon, H., Ghirlando, R., Guttman, S.B., Minsky, A. (1993) Mode of formation and structural features of DNA-cationic liposome complexes used for transfection, *Biochemistry* **32**, 7143–7151.

Giladi, E., Raz, E., Karmeli, F., Okon, E., Rachmilewitz, D. (1995) Transforming growth factor-beta gene therapy ameliorates experimental colitis in rats, *Eur. J. Gastroenterol. Hepatol.* **7**, 341–347.

Gill, D.R., Southern, K.W., Mofford, K.A., Seddon, T., Huang, L., Sorgi, F., Thomson, A., MacVinish, L.J., Ratcliff, R., Bilton, D., Lane, D.J., Littlewood, J.M., Webb, A.K., Middleton, P.G., Colledge, W.H., Cuthbert, A.W., Evans, M.J., Higgins, C.F., Hyde, S.C. (1997) A placebo-controlled study of liposome-mediated gene transfer to the nasal epithelium of patients with cystic fibrosis, *Gene Ther.* **4**, 199–209.

Girard, F., Strausfeld, U., Fernandez, A., Lamb, N.J.C. (1991) Cyclin A is required for the onset of DNA replication in mammalian fibroblasts, *Cell* **67**, 1169–1179.

Godbey, W., Wu, K., Mikos, A. (1999) Size matters: molecular weight affects the efficiency of poly(ethylenimine) as a gene delivery vehicle, *J. Biomed. Mater. Res.* **45**, 268–275.

Gustafsson, J., Arvindson, G., Karlsson, G., Almgren, M.B. (1995) Complexes between cationic liposomes and DNA visualized by cryo-TEM, *Biochim. Biophys. Acta* **1235**, 305–312.

Hara, T., Tan, Y., Huang, L. (1997) In vivo gene delivery to the liver using reconstituted chylomicron remnants as a novel nonviral vector, *Proc. Natl. Acad. Sci. U.S.A.* **94**, 14547–14552.

He, Y., Huang, L. (1997) Growth inhibition of human papillomavirus 16 DNA-positive mouse tumor by antisense RNA transcribed from U6 promoter, *Cancer Res.* **57**, 3993–3999.

Hefeneider, S.H., Cornell, K.A., Brown, L.E., Bakke, A.C., McCoy, S.L., Bennett, R.M. (1992) Nucleosomes and DNA bind to specific cell-surface molecules on murine cells and induce cytokine production, *Clin. Immunol. Immunopathol.* **63**, 245–251.

Heller, L., Jaroszeski, M.J., Coppola, D., Pottinger, C., Gilbert, R., Heller, R. (2000) Electrically mediated plasmid DNA delivery to hepatocellular carcinomas in vivo, *Gene Ther.* **7**, 826–829.

Heller, R., Jaroszeski, M., Atkin, A., Moradpour, D., Gilbert, R., Wands, J., Nicolau, C. (1996) In vivo gene electroinjection and expression in rat liver, *FEBS Lett.* **389**, 225–228.

Herweijer, H., Zhang, G., Subbotin, V.M., Budker, V., Williams, P., Wolff, J.A. (2001) Time course of gene expression after plasmid DNA gene transfer to the liver, *J. Gene Med.* **3**, 280–291.

Hickman, M.A., Malone, R.W., Lehmann-Bruinsma, K., Sih, T.R., Knoell, D., Szoka, F.C., Walzem, R., Carlson, D.M., Powell, J.S. (1994) Gene expression following direct injection of DNA into liver, *Hum. Gene Ther.* **5**, 1477–1483.

Hofman, C.R., Dileo, J.P., Li, Z., Li, S., Huang, L. (2001) Efficient in vivo gene transfer by PCR amplified fragment with reduced inflammatory activity, *Gene Ther.* **8**, 71–74.

Hong, K., Zheng, W., Baker, A., Papahadjopoulos, D. (1997) Stabilization of cationic liposome-plasmid DNA complexes by polyamines and poly(ethylene glycol)-phospholipid conjugates for efficient in vivo gene delivery, *FEBS Lett.* **400**, 233–237.

Hsu, D.H., de Waal Malefyt, R., Fiorentino, D.F., Dang, M.N., Vieira, P., de Vries, J., Spits, H., Mosmann, T.R., Moore, K.W. (1990) Expression of interleukin-10 activity by Epstein-Barr virus protein BCRF1, *Science* **250**, 830–832.

Hudde, T., Rayner, S.A., Comer, R.M., Weber, M., Isaacs, J.D., Waldmann, H., Larkin, D.F., George, A.J. (1999) Activated polyamidoamine dendrimers, a non-viral vector for gene transfer to the corneal endothelium, *Gene Ther.* **6**, 939–943.

Huettinger, M., Retzek, H., Eder, M., Goldenberg, H. (1988) Characteristics of chylomicron remnant uptake into rat liver, *Clin. Biochem.* **21**, 87–92.

Hussain, M.M., Maxfield, F.R., Mas-Oliva, J., Tabas, I., Ji, Z.S., Innerarity, T.L., Mahley, R.W. (1991) Clearance of chylomicron remnants by the low density lipoprotein receptor-related protein/alpha 2-macroglobulin receptor, *J. Biol. Chem.* **266**, 13936–13940.

Hwang, S.J., Bellocq, N.C., Davis, M.E. (2001) Effects of structure of beta-cyclodextrin-containing polymers on gene delivery, *Bioconjugate Chem.* **12**, 280–290.

Hwang, S.H., Hayashi, K., Takayama, K., Maitani, Y. (2001) Liver-targeted gene transfer into a human hepatoblastoma cell line and in vivo by sterylglucoside-containing cationic liposomes, *Gene Ther.* **8**, 1276–1280.

Jakob, T., Walker, P.S., Krieg, A.M., Udey, M.C., Vogel, J.C. (1998) Activation of cutaneous dendritic cells by CpG-containing oligodeoxynucleotides: a role for dendritic cells in the augmentation of Th1 responses by immunostimulatory DNA, *J. Immunol.* **161**, 3042–3049.

Jarnagin, W.R., Debs, R.J., Wang, S.S., Bisell, D.M. (1992) Cationic lipid-mediated transfection of liver cells in primary culture, *Nucleic Acids Res.* **20**, 4205–4211.

Kabakov, A.E., Saenko, V.A., Poverenny, A.M. (1991) LDL-mediated interaction of DNA and DNA-anti-DNA immune complexes with cell surface, *Clin. Exp. Immunol.* **83**, 359–363.

Kalderon, D., Roberts, B.L., Richardson, W.D., Smith, A.E. (1994) A short amino acid sequence able to specify nuclear location, *Cell* **39**, 499–509.

Kim, T.W., Chung, H., Kwon, I.C., Sung, H.C., Jeong, S.Y. (2000) In vivo gene transfer to the mouse nasal cavity mucosa using a stable cationic lipid emulsion, *Mol. Cells* **10**, 142–147.

Kircheis, R., Schüller, S., Brunner, S., Ogris, M., Heider, K.H., Zauner, W., Wagner, E. (1999) Polycation-based DNA complexes for tumor-targeted gene delivery in vivo, *J. Gene Med.* **1**, 111–120.

Kircheis, R., Kichler, A., Wallner, G., kursa, M., Ogris, M., Felzmann, T., Buchberger, M., Wagner, E. (1997) Coupling of cell-binding ligands to polyethylenimine for targeted gene delivery, *Gene Ther.* **4**, 409–418.

Kitsis, R.N., Buttrick, P.M., McNally, E.M., Kaplan, M.L., Leinwand, L.A. (1991) Hormonal modulation of a gene injected into rat heart in vivo, *Proc. Natl. Acad. Sci. U.S.A.* **88**, 4138–4142.

Klinman, D.M., Yamshchikov, G., Ishigatsubo, Y. (1997) Contribution of CpG motifs to the immunogenicity of DNA vaccines, *J. Immunol.* **158**, 3635–3639.

Krieg, A.M., Yi, A.K., Matson, S., Waldschmidt, T.J., Bishop, G.A., Teasdale, R., Koretzky, G.A., Klinman, D.M. (1995) CpG motifs in bacterial DNA trigger direct B-cell activation, *Nature* **374**, 546–549.

Kukowska-Latallo, J.F., Bielinska, A.U., Johnson, J., Spindler, R., Tomalia, D.A., Baker, J.R., Jr. (1996) Efficient transfer of genetic material into mammalian cells using Starburst polyamidoamine dendrimers, *Proc. Natl. Acad. Sci. U.S.A.* **93**, 4897–4902.

Kukowska-Latallo, J.F., Raczka, E., Quintana, A., Chen, C., Rymaszewski, M., Baker, J.R., Jr. (2000) Intravascular and endobronchial DNA delivery to murine lung tissue using a novel, nonviral vector, *Hum. Gene Ther.* **11**, 1385–1395.

Kuriyama, S., Mitoro, A., Tsujinoue, H., Nakatani, T., Yoshiji, H., Tsujimoto, T., Yamazaki, M., Fukui, H. (2000) Particle-mediated gene transfer into murine livers using a newly developed gene gun, *Gene Ther.* **7**, 1132–1136.

Labat-Moleur, F., Steffan, A.M., Brisson, C., Perron, H., Feugeas, O., Furstenberger, P.,

Oberling, F., Brambilla, E., Behr, J.P. (1996) An electron microscopy study into the mechanism of gene transfer with lipopolyamines, *Gene Ther.* **3**, 1010–1017.

Larsen, D.L., Dybdahl-Sissoko, N., McGregor, M.W., Drape, R., Neumann, V., Swain, W.F., Lunn, D.P., Olsen, C.W. (1998) Coadministration of DNA encoding interleukin-6 and hemagglutinin confers protection from influenza virus challenge in mice, *J. Virol.* **72**, 1704–17048.

Lee, R.J., Huang, L. (1996) Folate-targeted, anionic liposome-entrapped polylysine-condensed DNA for tumor cell-specific gene transfer, *J. Biol. Chem.* **271**, 8481–8487.

Lee, P.Y., Chesnoy, S., Huang, L. (2004) Electroporatic delivery of TGF-beta1 gene works synergistically with electric therapy to enhance diabetic wound healing in db/db mice, *J. Invest. Dermatol.* **123**, 791–798.

Lee, K.D., Hong, K., Papahadjopoulos, D. (1992) Recognition of liposomes by cells: in vitro binding and endocytosis mediated by specific lipid headgroups and surface charge density, *Biochim. Biophys. Acta* **1103**, 185–197.

Lee, E.R., Marshall, J., Siegel, C.S., Jiang, C., Yew, N.S., Nichols, M.R., Nietupski, J.B., Ziegler, R.J., Lane, M.B., Wang, k.X., Scheule, R.K., Harris, D.J., Smith, A.E., Cheng, S.H. (1996) Detailed analysis of structures and formulations of cationic lipids for efficient gene transfer to the lung, *Hum. Gene Ther.* **7**, 1701–1717.

Leong, K.W., Mao, H.-Q., Truong-Le, V.L., Roy, K., Walsh, S.M., August, J.T. (1998) DNA-polycation nanospheres as non-viral gene delivery vehicles, *J. Control Release* **53**, 183–193.

Leventis, R., Silvius, J.R. (1990) Interactions of mammalian cells with lipid dispersions containing novel metabolizable cationic amphiphiles, *Biochim. Biophys. Acta* **1023**, 124–132.

Li, S., Huang, L. (1997) In vivo gene transfer via intravenous administration of cationic lipid-protamine-DNA (LPD) complexes, *Gene Ther.* **4**, 891–900.

Li, L.H., McCarthy, P., Hui, S.W. (2001) High-efficiency electrotransfection of human primary hematopoietic stem cells, *FASEB J.* **15**, 586–588.

Li, S., Tan, Y., Viroonchatapan, E., Pitt, B.R., Huang, L. (2000) Targeted gene delivery to pulmonary endothelium by anti-PECAM antibody, *Am. J. Physiol. Lung Cell Mol. Physiol.* **278**, L504–L511.

Li, S., Tseng, W.C., Stolz, D.B., Wu, S.P., Watkins, S.C., Huang, L. (1999) Dynamic changes in the characteristics of cationic lipidic vectors after exposure to mouse serum: implications for intravenous lipofection, *Gene Ther.* **6**, 585–594.

Li, S., Wu, S.P., Whitmore, M., Loeffert, E.J., Wang, L., Watkins, S.C., Pitt, B.R., Huang, L. (1999) Effect of immune response on gene transfer to the lung via systemic administration of cationic lipidic vectors, *Am. J. Physiol.* **276**, L796–L804.

Lin, H., Parmacek, M.S., Morle, G., Bolling, S., Leiden, J.M. (1990) Expression of recombinant genes in myocardium in vivo after direct injection of DNA, *Circulation* **82**, 2217–2221.

Liu, F., Huang, L. (2001) Improving plasmid DNA-mediated liver gene transfer by prolonging its retention in the hepatic vasculature, *J Gene Med.* **3**, 569–576.

Liu, F., Huang, L. (2002) A syringe electrode device for simultaneous injection of DNA and electrotransfer, *Mol. Ther.* **5**, 323–328.

Liu, F., Song, Y., Liu, D. (1999) Hydrodynamics-based transfection in animals by systemic administration of plasmid DNA, *Gene Ther.* **6**, 1258–1266.

Liu, F., Nishikawa, M., Clemens, P.R., Huang, L. (2001) Transfer of full-length DMD to the diaphragm muscle of Dmd(mdx/mdx) mice through systemic administration of plasmid DNA, *Mol. Ther.* **4**, 45–51.

Liu, F., Qi, H., Huang, L., Liu, D. (1997) Factors controlling the efficiency of cationic lipid-mediated transfection in vivo via intravenous administration, *Gene Ther.* **4**, 517–523.

Liu, F., Yang, J., Huang, L., Liu, D. (1996) Effect of non-ionic surfactants on the formation of DNA/emulsion complexes and emulsion-mediated gene transfer, *Pharm. Res.* **13**, 1642–1646.

Lunn, D.P., Soboll, G., Schram, B.R., Quass, J., McGregor, M.W., Drape, R.J., Macklin, M.D., McCabe, D.E., Swain, W.F., Olsen, C.W. (1999) Antibody responses to DNA vaccination of horses using the influenza virus hemagglutinin gene, *Vaccine* **17**, 2245–2258.

Macklin, M.D., McCabe, D., McGregor, M.W., Neumann, V., Meyer, T., Callan, R., Hinshaw, V.S., Swain, W.F. (1998) Immunization of pigs with a particle-mediated DNA vaccine to influenza A virus protects against challenge with homologous virus, *J. Virol.* **72**, 1491–1496.

Mahvi, D.M., Burkholder, J.K., Turner, J., Culp, J., Malter, J.S., Sondel, P.M., Yang, N.S. (1996) Particle-mediated gene transfer of granulocyte-macrophage colony-stimulating factor cDNA to tumor cells: implications for a clinically relevant tumor vaccine, *Hum. Gene Ther.* **7**, 1535–1543.

Maruyama-Tabata, H., Harada, Y., Matsumura, T., Satoh, E., Cui, F., Iwai, M., Kita, M., Hibi, S., Imanishi, J., Sawada, T., Mazda, O. (2000) Effective suicide gene therapy in vivo by EBV-based plasmid vector coupled with polyamidoamine dendrimer, *Gene Ther.* **7**, 53–60.

Matsubara, H., Maeda, T., Gunji, Y., Koide, Y., Asano, T., Ochiai, T., Sakiyama, S., Tagawa, M. (2001) Combinatory antitumor effects of electroporation-mediated chemotherapy and wild-type p53 gene transfer to human esophageal cancer cells, *Int. J. Oncol.* **18**(:) 825–829.

Matsui, H., Johnson, L.G., Randell, S.H., Boucher, R.C. (1997) Loss of binding and entry of liposome-DNA complexes decreases transfection efficiency in differentiated airway epithelial cells, *J. Biol. Chem.* **272**, 1117–1126.

McDonald, P., Hicks, M.N., Cobbe, S.M., Prentice, H. (1995) Gene transfer in models of myocardial ischemia, *Ann. N.Y. Acad. Sci.* **752**, 455–459.

McNeil, P.L., Khakee, R. (1992) Disruptions of muscle fiber plasma membranes. Role in exercise-induced damage, *Am. J. Pathol.* **140**, 1097–1109.

Meyer, O., Schughart, K., Pavirani, A., Kolbe, H.V. (2000) Multiple systemic expression of human interferon-beta in mice can be achieved upon repeated administration of optimized pcTG90-lipoplex, *Gene Ther.* **7**, 1606–1611.

Miao, C.H., Thompson, A.R., Loeb, K., Ye, X. (2001) Long-term and therapeutic-level hepatic gene expression of human factor IX after naked plasmid transfer in vivo, *Mol. Ther.* **3**, 947–957.

Middleton, P., Caplen, G.N.J., Gao, X., Huang, L., Gaya, H., Geddes, D.M., Alton, E.W. (1994) Nasal application of the cationic liposome DC-Chol:DOPE does not alter ion transport, lung function or bacterial growth, *Eur. Respir. J.* **7**, 442–445.

Mislick, K.A., Baldeschweiler, J.D. (1996) Evidence for the role of proteoglycans in cation-mediated gene transfer, *Proc. Natl. Acad. Sci. U.S.A.* **93**, 12349–12354.

Mohr, L., Yoon, S.K., Eastman, S.J., Chu, Q., Scheule, R.K., Scaglioni, P.P., Geissler, M., Heintges, T., Blum, H.E., Wands, J.R. (2001) Cationic liposome-mediated gene delivery to the liver and to hepatocellular carcinomas in mice, *Hum. Gene Ther.* **12**, 799–809.

Momose, T., Tonegawa, A., Takeuchi, J., Ogawa, H., Umesono, K., Yasuda, K. (1999) Efficient targeting of gene expression in chick embryos by microelectroporation, *Dev. Growth Differ.* **41**, 335–344.

Monroe, W.T., McQuain, M.M., Chang, M.S., Alexander, J.S., Haselton, F.R. (1999) Targeting expression with light using caged DNA, *J. Biol. Chem.* **274**, 20895–20900.

Moore, K.W., Vieira, P., Fiorentino, D.F., Trounstine, M.L., Khan, T.A., Mosmann, T.R. (1990) Homology of cytokine synthesis inhibitory factor (IL-10) to the Epstein-Barr virus gene BCRFI, *Science* **248**, 1230–1234.

Moradpour, D., Schauer, J.I., Zurawski, V.R., Wands, J.R., Boutin, R.H. (1996) Efficient gene transfer into mammalian cells with cholesteryl-spermidine, *Biochem. Biophys. Res. Commun.* **221**, 82–88.

Mounkes, L.C., Zhong, W., Palacin, G.C., Heath, T.D., Debs, R.J. (1998) Proteoglycans mediate cationic liposome-DNA complex-based gene delivery in vitro and in vivo, *J. Biol. Chem.* **273**, 26164–26170.

Mukherjee, A., Prasad, T.K., Rao, N.M., Banerjee, R. (2005) Haloperidol associated stealth liposomes: a potent carrier for delivering genes to human breast cancer cells, *J. Biol. Chem.* (Article in Press).

Muramatsu, T., Shibata, O., Ryoki, S., Ohmori, Y., Okumura, J. (1997) Foreign gene expression in the mouse testis by localized in vivo gene transfer, *Biochem. Biophys. Res. Commun.* **233**, 45–49.

Nabel, G.J., Gordon, D., Bishop, D.K., Nickoloff, B.J., Yang, Z., Aruga, A., Cameron, M.J., Nabel, E.G., Chang, A.E. (1996) Immune response in human melanoma after transfer of an allogeneic class I major histocompatibility complex gene with DNA-liposome complexes, *Proc. Natl. Acad. Sci. U.S.A.* **93**, 15388–15393.

Nabel, E.G., Gordon, D., Yang, Z.Y., Xu, L., San, H., Plautz, G.E., Wu, B.Y., Gao, X., Huang, L., Nabel, G.J. (1992) Gene transfer in vivo with DNA-liposome complexes: lack of autoimmunity and gonadal localization, *Hum. Gene Ther.* **3**, 649–656.

Nakamura, H., Watanabe, Y., Funahashi, J.I. (2000) Misexpression of genes in brain vesicles by in ovo electroporation, *Dev. Growth Differ.* **42**, 199–201.

Nanney, L.B., Paulsen, S., Davidson, M.K., Cardwell, N.L., Whitsitt, J.S., Davidson, J.M. (2000) Boosting epidermal growth factor receptor expression by gene gun transfection stimulates epidermal growth in vivo, *Wound Rep. Reg.* **8**, 117–127.

Nitta, Y., Tashiro, F., Tokui, M., Shimada, A., Takei, I., Tabayashi, K., Miyazaki, J. (1998) Systemic delivery of interleukin 10 by intramuscular injection of expression plasmid DNA prevents autoimmune diabetes in nonobese diabetic mice, *Hum. Gene Ther.* **9**, 1701–1707.

Ogino, H., Yasuda, K. (1998) Induction of lens differentiation by activation of a bZIP transcription factor, L-Maf, *Science* **280**, 115–118.

Ogris, M., Brunner, S., Schuller, S., Kircheis, R., Wagner, E. (1999) PEGylated DNA/trans-ferrin-PEI complexes: reduced interaction with blood components, extended circulation in blood and potential for systemic gene delivery, *Gene Ther.* **6**, 595–605.

Olivares, E.C., Hollis, R.P., Chalberg, T.W., Meuse, L., Kay, M.A., Calos, M.P. (2002) Site-specific genomic integration produces therapeutic Factor IX levels in mice, *Nat. Biotechnol.* **20**, 1124–1128.

Ortiz-Urda, S., Thyagarajan, B., Keene, D.R., Lin, Q., Fang, M., Calos, M.P., Khavari, P.A. (2002) Stable nonviral genetic correction of inherited human skin disease, *Nat. Med.* **8**, 1166–1170.

Parker, S.E., Khatibi, S., Margalith, M., Anderson, D., Yankauckas, M., Gromkowski, S.H., Latimer, T., Lew, D., Marquet, M., Manthorpe, M., Hobart, P., Hersh, E., Stopeck, A.T., Norman, J. (1996) Plasmid DNA gene therapy: studies with the human interleukin-2 gene in tumor cells in vitro and in the murine B16 melanoma model in vivo, *Cancer Gene Ther.* **3**, 175–185.

Parmacek, M.S., Ip, H.S., Jung, F., Shen, T., Martin, J.F., Vora, A.J., Olson, E.N., Lei-den, J.M. (1994) A novel myogenic regulatory circuit controls slow/cardiac troponin C gene

transcription in skeletal muscle, *Mol. Cell. Biol.* **14**, 1870–1875.

Piccirillo, C.A., Prud'homme, G.J. (1999) Prevention of experimental allergic encephalomyelitis by intramuscular gene transfer with cytokine-encoding plasmid vectors, *Hum. Gene Ther.* **10**, 1915–1922.

Piccirillo, C.A., Chang, Y., Prud'homme, G.J. (1998) TGF-beta1 somatic gene therapy prevents autoimmune disease in nonobese diabetic mice, *J. Immunol.* **161**, 3950–3956.

Pollard, H., Remy, J.S., Loussouarn, G., Demolombe, S., Behr, J.-P., Escande, D. (1998) Polyethylenimine but not cationic lipids promotes transgene delivery to the nucleus in mammalian cells, *J. Biol. Chem.* **273**, 7507–7511.

Porteous, D.J., Dorin, J.R., McLachlan, G., Davidson-Smith, H., Davidson, H., Stevenson, B.J., Carothers, A.D., Wallace, W.A., Moralee, S., Hoenes, C., Kallmeyer, G., Michaelis, U., Naujoks, K., Ho, L.P., Samways, J.M., Imrie, M., Greening, A.P., Innes, J.A. (1997) Evidence for safety and efficacy of DOTAP cationic liposome mediated CFTR gene transfer to the nasal epithelium of patients with cystic fibrosis, *Gene Ther.* **4**, 210–218.

Prabhakar, B.S., Allaway, G.P., Srinivasappa, J., Notkins, A.L. (1990) Cell surface expression of the 70-kD component of Ku, a DNA-binding nuclear autoantigen, *J. Clin. Invest.* **86**, 1301–1305.

Prentice, H., Kloner, R.A., Li, Y., Newman, L., Kedes, L. (1996) Ischemic/reperfused myocardium can express recombinant protein following direct DNA or retroviral injection, *J. Mol. Cell Cardiol.* **28**, 133–140.

Prentice, H., Bishopric, N.H., Hicks, M.N., Discher, D.J., Wu, X., Wylie, A.A., Webster, K.A. (1997) Regulated expression of a foreign gene targeted to the ischaemic myocardium, *Cardiovasc. Res.* **35**, 567–574.

Prud'homme, G.J. (2000) Gene therapy of autoimmune diseases with vectors encoding regulatory cytokines or inflammatory cytokine inhibitors, *J. Gene Med.* **2**, 222–232.

Qin, L., Ding, Y., Bromberg, J.S. (1996) Gene transfer of transforming growth factor-beta 1 prolongs murine cardiac allograft survival by inhibiting cell-mediated immunity, *Hum. Gene Ther.* **7**, 1981–1988.

Qin, L., Ding, Y., Pahud, D.R., Chang, E., Imperiale, M.J., Bromberg, J.S. (1997) Promoter attenuation in gene therapy: interferon-gamma and tumor necrosis factor-alpha inhibit transgene expression, *Hum. Gene Ther.* **8**, 2019–2029.

Qin, L., Pahud, D.R., Ding, Y., Bielinska, A.U., Kukowska-Latallo, J.F., Baker, J.R., Jr., Bromberg, J.S. (1998) Efficient transfer of genes into murine cardiac grafts by Starburst polyamidoamine dendrimers, *Hum. Gene Ther.* **9**, 553–560.

Qin, L., Chavin, K.D., Ding, Y., Tahara, H., Favaro, J.P., Woodward, J.E., Suzuki, T., Robbins, P.D., Lotze, M.T., Bromberg, J.S. (1996) Retrovirus-mediated transfer of viral IL-10 gene prolongs murine cardiac allograft survival, *J. Immunol.* **156**, 2316–2323.

Radler, J.O., Koltover, I., Salditt, T., Safinya, C.R. (1997) Structure of DNA-cationic liposome complexes: DNA intercalation in multilamellar membranes in distinct interhelical packing regimes, *Science* **275**, 810–814.

Rakhmilevich, A.L., Turner, J., Ford, M.J., McCabe, D., Sun, W.H., Sondel, P.M., Grota, K., Yang, N.S. (1996) Gene gun-mediated skin transfection with interleukin 12 gene results in regression of established primary and metastatic murine tumors, *Proc. Natl. Acad. Sci. U.S.A.* **93**, 6291–6296.

Raz, E., Duddler, J., Lotz, M., Bairs, S.M., Berry, C.C., Eisenberg, R.A., Carson, D. (1995) Modulation of disease activity in murine systemic lupus erythematosus by cytokine gene delivery, *Lupus* **4**, 286–292.

Regnier, V., De Morre, N., Jadoul, A., Preat, V. (1999) Mechanisms of a phosphorothioate oligonucleotide delivery by skin electroporation, *Int. J. Pharm.* **184**, 147–156.

Rensen, P.C., van Dijk, M.C., Havenaar, E.C., Bijsterbosch, M.K., Kruijt, J.K., van Berkel, T.J. (1995) Selective liver targeting of antivirals by recombinant chylomicrons–a new therapeutic approach to hepatitis B, *Nat. Med.* **1**, 221–225.

Ritchie, M.E. (1996) Characterization of human B creatine kinase gene regulation in the heart in vitro and in vivo, *J. Biol. Chem.* **271**, 25485–25491.

Rizzuto, G., Cappelletti, M., Mennuni, C., Wiznerowicz, M., DeMartis, A., Maione, D., Ciliberto, G., La Monica, N., Fattori, E. (2000) Gene electrotransfer results in a high-level transduction of rat skeletal muscle and corrects anemia of renal failure, *Hum. Gene Ther.* **11**, 1891–1900.

Rizzuto, G., Cappelletti, M., Maione, D., Savino, R., Lazzaro, D., Costa, P., Mathiesen, I., Cortese, R., Ciliberto, G., Laufer, R., La Monica, N., Fattori, E. (1999) Efficient and regulated erythropoietin production by naked DNA injection and muscle electroporation, *Proc. Natl. Acad. Sci. U.S.A.* **96**, 6417–6422.

Rols, M.P., Delteil, C., Golzio, M., Dumond, P. (1998) In vivo electrically mediated protein and gene transfer in murine melanoma, *Nat. Biotechnol.* **16**, 168–171.

Rols, M.P., Bachaud, J.M., Giraud, P., Chevreau, C., Roche, H., Teissie, J. (2000) Electrochemotherapy of cutaneous metastases in malignant melanoma, *Melanoma Res.* **10**, 468–474.

Ruysschaert, J.M., El Quahabi, A., Willeaume, V., Huez, G., Fuks, R., Vandenbremden, M., Di Stefano, P. (1994) A novel cationic amphiphile for transfection of mammalian cells, *Biochem. Biophys. Res. Commun.* **103**, 1622–1628.

Sakurai, F., Nishioka, T., Saito, H., Baba, T., Okuda, A., Matsumoto, O., Taga, T., Yamashita, F., Takakura, Y., Hashida, M. (2001) Interaction between DNA-cationic liposome complexes and erythrocytes is an important factor in systemic gene transfer via the intravenous route in mice: the role of the neutral helper lipid, *Gene Ther.* **8**, 677–686.

San, H., Yang, Z.Y., Pompili, V.J., Jaffe, M.L., Plautz, G.E., Xu, L., Felgner, J.H., Wheeler, C.J., Felgner, P.L., Gao, X., et al. (1993) Safety and short-term toxicity of a novel cationic lipid formulation for human gene therapy, *Hum. Gene Ther.* **4**, 781–788.

Schwartz, B., Benoist, C., Abdallah, B., Rangara, R., Hassan, A., Scherman, D., Demeneix, B.A. (1996) Gene transfer by naked DNA into adult mouse brain, *Gene Ther.* **3**, 405–411.

Sebestyen, M.G., Ludtke, J.J., Bassik, M.C., Zhang, G., Budker, V., Lukhtanov, E.A., Hagstrom, J.E., Wolff, J.A. (1998) DNA vector chemistry: the covalent attachment of signal peptides to plasmid DNA, *Nat. Biotechnol.* **16**, 80–85.

Shi, N., Pardridge, W.M. (2000) Noninvasive gene targeting to the brain, *Proc. Natl. Acad. Sci. U.S.A.* **97**, 7567–7572.

Siess, D.C., Vedder, C.T., Merkens, L.S., Tanaka, T., Freed, A.C., McCoy, S.L., Heinrich, M.C., Deffebach, M.E., Bennett, R.M., Hefeneider, S.H. (2000) A human gene coding for a membrane-associated nucleic acid-binding protein, *J. Biol. Chem.* **275**, 33655–33662.

Sikes, M.L., O'Malley, B.W., Jr., Finegold, M.J., Ledley, F.D. (1994) In vivo gene transfer into rabbit thyroid follicular cells by direct DNA injection, *Hum. Gene Ther.* **5**, 837–844.

Simovic, D., Isner, J.M., Ropper, A.H., Pieczek, A., Weinberg, D.H. (2001) Improvement in chronic ischemic neuropathy after intramuscular phVEGF165 gene transfer in patients with critical limb ischemia, *Arch. Neurol.* **58**, 761–768.

Smith, J.G., Walzem, R.L., German, J.B. (1993) Liposomes as agents of DNA transfer, *Biochim. Biophys. Acta.* **1154**, 327–340.

Soler, M.N., Bobe, P., Benihoud, K., Lemaire, G., Roos, B.A., Lausson, S. (2000) Gene therapy of rat medullary thyroid cancer by naked nitric oxide synthase II DNA injection, *J. Gene Med.* **2**, 344–352.

Solodin, I., Brown, C.S., Bruno, M.S., Chow, C.-Y., Jang, E.-H., Debs, R.J., Heath, T.D. (1995) A novel series of amphiphilic imidazolinium compounds for in vitro and in vivo gene delivery, *Biochemistry* **34**, 13537–13544.

Song, Y.K., Liu, F., Liu, D. (1998) Enhanced gene expression in mouse lung by prolonging the retention time of intravenously injected plasmid DNA, *Gene Ther.* **5**, 1531–1537.

Song, X.Y., Gu, M., Jin, W.W., Klinman, D.M., Wahl, S.M. (1998) Plasmid DNA encoding transforming growth factor-beta1 suppresses chronic disease in a streptococcal cell wall-induced arthritis model, *J. Clin. Invest.* **101**, 2615–26121.

Sorgi, F.L., Bhattacharya, S., Huang, L. (1997) Protamine sulfate enhances lipid-mediated gene transfer, *Gene Ther.* **4**, 961–968.

Sparwasser, T., Koch, E.S., Vabulas, R.M., Heeg, K., Lipford, G.B., Ellwart, J.W., Wagner, H. (1998) Bacterial DNA and immunostimulatory CpG oligonucleotides trigger maturation and activation of murine dendritic cells, *Eur. J. Immunol.* **28**, 2045–2054.

Stamatos, L., Leventis, R., Zuckermann, M.J., Silvius, J.R. (1988) Interactions of cationic lipid vesicles with negatively charged phospholipid vesicles and biological membranes, *Biochemistry* **27**, 3917–3925.

Stein, C.A., Tonkinson, J.L., Zhang, L.M., Yakubov, L., Gervasoni, J., Taub, R., Rotenberg, S.A. (1993) Dynamics of the internalization of phosphodiester oligodeoxynucleotides in HL60 cells, *Biochemistry* **32**, 4855–4861.

Sternberg, B., Sorgi, F.L., Huang, L. (1994) New structures in complex formation between DNA and cationic liposomes visualized by freeze-fracture electron microscopy, *FEBS Lett.* **356**, 361–366.

Stewart, M.J., Plautz, G.E., Del Buono, L., Yang, Z.Y., Xu, L., Gao, X., Huang, L., Nabel, E.G., Nabel, G.J. (1992) Gene transfer in vivo with DNA-liposome complexes: safety and acute toxicity in mice, *Hum. Gene Ther.* **3**, 267–275.

Straubinger, R.M., Papahadjopoulos, D., Hong, K.L. (1990) Endocytosis and intracellular fate of liposomes using pyranine as a probe, *Biochemistry* **29**, 4929–4939.

Straubinger, R.M., Hong, K., Friend, D.S., Papahadjopoulos, D. (1983) Endocytosis of liposomes and intracellular fate of encapsulated molecules: encounter with a low pH compartment after internalization in coated vesicles, *Cell* **32**, 1069–1079.

Sukharev, S.I., Klenchin, V.A., Serov, S.M., Chernomordik, L.V., Chizmadzhev, Y.A. (1992) Electroporation and electrophoretic DNA transfer into cells. The effect of DNA interaction with electropores, *Biophys. J.* **63**, 1320–1327.

Suzuki, T., Shin, B.C., Fujikura, K., Matsuzaki, T. (1998) Direct gene transfer into rat liver cells by in vivo electroporation, *FEBS Lett.* **425**, 436–440.

Tabata, H., Nakajima, K. (2001) Efficient in utero gene transfer system to the developing mouse brain using electroporation: visualization of neuronal migration in the developing cortex, *Neuroscience* **103**, 865–872.

Takagi, T., Hashiguchi, M., Mahato, R.I., Tokuda, H., Takakura, Y., Hashida, M. (1998) Involvement of specific mechanism in plasmid DNA uptake by mouse peritoneal macrophages, *Biochem. Biophys. Res. Commun.* **245**, 729–733.

Takeuchi, J., Koshiba-Takeuchi, K., Matsumoto, K., Vogel-Hopker, A., Naitoh-Matsuo, M., Ogura, K., Takahashi, N., Yasuda, K., Ogura, T. (1999) Tbx5 and Tbx4 genes determine the wing/leg identity of limb buds, *Nature* **398**, 810–814.

Tan, Y., Li, S., Pitt, B.R., Huang, L. (1999) The inhibitory role of CpG immunostimulatory motifs in cationic lipid vector-mediated transgene expression in vivo, *Hum. Gene Ther.* **10**, 2153–2161.

Tang, M.X., Szoka, F.C., Jr. (1997) The influence of polymer structure on the interactions of cationic polymers with DNA and morphology of the resulting complexes, *Gene Ther.* **4**, 823–832.

Tang, M.X., Redeman, C.T., Szoka, F.C., Jr. (1996) In vitro gene delivery by degraded polyamidoamine dendrimers, *Bioconjugate Chem.* **7**, 703–714.

Templeton, N.S., Lasic, D.D., Frederik, P.M., Strey, H.H., Roberts, D.D., Pavlakis, G.N. (1997) Improved DNA: liposome complexes for increased systemic delivery and gene expression, *Nat. Biotechnol.* **15**, 647–652.

Tousignant, J.D., Gates, A.L., Ingram, L.A., Johnson, C.L., Nietupski, J.B., Cheng, S.H., Eastman, S.J., Scheule, R.K. (2000) Comprehensive analysis of the acute toxicities induced by systemic administration of cationic lipid:plasmid DNA complexes in mice, *Hum. Gene Ther.* **11**, 2493–2513.

Tsujie, M., Isaka, Y., Nakamura, H., Imai, E., Hori, M. (2001) Electroporation-mediated gene transfer that targets glomeruli, *J. Am. Soc. Nephrol.* **12**, 949–954.

Tsurumi, Y., Takeshita, S., Chen, D., Kearney, M., Rossow, S.T., Passeri, J., Horowitz, J.R., Symes, J.F., Isner, J.M. (1996) Direct intramuscular gene transfer of naked DNA encoding vascular endothelial growth factor augments collateral development and tissue perfusion, *Circulation* **94**, 3281–3290.

Turunen, M.P., Hiltunen, M.O., Ruponen, M., Virkamaki, L., Szoka, F.C., Jr., Urtti, A., Yla-Herttuala, S. (1999) Efficient adventitial gene delivery to rabbit carotid artery with cationic polymer-plasmid complexes, *Gene Ther.* **6**, 6–11.

Uyechi, L.S., Gagne, L., Thurston, G., Szoka, F.C., Jr. (2001) Mechanism of lipoplex gene delivery in mouse lung: binding and internalization of fluorescent lipid and DNA components, *Gene Ther.* **8**, 828–836.

Vigneron, J.P., Oudrhiri, N., Fauquet, M., Vergely, L., Bradley, J.C., Basseville, M., Lehn, P., Lehn, J.-M. (1996) Guanidinium-cholesterol cationic lipids: efficient vectors for the transfection of eukaryotic cells, *Proc. Natl. Acad. Sci. U.S.A.* **93**, 9682–9686.

Vrancken Peeters, M.J., Perkins, A.L., Kay, M.A. (1996) Method for multiple portal vein infusions in mice: quantitation of adenovirus-mediated hepatic gene transfer, *Biotechniques* **20**, 278–285.

Wagner, E., Zenke, M., Cotten, M., Beug, H., Birnsteil, M.L. (1990) Transferrin-polycation conjugates as carriers for DNA uptake into cells, *Proc. Natl. Acad. Sci. U.S.A.* **87**, 3410–3414.

Walker, S., Sofia, M.J., Kokarla, R., Kogan, N.A., Wierichs, L., Longley, C.B., Bruku, K., Axelrod, H.R., Midha, S., Babu, S., Kahne, D. (1996) Cationic facial amphiphiles: a promising class of transfection agents, *Proc. Natl. Acad. Sci. U.S.A.* **93**, 1585–1590.

Wang, C.Y., Huang, L. (1987) pH-sensitive immunoliposomes mediate target-cell-specific delivery and controlled expression of a foreign gene in mouse, *Proc. Natl. Acad. Sci. U.S.A.* **84**, 7851–7855.

Wang, C., Chao, C., Madeddu, P., Chao, L., Chao, J. (1998) Central delivery of human tissue kallikrein gene reduces blood pressure in hypertensive rats, *Biochem. Biophys. Res. Commun.* **244**, 449–454.

Wang, J., Guo, X., Xu, Y., Barron, L., Szoka, F.C., Jr. (1998) Synthesis and characterization of long chain alkyl acyl carnitine esters. Potentially biodegradable cationic lipids for use in gene delivery, *J. Med. Chem.* **41**, 2207–2215.

Warrant, R.W., Kim, S.H. (1978) alpha-Helix-double helix interaction shown in the structure of a protamine-transfer RNA complex and a nucleoprotamine model, *Nature* **271**, 130–135.

Wells, D.J. (1993) Improved gene transfer by direct plasmid injection associated with regeneration in mouse skeletal muscle, *FEBS Lett.* **332**, 179–182.

Wheeler, C.J., Felgner, P.L., Tsai, Y.J., Marshall, J., Sukhu, L., Doh, S.J., Hartikka, J., Nieptupski, J., Manthorpe, M., Nichols, M., Plewe, M., Liang, X., Norman, J., Smith, A., Cheng, S.J. (1996) A novel cationic lipid greatly enhances plasmid DNA delivery and expression in mouse lung, *Proc. Natl. Acad. Sci. U.S.A.* **93**, 11454–11459.

Whitmore, M., Li, S., Huang, L. (1999) LPD lipopolyplex initiates a potent cytokine response and inhibits tumor growth, *Gene Ther.* **6**, 1867–1875.

Wilson, R.W., Bloomfield, V.A. (1979) Counterion-induced condensation of deoxyribonucleic acid. a light-scattering study, *Biochemistry* **18**, 2192–2196.

Wolff, J.A., Ludtke, J.J., Acsadi, G., Williams, P., Jani, A. (1992) Long-term persistence of plasmid DNA and foreign gene expression in mouse muscle, *Hum. Mol. Genet.* **1**, 363–369.

Wolff, J.A., Williams, P., Acsadi, G., Jiao, S., Jani, A., Chong, W. (1991) Conditions affecting direct gene transfer into rodent muscle in vivo, *Biotechniques* **11**, 474–485.

Wolff, J.A., Malone, R.W., Williams, P., Chong, W., Acsadi, G., Jani, A., Felgner, P.L. (1990) Direct gene transfer into mouse muscle in vivo, *Science* **247**, 1465–1468.

Wu, G.Y., Wu, C.H. (1988) Receptor-mediated gene delivery and expression in vivo, *J. Biol. Chem.* **263**, 14621–14624.

Xie, K., Huang, S., Dong, Z., Juang, S.H., Wang, Y., Fidler, I.J. (1997) Destruction of bystander cells by tumor cells transfected with inducible nitric oxide (NO) synthase gene, *J. Natl. cancer Inst.* **89**, 421–427.

Xie, K., Huang, S., Dong, Z., Juang, S.H., Gutman, M., Xie, Q.W., Nathan, C., Fidler, I.J. (1995) Transfection with the inducible nitric oxide synthase gene suppresses tumorigenicity and abrogates metastasis by K-1735 murine melanoma cells, *J. Exp. Med.* **181**, 1333–1343.

Xu, F., Szoka, F.C. Jr (1996) Mechanism of DNA release from cationic liposome/DNA complexes used in cell transfection, *Biochemistry* **35**, 5616–5623.

Yamamoto, S., Kuramoto, E., Shimada, S., Tokunaga, T. (1988) In vitro augmentation of natural killer cell activity and production of interferon-alpha/beta and -gamma with deoxyribonucleic acid fraction from Mycobacterium bovis BCG, *Jpn. J. Cancer Res.* **79**, 866–873.

Yanai, K., Hirota, K., Taniguchi-Yanai, K., Shigematsu, Y., Shimamoto, Y., Saito, T., Chowdhury, S., Takiguchi, M., Arakawa, M., Nibu, Y., Sugiyama, F., Yagami, K., Fukamizu, A. (1999) Regulated expression of human angiotensinogen gene by hepatocyte nuclear factor 4 and chicken ovalbumin upstream promoter-transcription factor, *J. Biol. Chem.* **274**, 34605–34612.

Yew, N.S., Zhao, H., Wu, I.H., Song, A., Tousignant, J.D., Przybylska, M., Cheng, S.H. (2000) Reduced inflammatory response to plasmid DNA vectors by elimination and inhibition of immunostimulatory CpG motifs, *Mol. Ther.* **1**, 255–262.

Yew, N.S., Wang, K.X., Przybylska, M., Bagley, R.G., Stedman, M., Marshall, J., Scheule, R.K., Cheng, S.H. (1999) Contribution of plasmid DNA to inflammation in the lung after administration of cationic lipid:pDNA complexes, *Hum. Gene Ther.* **10**, 223–234.

Yi, A.K., Chace, J.H., Cowdery, J.S., Krieg, A.M. (1996) IFN-gamma promotes IL-6 and IgM secretion in response to CpG motifs in bacterial DNA and oligodeoxynucleotides, *J. Immunol.* **156**, 558–564.

Yi, S.W., Yune, T.Y., Kim, T.W., Chung, H., Choi, Y.W., Kwon, I.C., Lee, E.B., Jeong, S.Y. (2000) A cationic lipid emulsion/DNA complex as a physically stable and serum-resistant gene delivery system, *Pharm. Res.* **17**, 314–320.

Yoo, J.J., Soker, S., Lin, L.F., Mehegan, K., Guthrie, P.D., Atala, A. (1999) Direct in vivo gene transfer to urological organs, *J. Urol.* **162**, 1115–1118.

Yoshida, S., Kashiwamura, S.I., Hosoya, Y., Luo, E., Matsuoka, H., Ishii, A., Fujimura, A., Kobayashi, E. (2000) Direct immunization of malaria DNA vaccine into the liver by gene gun protects against lethal challenge of Plasmodium berghei sporozoite, *Biochem. Biophys. Res. Commun.* **271**, 107–115.

Yoshimura, T., Shono, M., Imai, K., Hong, K. (1995) Kinetic analysis of endocytosis and intracellular fate of liposomes in single macrophages, *J. Biochem.* **117**, 34–41.

Yoshimura, K., Rosenfeld, M.A., Nakamura, H., Scherer, E.M., Pavirani, A., Lecocq, J.P., Crystal, R.G. (1992) Expression of the human cystic fibrosis transmembrane conductance regulator gene in the mouse lung after in vivo intratracheal plasmid-mediated gene transfer, *Nucleic Acids Res.* **20**, 3233–3240.

Yu, D., Matin, A., Xia, W., Sorgi, F., Huang, L., Hung, M.C. (1995) Liposome-mediated in vivo E1A gene transfer suppressed dissemination of ovarian cancer cells that overexpress HER-2/neu, *Oncogene* **11**, 1383–1388.

Zabner, J., Fasbender, A.J., Moninger, T., Poellinger, K.A., Welsh, M.J. (1995) Cellular and molecular barriers to gene transfer by a cationic lipid, *J. Biol. Chem.* **270**, 18997–19007.

Zabner, J., Cheng, S.H., Meeker, D., Launspach, J., Balfour, R., Perricone, M.A., Morris, J.E., Marshall, J., Fasbender, A., Smith, A.E., Welsh, M.J. (1997) Comparison of DNA-lipid complexes and DNA alone for gene transfer to cystic fibrosis airway epithelia in vivo, *J. Clin. Invest.* **100**, 1529–1537.

Zelphati, O., Szoka, F.C., Jr. (1996) Intracellular distribution and mechanism of delivery of oligonucleotides mediated by cationic lipids, *Pharm. Res.* **13**, 1367–1372.

Zhang, G., Budker, V., Wolff, J.A. (1999) High levels of foreign gene expression in hepatocytes after tail vein injections of naked plasmid DNA, *Hum. Gene Ther.* **10**, 1735–1737.

Zhang, G., Budker, V., Williams, P., Subbotin, V., Wolff, J.A. (2001) Efficient expression of naked DNA delivered intraarterially to limb muscles of nonhuman primates, *Hum. Gene Ther.* **12**, 427–438.

Zhang, Y., Jiang, Q., Dudus, L., Yankaskas, J.R., Engelhardt, J.F. (1998) Vector-specific complementation profiles of two independent primary defects in cystic fibrosis airways, *Hum. Gene Ther.* **9**, 635–648.

Zheng, Q.A., Chang, D.C. (1991) High-efficiency gene transfection by in situ electroporation of cultured cells, *Biochim. Biophys. Acta* **1088**, 104–110.

Zhou, X., Huang, L. (1994) DNA transfection mediated by cationic liposomes containing lipopolylysine: characterization and mechanism of action, *Biochim. Biophys. Acta* **1189**, 195–203.

Zhu, N., Liggitt, D., Liu, Y., Debs, R. (1993) Systemic gene expression after intravenous DNA delivery into adult mice, *Science* **261**, 209–211.

Ziady, A., Ferkol, T., Dawson, D., Perlmutter, D., Davis, P. (1999) Chain length of the polylysine in receptor-targeted gene transfer complexes affects duration of reporter gene expression both in vitro and in vivo, *J. Biol. Chem.* **274**, 4908–4916.

Zuidam, N.J., Barenholz, Y. (1998) Electrostatic and structural properties of complexes involving plasmid DNA and cationic lipids commonly used for gene delivery, *Biochim. Biophys. Acta* **1368**, 115–128.

33

Vector Targeting in Gene Therapy

Yosuke Kawakami and David T. Curiel
University of Alabama at Birmingham, Birmingham, UK

1   Introduction   1047

2   **Transcriptional Targeting   1048**
2.1   Gastrointestinal Cancers   1049
2.2   Hepatocellular Carcinoma   1050
2.3   Pancreas/Pancreatic Carcinoma   1050
2.4   Lung Cancers/Mesothelioma   1051
2.5   Breast Cancer   1052
2.6   Urological Cancers   1053
2.7   Gynecological Cancers   1054
2.8   Brain Tumors   1054
2.9   Thyroid Tumors   1055
2.10   Malignant Melanoma   1055
2.11   Other Cancers   1056
2.12   Normal Tissue/Organs   1056
2.13   Transcriptional Targeting of Replication-competent Ad   1056
2.14   Summary   1057

3   **Transductional Targeting   1059**
3.1   Genetic Capsid Modification   1060
3.1.1   Chimeric Ad Vector with Different Serotype or Species Fiber   1060
3.1.2   Ad Vector with Modified Fiber Proteins   1061
3.2   Adaptor Molecules   1061
3.3   Genetic Capsid Modification Combined with Adaptor
           Molecules   1062
3.4   Genetic Capsid Modification with Incorporation of Larger-sized
           Targeting Molecules   1064

Pharmacology. From Drug Development to Gene Therapy. Edited by Robert A. Meyers.
Copyright © 2008 Wiley-VCH Verlag GmbH & Co. KGaA, Weinheim
ISBN: 978-3-527-32343-2

4   **Transductional and Transcriptional Dual Targeting   1064**
4.1   Combination of Targeting with Adaptor Molecule and
             Transcriptional Targeting   1065
4.2   Genetic Capsid Modification Coupled with Transcriptional
             Targeting   1065

5   **Conclusions   1066**

             Acknowledgments   1067

             Bibliography   1067
             Books and Reviews   1067
             Primary Literature   1067

Keywords

Fiber (of Viruses)
Extracellular structure protruding from each vertex of the virus capsid, which plays an important role in virus infection by binding to its primary receptor.

Promoter
A DNA sequence recognized by RNA polymerase, which initiates transcription and contributes to specific transgene expression by regulation of viral DNA transcription process.

Transcription
The process of copying DNA to RNA by RNA polymerase, in which protein expression level can be controlled for specificity.

Transcriptional Targeting
To achieve selective transgene expression by placing the therapeutic gene under the control of specific promoters that are activated in target cells but not in untarget cells.

Transductional Targeting
To achieve selective transgene expression by redirecting binding of the fiber capsid protein away from a native receptor to an alternative cell-selective receptor.

Tropism
Movement in an organism in response to some environmental stimulus, which is utilized as affinity of adenovirus vectors to the cells representing infectivity in vector targeting.

In gene therapy, current vector systems demonstrate insufficient expression and lack of specificity, resulting in poor curative effects in target cells and/or high toxicity to nontarget cells. Thus, vector optimization is critical for the derivation of efficient clinical gene therapeutics. Recently, adenoviral vectors have been targeted at the level of transduction and transcription to overcome these issues. Using genetic capsid modification techniques, adapter molecules with tissue-specific antibodies and tissue-specific promoters (TSPs), these vectors can be efficiently targeted. These strategies are applicable for many types of target cells and are compatible with a variety of targeting molecules. These combinations are aimed at improving therapeutic index of diseases such as cancers, as well as nonmalignant diseases such as pulmonary hypertension.

1
Introduction

Genetic-based therapies, such as gene therapy, represent a novel approach under investigation for the diagnosis and treatment of a wide variety of diseases. As with most conventional therapies, the balance between target cell and nontarget cell toxicity determines the therapeutic index of gene therapy. All gene therapy strategies are fundamentally based on the expression of transgenes and require efficient delivery of the therapeutic gene. However, correlative laboratory studies have demonstrated the limited ability of current generation vector systems to efficiently transduce targeted cells. In addition, limitations in vector specificity can lead to transduction of normal cells and untoward toxicity even in the setting of compartmental dosing. Thus, vector optimization is critical for the derivation of efficient clinical gene therapeutics. In this regard, adenovirus (Ad) serotype 5 (Ad5) is the predominant adenovirus vector for gene therapy, since it can transduce both dividing and nondividing cells and infect a wide variety of cell types. However, an increasing number of tumor types have been reported to be relatively refractory to Ad5 infection due to the paucity of the native Ad5 receptor, coxsackievirus-adenovirus receptor (CAR). On the other hand, its wide tropism, which is mediated by Ad5 fiber protein and CAR, allows infection of many types of cells expressing CAR in normal human tissues such as hepatocytes, precluding *in vivo* targeting and provoking immune responses that can prevent repeated administration and even shorten the duration of therapeutic gene expression.

In the last two decades, Ad5 has been well characterized in its life cycle, capsid proteins function and, more importantly, the biology of infection in cells. Thus, there is much data on which to base Ad vector targeting strategies. Briefly, three distinct sequential steps are required for Ad infection and transgene expression: (1) binding of the Ad to specific receptors on the surface of the target cell; (2) internalization of the virus; and (3) transfer of the viral genome to the nucleus in which the transgene is expressed through transcription and translation (Fig. 1). On the basis of these steps, three opportunities for targeting intervention are implied: (1) Ad delivery to targeted organs/sites; (2) Ad binding

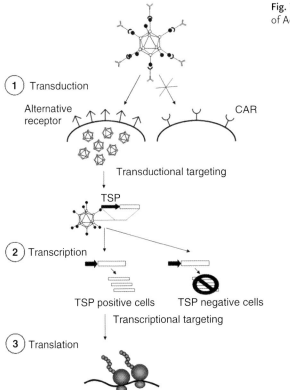

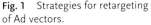

Fig. 1 Strategies for retargeting of Ad vectors.

and entry in targeted cells through primary and/or secondary Ad receptor; (3) protein expression of the transgene in the targeted cells through transcription and translation. This review outlines a series of Ad vectors that have addressed the issue of the vector targeting of gene therapy.

2
Transcriptional Targeting

To date, vectors employed for cancer gene therapy have included constitutively active promoters such as the cytomegalovirus (CMV) promoter, simian virus 40 (SV40) promoter and cytomegalovirus immediate-early enhancer, chicken β-actin promoter and the rabbit β-globin polyadenylation

signal (CAG) promoter. The CMV promoter is a strongly positive regulator but lacks expression specificity. Owing to this and other reasons, mammalian cellular promoters are being explored for cancer gene therapy; the goal is specific and it is the persistent expression of therapeutic genes in tumors or target tissues.

One goal of targeting is to minimize the ectopic transgene expression in order to prevent toxicity when the therapeutic gene is cytocidal or an enzyme that activates a prodrug. Adverse effects due to gene expression in nontarget cells, most abundantly liver toxicity and toxicity to the bone marrow, have been reported in preclinical studies. Furthermore, ectopic gene expression in immune cells may be responsible for an immune response to the transgene, thus limiting therapeutic efficacy. Target cell–specific gene expression may be accomplished through restriction of gene expression by using tissue-specific promoters (TSPs). To achieve this, efficient gene therapy regimens require transgene expression in the tumor, which has been denoted as the "on" status, and absence of expression in the relevant normal tissues, particularly in liver, which has been denoted as the "off" status.

Most TSPs reflect the natural property of the normal cells in target tissue/organs. Pathological changes in target tissues/organs, such as degeneration or malignant transformation, can alter expression of TSPs (i.e. activation of TSPs may be caused by these pathological changes). Thus, utilizing TSPs can enable a successful transcriptional targeting by maintaining higher transductional activity and specificity. To identify the best TSP for targeting cancer, one approach is to use "organ specific" promoters. Some of the targeted organs such as thyroid, breast, and pancreas secrete organ-specific proteins, such as thyroglobulin (TG), lactalbumin, and insulin. Promoters of these proteins are candidates of TSP and promoter activities can be predicted via monitoring these proteins. On the other hand, ectopic expression of these TSPs in normal cells in the organ must also be considered, except in particular cancers in which the function of the organ does not require preservation, such as uterus and prostate. However, TSPs often become overexpressed during transformation and may have a high therapeutic index without damaging normal cells/tissues. Another approach is to use "cancer specific" promoters, the genes of which are linked to malignant transformation and are expressed in a variety of cancers. In this case, promoter activity should also be analyzed in normal cells, such as stem cells and germ cells.

2.1
Gastrointestinal Cancers

Advanced gastrointestinal cancers, especially those associated with distant metastatic disease, are excellent candidates for gene therapy. A number of colon cancer targeting strategies have been reported. Carcinoembryonic antigen (CEA) promoter is the most frequently used TSP for colon cancer targeting. CEA is an oncofetal protein and is often detected at high levels in the serum of patients with colon cancers. Cytosine deaminase (CD), herpes simplex virus-thymidine kinase (HSV-tk), and diphtheria toxin are common therapeutic genes, and suicide gene therapy strategies using Ad vector constructed with *HSV-tk* or *CD* gene driven by the CEA promoter have been reported. One approach utilized the Cre/*loxP* recombination system, consisting of a Cre-producing Ad driven by the CEA promoter (Ad.CEA-Cre) and another Ad designed for inducible expression of the *HSV-TK* gene by Cre (Ad.lox-TK), to overcome the low activity of CEA promoter.

Human telomerase reverse transcriptase (hTERT) promoter, which is the catalytic subunit of the telomerase, is another promoter widely used for colon cancer and other cancers. It is expressed in most cancer cells but is quiescent in normal cells. Ad vectors with hTERT promoter driving expression of *CD* or *Bax* gene have been currently used in colon cancer models. Cyclooxygenase-2 (cox-2), an inducible isoform of the cyclooxygenase family, is closely linked to carcinogenesis and progression of colon cancers and about half of benign colon polyps. An Ad vector constructed with a cox-2 driven

HSV-tk gene demonstrated specific tumor cell killing with reduced liver toxicity using *in vitro* and *in vivo* models. Other colon cancer–specific promoters such as, the CTP1 promoter (beta-catenin-dependent promoter), the EGP-2 promoter (human epithelial glycoprotein-2 promoter), and the p21/WAF-1 promoter can also drive CD, HSV-tk or iNOS; these are useful promoters for carcinoma directed treatment modalities. For example, the EGP-2 promoter is epithelium specific, but there is highly abundant expression in the human epithelium, while the p21/WAF-1 promoter is an X-ray inducible promoter.

Gastric cancer is one of the leading causes of cancer-related death, and it remains endemic, especially in Asia, Africa, and parts of Europe. Targeted gene therapy could be one of the candidates for an innovative therapeutic approach in the treatment of advanced gastric cancer. The majority of gastric as well as colon cancers have been reported to show increased expression of cox-2 and CEA. Ad vectors with cox-2 or CEA-driven *HSV-tk* or *CD* genes showed specific cell killing for the treatment of gastric cancer. Nakaya et al. reported that suicide gene therapy with α-fetoprotein (AFP) promoter-driven HSV-tk was useful for the treatment of AFP-producing gastric cancer.

2.2
Hepatocellular Carcinoma

Hepatocellular carcinoma (HCC) is one of the most common malignancies worldwide. Since most conventional therapies have shown no survival benefit, gene therapy may provide an alternative therapeutic approach for the treatment of HCC. Many trials for targeting HCC have been reported and most of these were targeted

using the AFP promoter. AFP is a glycoprotein that is similar to albumin and is produced by the fetal liver. The AFP gene is normally expressed in fetal liver and is transcriptionally silent in adult liver but is overexpressed in HCC. The level of AFP elevation in HCC has been shown to correlate with poor tumor differentiation, increased tumor burden, early recurrence following tumor resection, and unfavorable prognosis. A number of strategies using AFP promoter driving the suicide genes, CD or HSV-tk, have been reported, some of which were constructed in combination with the Cre/*loxP* system or with the phosphoglycerate kinase (PKG) promoter to overcome the low transcriptional activity of the AFP promoter. Other TSPs for HCC have not been reported yet in the context of Ad-based gene therapy. However, Onishi et al. demonstrated hTERT transcripts in surgically resected HCC by *in situ* hybridization and suggested that the hTERT promoter is a good candidate as a target for HCC.

2.3
Pancreas/Pancreatic Carcinoma

The pancreas is both an exocrine and an endocrine organ. Amylase and insulin are representative proteins that are secreted from this organ. Therefore, targeting pancreatic carcinoma using these promoters is a rational strategy. The homeodomain transcription factor activating the insulin promoter, the pancreatic duodenal homeobox-1 (PDX-1), is an essential regulator of pancreatic endocrine cell development and adult islet β-cell function. Recently, expression of PDX-1 was found in several human pancreatic cancer cell lines. Wang et al. showed that the rat insulin promoter (RIP), used to drive the

HSV-tk and *CD* genes, resulted in cytotoxicity of PDX-1–positive insulinoma cells. The murine pancreatic amylase promoter was also tested for LacZ reporter gene expression in the pancreas for the treatment of metabolic disease therapy. In approximately one-third of pancreatic cancers, the proto-oncogene, *erbB2*, is overexpressed due to transcriptional upregulation of the *erbB2* gene with or without amplification. Harris et al. constructed an Ad vector with the *CD* gene driven by the erbB2 promoter, which demonstrated pancreatic cell–specific killing. Several other cancer-specific promoters such as the midkine, cox-2, and hTERT promoters, driving either reporter or suicide genes have shown specific transduction and therapeutic effect in pancreatic carcinoma.

2.4
Lung Cancers/Mesothelioma

Lung cancer has the highest mortality rate of all malignancies in developed countries; thus, novel therapeutic approaches such as gene therapy is required in this field. Small-cell lung cancer (SCLC), which comprises about 25% of lung cancers, characteristically secretes a variety of neuropeptides, such as adrenocorticotrophin hormone (ACTH), gastrin-releasing peptide (GRP), gastrin, neuron-specific enolase (NSE), cholecystokinin, and arginine vasopressin promoter (AVP). Many of these peptides can act as autocrine growth factors to the tumor. Yoshizawa et al. constructed vectors with HSV-tk driven by the NSE or GRP promoter and demonstrated a therapeutic effect in SCLC in an *in vitro* or *in vivo* model. Coulson et al. showed specific reporter gene transduction in SCLC cells using an AVP driven vector, indicating that AVP is also a candidate TSP for SCLC targeting.

Carcinogenesis related promoters, which are also candidate TSPs for other cancers, demonstrate lung cancer–specific transduction. For example, vascular endothelial growth factor (VEGF), which is one of the most effective mitogens specific for endothelial cells (EC), has been implicated in the neovascularization of a variety of tumors including lung cancers, especially in hypoxic conditions such as that found inside solid tumors. The mouse lung cancer cell line, A11, which was transfected with a vector harboring the VEGF promoter fused to the *HSV-tk* gene were demonstrated to give specific sensitivity to ganciclovir (GCV). This effect was enhanced by exposure to hypoxia followed by reoxygenation. The cytotoxic effect of the proapoptotic gene, *Bax*, was evaluated using an Ad vector expressing the human *Bax* gene under the control of the human VEGF promoter, suggesting a possible therapeutic application using this cancer-specific proapoptotic gene. Hexokinase type II (HKII), one of the hexokinases (HKs; ATP: D-hexose-6-phosphotransferase) that catalyzes the first committed step of glycolysis, is found in insulin-responsive tissues such as skeletal muscle, adipose tissue, and heart. In addition, tumors at various stages of malignancies show an increase in HK II activity compared with normal tissues. Katabi et al. reported that HKII promoter is another candidate TSP for non–small cell lung cancer by showing specific reporter gene expression and therapeutic effect of suicide gene therapy in an *in vivo* model.

Other TSPs, such as EGP-2/Ep-CAM and hTERT, which were previously utilized in gastrointestinal cancers and HCCs, were also successful for targeting lung cancer. Ad vectors with HSV-tk, CD and Bax, driven by these promoters demonstrated specific gene transfer and therapeutic effects using both *in vitro* and *in vivo* models. Fukazawa et al. reported that a dual promoter system using the human surfactant protein A1 (hSPA1) promoter and the hTERT promoter were useful for targeting lung cancer as demonstrated by reporter gene analysis.

2.5
Breast Cancer

Breast cancer remains one of the most common malignancies in women today and many gene therapy strategies are studied in this field. In some women, breast cancer is a local disease without distant spread. However, most women with primary breast cancer have subclinical metastases. Therefore, systemic administration of targeted Ad vector is a reasonable approach in the treatment of breast cancer patients with metastasis.

Human α-lactalbumin (ALA) is an enzyme involved in lactose production and the breast cancer antigen ALA, which is normally expressed in the fully differentiated lactating mammary gland at the onset of parturition. ALA was shown to be expressed in more than 60% of breast cancer tissues in the clinical cases tested. The ovine β-lactoglobulin (BLG) protein is the most abundant whey protein in the milk of ruminants and it is regulated in a hormone-dependent manner similar to ALA, although it is not normally expressed in mice or humans. Leonard et al. constructed a series of Ad vectors that express *CD* gene under the transcriptional control of either the ALA or the BLG promoter, and demonstrated a therapeutic effect in a breast cancer xenograft model. CEA, previously mentioned as a TSP for GI cancers, is also a tumor marker of breast cancers, and increased CEA level in the

serum has been observed in approximately 10% of the total breast cancer patients and 40 to 70% of recurrent ones. Qiao et al. reported that an Ad vector with *HSV-tk* gene driven by the CEA promoter demonstrated CEA-specific breast cancer cell killing using both *in vitro* and *in vivo* models.

Highly malignant cancers, such as breast cancer, are usually thermoresistant because they produce heat shock protein 70 (hsp70). Braiden et al. examined the effects of hsp promoter-mediated suicide gene therapy using the HSV-tk/GCV system for breast cancer in combination with hyperthermia. This report demonstrated that combination strategies were synergistically effective in mediating Fas-dependent apoptosis for breast cancer–specific gene therapy. Another stress-inducible chaperone protein with antiapoptotic properties is GRP78. GRP78 is overexpressed in transformed cells and during glucose starvation, acidosis, and hypoxic conditions, characteristic of poorly vascularized tumors. Dong et al. demonstrated that the GRP78 promoter is able to eradicate tumors using murine cells in immunocompetent models by driving expression of the *HSV-tk* suicide gene. Further, this system offers the advantage of positron-emission tomography (PET) imaging in combination with the suicide gene therapy in a breast cancer model.

Breast cancers usually arise from epithelial cells, and epithelial-based cancers have a variety of target specific TSPs. L-plastin (*LP*), which gene codes for an actin-binding protein, has been shown to be expressed at high levels in human epithelial cancer cells, but not in normal cells. Thus, LP is also a candidate TSP for targeting breast cancer. An Ad vector with an LP-driven *CD* or *E1* gene demonstrated a therapeutic effect in breast cancer xenograft model. Additionally, the chemokine receptor, CXCR4, was recently reported to be markedly upregulated in breast cancer cells, but undetectable in normal mammary epithelial cells. An Ad vector with a CXCR4 promoter-driven reporter gene showed breast cancer–specific transduction, indicating that it is also a candidate TSP for targeting breast cancer. In breast cancer, overexpression of *erb*B-2 has been observed in approximately 20% and has been associated with reduced relapse-free patients and overall poor patient survival. Pandha et al. have shown that the tumor-specific *erb*B-2 promoter driving the *CD* gene resulted in levels of CD expression in a phase I clinical trial of breast cancer patients. Finally, two promoters of note are the hTERT and hexokinase promoters. The analysis of reporter gene expression driven by hTERT promoter or hexokinase promoter has demonstrated breast cancer–specific transduction, indicating that they are candidate TSPs for targeting breast cancer.

2.6
Urological Cancers

Gene therapy studies in urological diseases have been performed in prostate, bladder, and renal cell cancers. A variety of clinical gene therapy trials for prostate cancer have been reported, because of the large numbers of patients that are available and regional localization allowing a variety of direct intratumoral approaches. Prostate-specific antigen (PSA), a 34-kDa chymotrypsin-like serine protease and its promoter are known to be highly specific to prostate tissue and multiple PSA-targeted gene therapy strategies have been utilized for prostate cancer using reporter genes and suicide genes. However, due to low activity, some PSA promoter approaches have used a Cre/*loxP* system to enhance promoter activity. Prostate-specific membrane antigen (PSMA) is a type-2 membrane protein expressed in the prostate, and it is highly expressed in metastatic or poorly differentiated adenocarcinomas. Ad vectors with *HSV-tk* or *CD* gene driven by PSMA promoter, demonstrated a therapeutic effect using *in vitro* and *in vivo* models. These results illustrate that PSMA is also a candidate TSP for targeting prostate cancer.

Dihydrotestosterone (DHT)-inducible third-generation probasin-derived promoter, ARR(2)PB, which has been modified to contain two androgen response elements, has also been one of the prostate cancer–specific promoters used. Therapeutic viruses constructed with the Bax or Bad apoptotic protein gene driven by ARR(2)PB induced specific overexpression of these gene and apoptosis in prostate cancer cells. The T-cell receptor γ-chain alternate reading frame protein (TARP), is a protein that is uniquely expressed in prostate epithelial cells and prostate cancer cells. Cheng et al. showed that the transcriptional activity of an Ad vector with a chimeric sequence comprising of the TARP promoter and the PSA enhancer is highly active in testosterone-deprived prostate cancer cells. Caveolin-1 (a structural component of caveolae), human glandular kallikrein 2 (hK2) and osteocalcin (a major noncollagenous bone matrix protein) are upregulated in higher-grade stage, androgen resistant or metastatic prostate cancer. Ad vectors with these promoters have been demonstrated to possess prostate cancer cell–specific transduction or killing with reporter gene expression or suicide gene therapy.

Compared to prostate cancer, very few gene therapy strategies have been studied in bladder cancer or renal cell carcinoma

(RCC). In bladder cancer gene therapy, Ad vectors with either an *LacZ* or a *CD* gene driven by the L-plastin promoter demonstrated specific reporter gene expression and therapeutic effect, respectively. An Ad vector with the luciferase reporter gene driven by CXCR4 (one of the chemokine receptors), showed specific transduction of RCC cells with liver off status *in vivo*, indicating that the CXCR4 promoter is a novel candidate for transcriptional targeting of RCC.

2.7
Gynecological Cancers

In the gynecological field, ovarian and cervical cancers are good candidates for gene therapy. A number of targeting strategies for ovarian cancer have been reported, with targeting using hTERT promoter being utilized most frequently. Ad vectors in combination with luciferase, *HSV-tk* and *Bax* gene demonstrated ovarian cancer–specific transduction and cell killing. KDR/flk-1 and flt-1 are receptors of VEGF and are known to display dysregulated expression in both tumor vasculature and their progressions. These promoters were used for Ad construction with reporter and *CD* genes, showing usefulness for targeting certain ovarian cancers, such as nonendothelial originated ovarian cancer and teratocarcinomas.

The whey-acidic protein human epididymis protein 4 (HE4) is frequently overexpressed in ovarian cancer, suggesting that the HE4 promoter is highly transcriptionally active in this disease. Luciferase expression Ad vector driven by the HE4 promoter exhibited significant expression in ovarian cancer cells, but not in normal cells. Secretory leukoprotease inhibitor (SLPI) is a 12-kDa serine

protease inhibitor expressed in some human carcinomas, including breast, lung, endometrium, and ovary. Selective Ad-mediated transgene expression could be achieved through the use of the SLPI promoter in the context of ovarian cancer. Mesothelin (MSLN), a cell surface glycoprotein, is overexpressed in ovarian cancer, but not in normal tissues with the exception of mesothelial cells. MSLN-driven luciferase expression Ad vector achieved transcriptional targeting in the context of ovarian cancer cells. Cox-2, midkine, hK2 and LP promoters have also been used for targeting ovarian cancer cells in the context of Ad vectors with reporter genes and suicide genes, demonstrating their utility as candidate TSPs for ovarian cancer.

For targeting cervical cancer cells, several TSPs, such as SLPI, cox-2, midkine, flt-1, VEGF, Survivin, and CXCR4 promoters have recently been screened using luciferase reporters in Ad vectors, with results demonstrating that VEGF and midkine are the most promising TSPs. Ad vectors with hTERT promoter-driven Bax and monocyte chemoattractant protein-1 (*MCP-1*) gene have also demonstrated tumor-specific cell killing in cervical cancer cells.

2.8
Brain Tumors

Brain tumors are some of the most fatal malignancies, and do not respond to conventional therapies, such as chemotherapy and radiotherapy. A number of gene therapy strategies, such as suicide gene therapy, have been performed with respect to these types of cancers. However, few systemic transcriptional targeting strategies have been studied in this field, because brain tumors exist in a compartment protected by a blood-brain barrier. This fact also means that little amounts of virus flowing out from the compartment would occur in the context of local administration of therapeutic Ad vectors. Glial fibrillary acidic protein, GFA2, is an intermediate filament protein expressed primarily in astrocytes. Vandier et al. constructed a recombinant Ad vector, Adgfa2TK, in which the HSV-tk was gene driven by GFA2 promoter, demonstrating inhibition of glioma cells growing *in vitro* and *in vivo*. Ad vectors with the hTERT promoter driving the caspase-8 or the Fas associated protein with death domain (*FADD*) genes showed specific cell killing, which indicated that hTERT is also a candidate TSP for targeting gliomas. Human glandular kallikrein 2 has also been reported to be useful for gliomas as well as cervical cancer mentioned earlier.

Pituitary tumors producing prolactin (PRL) were successfully treated using Ad vectors containing the *HSV-tk* gene driven by the PRL promoter both *in vitro* and *in vivo*. Proopiomelanocortin (*POMC*) gene encodes ACTH, which causes Cusing's syndrome, when overexpressed. The POMC promoter provided useful treatment of ACTH-producing pituitary tumors via Ad transduction.

2.9
Thyroid Tumors

The thyroid gland is a relatively common site of malignant neoplasms, giving rise to 90% of all endocrine cancers, and targeted therapy is especially important for this disease in regard to preserving normal thyroid function. Thyroid carcinomas are pathologically classified into papillary, follicular, anaplastic, and medullary cancers. The two most frequent entities, papillary and follicular thyroid cancers, are usually referred to as *differentiated thyroid carcinoma* and are always positive for TG immunohistochemical staining. The Ad vectors with *HSV-tk* gene driven by the TG promoter–mediated thyroid cancer–specific cell-killing ability, with less toxicity to normal cells. On the other hand, some poorly differentiated, metastatic or most anaplastic thyroid carcinomas show diminished TG expression, accompanied by loss of some thyroid-specific transcription factors. The promoter from the calcitonin/calcitonin gene-related peptide (*CT/CGRP*) gene was tested for targeting medullary thyroid carcinoma, and showed higher, specific transduction by reporter gene analysis. Undifferentiated thyroid carcinoma was successfully targeted using an hTERT promoter-driven luciferase Ad vector, and an hTERT-targeted HSV-tk Ad vectors demonstrated specific cell killing.

2.10
Malignant Melanoma

Melanoma is a relatively rare disease, but its biological characteristics are well investigated because of its accessibility. Melanoma inhibitory activity (MIA) protein, which is highly expressed in melanoma, plays an important role in melanoma metastasis and invasion, and MIA has been identified as a highly specific and sensitive marker for malignant melanoma. Tyrosinase, the enzyme catalyzing the rate-limiting step in melanin production, is exclusively expressed in melanocytes, pigment cells of the retina and melanoma cells. Rothfels et al. reported that MIA and tyrosinase promoters mediated suicide gene therapy of malignant melanoma, resulting in melanoma-specific cell killing. Survivin, a novel member of the inhibitor of apoptosis

(IAP) protein family, is expressed in human cancers, but is quiescent in normal differentiated tissues. A survivin-driven luciferase expression Ad vector showed high activity in melanoma cells with liver off status. Cox-2 is also reported to be expressed in melanoma cells and an Ad vector containing cox-2 promoter driving the luciferase gene, demonstrating activity of the cox-2 promoter in melanoma cell lines as well as in primary melanoma cells but not in normal cells.

2.11
Other Cancers

Several transcriptional targeting strategies have been reported in squamous cell cancer and pediatric tumors. Two inducible promoters, early growth response (Egr-1), which is radiation sensitive, and Hsp70 were demonstrated to induce squamous cell cancer–specific transduction. In pediatric tumors, tyrosine hydroxylase promoter and midkine promoter were tested using neuroblastoma and Wilms' tumor cells, demonstrating their usefulness for targeting these cancers. Osteocalcin (OS) is a major noncollagenous protein of bone regulated by 1,25dihydroxyvitamin DJ [1,25-(OH)pDa] and it is believed to be expressed only by differentiated osteoblasts. The OS promoter for osteosarcoma and the hTERT promoter for fibrosarcoma were reported as useful TSPs for specific cell killing or therapeutic effects.

2.12
Normal Tissue/Organs

Fewer numbers of gene therapy strategies have been studied for nonmalignant diseases for the following reasons. First, nonmalignant targeted cells, such as endothelial cells, muscle cells, neurons and hematopoietic cells, are relatively resistant to Ad infection. Further reduction of transgene expression through transcriptional targeting would result in insufficient therapeutic effects, since most transcriptional targeting involves the loss of transgene activity in exchange for specificity. Second, most therapeutic genes for nonmalignant diseases are nontoxic ones, such as enzymes, hormones, and other important factors of cell function, which do not cause nontargeting cell death that would have resulted in severe side effects. Some gene therapy strategies for nonmalignant diseases, which would be inappropriate for targeting by constitutively active promoters, utilize targeting by TSPs (see Table 1).

2.13
Transcriptional Targeting
of Replication-competent Ad

Conditionally replicative adenovirus (CRAd) agents have recently been applied for a variety of neoplastic diseases as a novel cancer gene therapy (see Fig. 2). In this approach, the virus replicates conditionally in transduced tumor cells, which lead to infection of neighboring cancer cells with progeny virus, resulting in virus-mediated oncolysis. Therefore, it is important to target CRAd agents more strictly than replication-incompetent Ad since even marginal levels of expression of TSP in untargeted normal cells could result in severe toxicity. Some TSPs that have been proved to be useful for targeting in the context of replication deficient Ad vectors have been studied in replication-competent CRAds agents (Table 2).

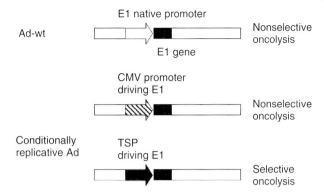

Fig. 2 Schematic representation of types of CRAd agents.

Tab. 1 Transcriptional targeting of nonmalignant cells.

Promoter	Target cells	Transgene	Investigator
Flt-1 (VEGFR-2)	Endothelial cells	Reporter gene	Nicklin
ICAM-1			
Von Willebrand factor			
KDR (VEGFR-1)	HUVEC	CD	Huang
Skeletal a-actin	Skeletal muscle	Reporter gene	Frauli
b-Enolase			
Creatine kinase			
Synapsin 1	Neuron	Reporter gene	Kugler
		BclX	Kilic
ICAM-2	Endothelial cells	Endoglin	Velasco
K18 (keratin 18)	Airway cells	Reporter gene	Toietta
Platelet-specific glycopron IIb	Platelets	Factor VIII	Shi
	Megakaryocytes		
Fascin	Dendritic cells (DC)	Reporter gene	Ross
Dectin-2	Langerhans cells (LC)	Reporter gene	Morita
Albumin	Hepatocytes	Reporter gene	Walther
α1-Antitrypsin		Reporter gene	Walther
Liver-type pyruvate kinase (LPK)		Reporter gene	Park

Notes: DC: dendritic cells; LC: Langerhans cells; LPK: liver-type pyruvate kinase.

2.14
Summary

A number of promoters have already been and will be reported as TSPs for transcriptional targeting, allowing us to choose a variety of targeting strategies that would be the best for the patients or diseases. In addition, transcriptional targeting is more advantageous compared to transductional targeting in respect to a "liver off" phenotype. However, the use of many TSPs results in reduced transgene expression in exchange for excellent specificity, which often causes insufficient therapeutic effect. Transductional augmentation, such

Tab. 2 Transcriptional targeting of replication-competent Ad.

Promoter	Driving gene	Target disease/cells	Investigator
Calcitonin	ICP4	Leiomyosarcoma	Yamamura
Cyclooxygenase-2	E1A	Pancreatic cancer	Yamamoto
	E1A	Ovarian cancer	Kanerva
	E1A	Esophageal cancer	Davydova
	E1A	Bladder cancer	Shirakawa
Flk-1	E1A	Endothelial cells	Savontaus
Human telomerase reverse transcriptase (hTERT)	E4	Breast cancer	Hernandez-Alcoceba
	E1A	Gastric cancer Cervical cancer Hepatocellular carcinoma Renal cell carcinoma	Wirth
	E1A	Hepatocellular carcinoma	Huang
	E1A	Lung cancer Hepatocellular carcinoma Cervical cancer Brain tumor	Kim
	E1A, E1B	Lung cancer	Kawashima
	E1A	Breast cancer Ovarian cancer Colon cancer	Huang
	E1A	Lung cancer Hepatocellular carcinoma Prostate cancer Colon cancer Pancreatic cancer Breast cancer	Irving
IAI.3B	E1A	Ovarian cancer	Hamada
L-plastin	E1A	Breast cancer Melanoma	Zhang
Midkine	E1A	Neuroblastoma Ewing's sarcoma	Adachi
	E1A	Glioma	Kohno
	E1A	Hepatocellular carcinoma	Yu
MN/CA9	E1A	Cervical cancer	Lim
Secretory laukoprotease inhibitor (SLPI)	E1A	Lung cancer	Maemondo
Surfactant protein B (SPB)	E4	Hepatocellular carcinoma Cervical cancer Colon cancer Prostate cancer	Doronin
Tyrosinase	E1A	Melanoma	Nettelbeck
	E1A	Melanoma	Peter
	E1A	Melanoma	Liu
	E1A, E4	Melanoma	Banerjee
Vascular endothelium growth factor (VEGF)	E1A	Ovarian cancer	Lam

Notes: SPB: Surfactant protein B.

as high dosage of the vector in combination with transductional targeting may result in a good therapeutic index.

3
Transductional Targeting

The extensively characterized capsid structure, genome, and replication cycle of Ad, particularly of the most commonly employed serotype 5, have allowed the molecular modifications required for their utilization of Ads as gene transfer vectors. Adenoviral infection is initiated by the recognition of the primary cellular receptor the CAR on target cells by the C-terminal portion of the fiber protein, termed the *knob*. After binding of the fiber knob domain, entry of the virus into the cell occurs via interaction of the Arg-Gly-Asp (RGD) sequence located in the viral penton base protein with cellular integrins (see Fig. 3). The development of genetically modified adenovirus (Ad) vectors with specificity for a single-cell type will require both the introduction of novel tropism determinants and the ablation of

endogenous tropism. Consequently, it will not be possible to exploit the native cellular entry pathway in the propagation of these targeted Ad vectors. On this basis, Ad vector can be targeted at the level of transduction through CAR-independent infection pathways by both ablation of its wide native tropism and introduction of novel infectivity preference for target cells, a concept that is otherwise known as *retargeting*.

As most transductional targeting strategies have shown, the advantage of transductional targeting is that the retargeted Ad vector would function not only with respect to enhanced specificity but also with respect to enhanced activity of transgene expression due to improved infectivity via the receptor of interest that would typically be sacrificed in exchange for specificity in most cases of transcriptional targeting. Retargeting of Ad vectors was originally initiated with two different approaches, genetic Ad capsid modification and adaptor targeting molecules, both of which are designed to attain CAR-independent transduction pathway while forgoing the native CAR pathway. Recently, the combination

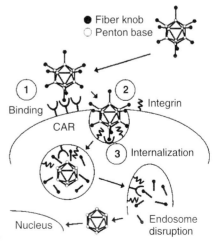

Fig. 3 The pathway of Ad entry.

of these two distinct methods was successfully achieved in an Ad vector by using the phage T4 fibritin motif.

3.1
Genetic Capsid Modification

3.1.1 Chimeric Ad Vector with Different Serotype or Species Fiber

The adenovirus fiber protein is responsible for attachment of the virion to cell surface receptors. The identity of the cellular receptor with which subgroup C adenoviruses, including Ad5 and Ad2, interact is CAR. Other subgroups including A–F except B also share this common CAR receptor for primary attachment. There is also evidence that suggests that Ad5 can also associate with other receptors including MHC class I proteins, heparin sulfate. Subgroup B adenoviruses, such as Ad3, Ad7, Ad11, Ad16, and Ad35 do not utilize CAR for cell entry. Several putative receptors for these viruses have been identified including CD46 for Ad35 and CD80/86 for Ad3. Stevenson et al. carried out a series of competition binding experiments using recombinant native fiber polypeptides from Ad5 and Ad3 and chimeric fiber proteins in which the head domains of Ad5 and Ad3 were exchanged. The results demonstrated that the determinants of Ad receptor binding are located in the knob (head) domain of the fiber, suggesting the possibility of altering the receptor specificity of the fiber protein by manipulation of sequences contained in the head domain. This very concept was initially tested by Krasnykh et al. and Stevenson et al., whereby an Ad vector containing chimeric fibers composed of the Ad3 fiber knob domain fused to the Ad5 fiber tail and shaft (Ad5/3). Ad5/3, which targets the Ad3 receptor, displayed high efficiency

in circumventing CAR deficiency and enhancing gene delivery into neuroblastoma, B-lymphocytes, ovarian cancer, RCC, squamous cell carcinoma of the head and neck and melanoma cells.

Shayakhmetov et al. screened different Ad serotypes, namely, Ad3, Ad4, Ad5, Ad9, Ad35, and Ad41, for interaction with noncycling human CD34(+) cells and K562 cells at the level of virus attachment, internalization, and replication. Ad serotype 35 emerged as the variant with the highest tropism for CD34(+) cells, resulting in the completion of the chimeric Ad vector Ad5/F35, the fiber of which consists of the tail and shaft domains of Ad5 and the knob domain of Ad35. Ad5/F35 demonstrated enhanced transduction in many nonmalignant cells, such as hematopoietic cells, bone marrow cells, endothelial cells, fibroblasts, DCs, and retinal cells as well as glioma, leukemia, osteosarcoma, melanoma, colon cancer, and cervical cancer cells.

Various other chimeric Ad vectors have been reported, including Ad2 with Ad17 fiber (Ad2(17f)), Ad5 with Ad16 fiber (Ad5.Fib16) and Ad5 with Ad11 fiber (Ad5/11), demonstrating efficient transduction in airway epithelia, cardiovascular tissue, and hematopoietic cells, respectively. Interestingly, Schoggins et al. demonstrated that a chimeric Ad5 vector with the Ad41 fiber decreases transduction to hepatocytes and is useful for liver nontargeting. The Toronto strain of canine adenovirus type 2 (CAV2) exhibits native tropism and it has been evaluated as a gene therapy vector. An Ad5 vector containing the nonhuman CAV2 knob can efficiently bind to and enter CAR-deficient cells, with up to 30-fold augmentation in gene delivery in comparison to the Ad5 control vector.

3.1.2 Ad Vector with Modified Fiber Proteins

Retargeting approaches based on genetic alternation of the virion capsid via fiber knob modification with small peptides have achieved cell-specific gene delivery. Certain targeting motifs may be incorporated in this manner to route the virus toward nonnative cellular entry pathways. Wickham et al. constructed two Ad vectors that contained insertions in the Ad fiber coat protein to redirect virus binding to either $\alpha(v)$ integrin or heparan sulfate cellular receptors by inserting Arg-Gly-Asp (RGD) or polylysin (pK7) at the C terminus of the fiber knob region respectively. These vectors demonstrated increased transduction 5- to 500-fold in numerous cell types lacking sufficient levels of the primary Ad receptor including macrophage, endothelial, smooth muscle, fibroblast, and T cells. Krasnykh and Dmitriev et al. have shown that peptides incorporated into the HI loop of the fiber knob remains available for binding in the context of mature virions containing modified fibers, suggesting that heterologous ligands, such as RGD, could be incorporated into the HI loop of the fiber knob and that this locale possesses properties consistent with its employment in adenovirus retargeting strategies. These integrin- and/or heparan sulfate-targeting Ad vector demonstrated enhanced transgene expression in dendritic, leukemic, myeloma, head and neck cancer, ovarian cancer, and renal cell cancer cells.

Douglas et al. demonstrated retargeting of an Ad vector via nonadenoviral, artificial receptor with six histidine (6His) incorporated Ad in the knob and anti-6His single-chain antibody (scFv) expressing cells. Nicklin et al. generated genetically modified Ad fiber proteins with selective tropism to EC by engineering human endothelial cell-binding peptides SIGYPLP into the HI loop of the Ad fiber, demonstrating efficient and selective tropism for EC compared with control Ad vectors.

In summary, genetic capsid modification allows progeny virions to maintain the same physical and genome structure as their parent viruses. This property is essential when applying targeting methods to replication. Genetic capsid modification has proven to be a useful method for enhancing the infectivity of CRAds as described below. Despite the gains that have been achieved with transductional targeting via genetic methods, challenges still remain. In designing serotype or xenotype chimeras, it is difficult to predict the targeting effect in advance since cellular receptors and therefore the viral tropism of Ads other than those conventionally applied as vectors are unknown. Genetic fiber modification is complicated by the limited size restriction of peptides that can be incorporated due to the structural incompatibility between the fiber and the targeting ligand. Moreover, RGD and pK7, which are recognized by integrins and heparan sulfate that are broadly expressed in many types of cells, may contribute to enhance transductional activity but not its specificity. Combination with the other control mechanisms, such as transcriptional targeting, may be recommended to achieve more selective results.

3.2 Adaptor Molecules

Several retargeting strategies to abrogate native tropism and redirect Ad uptake through defined receptors have been attempted using bifunctional adaptor molecules. In this strategy, one element of the bispecific adaptor binds to the

Ad knob, blocking its interaction with CAR and hence its native tropism. Such attachment may be accomplished with anti-adenovirus knob Fab, single-chain Fv fragments (scFv), and the extracellular domain of CAR. The second component of the bispecific adaptor is chemically or genetically conjugated to the knob-binding portion, introducing specificity for the target cells. Some of these molecules have been antibodies (Fab, scFv) or ligands that bind to specific receptors expressed on target cells.

Particularly, these candidate molecules have included fibroblast growth factor (FGF) for Kaposi'e sarcoma, melanoma, and ovarian cancer cells; epidermal growth factor (EGF) for glioma, head and neck, skin, ovarian, and lung cancer cells; CD40 ligand for DC and ovarian cancer cells; epithelial cell adhesion molecule (Ep-CAM) for head and neck, ovarian, hepatocellular, and prostate cancer cells; angiotensin converting enzyme (ACE) for pulmonary ECs; CEA for breast cancer cells; PSMA for prostate cancer cells; MSLN for ovarian cancer cells; and high molecular weight melanoma-associated antigen (HMWMAA) for melanoma cells and the pancarcinoma antigen tumor-associated glycoprotein 72 (TAG-72), for ovarian cancer. (Table 3)

Transductional targeting with adaptor molecules was originally developed using a chemical conjugate comprising the Fab fragment of a monoclonal antibody directed against the Ad5 fiber and a full monoclonal antibody against the target molecules. However, chemical conjugates consisting of two individual portions may be difficult to manufacture as they have homogeneity property, which is undesirable in a product intended for clinical use. Recombinant fusion proteins offer a number of technological advantages

including simplified production and purification when compared with chemical conjugates. Therefore, using bispecific adaptor-based Ad targeting with a recombinant fusion protein consisting of an extracellular portion of the Ad receptor CAR linked to an scFv or ligand to the targeting molecule may be a more rational approach (Table 3).

The use of bifunctional adaptors allows a myriad of molecules to be considered as candidates for rational vector targeting design. This method may be accomplished without concerns regarding size restrictions or perturbation of virus function that are commonly encountered in genetic modification techniques. With specific, defined targets incorporated into the design, cell receptor levels may be examined beforehand with flow cytometry or PCR analyses. Also, a great advantage is the fact that bispecific conjugates may be applied to the multitude of available Ad5-based vectors that have already been constructed for specific disease contexts. These vectors contain the unmodified Ad5 knob with which the conjugates can interact. On the other hand, retargeting in this case is successful only during the initial transduction, but not in replication-dependent situations involving subsequent infection by progeny virions, unless the adaptor molecules are continuously and appropriately provided *in situ*. Therefore, it is unclear how feasible this method would be in the context of replication-competent Ad vectors.

3.3
Genetic Capsid Modification Combined with Adaptor Molecules

A potential barrier to the development of Ad targeting with the aforementioned adaptor molecules for cell-specific delivery lies in the fact that several types of targeting

Tab. 3 Transductional targeting with adaptor molecules.

Targeting molecule	Target cell recognition site	Ad recognition site	Type of molecule	Target cell	Investigator
Anti-6 Histidine Fab	Six histidine	Anti-Ad5 fiber scFv	Fusion protein	Glioma expressing anti-His tag sFv	Douglas
Fibroblast growth factor (FGF)	Anti-FGF Fab	Anti-Ad5 knob Fab	Chemical conjugate	Kaposi's sarcoma Melanoma Ovarian cancer	Goldman Gu Rancourt
Epidermal growth factor receptor (EGFR)	Anti-EGFR Fab	Anti-Ad5 knob Fab	Chemical conjugate	Glioma Head and neck cancer	Miller Blackwell
	Anti-EGFR scFv	Anti-Ad5 fiber scFv	Fusion protein	Glioma Ovarian cancer Skin cancer Lung cancer	Haisma
	Anti-EGFR scFv	Soluble CAR	Fusion protein	Head and neck cancer Ovarian cancer Skin cancer Skin cancer	Dmitriev
c-erbB-2	Anti-c-erbB-2 scFv	Soluble CAR	Fusion protein	Breast cancer Ovarian cancer	Hemminki Kashentseva
CD40	Anti-CD40 Fab	Anti-Ad5 knob Fab	Chemical conjugate	Dendritic cells	de Gruijl
	Anti-CD40 scFv	Soluble CAR	Fusion protein	Dendritic cells Ovarian cancer	Pereboev Hakkarainen
Angiotensin converting enzyme (ACE)	CD40 ligand	Soluble CAR	Fusion protein	Dendritic cells	Pereboev
	Anti-ACE Fab	Anti-Ad5 knob Fab	Chemical conjugate	Pulmonary epithelial cells	Reynolds
Epithelial cell adhesion molecule (Ep-CAM)	Anti-EpCAM Fab	Anti-Ad5 knob Fab	Chemical conjugate	Head and neck cancer Ovarian cancer Hepatocellular carcinoma	Haisma
Prostate-specific membrane antigen (PSMA)	Anti-PSMA Fab	Anti-Ad5 knob Fab	Chemical conjugate	Prostate cancer	Kraaji
Carcinoembryonic antigen (CEA)	Anti-CEA scFv	Anti-Ad5 fiber scFv	Fusion protein	Breast cancer	Korn
High molecular weight melanoma-associated antigen (HMWMAA)	Anti-HMWMAA	Anti-Ad5 fiber scFv	Fusion protein	Melanoma	Nettelbeck

protein ligands require posttranslational modifications, such as the formation of disulfide bonds. This fact poses a problem especially for Ad capsid proteins that do not undergo such posttranslational modifications and are mostly localized in the nucleus during assembly of the virions. In addition, recombinant or chemically engineered adaptor molecules have to be specifically tailored for each particular targeting situation. To overcome these problems, a new general targeting strategy, which combines genetic modifications of the Ad capsid with a protein bridge approach, was recently developed, allowing the direct formation of vector–ligand complexes with monoclonal antibodies against cell surface antigens for targeting of Ad vectors. This capsid modification method entails the genetic incorporation of the Fc-binding domain derived from staphylococcal protein A into the Ad fiber protein. Significant augmentation of transduction efficiency using EGFR or CD40 specific monoclonal antibodies was achieved by applying this scheme.

Another approach of capsid modification with a protein bridge is avidin-based targeting with metabolically biotinylated Ad vector. In this strategy, a biotin acceptor peptide (BAP) was genetically fused to the Ad capsid fiber protein, which, during propagation would be biotinylated by the endogenous biotin ligase in 293 cells to produce covalently biotinylated virions. The resulting biotinylated vector could be retargeted to new receptors by conjugation to biotinylated antibodies via tetrameric avidin, resulting in increased transduction 10- to 30-fold over untargeted Ad-Fiber-BAP-TR in the case of biotinylated anti-CD59 or anti-CD71 antibodies in HeLa cells. In addition to the many advantages of targeting with adaptor molecules,

the combination of genetic capsid modification and adaptor proteins is useful especially for the screening of targeting molecules and would enable dual targeting with plural antibodies.

3.4
Genetic Capsid Modification with Incorporation of Larger-sized Targeting Molecules

Transductional targeting using adaptor molecules requires a more complicated procedure, especially for clinical usage. However, as noted above, attempts to alter Ad tropism by genetic modification of the Ad fiber have had limited success due to structural conflicts between the fiber and the targeting ligand. Additionally, adaptor molecule systems may only work effectively in situations not requiring virus replication. Therefore, novel approaches compatible with adenovirus replication are required to apply targeting to oncolytic Ad vectors. Krasnykh and Belousova et al. reported the use of the phage T4 fibritin trimerization motif to facilitate the genetic incorporation of larger targeting ligands into the Ad fiber. They validated this strategy with the human CD40 ligand (CD40L), demonstrating the incorporation of a large sized targeting molecule in the modified Ad5 fiber that had not been accomplished previously. This complex chimera was fully functional, conferring specific transgene expression in CD40 expressing cells.

4
Transductional and Transcriptional Dual Targeting

As stated above, various transductional and transcriptional approaches have been devised to improve targeting of Ad vectors. Transductional targeting alters the natural infection pathway of the Ad vector to enhance gene delivery to the target tissue and to reduce transgene expression in the liver. However, genetic modifications of Ad to ablate CAR recognition have not reduced hepatic transgene expression. Secondary interactions between the RGD motif in the Ad penton base and cell surface integrins, which normally mediate internalization of the virion after primary attachment to CAR, may account for some of the residual hepatocyte transduction. These findings suggest the need for complementary approaches to achieve improved targeting.

Transcriptional targeting has achieved exceptional specificity to the target cells while maintaining a "liver off" profile. However, transcriptional targeting alone is of little merit if the target cells are poorly transduced. Also, no promoter is entirely specific without having to sacrifice promoter strength. On the basis of these considerations, combining the complementary approaches of transductional and transcriptional targeting, neither of which is perfect or "non-leaky" by itself may be a rational approach.

4.1
Combination of Targeting with Adaptor Molecule and Transcriptional Targeting

The first report of dual targeting by combining both transductional and transcriptional targeting was accomplished in the pulmonary endothelium. The transductional targeting utilized was on the basis of a bispecific antibody consisting of anti-ACE (pulmonary endothelium marker) and anti-Ad5 knob Fabs while transcriptional targeting was achieved with the endothelial-specific promoter flt-1. Transcriptionally targeted Ad vectors were complexed with transductional targeting proteins to redirect the transduction of cells in a specific manner. This approach resulted in a synergistic, 300 000-fold improvement in the selectivity of transgene expression for the lungs in comparison to the usual site of vector sequestration, the liver. For targeting brain tumors and osteosarcoma cells, the bispecific antibody consisting of anti-EGFR and anti-Ad5 knob Fabs was utilized for transductional and OS promoter, which is TSP for osteosarcoma, was utilized for transcriptional targeting, respectively, showing enhanced transduction of reporter genes while retaining specificity. The aforementioned fusion protein consisting of EGF, one of the EGFR ligands, and sCAR was also utilized for dual targeting. Ad vectors constructed with a reporter or the *HSV-tk* gene driven by the SLPI promoter, which is one of the TSPs for ovarian cancer, demonstrated enhanced transduction and therapeutic effect in ovarian cancer both *in vitro* and *in vivo*.

4.2
Genetic Capsid Modification Coupled with Transcriptional Targeting

Genetic capsid modification has demonstrated the ability of the cyclic RGD-4C peptide to retarget Ad tropism toward αv integrins, leading to enhanced gene delivery to a repertoire of cell types. However, vectors modified in this manner are not selective in that they can transduce a wide variety of cells. In fact, RGD-modified vectors were originally developed to broaden the tropism of Ad-based vectors and achieve enhanced infectivity. Strategies to maintain the increased transduction afforded by RGD modification, but on a more cell-selective basis, have been exploited by combination with transcriptional targeting using TSPs. Work et al. combined transcriptional targeting using the endothelial-specific promoter, flt-1, with genetic fiber modification using the RGD motif for targeting endothelial cells, showing that double modification substantially shifted transduction profiles toward vascular endothelial cells in rat hepatocytes and endothelial cells. Nicklin et al. also combined transcriptional targeting on the basis of the flt-1 promoter with genetic fiber modification using the human endothelial cell-binding peptide SIGYPLP, demonstrating efficient and selective transduction of some cancer cell lines.

The combination of genetic capsid modification and transcriptional targeting with TSP gives full play to its abilities in CRAd, since the enhanced infectivity achieved by transductional targeting with capsid modification would lead to robust replication in target cancer cells, producing progeny virus that can go on to infect the surrounding cells. These replication and lateralization functions of CRAds greatly influence their efficacy. As noted in the previous section, fiber-modified Ad vectors, such as Ad5RGD and Ad5/3, show enhanced infectivity in various cancer cells by exploiting CAR-independent infection pathways. Cox-2 promoter-based CRAds with RGD fibers or Ad5/3 chimeric fibers have been constructed, demonstrating dramatic improvements in oncolysis of pancreatic, esophageal, and ovarian cancer cells both *in vitro* and *in vivo*. For melanoma treatment, a tyrosinase promoter–based CRAd was generated with an Ad5/3 chimeric fiber, also resulting in enhanced oncolysis.

5
Conclusions

In any treatment modality, a low therapeutic index resulting from poor curative effects in target cells and/or high toxicity to nontarget cells presents great obstacles hindering successful treatment of the disease. In this regard, Ad vectors can be targeted at the level of transduction and transcription to overcome these issues, contributing enhanced specificity and efficiency of therapeutic transgene expression. Transcriptional targeting is practical only for specificity, while transductional targeting can achieve both increased efficiency and specificity. Each targeting strategy possesses both advantages and disadvantages, perhaps making neither one alone adequate for gene therapy goals.

On the basis of the above considerations, combined transductional and transcriptional targeting represents a viable targeting method for the following two reasons. First, combined targeting enables both efficient and specific transduction that is essential for effective therapy. Additionally, increased transgene expression resulting from transductional targeting approaches that provide enhanced gene delivery would make it possible to apply TSPs that show high specificity, but have been disregarded due to their low promoter activity. Second, transgenes were screened stringently for specificity through both transductional and transcriptional targeting.

The number of gene therapy strategies carried out to date, however, has fallen short of expectations. It is obvious that seeking better efficiency and specificity are major considerations that need to be addressed. Current methodology for dual targeting may be too complicated at present for clinical usage. As introduced above, radically modified Ad vectors with large-sized targeting molecules have been generated and they mainly contribute to simplifying clinical protocols through the combination of transcriptional targeting portion inside the capsid. Further investigation of Ad biology and identification of novel targeting molecules will lead to an improvement of current gene therapy approaches.

Acknowledgments

The authors thank Dr. J. Michael Mathis, Director, Gene Therapy Program, LSU Health Sciences Center, Shreveport, for critical reading of the manuscript. This work was supported by the following grants: National Institutes of Health R01 CA86881 (D.T.C.), R01 HL67962 (D.T.C.), Muscular Dystrophy Association MDA359 (D.T.C.) and The Department of Defense W81XWH-05-1-0035 (D.T.C.).

See also Liposome Gene Transfection; Medicinal Chemistry; Molecular Oncology; Somatic Gene Therapy.

Bibliography

Books and Reviews

Alemany, R., Balague, C. (2000) Replicative adenoviruses for cancer therapy, *Nat. Biotechnol.* **18**, 723–727.
Culver, K.W., Blaese, R.M. (1994) Gene therapy for cancer, *Trends Genet.* **10**, 174–178.
DeGroot, L.J., Jameson, J.L. (2001) *Endocrinology*, 4th edition, Saunders, Philadelphia, PA.
Fengzhi, L. (2003) Survivin study: what is the next wave? *J. Cell. Physiol.* **197**, 8–29.
Freeman, S.M., Zwiebel, J.A. (1993) Gene therapy of cancer, *Cancer Invest.* **11**, 676–688.

Haviv, Y.S., Curiel, D.T. (2003) Engineering regulatory elements for conditionally-replicative adeno-viruses, *Curr. Gene Ther.* **3**, 357–385.
Herrmann, F. (1995) Cancer gene therapy: principles, problems, and perspectives, *J. Mol. Med.* **73**, 157–163.
Kirn, D., Martuza, R.L., Zwiebel, J. (2001) Replication-selective virotherapy for cancer: biological principles, risk management and future directions, *Nat. Med.* **7**, 781–787.
Kruyt, F.A., Curiel, D.T. (2002) Toward a new generation of conditionally replicating adenoviruses: pairing tumor selectivity with maximal oncolysis, *Hum. Gene Ther.* **13**, 485–495.
Nettelbeck, D.M. (2003) Virotherapeutics: conditionally replicative adenoviruses for viral oncolysis, *Anticancer Drugs* **14**, 577–584.
Oosterhoff, D., van Beusechem, V.W. (2004) Conditionally replicating adenoviruses as anticancer agents and ways to improve their efficacy, *J. Exp. Ther. Oncol.* **4**, 37–57.
Schmidt-Wolf, G., Schmidt-Wolf, I.G. (1994) Human cancer and gene therapy, *Ann. Hematol.* **69**, 273–279.
Shively, J.E., Beatty, J.D. (1985) CEA-related antigens: molecular biology and clinical significance, *Crit. Rev. Oncol. Hematol.* **2**, 355–399.
Thean, E.T., Toh, B. (1990) Serum human alpha-lactalbumin as a marker for breast cancer, *Br. J. Cancer* **61**, 773–775.
Verma, I.M., Somia, N. (1997) Gene therapy – promises, problems and prospects, *Nature* **389**, 239–242.
Williams, C., Shattuck-Brandt, R.L., DuBois, R.N. (1999) The role of COX-2 in intestinal cancer, *Ann. N. Y. Acad. Sci.* **899**, 72–83.
Wilson, J.E. (1995) Hexokinases, *Rev. Physiol. Biochem. Pharmacol.* **126**, 65–198.
Woll, P.J. (1996) *Growth Factors and Lung Cancer*, Lippincott-Raven, Philadelphia, PA.

Primary Literature

Adachi, Y., Matsubara, S., Muramatsu, T., Curiel, D.T., Reynolds, P.N. (2002) Midkine promoter-based adenoviral suicide gene therapy to midkine-positive pediatric tumor, *J. Pediatr. Surg.* **37**, 588–592.
Adachi, Y., Reynolds, P.N., Yamamoto, M., Wang, M., Takayama, K., Matsubara, S.,

Muramatsu, T., Curiel, D.T. (2001) A midkine promoter-based conditionally replicative adenovirus for treatment of pediatric solid tumors and bone marrow tumor purging, *Cancer Res.* **61**, 7882–7888.

Adams, V., Kempf, W., Hassam, S., Briner, J. (1995) Determination of hexokinase isoenzyme I and II composition by RTPCR: increased hexokinase isoenzyme II in human renal cell carcinoma, *Biochem. Mol. Med.* **54**, 53–58.

Akbulut, H., Zhang, L., Tang, Y., Deisseroth, A. (2003) Cytotoxic effect of replication-competent adenoviral vectors carrying L-plastin promoter regulated E1A and cytosine deaminase genes in cancers of the breast, ovary and colon, *Cancer Gene Ther.* **10**, 388–395.

Alemany, R., Curiel, D.T. (2001) CAR-binding ablation does not change biodistribution and toxicity of adenoviral vectors, *Gene Ther.* **8**, 1347–1353.

Ali, S., McClenaghan, M., Simons, P.J., Clark, J.A. (1990) Characterization of the alleles encoding ovine beta-lactoglobulins A and B, *J. Mol. Biol.* **91**, 201–207.

Anderson, L.M., Krotz, S., Weitzman, S.A., Thimmapaya, B. (2000) Breast cancer-specific expression of the Candida albicans cytosine deaminase gene using a transcriptional targeting approach, *Cancer Gene Ther.* **7**, 845–852.

Banerjee, N.S., Rivera, A.A., Wang, M., Chow, L.T., Broker, T.R., Curiel, D.T., Nettelbeck, D.M. (2004) Analyses of melanoma-targeted oncolytic adenoviruses with tyrosinase enhancer/promoter-driven E1A, E4, or both in submerged cells and organotypic cultures, *Mol. Cancer Ther.* **3**, 437–449.

Barbee, R.W., Stapleton, D.D., Perry, B.D., Re, R.N., Murgo, J.P., Valentino, V.A., Cook, J.L. (1993) Prior arterial injury enhances luciferase expression following in vivo gene transfer, *Biochem. Biophys. Res. Commun.* **190**, 70–78.

Barker, S.D., Dmitriev, I.P., Nettelbeck, D.M., Liu, B., Rivera, A.A., Alvarez, R.D., Curiel, D.T., Hemminki, A. (2003) Combined transcriptional and transductional targeting improves the specificity and efficacy of adenoviral gene delivery to ovarian carcinoma, *Gene Ther.* **10**, 1198–1204.

Barker, S.D., Coolidge, C.J., Kanerva, A., Hakkarainen, T., Yamamoto, M., Liu, B., Rivera, A.A., Bhoola, S.M., Barnes, M.N.,

Alvarez, R.D., Curiel, D.T., Hemminki, A. (2003) The secretory leukoprotease inhibitor (SLPI) promoter for ovarian cancer gene therapy, *J. Gene Med.* **5**, 300–310.

Barnett, B.G., Tillman, B.W., Curiel, D.T., Douglas, J.T. (2002) Dual targeting of adenoviral vectors at the levels of transduction and transcription enhances the specificity of gene expression in cancer cells, *Mol. Ther.* **6**, 377–385.

Bauerschmitz, G.J., Nettelbeck, D.M., Kanerva, A., Baker, A.H., Hemminki, A., Reynolds, P.N., Curiel, D.T. (2002) The flt-1 promoter for transcriptional targeting of teratocarcinoma, *Cancer Res.* **62**, 1271–1274.

Belousova, N., Korokhov, N., Krendelshchikova, V., Simonenko, V., Mikheeva, G., Triozzi, P.L., Aldrich, W.A., Banerjee, P.T., Gillies, S.D., Curiel, D.T., Krasnykh, V. (2003) Genetically targeted adenovirus vector directed to CD40-expressing cells, *J. Virol.* **77**, 11367–11377.

Berry, N.B., Cho, Y.M., Harrington, M.A., Williams, S.D., Foley, J., Nephew, K.P. (2004) Transcriptional targeting in ovarian cancer cells using the human epididymis protein 4 promoter, *Gynecol. Oncol.* **92**, 896–904.

Bilbao, R., Gerolami, R., Bralet, M.P., Qian, C., Tran, P.L., Tennant, B., Prieto, J., Brechot, C. (2000) Transduction efficacy, antitumoral effect, and toxicity of adenovirus-mediated herpes simplex virus thymidine kinase/ganciclovir therapy of hepatocellular carcinoma: the woodchuck animal model, *Cancer Gene Ther.* **7**, 657–662.

Blackwell, J.L., Li, H., Gomez-Navarro, J., Dmitriev, I., Krasnykh, V., Richter, C.A., Shaw, D.R., Alvarez, R.D., Curiel, D.T., Strong, T.V. (2000) Using a tropism-modified adenoviral vector to circumvent inhibitory factors in ascites fluid, *Hum. Gene Ther.* **11**, 1657–1669.

Braiden, V., Ohtsuru, A., Kawashita, Y., Miki, F., Sawada, T., Ito, M., Cao, Y., Kaneda, Y., Koji, T., Yamashita, S. (2000) Eradication of breast cancer xenografts by hyperthermic suicide gene therapy under the control of the heat shock protein promoter, *Hum. Gene Ther.* **11**, 2453–2463.

Breidenbach, M., Rein, D.T., Everts, M., Glasgow, J.N., Wang, M., Passineau, M.J., Alvarez, R.D., Korokhov, N., Curiel, D.T. (2005) Mesothelin-mediated targeting of adenoviral vectors for ovarian cancer gene therapy, *Gene Ther.* **12**, 187–193.

Cao, G.W., Qi, Z.T., Pan, X., Zhang, X.Q., Miao, X.H., Feng, Y., Lu, X.H., Kuriyama, S., Du, P. (1998) Gene therapy for human colorectal carcinoma using human CEA promoter contro led bacterial ADP-ribosylating toxin genes human CEA: PEA & DTA gene transfer, *World J. Gastroenterol.* **4**, 388–391.

Cao, G., Kuriyama, S., Gao, J., Nakatani, T., Chen, Q., Yoshiji, H., Zhao, L., Kojima, H., Dong, Y., Fukui, H., Hou, J. (2001) Gene therapy for hepatocellular carcinoma based on tumour-selective suicide gene expression using the alpha-fetoprotein (AFP) enhancer and a housekeeping gene promoter, *Eur. J. Cancer* **37**, 140–147.

Casado, E., Gomez-Navarro, J., Yamamoto, M., Adachi, Y., Coolidge, C.J., Arafat, W.O., Barker, S.D., Wang, M.H., Mahasreshti, P.J., Hemminki, A., Gonzalez-Baron, M., Barnes, M.N., Pustilnik, T.B., Siegal, G.P., Alvarez, R.D., Curiel, D.T. (2001) Strategies to accomplish targeted expression of transgenes in ovarian cancer for molecular therapeutic applications, *Clin. Cancer Res.* **7**, 2496–2504.

Cheng, W.S., Kraaij, R., Nilsson, B., van der Weel, L., de Ridder, C.M., Totterman, T.H., Essand, M. (2004) A novel TARP-promoter-based adenovirus against hormone-dependent and hormone-refractory prostate cancer, *Mol. Ther.* **10**, 355–364.

Coulson, J.M., Stanley, J., Woll, P.J. (1999) Tumour-specific arginine vasopressin promoter activation in small-cell lung cancer, *Br. J. Cancer* **80**, 1935–1944.

Daniele, B., Bencivenga, A., Megna, A.S., Tinessa, V. (2004) Alpha-fetoprotein and ultrasonography screening for hepatocellular carcinoma, *Gastroenterology* **127**, S108–S112.

Davidoff, A.M., Stevenson, S.C., McClelland, A., Shochat, S.J., Vanin, E.F. (1999) Enhanced neuroblastoma transduction for an improved antitumor vaccine, *J. Surg. Res.* **83**, 95–99.

Davydova, J., Le, L.P., Gavrikova, T., Wang, M., Krasnykh, V., Yamamoto, M. (2004) Infectivity-enhanced cyclooxygenase-2-based conditionally replicative adenoviruses for esophageal adenocarcinoma treatment, *Cancer Res.* **64**, 4319–4327.

de Gruijl, T.D., Luykx-de Bakker, S.A., Tillman, B.W., van den Eertwegh, A.J., Buter, J., Lougheed, S.M., van der Bij, G.J., Safer, A.M., Haisma, H.J., Curiel, D.T., Scheper, R.J., Pinedo, H.M., Gerritsen, W.R. (2002) Prolonged maturation and enhanced transduction of dendritic cells migrated from human skin explants after in situ delivery of CD40-targeted adenoviral vectors, *J. Immunol.* **169**, 5322–5331.

Dematteo, R.P., McClane, S.J., Fisher, K., Yeh, H., Chu, G., Burke, C., Raper, S.E. (1997) Engineering tissue-specific expression of a recombinant adenovirus: selective transgene transcription in the pancreas using the amylase promoter, *J. Surg. Res.* **72**, 155–161.

Dmitriev, I., Kashentseva, E., Rogers, B.E., Krasnykh, V., Curiel, D.T. (2000) Ectodomain of coxsackievirus and adenovirus receptor genetically fused to epidermal growth factor mediates adenovirus targeting to epidermal growth factor receptor-positive cells, *J. Virol.* **74**, 6875–6884.

Dmitriev, I., Krasnykh, V., Miller, C.R., Wang, M., Kashentseva, E., Mikheeva, G., Belousova, N., Curiel, D.T. (1998) An adenovirus vector with genetically modified fibers demonstrates expanded tropism via utilization of a coxsackievirus and adenovirus receptor-independent cell entry mechanism, *J. Virol.* **72**, 9706–9713.

Dong, D., Dubeau, L., Bading, J., Nguyen, K., Luna, M., Yu, H., Gazit-Bornstein, G., Gordon, E.M., Gomer, C., Hall, F.L., Gambhir, S.S., Lee, A.S. (2004) Spontaneous and controllable activation of suicide gene expression driven by the stress-inducible grp78 promoter resulting in eradication of sizable human tumors, *Hum. Gene Ther.* **15**, 553–561.

Doronin, K., Kuppuswamy, M., Toth, K., Tollefson, A.E., Krajcsi, P., Krougliak, V., Wold, W.S. (2001) Tissue-specific, tumor-selective, replication-competent adenovirus vector for cancer gene therapy, *J. Virol.* **75**, 3314–3324.

Douglas, J.T., Rogers, B.E., Rosenfeld, M.E., Michael, S.I., Feng, M., Curiel, D.T. (1996) Targeted gene delivery by tropism-modified adenoviral vectors, *Nat. Biotechnol.* **14**, 1574–1578.

Douglas, J.T., Miller, C.R., Kim, M., Dmitriev, I., Mikheeva, G., Krasnykh, V., Curiel, D.T. (1999) A system for the propagation of adenoviral vectors with genetically modified receptor specificities, *Nat. Biotechnol.* **17**, 470–475.

Dvorak, H.F., Brown, L.F., Detmer, M., Dvrak, A.M. (1995) Vascular permeability factor/vascular endothelial growth factor, microvascular hyperpermeability, and angiogenesis, *Am. J. Pathol.* **146**, 1029–1039.

Eberhart, C.E., Coffey, R.J., Radhika, A., Giardiello, F.M., Ferrenbach, S., DuBois, R.N. (1994) Up-regulation of cyclooxygenase 2 gene expression in human colorectal adenomas and adenocarcinomas, *Gastroenterology* **107**, 1183–1188.

Findlay, J., Brew, K. (1972) The complete amino acid sequence of human alpha-lactalbumin, *Eur. J. Biochem.* **27**, 65–86.

Frauli, M., Ribault, S., Neuville, P., Auge, F., Calenda, V. (2003) Adenoviral-mediated skeletal muscle transcriptional targeting using chimeric tissue-specific promoters, *Med. Sci. Monit.* **9**, BR–78–84.

Fukazawa, T., Maeda, Y., Sladek, F.M., Owen-Schaub, L.B. (2004) Development of a cancer-targeted tissue-specific promoter system, *Cancer Res.* **64**, 363–369.

Gerrish, K., Gannon, M., Shih, D., Henderson, E., Stoffel, M., Wright, C.V., Stein, R. (2000) Pancreatic beta cell-specific transcription of the pdx-1 gene. The role of conserved upstream control regions and their hepatic nuclear factor 3beta sites, *J. Biol. Chem.* **275**, 3485–3492.

Glasgow, J.N., Kremer, E.J., Hemminki, A., Siegal, G.P., Douglas, J.T., Curiel, D.T. (2004) An adenovirus vector with a chimeric fiber derived from canine adenovirus type 2 displays novel tropism, *Virology* **324**, 103–116.

Goldberg, M.A., Schneider, T.J. (1994) Similarities between the oxygen-sensing mechanisms regulating the expression of vascular endothelial growth factor and erythropoietin, *J. Biol. Chem.* **269**, 4355–4359.

Goldman, C.K., Rogers, B.E., Douglas, J.T., Sosnowski, B.A., Ying, W., Siegal, G.P., Baird, A., Campain, J.A., Curiel, D.T. (1997) Targeted gene delivery to Kaposi's sarcoma cells via the fibroblast growth factor receptor, *Cancer Res.* **57**, 1447–1451.

Gonzalez, R., Vereecque, R., Wickham, T.J., Vanrumbeke, M., Kovesdi, I., Bauters, F., Fenaux, P., Quesnel, B. (1999) Increased gene transfer in acute myeloid leukemic cells by an adenovirus vector containing a modified fiber protein, *Gene Ther.* **6**, 314–320.

Gonzalez, R., Vereecque, R., Wickham, T.J., Facon, T., Hetuin, D., Kovesdi, I., Bauters, F.,

Fenaux, P., Quesnel, B. (1999) Transduction of bone marrow cells by the AdZ.F(pK7) modified adenovirus demonstrates preferential gene transfer in myeloma cells, *Hum. Gene Ther.* **10**, 2709–2717.

Gu, J., Andreeff, M., Roth, J.A., Fang, B. (2002) hTERT promoter induces tumor-specific Bax gene expression and cell killing in syngenic mouse tumor model and prevents systemic toxicity, *Gene Ther.* **9**, 30–37.

Gu, J., Kagawa, S., Takakura, M., Kyo, S., Inoue, M., Roth, J.A., Fang, B. (2000) Tumor-specific transgene expression from the human telomerase reverse transcriptase promoter enables targeting of the therapeutic effects of the Bax gene to cancers, *Cancer Res.* **60**, 5359–5364.

Gu, D.L., Gonzalez, A.M., Printz, M.A., Doukas, J., Ying, W., D'Andrea, M., Hoganson, D.K., Curiel, D.T., Douglas, J.T., Sosnowski, B.A., Baird, A., Aukerman, S.L., Pierce, G.F. (1999) Fibroblast growth factor 2 retargeted adenovirus has redirected cellular tropism: evidence for reduced toxicity and enhanced antitumor activity in mice, *Cancer Res.* **59**, 2608–2614.

Gugala, Z., Olmsted-Davis, E.A., Gannon, F.H., Lindsey, R.W., Davis, A.R. (2003) Osteoinduction by ex vivo adenovirus-mediated BMP2 delivery is independent of cell type, *Gene Ther.* **10**, 1289–1296.

Haisma, H.J., Grill, J., Curiel, D.T., Hoogeland, S., van Beusechem, V.W., Pinedo, H.M., Gerritsen, W.R. (2000) Targeting of adenoviral vectors through a bispecific single-chain antibody, *Cancer Gene Ther.* **7**, 901–904.

Haisma, H.J., Pinedo, H.M., Rijswijk, A., der Meulen-Muileman, I., Sosnowski, B.A., Ying, W., Beusechem, V.W., Tillman, B.W., Gerritsen, W.R., Curiel, D.T. (1999) Tumor-specific gene transfer via an adenoviral vector targeted to the pan-carcinoma antigen EpCAM, *Gene Ther.* **6**, 1469–1474.

Hakkarainen, T., Hemminki, A., Pereboev, A.V., Barker, S.D., Asiedu, C.K., Strong, T.V., Kanerva, A., Wahlfors, J., Curiel, D.T. (2003) CD40 is expressed on ovarian cancer cells and can be utilized for targeting adenoviruses, *Clin. Cancer Res.* **9**, 619–624.

Hamada, K., Kohno, S., Iwamoto, M., Yokota, H., Okada, M., Tagawa, M., Hirose, S., Yamasaki, K., Shirakata, Y., Hashimoto, K., Ito, M. (2003) Identification of the human IAI.3B promoter element and its use in the construction of a replication-selective adenovirus for ovarian cancer therapy, *Cancer Res.* **63**, 2506–2512.

Harris, J.D., Gutierrez, A.A., Hurst, H.C., Sikora, K., Lemoine, N.R. (1994) Gene therapy for cancer using tumour-specific prodrug activation, *Gene Ther.* **1**, 170–175.

Havenga, M.J., Lemckert, A.A., Grimbergen, J.M., Vogels, R., Huisman, L.G., Valerio, D., Bout, A., Quax, P.H. (2001) Improved adenovirus vectors for infection of cardiovascular tissues, *J. Virol.* **75**, 3335–3342.

Haviv, Y.S., van Houdt, W.J., Lu, B., Curiel, D.T., Zhu, Z.B. (2004) Transcriptional targeting in renal cancer cell lines via the human CXCR4 promoter, *Mol. Cancer Ther.* **3**, 687–691.

Haviv, Y.S., Blackwell, J.L., Kanerva, A., Nagi, P., Krasnykh, V., Dmitriev, I., Wang, M., Naito, S., Lei, X., Hemminki, A., Carey, D., Curiel, D.T. (2002) Adenoviral gene therapy for renal cancer requires retargeting to alternative cellular receptors, *Cancer Res.* **62**, 4213–4281.

Hemminki, A., Dmitriev, I., Liu, B., Desmond, R.A., Alemany, R., Curiel, D.T. (2001) Targeting oncolytic adenoviral agents to the epidermal growth factor pathway with a secretory fusion molecule, *Cancer Res.* **61**, 6377–6381.

Hernandez-Alcoceba, R., Pihalja, M., Qian, D., Clarke, M.F. (2002) New oncolytic adenoviruses with hypoxia- and estrogen receptor-regulated replication, *Hum. Gene Ther.* **13**, 1737–1750.

Huang, X., Zhang, W., Wakimoto, H., Hamada, H., Cao, X. (2002) Adenovirus-mediated tissue-specific cytosine deaminase gene therapy for human hepatocellular carcinoma with different AFP expression levels, *J. Exp. Ther. Oncol.* **2**, 100–106.

Huang, T.G., Savontaus, M.J., Shinozaki, K., Sauter, B.V., Woo, S.L. (2003) Telomerase-dependent oncolytic adenovirus for cancer treatment, *Gene Ther.* **10**, 1241–1247.

Huang, Z.H., Yang, W.Y., Gong, X.W., Qian, Y., Che, X.Y. (2004) Killing effect of suicide gene system under control by KDR promotor on human umbilical vein endothelial cells, *Di Yi Jun Yi Da Xue Xue Bao* **24**, 139–143.

Huang, Q., Zhang, X., Wang, H., Yan, B., Kirkpatrick, J., Dewhrist, M.W., Li, C.Y. (2004) A novel conditionally replicative adenovirus vector targeting telomerase-positive tumor cells, *Clin. Cancer Res.* **10**, 1203–1205.

Huard, J., Lochmuller, H., Acsadi, G., Jani, A., Massie, B., Karpati, G. (1995) The route of administration is a major determinant of the transduction efficiency of rat tissues by adenoviral recombinants, *Gene Ther.* **2**, 107–115.

Ido, A., Uto, H., Moriuchi, A., Nagata, K., Onaga, Y., Onaga, M., Hori, T., Hirono, S., Hayashi, K., Tamaoki, T., Tsubouchi, H. (2001) Gene therapy targeting for hepatocellular carcinoma: selective and enhanced suicide gene expression regulated by a hypoxia-inducible enhancer linked to a human alpha-fetoprotein promoter, *Cancer Res.* **61**, 3016–3021.

Ikegami, S., Tadakuma, T., Ono, T., Suzuki, S., Yoshimura, I., Asano, T., Hayakawa, M. (2004) Treatment efficiency of a suicide gene therapy using prostate-specific membrane antigen promoter/enhancer in a castrated mouse model of prostate cancer, *Cancer Sci.* **95**, 367–370.

Imamura, H., Matsuyama, Y., Tanaka, E., Ohkubo, T., Hasegawa, K., Miyagawa, S., Sugawara, Y., Minagawa, M., Takayama, T., Kawasaki, S., Makuuchi, M. (2003) Risk factors contributing to early and late phase intrahepatic recurrence of hepatocellular carcinoma after hepatectomy, *J. Hepatol.* **38**, 200–207.

Irving, J., Wang, Z., Powell, S., O'Sullivan, C., Mok, M., Murphy, B., Cardoza, L., Lebkowski, J.S., Majumdar, A.S. (2004) Conditionally replicative adenovirus driven by the human telomerase promoter provides broad-spectrum antitumor activity without liver toxicity, *Cancer Gene Ther.* **11**, 174–185.

Jiang, Q., Ge, K., Xu, D.H., Sun, L.Y., Zheng, Z.C., Liu, X.Y. (1998) Use of carcinoembryonic antigen gene promoter in colorectal carcinoma-specific suicidal gene therapy, *Sheng Wu Hua Xue Yu Sheng Wu Wu Li Xue Bao (Shanghai).* **30**, 1–8.

Kaliberov, S.A., Buchsbaum, D.J., Gillespie, G.Y., Curiel, D.T., Arafat, W.O., Carpenter, M., Stackhouse, M.A. (2002) Adenovirus-mediated transfer of BAX driven by the vascular endothelial growth factor promoter induces apoptosis in lung cancer cells, *Mol. Ther.* **6**, 190–198.

Kanerva, A., Bauerschmitz, G.J., Yamamoto, M., Lam, J.T., Alvarez, R.D., Siegal, G.P., Curiel, D.T., Hemminki, A. (2004) A cyclooxygenase-2 promoter-based conditionally replicating adenovirus with enhanced infectivity for treatment of ovarian adenocarcinoma, *Gene Ther.* **11**, 552–559.

Kanerva, A., Mikheeva, G.V., Krasnykh, V., Coolidge, C.J., Lam, J.T., Mahasreshti, P.J., Barker, S.D., Straughn, M., Barnes, M.N., Alvarez, R.D., Hemminki, A., Curiel, D.T. (2002) Targeting adenovirus to the serotype 3 receptor increases gene transfer efficiency to ovarian cancer cells, *Clin. Cancer Res.* **8**, 275–280.

Kashentseva, E.A., Seki, T., Curiel, D.T., Dmitriev, I.P. (2002) Adenovirus targeting to c-erbB-2 oncoprotein by single-chain antibody fused to trimeric form of adenovirus receptor ectodomain, *Cancer Res.* **62**, 609–616.

Kasono, K., Blackwell, J.L., Douglas, J.T., Dmitriev, I., Strong, T.V., Reynolds, P., Kropf, D.A., Carroll, W.R., Peters, G.E., Bucy, R.P., Curiel, D.T., Krasnykh, V. (1999) Selective gene delivery to head and neck cancer cells via an integrin targeted adenoviral vector, *Clin. Cancer Res.* **5**, 2571–2579.

Katabi, M.M., Chan, H.L., Karp, S.E., Batist, G. (1999) Hexokinase type II: a novel tumor-specific promoter for gene-targeted therapy differentially expressed and regulated in human cancer cells, *Hum. Gene Ther.* **10**, 155–164.

Katz, M.H., Spivack, D.E., Takimoto, S., Fang, B., Burton, D.W., Moossa, A.R., Hoffman, R.M., Bouvet, M. (2003) Gene therapy of pancreatic cancer with green fluorescent protein and tumor necrosis factor-related apoptosis-inducing ligand fusion gene expression driven by a human telomerase reverse transcriptase promoter, *Ann. Surg. Oncol.* **10**, 762–772.

Kawakami, Y., Li, H., Lam, J.T., Krasnykh, V., Curiel, D.T., Blackwell, J.L. (2003) Substitution of the adenovirus serotype 5 knob with a serotype 3 knob enhances multiple steps in virus replication, *Cancer Res.* **63**, 1262–1269.

Kawashima, T., Kagawa, S., Kobayashi, N., Shirakiya, Y., Umeoka, T., Teraishi, F., Taki, M., Kyo, S., Tanaka, N., Fujiwara, T. (2004) Telomerase-specific replication-selective virotherapy for human cancer, *Clin. Cancer Res.* **10**, 285–292.

Kelly, F.J., Miller, C.R., Buchsbaum, D.J., Gomez-Navarro, J., Barnes, M.N., Alvarez, R.D., Curiel, D.T. (2000) Selectivity of TAG-72-targeted adenovirus gene transfer to primary ovarian carcinoma cells versus autologous mesothelial cells in vitro, *Clin. Cancer Res.* **6**, 4323–4333.

Kijima, T., Osaki, T., Nishino, K., Kumagai, T., Funakoshi, T., Goto, H., Tachibana, I., Tanio, Y., Kishimoto, T. (1999) Application of the Cre recombinase/loxP system further enhances antitumor effects in cell type-specific gene therapy against carcinoembryonic antigen-producing cancer, *Cancer Res.* **59**, 4906–4911.

Kilic, E., Hermann, D.M., Kugler, S., Kilic, U., Holzmuller, H., Schmeer, C., Bahr, M. (2002) Adenovirus-mediated Bcl-X(L) expression using a neuron-specific synapsin-1 promoter protects against disseminated neuronal injury and brain infarction following focal cerebral ischemia in mice, *Neurobiol. Dis.* **11**, 275–284.

Kim, E., Kim, J.H., Shin, H.Y., Lee, H., Yang, J.M., Kim, J., Sohn, J.H., Kim, H., Yun, C.O. (2003) Ad-mTERT-delta19, a conditional replication-competent adenovirus driven by the human telomerase promoter, selectively replicates in and elicits cytopathic effect in a cancer cell-specific manner, *Hum. Gene Ther.* **14**, 1415–1428.

Kiwaki, K., Kanegae, Y., Saito, I., Komaki, S., Nakamura, K., Miyazaki, J.I., Endo, F., Matsuda, I. (1996) Correction of ornithine transcarbamylase deficiency in adult spf(ash) mice and in OTC-deficient human hepatocytes with recombinant adenoviruses bearing the CAG promoter, *Hum. Gene Ther.* **7**, 821–830.

Kohno, S., Nakagawa, K., Hamada, K., Harada, H., Yamasaki, K., Hashimoto, K., Tagawa, M., Nagato, S., Furukawa, K., Ohnishi, T. (2004) Midkine promoter-based conditionally replicative adenovirus for malignant glioma therapy, *Oncol. Rep.* **12**, 73–78.

Komata, T., Koga, S., Hirohata, S., Takakura, M., Germano, I.M., Inoue, M., Kyo, S., Kondo, S., Kondo, Y. (2001) A novel treatment of human malignant gliomas in vitro and in vivo: FADD gene transfer under the control of the human telomerase reverse transcriptase gene promoter, *Int. J. Oncol.* **19**, 1015–1020.

Komata, T., Kondo, Y., Kanzawa, T., Ito, H., Hirohata, S., Koga, S., Sumiyoshi, H., Takakura, M., Inoue, M., Barna, B.P., Germano, I.M., Kyo, S., Kondo, S. (2002) Caspase-8 gene therapy using the human telomerase reverse transcriptase promoter for malignant glioma cells, *Hum. Gene Ther.* **13**, 1015–1025.

Korn, T., Nettelbeck, D.M., Volkel, T., Muller, R., Kontermann, R.E. (2004) Recombinant bispecific antibodies for the targeting of adenoviruses to CEA-expressing tumour cells: a comparative analysis of bacterially expressed single-chain diabody and tandem scFv, *J. Gene Med.* **6**, 642–651.

Korokhov, N., Mikheeva, G., Krendelshchikov, A., Belousova, N., Simonenko, V., Krendelshchikova, V., Pereboev, A., Kotov, A., Kotova, O., Triozzi, P.L., Aldrich, W.A., Douglas, J.T., Lo, K.M., Banerjee, P.T., Gillies, S.D., Curiel, D.T., Krasnykh, V. (2003) Targeting of adenovirus via genetic modification of the viral capsid combined with a protein bridge, *J. Virol.* **77**, 12931–12940.

Koshikawa, N., Takenaga, K., Tagawa, M., Sakiyama, S. (2000) Therapeutic efficacy of the suicide gene driven by the promoter of vascular endothelial growth factor gene against hypoxic tumor cells, *Cancer Res.* **60**, 2936–2941.

Kraaij, R., Van Rijswijk, A.L., Oomen, M.H., Haisma, H.J., Bangma, C.H. (2005) Prostate specific membrane antigen (PSMA) is a tissue-specific target for adenoviral transduction of prostate cancer in vitro, *Prostate*, **62**, 253–259.

Krasnykh, V.N., Mikheeva, G.V., Douglas, J.T., Curiel, D.T. (1996) Generation of recombinant adenovirus vectors with modified fibers for altering viral tropism, *J. Virol.* **70**, 6839–6846.

Krasnykh, V., Belousova, N., Korokhov, N., Mikheeva, G., Curiel, D.T. (2001) Genetic targeting of an adenovirus vector via replacement of the fiber protein with the phage T4 fibritin, *J. Virol.* **75**, 4176–4183.

Krasnykh, V., Dmitriev, I., Mikheeva, G., Miller, C.R., Belousova, N., Curiel, D.T. (1998) Characterization of an adenovirus vector containing a heterologous peptide epitope in the HI loop of the fiber knob, *J. Virol.* **72**, 1844–1852.

Kremer, E.J., Boutin, S., Chillon, M., Danos, O. (2000) Canine adenovirus vectors: an alternative for adenovirus-mediated gene transfer, *J. Virol.* **74**, 505–512.

Kubo, H., Gardner, T.A., Wada, Y., Koeneman, K.S., Gotoh, A., Yang, L., Kao, C., Lim, S.D., Amin, M.B., Yang, H., Black, M.E., Matsubara, S., Nakagawa, M., Gillenwater, J.Y., Zhau, H.E., Chung, L.W. (2003) Phase I dose escalation clinical trial of adenovirus vector carrying osteocalcin promoter-driven herpes simplex virus thymidine kinase in localized and metastatic hormone-refractory prostate cancer, *Hum. Gene Ther.* **14**, 227–241.

Kugler, S., Kilic, E., Bahr, M. (2003) Human synapsin 1 gene promoter confers highly neuron-specific long-term transgene expression from an adenoviral vector in the adult rat brain depending on the transduced area, *Gene Ther.* **10**, 337–347.

Kutchera, W., Jones, D.A., Matsunami, N., Groden, J., McIntyre, T.M., Zimmerman, G.A., White, R.L., Prescott, S.M. (1996) Prostaglandin H synthase 2 is expressed abnormally in human colon cancer: Evidence for a transcriptional effect, *Proc. Natl. Acad. Sci. U.S.A.* **93**, 4816–4820.

Lam, J.T., Kanerva, A., Bauerschmitz, G.J., Takayama, K., Suzuki, K., Yamamoto, M., Bhoola, S.M., Liu, B., Wang, M., Barnes, M.N., Alvarez, R.D., Siegal, G.P., Curiel, D.T., Hemminki, A. (2004) Inter-patient variation in efficacy of five oncolytic adenovirus candidates for ovarian cancer therapy, *J. Gene Med.* **6**, 1333–1342.

Lee, E.J., Martinson, F., Kotlar, T., Thimmapaya, B., Jameson, J.L. (2001) Adenovirus-mediated targeted expression of toxic genes to adrenocorticotropin-producing pituitary tumors using the proopiomelanocortin promoter, *J. Clin. Endocrinol. Metab.* **86**, 3400–3409.

Lee, A.K., Delellis, R.A., Rosen, P.P., Herbert-Stanton, T., Tallberg, K., Garcia, C., Wolfe, H. (1984) Alpha-lactalbumin as an immunohistochemical marker for metastatic breast carcinomas, *Am. J. Surg. Pathol.* **8**, 93–100.

Lim, H.Y., Ahn, M., Chung, H.C., Gardner, T.A., Kao, C., Lee, S.J., Kim, S.J. (2004) Tumor-specific gene therapy for uterine cervical cancer using MN/CA9-directed replication-competent adenovirus, *Cancer Gene Ther.* **11**, 532–538.

Lin, T., Huang, X., Gu, J., Zhang, L., Roth, J.A., Xiong, M., Curley, S.A., Yu, Y., Hunt, K.K., Fang, B. (2002) Long-term tumor-free survival from treatment with the GFP-TRAIL fusion gene expressed from the hTERT promoter in breast cancer cells, *Oncogene* **21**, 8020–8028.

Liu, Y., Ye, T., Sun, D., Maynard, J., Deisseroth, A. (2004) Conditionally replication-competent adenoviral vectors with enhanced infectivity for use in gene therapy of melanoma, *Hum. Gene Ther.* **15**, 637–647.

Liu, J., Zou, W.G., Lang, M.F., Luo, J., Sun, L.Y., Wang, X.N., Qian, Q.J., Liu, X.Y. (2002)

Cancer-specific killing by the CD suicide gene using the human telomerase reverse transcriptase promoter, *Int. J. Oncol.* **21**, 661–666.

Liu, F.F., Miller, N., Levin, W., Zanke, B., Cooper, B., Henry, M., Sherar, M.D., Pintilie, M., Hunt, J.W., Hill, R.P. (1996) The potential role of HSP70 as an indicator of response to radiation and hyperthermia treatments for recurrent breast cancer, *Int. J. Hyperthermia* **12**, 197–208.

Lovekin, C., Ellis, I.O., Locker, A., Robertson, J.F., Bell, J., Nicholson, R., Gullick, W.J., Elston, C.W., Blamey, R.W. (1991) c-erbB-2 oncoprotein expression in primary and advanced breast cancer, *Br. J. Cancer* **63**, 439–443.

Maemondo, M., Saijo, Y., Narumi, K., Kikuchi, T., Usui, K., Tazawa, R., Matsumoto, K., Nakamura, T., Sasaki, K., Takahashi, M., Niitsu, Y., Nukiwa, T. (2004) Gene therapy with secretory leukoprotease inhibitor promoter-controlled replication-competent adenovirus for non-small cell lung cancer, *Cancer Res.* **64**, 4611–4620.

Mallam, J.N., Hurwitz, M.Y., Mahoney, T., Chevez-Barrios, P., Hurwitz, R.L. (2004) Efficient gene transfer into retinal cells using adenoviral vectors: dependence on receptor expression, *Invest. Ophthalmol. Vis. Sci.* **45**, 1680–1687.

Matsumoto, K., Yoshimoto, J., Sugo, H., Kojima, K., Futagawa, S., Matsumoto, T. (2002) Relationship between the histological degrees of hepatitis and the postoperative recurrence of hepatocellular carcinoma in patients with hepatitis C, *Hepatol. Res.* **23**, 196–201.

McLaughlin, P.M., Trzpis, M., Kroesen, B.J., Helfrich, W., Terpstra, P., Dokter, W.H., Ruiters, M.H., de Leij, L.F., Harmsen, M.C. (2004) Use of the EGP-2/Ep-CAM promoter for targeted expression of heterologous genes in carcinoma derived cell lines, *Cancer Gene Ther.* **11**, 603–612.

Messina, M., Yu, D.M., Learoyd, D.L., Both, G.W., Molloy, P.L., Robinson, B.G. (2003) High level, tissue-specific expression of a modified calcitonin/calcitonin gene-related peptide promoter in a human medullary thyroid carcinoma cell line, *Mol. Cell. Endocrinol.* **164**, 219–224.

Miller, C.R., Buchsbaum, D.J., Reynolds, P.N., Douglas, J.T., Gillespie, G.Y., Mayo, M.S., Raben, D., Curiel, D.T. (1998) Differential susceptibility of primary and established human glioma cells to adenovirus infection: targeting via the epidermal growth factor receptor achieves fiber receptor-independent gene transfer, *Cancer Res.* **58**, 5738–5748.

Mink, S., Hartig, E., Jennewein, P., Doppler, W., Cato, A.C. (1992) A mammary cell-specific enhancer in mouse mammary tumor virus DNA is composed of multiple regulatory elements including binding sites for CTF/NFI and a novel transcription factor, mammary cell-activating factor, *Mol. Cell. Biol.* **12**, 4906–4918.

Mizuguchi, H., Hayakawa, T. (2002) Adenovirus vectors containing chimeric type 5 and type 35 fiber proteins exhibit altered and expanded tropism and increase the size limit of foreign genes, *Gene* **285**, 69–77.

Molina, R., Filella, X., Zanon, G., Pahisa, J., Alicarte, J., Munoz, M., Farrus, B., Ballesta, A.M. (2003) Prospective evaluation of tumor markers (c-erbB-2 oncoprotein, CEA and CA 15.3) in patients with locoregional breast cancer, *Anticancer Res.* **23**, 1043–1050.

Morimoto, E., Inase, N., Miyake, S., Yoshizawa, Y. (2001) Adenovirus-mediated suicide gene transfer to small cell lung carcinoma using a tumor-specific promoter, *Anticancer Res.* **21**, 329–331.

Morita, A., Ariizumi, K., Ritter, R. III, Jester, J.V., Kumamoto, T., Johnston, S.A., Takashima, A., (2001) Development of a Langerhans cell-targeted gene therapy format using a dendritic cell-specific promoter, *Gene Ther.* **8**, 1729–1737.

Muller, A., Homey, B., Soto, H., Ge, N., Catron, D., Buchanan, M.E., McClanahan, T., Murphy, E., Yuan, W., Wagner, S.N., Barrera, J.L., Mohar, A., Verastegui, E., Zlotnik, A. (2001) Involvement of chemokine receptors in breast cancer metastasis, *Nature* **410**, 50–56.

Nakamura, M., Kyo, S., Kanaya, T., Yatabe, N., Maida, Y., Tanaka, M., Ishida, Y., Fujii, C., Kondo, T., Inoue, M., Mukaida, N. (2004) hTERT-promoter-based tumor-specific expression of MCP-1 effectively sensitizes cervical cancer cells to a low dose of cisplatin, *Cancer Gene Ther.* **11**, 1–7.

Nakaya, H., Ishizu, A., Ikeda, H., Tahara, M., Shindo, J., Itoh, R., Takahashi, T., Asaka, M., Ishikura, H., Yoshiki, T. (2003) In vitro model of suicide gene therapy for alpha-fetoprotein-producing gastric cancer, *Anticancer Res.* **23**, 3795–3800.

Nettelbeck, D.M., Rivera, A.A., Balague, C., Alemany, R., Curiel, D.T. (2002) Novel oncolytic adenoviruses targeted to melanoma: specific viral replication and cytolysis by expression of E1A mutants from the tyrosinase enhancer/promoter, *Cancer Res.* **62**, 4663–4670.

Nettelbeck, D.M., Rivera, A.A., Davydova, J., Dieckmann, D., Yamamoto, M., Curiel, D.T. (2003) Cyclooxygenase-2 promoter for tumour-specific targeting of adenoviral vectors to melanoma, *Melanoma Res.* **13**, 287–292.

Nettelbeck, D.M., Rivera, A.A., Kupsch, J., Dieckmann, D., Douglas, J.T., Kontermann, R.E., Alemany, R., Curiel, D.T. (2004) Retargeting of adenoviral infection to melanoma: combining genetic ablation of native tropism with a recombinant bispecific single-chain diabody (scDb) adapter that binds to fiber knob and HMWMAA, *Int. J. Cancer* **108**, 136–145.

Nicklin, S.A., Reynolds, P.N., Brosnan, M.J., White, S.J., Curiel, D.T., Dominiczak, A.F., Baker, A.H. (2001) Analysis of cell-specific promoters for viral gene therapy targeted at the vascular endothelium, *Hypertension* **38**, 65–70.

Nicklin, S.A., Von Seggern, D.J., Work, L.M., Pek, D.C., Dominiczak, A.F., Nemerow, G.R., Baker, A.H. (2001) Ablating adenovirus type 5 fiber-CAR binding and HI loop insertion of the SIGYPLP peptide generate an endothelial cell-selective adenovirus, *Mol. Ther.* **4**, 534–542.

Nicklin, S.A., Dishart, K.L., Buening, H., Reynolds, P.N., Hallek, M., Nemerow, G.R., Von Seggern, D.J., Baker, A.H. (2003) Transductional and transcriptional targeting of cancer cells using genetically engineered viral vectors, *Cancer Lett.* **201**, 165–173.

Nishimura, R., Nagao, K., Miyayama, H., Matsuda, M., Baba, K., Matsuoka, Y., Yamashita, H. (2003) Elevated serum CA15-3 levels correlate with positive estrogen receptor and initial favorable outcome in patients who died from recurrent breast cancer, *Breast Cancer* **10**, 220–227.

Nyati, M.K., Sreekumar, A., Li, S., Zhang, M., Rynkiewicz, S.D., Chinnaiyan, A.M., Rehemtulla, A., Lawrence, T.S. (2002) High and selective expression of yeast cytosine deaminase under a carcinoembryonic antigen promoter-enhancer, *Cancer Res.* **62**, 2337–2342.

Okada, N., Mori, N., Koretomo, R., Okada, Y., Nakayama, T., Yoshie, O., Mizuguchi, H., Hayakawa, T., Nakagawa, S., Mayumi, T., Fujita, T., Yamamoto, A. (2005) Augmentation of the migratory ability of DC-based vaccine into regional lymph nodes by efficient CCR7 gene transduction, *Gene Ther.* **12**, 129–139.

Olmsted-Davis, E.A., Gugala, Z., Gannon, F.H., Yotnda, P., McAlhany, R.E., Lindsey, R.W., Davis, A.R. (2002) Use of a chimeric adenovirus vector enhances BMP2 production and bone formation, *Hum. Gene Ther.* **13**, 1337–1347.

Onishi, T., Nouso, K., Higashi, T., Toshikuni, N., Nakatsukasa, H., Kobayashi, Y., Uemura, M., Yumoto, E., Fujiwara, K., Sato, S., Nakamura, S., Yokoyama, J., Hanafusa, T., Shiratori, Y. (2003) Cellular distribution of telomerase reverse transcriptase in human hepatocellular carcinoma, *J. Gastroenterol. Hepatol.* **18**, 1168–1174.

Pandha, H.S., Martin, L.A., Rigg, A., Hurst, H.C., Stamp, G.W., Sikora, K., Lemoine, N.R. (1999) Genetic prodrug activation therapy for breast cancer: a phase I clinical trial of erbB-2-directed suicide gene expression, *J. Clin. Oncol.* **17**, 2180–2189.

Park, H.S., Cheon, J., Cho, H.Y., Ko, Y.H., Bae, J.H., Moon, D.G., Kim, J.J. (2003) In vivo characterization of a prostate-specific antigen promoter-based suicide gene therapy for the treatment of benign prostatic hyperplasia, *Gene Ther.* **10**, 1129–1134.

Park, C.W., Park, Y.M., Lee, G.T., Lee, Y., Woo, S., Cha, J.Y., Ahn, C.W., Cha, B.S., Kim, K.S., Ahn, Y.H., Lee, H.C. (2004) Targeting of therapeutic gene expression to the liver by using liver-type pyruvate kinase proximal promoter and the SV40 viral enhancer active in multiple cell types, *Biochem. Biophys. Res. Commun.* **314**, 131–137.

Parrott, M.B., Adams, K.E., Mercier, G.T., Mok, H., Campos, S.K., Barry, M.A. (2003) Metabolically biotinylated adenovirus for cell targeting, ligand screening, and vector purification, *Mol. Ther.* **8**, 688–700.

Peng, S.Y., Lai, P.L., Chu, J.S., Lee, P.H., Tsung, P.T., Chen, D.S., Hsu, H.C. (1993) Expression and hypomethylation of alpha-fetoprotein gene in unicentric and multicentric human hepatocellular carcinomas, *Hepatology* **17**, 35–41.

Peng, X.Y., Won, J.H., Rutherford, T., Fujii, T., Zelterman, D., Pizzorno, G., Sapi, E., Leavitt, J., Kacinski, B., Crystal, R., Schwartz, P., Deisseroth, A. (2001) The use of the L-plastin promoter for adenoviral-mediated, tumor-specific gene expression in ovarian and bladder cancer cell lines, *Cancer Res.* **61**, 4405–4413.

Pereboev, A.V., Nagle, J.M., Shakhmatov, M.A., Triozzi, P.L., Matthews, Q.L., Kawakami, Y., Curiel, D.T., Blackwell, J.L. (2004) Enhanced gene transfer to mouse dendritic cells using adenoviral vectors coated with a novel adapter molecule, *Mol. Ther.* **9**, 712–720.

Pereboev, A.V., Asiedu, C.K., Kawakami, Y., Dong, S.S., Blackwell, J.L., Kashentseva, E.A., Triozzi, P.L., Aldrich, W.A., Curiel, D.T., Thomas, J.M., Dmitriev, I.P. (2002) Coxsackie-virus-adenovirus receptor genetically fused to anti-human CD40 scFv enhances adenoviral transduction of dendritic cells, *Gene Ther.* **9**, 1189–1193.

Peshavaria, M., Henderson, E., Sharma, A., Wright, C.V., Stein, R. (1997) Functional characterization of the transactivation properties of the PDX-1 homeodomain protein, *Mol. Cell. Biol.* **17**, 3987–3996.

Peter, I., Graf, C., Dummer, R., Schaffner, W., Greber, U.F., Hemmi, S. (2003) A novel attenuated replication-competent adenovirus for melanoma therapy, *Gene Ther.* **10**, 530–539.

Plate, K.H., Breier, G., Weich, H.A., Risau, W. (1992) Vascular endothelial growth factor is a potential tumour angiogenesis factor in human gliomas in vivo, *Nature* **359**, 276–280.

Pollmann, A., Kabisch, H., Block, A., Muller, J., Hellwinkel, O.J. (2004) Limited specificity of promoter constructs for gene therapy in osteosarcoma, *Int. J. Mol. Med.* **14**, 737–742.

Pramudji, C., Shimura, S., Ebara, S., Yang, G., Wang, J., Ren, C., Yuan, Y., Tahir, S.A., Timme, T.L., Thompson, T.C. (2001) In situ prostate cancer gene therapy using a novel adenoviral vector regulated by the caveolin-1 promoter, *Clin. Cancer Res.* **7**, 4272–4279.

Qiao, J., Doubrovin, M., Sauter, B.V., Huang, Y., Guo, Z.S., Balatoni, J., Akhurst, T., Blasberg, R.G., Tjuvajev, J.G., Chen, S.H., Woo, S.L. (2002) Tumor-specific transcriptional targeting of suicide gene therapy of suicide gene therapy, *Gene Ther.* **9**, 168–175.

Quirk, S.J., Gannell, J.E., Funder, J.W. (1988) Alpha-lactalbumin production by rat mammary gland: prepartum emergence of resistance to glucocorticoids and progestins, *Mol. Cell. Biol.* **58**, 183–189.

Rancourt, C., Rogers, B.E., Sosnowski, B.A., Wang, M., Piche, A., Pierce, G.F., Alvarez, R.D., Siegal, G.P., Douglas, J.T., Curiel, D.T. (1998) Basic fibroblast growth factor enhancement of adenovirus-mediated delivery of the herpes simplex virus thymidine kinase gene results in augmented therapeutic benefit in a murine model of ovarian cancer, *Clin. Cancer Res.* **4**, 2455–2461.

Rasmussen, H., Rasmussen, C., Lempicki, M., Durham, R., Brough, D., King, C.R., Weichselbaum, R. (2002) TNFerade Biologic: preclinical toxicology of a novel adenovector with a radiation-inducible promoter, carrying the human tumor necrosis factor alpha gene, *Cancer Gene Ther.* **9**, 951–957.

Rea, D., Havenga, M.J., van Den Assem, M., Sutmuller, R.P., Lemckert, A., Hoeben, R.C., Bout, A., Melief, C.J., Offringa, R. (2001) Highly efficient transduction of human monocyte-derived dendritic cells with subgroup B fiber-modified adenovirus vectors enhances transgene-encoded antigen presentation to cytotoxic T cells, *J. Immunol.* **166**, 5236–5244.

Rein, D.T., Breidenbach, M., Nettelbeck, D.M., Kawakami, Y., Siegal, G.P., Huh, W.K., Wang, M., Hemminki, A., Bauerschmitz, G.J., Yamamoto, M., Adachi, Y., Takayama, K., Dall, P., Curiel, D.T. (2004) Evaluation of tissue-specific promoters in carcinomas of the cervix uteri, *J. Gene Med.* **6**, 1281–1289.

Rempel, A., Bannasch, P., Mayer, D. (1994) Differences in expression and intracellular distribution of hexokinase isoenzymes in rat liver cells of different transformation stages, *Biochim. Biophys. Acta* **1219**, 660–668.

Reynolds, P.N., Dmitriev, I., Curiel, D.T. (1999) Insertion of an RGD motif into the HI loop of adenovirus fiber protein alters the distribution of transgene expression of the systemically administered vector, *Gene Ther.* **6**, 1336–1339.

Reynolds, P.N., Nicklin, S.A., Kaliberova, L., Boatman, B.G., Grizzle, W.E., Balyasnikova, I.V., Baker, A.H., Danilov, S.M., Curiel, D.T. (2001) Combined transductional and transcriptional targeting improves the specificity of transgene expression in vivo, *Nat. Biotechnol.* **19**, 838–842.

Reynolds, P.N., Zinn, K.R., Gavrilyuk, V.D., Balyasnikova, I.V., Rogers, B.E., Buchsbaum, D.J., Wang, M.H., Miletich, D.J., Grizzle, W.E., Douglas, J.T., Danilov, S.M., Curiel, D.T. (2000) A targetable, injectable adenoviral vector for selective gene delivery to pulmonary endothelium in vivo, *Mol. Ther.* **2**, 562–578.

Ristimaki, A., Honkanen, N., Jankala, H., Sipponen, P., Harkonen, M. (1997) Expression of cyclooxygenase-2 in human gastric carcinoma, *Cancer Res.* **57**, 1276–1280.

Rivera, A.A., Davydova, J., Schierer, S., Wang, M., Krasnykh, V., Yamamoto, M., Curiel, D.T., Nettelbeck, D.M. (2004) Combining high selectivity of replication with fiber chimerism for effective adenoviral oncolysis of CAR-negative melanoma cells, *Gene Ther.* **11**, 1694–1702.

Ross, R., Sudowe, S., Beisner, J., Ross, X.L., Ludwig-Portugall, I., Steitz, J., Tuting, T., Knop, J., Reske-Kunz, A.B. (2003) Transcriptional targeting of dendritic cells for gene therapy using the promoter of the cytoskeletal protein fascin, *Gene Ther.* **10**, 1035–1040.

Rothfels, H., Paschen, A., Schadendorf, D. (2003) Evaluation of combined gene regulatory elements for transcriptional targeting of suicide gene expression to malignant melanoma, *Exp. Dermatol.* **12**, 799–810.

Sakai, Y., Kaneko, S., Sato, Y., Kanegae, Y., Tamaoki, T., Saito, I., Kobayashi, K. (2001) Gene therapy for hepatocellular carcinoma using two recombinant adenovirus vectors with alpha-fetoprotein promoter and Cre/lox P system, *J. Virol. Methods* **92**, 5–17.

Savontaus, M.J., Sauter, B.V., Huang, T.G., Woo, S.L. (2002) Transcriptional targeting of conditionally replicating adenovirus to dividing endothelial cells, *Gene Ther.* **9**, 972–979.

Schmidt, M., Heimberger, T., Gruensfelder, P., Schler, G., Hoppe, F. (2004) Inducible promoters for gene therapy of head and neck cancer: an in vitro study, *Eur. Arch. Otorhinolaryngol.* **261**, 208–215.

Schoggins, J.W., Gall, J.G., Falck-Pedersen, E. (2003) Subgroup B and F fiber chimeras eliminate normal adenovirus type 5 vector transduction in vitro and in vivo, *J. Virol.* **77**, 1039–1048.

Shayakhmetov, D.M., Papayannopoulou, T., Stamatoyannopoulos, G., Lieber, A. (2000) Efficient gene transfer into human CD34(+)

cells by a retargeted adenovirus vector, *J. Virol.* **74**, 2567–2583.

Shayakhmetov, D.M., Li, Z.Y., Ternovoi, V., Gaggar, A., Gharwan, H., Lieber, A. (2003) The interaction between the fiber knob domain and the cellular attachment receptor determines the intracellular trafficking route of adenoviruses, *J. Virol.* **77**, 3712–3723.

Shen, L.Z., Wu, W.X., Xu, D.H., Zheng, Z.C., Liu, X.Y., Ding, Q., Hua, Y.B., Yao, K. (2002) Specific CEA-producing colorectal carcinoma cell killing with recombinant adenoviral vector containing cytosine deaminase gene, *World J. Gastroenterol.* **8**, 270–275.

Shi, Q., Wilcox, D.A., Fahs, S.A., Kroner, P.A., Montgomery, R.R. (2003) Expression of human factor VIII under control of the platelet-specific alphaIIb promoter in megakaryocytic cell line as well as storage together with VWF, *Mol. Genet. Metab.* **79**, 25–33.

Shirakawa, T., Hamada, K., Zhang, Z., Okada, H., Tagawa, M., Kamidono, S., Kawabata, M., Gotoh, A. (2004) A cox-2 promoter-based replication-selective adenoviral vector to target the cox-2-expressing human bladder cancer cells, *Clin. Cancer Res.* **10**, 4342–4348.

Singh, J., Hamid, R., Reddy, B.S. (1997) Dietary fat and colon cancer: modulation of cyclooxygenase-2 by types and amount of dietary fat during the postinitiation stage of colon carcinogenesis, *Cancer Res.* **57**, 3465–3470.

Slager, E.H., van der Minne, C.E., Goudsmit, J., van Oers, J.M., Kostense, S., Havenga, M.J., Osanto, S., Griffioen, M. (2004) Induction of CAMEL/NY-ESO-ORF2-specific CD8+ T cells upon stimulation with dendritic cells infected with a modified Ad5 vector expressing a chimeric Ad5/35 fiber, *Cancer Gene Ther.* **11**, 227–236.

Song, J.S., Kim, H.P., Yoon, W.S., Lee, K.W., Kim, M.H., Kim, K.T., Kim, H.S., Kim, Y.T. (2003) Adenovirus-mediated suicide gene therapy using the human telomerase catalytic subunit (hTERT) gene promoter induced apoptosis of ovarian cancer cell line, *Biosci. Biotechnol. Biochem.* **67**, 2344–2350.

Soudais, C., Laplace-Builhe, C., Kissa, K., Kremer, E.J. (2001) Preferential transduction of neurons by canine adenovirus vectors and their efficient retrograde transport in vivo, *FASEB J.* **15**, 2283–2285.

Southgate, T.D., Windeatt, S., Smith-Arica, J., Gerdes, C.A., Perone, M.J., Morris, I., Davis,

J.R., Klatzmann, D., Lowenstein, P.R., Castro, M.G. (2000) Transcriptional targeting to anterior pituitary lactotrophic cells using recombinant adenovirus vectors in vitro and in vivo in normal and estrogen/sulpiride-induced hyperplastic anterior pituitaries, *Endocrinology* **141**, 3493–3505.

Stahlecker, J., Gauger, A., Bosserhoff, A., Buttner, R., Ring, J., Hein, R. (2000) MIA as a reliable tumor marker in the serum of patients with malignant melanoma, *Anticancer Res.* **20**, 5041–5044.

Stecher, H., Shayakhmetov, D.M., Stamatoyannopoulos, G., Lieber, A. (2001) A capsid-modified adenovirus vector devoid of all viral genes: assessment of transduction and toxicity in human hematopoietic cells, *Mol. Ther.* **4**, 36–44.

Steffens, S., Sandquist, A., Frank, S., Fischer, U., Lex, C., Rainov, N.G., Kramm, C.M. (2004) A neuroblastoma-selective suicide gene therapy approach using the tyrosine hydroxylase promoter, *Pediatr. Res.* **56**, 268–277.

Stevenson, S.C., Rollence, M., Marshall-Neff, J., McClelland, A. (1997) Selective targeting of human cells by a chimeric adenovirus vector containing a modified fiber protein, *J. Virol.* **71**, 4782–4790.

Stevenson, S.C., Rollence, M., White, B., Weaver, L., McClelland, A. (1995) Human adenovirus serotypes 3 and 5 bind to two different cellular receptors via the fiber head domain, *J. Virol.* **69**, 2850–2857.

Stoffers, D.A., Zinkin, N.T., Stanojevic, V., Clarke, W.L., Habener, J.F. (1997) Pancreatic agenesis attributable to a single nucleotide deletion in the human IPF1 gene coding sequence, *Nat. Genet.* **15**, 106–110.

Szary, J., Kalita, K., Przybyszewska, M., Dus, D., Kieda, C., Janik, P., Szala, S. (2001) KDR promoter can transcriptionally target cytosine deaminase suicide gene to cancer cells of nonendothelial origin, *Anticancer Res.* **21**, 3471–3475.

Takeda, T., Inaba, H., Yamazaki, M., Kyo, S., Miyamoto, T., Suzuki, S., Ehara, T., Kakizawa, T., Hara, M., DeGroot, L.J., Hashizume, K. (2003) Tumor-specific gene therapy for undifferentiated thyroid carcinoma utilizing the telomerase reverse transcriptase promoter, *J. Clin. Endocrinol. Metab.* **88**, 3531–3538.

Takeda, T., Yamazaki, M., Minemura, K., Imai, Y., Inaba, H., Suzuki, S., Miyamoto, T.,

Ichikawa, K., Kakizawa, T., Mori, J., DeGroot, L.J., Hashizume, K. (2002) A tandemly repeated thyroglobulin core promoter has potential to enhance efficacy for tissue-specific gene therapy for thyroid carcinomas, *Cancer Gene Ther.* **9**, 864–874.

Tanaka, M., Inase, N., Miyake, S., Yoshizawa, Y. (2001) Neuron specific enolase promoter for suicide gene therapy in small cell lung carcinoma, *Anticancer Res.* **21**, 291–294.

Tanyi, J.L., Lapushin, R., Eder, A., Auersperg, N., Tabassam, F.H., Roth, J.A., Gu, J., Fang, B., Mills, G.B., Wolf, J. (2002) Identification of tissue- and cancer-selective promoters for the introduction of genes into human ovarian cancer cells, *Gynecol. Oncol.* **85**, 451–458.

Tillman, B.W., de Gruijl, T.D., Luykx-de Bakker, S.A., Scheper, R.J., Pinedo, H.M., Curiel, T.J., Gerritsen, W.R., Curiel, D.T. (1999) Maturation of dendritic cells accompanies high-efficiency gene transfer by a CD40-targeted adenoviral vector, *J. Immunol.* **162**, 6378–6383.

Tirone, T., Fagan, S.P., Templeton, N.S., Wang, X., Brunicardi, F.C. (2001) Insulinoma-induced hypoglycemic death in mice is prevented with beta cell specific gene therapy, *Ann. Surg. Oncol.* **233**, 603–611.

Toietta, G., Koehler, D.R., Finegold, M.J., Lee, B., Hu, J., Beaudet, A.L. (2003) Reduced inflammation and improved airway expression using helper-dependent adenoviral vectors with a K18 promoter, *Mol. Ther.* **7**, 649–658.

Torbenson, M., Kannangai, R., Abraham, S., Sahin, F., Choti, M., Wang, J. (2004) Concurrent evaluation of p53, beta-catenin, and alpha-fetoprotein expression in human hepatocellular carcinoma, *Am. J. Clin. Pathol.* **122**, 377–382.

Tsujii, M., DuBois, R.N. (1995) Alterations in cellular adhesion and apoptosis in epithelial cells overexpressing prostaglandin endoperoxide synthase 2, *Cell* **83**, 493–501.

Uchida, A., O'Keefe, D.S., Bacich, D.J., Molloy, P.L., Heston, W.D. (2001) In vivo suicide gene therapy model using a newly discovered prostate-specific membrane antigen promoter/enhancer: a potential alternative approach to androgen deprivation therapy, *Urology* **58**, 132–139.

Ueda, K., Iwahashi, M., Nakamori, M., Nakamura, M., Matsuura, I., Yamaue, H., Tanimura, H. (2001) Carcinoembryonic antigen-specific suicide gene therapy of cytosine deaminase/5-fluorocytosine enhanced by the cre/loxP system in the orthotopic gastric carcinoma model, *Cancer Res.* **61**, 6158–6162.

Ueda, K., Iwahashi, M., Nakamori, M., Nakamura, M., Matsuura, I., Ojima, T., Yamaue, H. (2003) Improvement of carcinoembryonic antigen-specific prodrug gene therapy for experimental colon cancer, *Surgery* **133**, 309–317.

van der Eb, M.M., Cramer, S.J., Vergouwe, Y., Schagen, F.H., van Krieken, J.H., van der Eb, A.J., Rinkes, I.H., van de Velde, C.J., Hoeben, R.C. (1998) Severe hepatic dysfunction after adenovirus-mediated transfer of the herpes simplex virus thymidine kinase gene and ganciclovir administration, *Gene Ther.* **5**, 451–458.

Vandier, D., Rixe, O., Besnard, F., Kim, M., Rikiyama, T., Goldsmith, M., Brenner, M., Gouyette, A., Cowan, K.H. (2000) Inhibition of glioma cells in vitro and in vivo using a recombinant adenoviral vector containing an astrocyte-specific promoter, *Cancer Gene Ther.* **7**, 1120–1126.

Varga, M.J., Weibull, C., Everitt, E. (1991) Infectious entry pathway of adenovirus type 2, *J. Virol.* **65**, 6061–6070.

Varnavski, A.N., Calcedo, R., Bove, M., Gao, G., Wilson, J.M. (2005) Evaluation of toxicity from high-dose systemic administration of recombinant adenovirus vector in vector-naive and pre-immunized mice, *Gene Ther.* **12**, 427–436.

Velasco, B., Ramirez, J.R., Relloso, M., Li, C., Kumar, S., Lopez-Bote, J.P., Perez-Barriocanal, F., Lopez-Novoa, J.M., Cowan, P.J., d'Apice, A.J., Bernabeu, C. (2001) Vascular gene transfer driven by endoglin and ICAM-2 endothelial-specific promoters, *Gene Ther.* **8**, 897–904.

Volk, A.L., Rivera, A.A., Kanerva, A., Bauerschmitz, G., Dmitriev, I., Nettelbeck, D.M., Curiel, D.T. (2003) Enhanced adenovirus infection of melanoma cells by fiber-modification: incorporation of RGD peptide or Ad5/3 chimerism, *Cancer Biol. Ther.* **2**, 511–515.

Volpers, C., Thirion, C., Biermann, V., Hussmann, S., Kewes, H., Dunant, P., von der Mark, H., Herrmann, A., Kochanek, S., Lochmuller, H. (2003) Antibody-mediated targeting of an adenovirus vector modified to contain a synthetic immunoglobulin g-binding domain in the capsid, *J. Virol.* **77**, 2093–2104.

Von Seggern, D.J., Huang, S., Fleck, S.K., Stevenson, S.C., Nemerow, G.R. (2000) Adenovirus vector pseudotyping in fiber-expressing cell lines: improved transduction of epstein-barr virus-transformed B cells, *J. Virol.* **74**, 354–362.

Walther, W., Stein, U. (1996) Cell type specific and inducible promoters for vectors in gene therapy as an approach for cell targeting, *J. Mol. Med.* **74**, 379–392.

Wang, X.P., Yazawa, K., Yang, J., Kohn, D., Fisher, W.E., Brunicardi, F.C. (2004) Specific gene expression and therapy for pancreatic cancer using the cytosine deaminase gene directed by the rat insulin promoter, *J. Gastrointest. Surg.* **8**, 98–108.

Wesseling, J.G., Yamamoto, M., Adachi, Y., Bosma, P.J., van Wijland, M., Blackwell, J.L., Li, H., Reynolds, P.N., Dmitriev, I., Vickers, S.M., Huibregtse, K., Curiel, D.T. (2001) Midkine and cyclooxygenase-2 promoters are promising for adenoviral vector gene delivery of pancreatic carcinoma, *Cancer Gene Ther.* **8**, 990–996.

Wickham, T.J., Mathias, P., Cheresh, D.A., Nemerow, G.R. (1993) Integrins alpha v beta 3 and alpha v beta 5 promote adenovirus internalization but not virus attachment, *Cell* **73**, 309–319.

Wickham, T.J., Tzeng, E., Shears, L.L. II, Roelvink, P.W., Li, Y., Lee, G.M., Brough, D.E., Lizonova, A., Kovesdi, I. (1997) Increased in vitro and in vivo gene transfer by adenovirus vectors containing chimeric fiber proteins, *J. Virol.* **71**, 8221–8229.

Wirth, T., Zender, L., Schulte, B., Mundt, B., Plentz, R., Rudolph, K.L., Manns, M., Kubicka, S., Kuhnel, F. (2003) A telomerase-dependent conditionally replicating adenovirus for selective treatment of cancer, *Cancer Res.* **63**, 3181–3188.

Work, L.M., Ritchie, N., Nicklin, S.A., Reynolds, P.N., Baker, A.H. (2004) Dual targeting of gene delivery by genetic modification of adenovirus serotype 5 fibers and cell-selective transcriptional control, *Gene Ther.* **11**, 1296–1300.

Worthington, J., McCarthy, H.O., Barrett, E., Adams, C., Robson, T., Hirst, D.G. (2004) Use of the radiation-inducible WAF1 promoter to drive iNOS gene therapy as a novel anti-cancer treatment, *J. Gene Med.* **6**, 673–680.

Wu, H., Han, T., Lam, J.T., Leath, C.A., Dmitriev, I., Kashentseva, E., Barnes, M.N., Alvarez, R.D., Curiel, D.T. (2004) Preclinical evaluation of a class of infectivity-enhanced adenoviral vectors in ovarian cancer gene therapy, *Gene Ther.* **11**, 874–878.

Xie, X., Zhao, X., Liu, Y., Young, C.Y., Tindall, D.J., Slawin, K.M., Spencer, D.M. (2001) Robust prostate-specific expression for targeted gene therapy based on the human kallikrein 2 promoter, *Hum. Gene Ther.* **12**, 549–561.

Yamamoto, M., Alemany, R., Adachi, Y., Grizzle, W.E., Curiel, D.T. (2001) Characterization of the cyclooxygenase-2 promoter in an adenoviral vector and its application for the mitigation of toxicity in suicide gene therapy of gastrointestinal cancers, *Mol. Ther.* **3**, 385–394.

Yamamoto, M., Davydova, J., Wang, M., Siegal, G.P., Krasnykh, V., Vickers, S.M., Curiel, D.T. (2003) Infectivity enhanced, cyclooxygenase-2 promoter-based conditionally replicative adenovirus for pancreatic cancer, *Gastroenterology* **125**, 1203–1218.

Yamamura, H., Hashio, M., Noguchi, M., Sugenoya, Y., Osakada, M., Hirano, N., Sasaki, Y., Yoden, T., Awata, N., Araki, N., Tatsuta, M., Miyatake, S.I., Takahashi, K. (2001) Identification of the transcriptional regulatory sequences of human calponin promoter and their use in targeting a conditionally replicating herpes vector to malignant human soft tissue and bone tumors, *Cancer Res.* **61**, 3969–3977.

Yoshimura, I., Ikegami, S., Suzuki, S., Tadakuma, T., Hayakawa, M. (2002) Adenovirus mediated prostate specific enzyme prodrug gene therapy using prostate specific antigen promoter enhanced by the Cre-loxP system, *J. Urol.* **168**, 2659–2664.

Yotnda, P., Onishi, H., Heslop, H.E., Shayakhmetov, D., Lieber, A., Brenner, M., Davis, A. (2001) Efficient infection of primitive hematopoietic stem cells by modified adenovirus, *Gene Ther.* **8**, 930–937.

Yu, L., Hamada, K., Namba, M., Kadomatsu, K., Muramatsu, T., Matsubara, S., Tagawa, M. (2004) Midkine promoter-driven suicide gene expression and -mediated adenovirus replication produced cytotoxic effects to immortalized and tumour cells, *Eur. J. Cancer* **40**, 1787–1794.

Zabner, J., Chillon, M., Grunst, T., Moninger, T.O., Davidson, B.L., Gregory, R., Armentano, D. (1999) A chimeric type 2 adenovirus vector with a type 17 fiber enhances gene transfer to human airway epithelia, *J. Virol.* **73**, 8689–8695.

Zhang, R., Straus, F.H., DeGroot, L.J. (2001) Adenoviral-mediated gene therapy for thyroid carcinoma using thymidine kinase controlled by thyroglobulin promoter demonstrates high specificity and low toxicity, *Thyroid* **11**, 115–123.

Zhang, L., Akbulut, H., Tang, Y., Peng, X., Pizzorno, G., Sapi, E., Manegold, S., Deisseroth, A. (2002) Adenoviral vectors with E1A regulated by tumor-specific promoters are selectively cytolytic for breast cancer and melanoma, *Mol. Ther.* **6**, 386–393.

Zhang, Y., Yu, J., Unni, E., Shao, T.C., Nan, B., Snabboon, T., Kasper, S., Andriani, F., Denner, L., Marcelli, M. (2002) Monogene and polygene therapy for the treatment of experimental prostate cancers by use of apoptotic genes bax and bad driven by the prostate-specific promoter ARR(2)PB, *Hum. Gene Ther.* **13**, 2051–2064.

Zhu, Z.B., Makhija, S.K., Lu, B., Wang, M., Kaliberova, L., Liu, B., Rivera, A.A., Nettelbeck, D.M., Mahasreshti, P.J., Leath, C.A., III, Yamaoto, M., Alvarez, R.D., Curiel, D.T. (2004) Transcriptional targeting of adenoviral vector through the CXCR4 tumor-specific promoter, *Gene Ther.* **11**, 645–658.

Zhu, Z.B., Makhija, S.K., Lu, B., Wang, M., Kaliberova, L., Liu, B., Rivera, A.A., Nettelbeck, D.M., Mahasreshti, P.J., Leath, C.A., Barker, S., Yamaoto, M., Li, F., Alvarez, R.D., Curiel, D.T. (2004) Transcriptional targeting of tumors with a novel tumor-specific survivin promoter, *Cancer Gene Ther.* **11**, 256–262.

Index

a

A-ring   782
A-ring complexion   786–787
AAV, *see* adeno-associated virus
ABC transporter   93, 432
ABCA1   970, 981, 984
Abraham   91
absolv   74
absorption   113
absorption, distribution, metabolism and
   excretion, *see* ADME
accommodation   589
   antidonor antibody   589
ACE, *see* angiotensin converting enzyme
acetaminophen   50, 55
acetylation   52
   xenobiotic amino group   52
acetylcholinesterase   19ff
α 1-acid glycoprotein   97
acrylaldehyde   56
active targeting   152–155
acute lymphoblastic leukemia (ALL)   758
acute myeloid leukemia (AML)   165
acute vascular rejection   587
N-acyl transferase   41
ADA, *see* adenosine deaminase
Ad vector   1061
adaptor molecule   1061–1062
ADCC, *see* antibody-dependent cellular
   cytotoxicity
adeno-associated virus (AAV)   892f., 941
adenomatous polyposis coli   427
adenosine deaminase (ADA)   886, 953
adenovirus   836f., 890f
adenylyl cyclase   9
adherens junction (AJ)   735
adhesion molecule   970, 977, 987–988
ADME   65, 319, 339, 345, 355
adrenaline   397
adrenoleukodystrophy   907

β-adrenoceptor blocker   397
β$_2$-adrenergic receptor   183ff
adverse event   913
AEX, *see* anion exchange chromatography
affinity NMR   292, 300
aflatoxin   56
aging   499
agonist   316, 319
AJ, *see* adherens junction
alcohol   45
aldehyde dehydrogenase   41ff, 45
ALL, *see* acute lymphoblastic leukemia
allogeneic bone marrow transplant   910
allometric scaling   120
allosteric binding site   321, 327, 556, 562
allosteric inhibitor   725
allosteric ligand   327
allosteric modulation   326–329
allosteric transition   329
allyl alcohol   56
Alzheimer's diseases   496, 908
American Society of Clinical Oncology (ASCO)
   737
amidase   41, 47
amide-exchange   232, 243
12 amino acid–long oligopeptide   960
γ-amino butyric acid   911
amino acid conjugate   52
amino acids   193, 206
AML, *see* acute myeloid leukemia
AML-ETO   431
amphiphilic drug   162
amplicon   898
analog-based design   255
anandamide   367
angina pectoris   970, 990
angiogenesis   138, 148, 165, 502, 640ff., 703,
   729, 733–734, 756, 766, 970, 987
   blocking through inhibiting HIF1 activity
   766–768

Pharmacology. From Drug Development to Gene Therapy. Edited by Robert A. Meyers.
Copyright © 2008 Wiley-VCH Verlag GmbH & Co. KGaA, Weinheim
ISBN: 978-3-527-32343-2

angiogenic response   912
angioplasty   970, 987
angiopoietin   654
angiotensin-converting enzyme (ACE)   11, 20,
    208, 396
    inhibitor   20
anion exchange chromatography (AEX)   948
ANN (artificial neural net)   79
ANP, *see* atrial natriuretic peptide
antagonist   316, 322, 323, 326, 329, 330, 342
anthracycline   163
α1-antitrypsin   906
antiasthma drug   399–402
    contignasterol   402
    ephedrine   401
    isoprenaline   401
    Khellin   399
    salbutamol   401
    sodium cromoglycate   399
antibiotic   384–393
    β-lactam   384
    echinocandin   392
    erythromycin macrolide   390
    streptogramin   391
antibody   110, 113f., 121, 126f., 164–166, 471,
    472, 480
    classes of   472–474
    complexation   121
    engineering of   471–474
    fusion proteins   484–486
    genetic modifications of   480–486
    molecules   469, 486
        expression systems   486
        genetic engineering   469–486
    structure of   471–474
    subclasses of   472–474
antibody-based therapeutics   631
antibody-dependent cellular cytotoxicity (ADCC)
    470, 472
anticancer drug   373–384
    camptothecin   375
    catharanthus (vinca) alkaloids   373
    docetaxel   376
    epothilone   379
    etoposide   380
    marine source   383
    paclitaxel   376
    podophyllotoxin   380
    teniposide   380
antifungal   507
antigen-producing cell   892
antigen   471, 909
antimicrobial agents   405f.
antiparasitic drug   402–410

antisense oligonucleotide   35, 122, 142, 499,
    695–696
antisense RNA   539
antitumor estrogens   781–793
antitumor steroid   775–793
antiviral immunity   898
APC   428
apical membrane   970, 980
apoA1   971, 984
apoA2   984
apoA5   986
apoB100   971, 982
apoB48   971
apoE   971, 986
apolipoprotein   971, 979
    prevention of atherosclerosis   985–986
apoptosis   426, 499, 525, 703, 734, 912, 971,
    990, 1007f.
    FasL   1008
    lymphocytes   1008
aptamer   520
arteether   402–404
artemether   402–404
artemisinin   402–404
arteriogenesis   640ff
artificial neural net, *see* ANN
aryl hydrocarbon receptor   42
ascomycin   279–281
ascomycin-FKBP complex   281
asialoglycoprotein receptor   841ff
aspartyl protease   184
asperlicin   368–370
assembly   836ff
assignment protocol   257
asthma   183, 505
atenolol   397
atheroma   910
atherosclerosis   502, 971, 975–979, 984
atracurium   370–373
atrial natriuretic peptide (ANP)   114
AUC   84
autoimmune reaction   919
automated drug design   185
automation   494
avermectin   408–410
axin   427
axonal transport   907

b

B-cell (antibody) response   870
B-ring   782
bacterial or phage attachment site   1007

bacterial toxin   802, 803
   DT and DT derivatives   802–803
   PE and PE derivatives   803–804
bacteriophage   470, 478
barrier   833ff
basal (nonairway) surface   907
basolateral membrane   971
BBB, *see* blood brain barrier
BCR-ABL   184, 429, 430, 433
Beckmann rearrangement   390
behavior   499
benzo[a]pyrene   48
   epoxidation of   48
benzodiazepine   13, 27
beta-amyloid   502
bilamellar invaginated vesicle (BIV)   834ff
bile acid   971, 980
biliary excretion   116
binary state (of regulatory molecules)   704
binding kinetic   269
binding parameter   265
binding site   275
BIO, *see* biotechnology industry organization
bioanalytic   112
bioassay   112
bioavailability   113, 114, 122
bioballistical gene transfer method   956
bioballistic   956
biodistribution   113, 833ff
biological barrier   141
biological system   956
biomarker   628, 633
biomimetic polymer   138
bioreactor   442, 444
biotechnology industry organization (BIO)   448
biotechnology regulatory service (BRS)   448
bispecific antibody   482
BIV, *see* bilamellar invaginated vesicle
blast cell   735
blood   499
blood pressure
   regulators of   995
blood–brain barrier (BBB)   98, 148
bmi-1   426
bone   499
bone marrow stem cell   907
brain tumor   1054–1055
breast cancer   729, 1052–1053
bronchial airway epithelial cell   906
bronchiectasis   906
bronchoscopic instillation   906
budding   885

c
c-GMP phosphodiesterase   9
c-myc   426, 428
C-ring   782
C. elegans   495
CaCo-2   92
calcineurin   507
calcitonin   117
camptothecin   375
cancer   183, 503, 707, 713, 746, 756, 757, 763,
   1012
   clonal evolution   707–713
   hallmark traits   746
   key regulatory pathway   713–721
   molecular evolution   707–713
   targeting chromatin control   763–764
cancer cell cycle   761–763
cancer cell   721, 722
   molecular markers   721–726
cancer chemotherapy   755–768
cancer gene therapy   912
cancer genome anatomy project (CGAP)   628
cancer metastasis   917f
cancer stem cell   421, 424, 426, 428–433
cancer therapy   755, 757, 795, 796
   recombinant immunotoxins in   795–818
cannabinoids (CB)   362, 366–368
capsid   900, 1060–1066
captopril   396–397
capture step   948
carcinogenesis   704, 708
cardiac electrophysiology   102
cardiomyopathy   504
cardiovascular disease   944, 969–996
cardiovascular drug   393–399
caspase   187
cassette dosing   66
catechol *O*-methyltransferase   53
β-catenin   427, 428, 430
catharanthus (Vinca) alkaloids   373–375
cationic formulation   832ff
cationic gene transfer system   962
cationic lipid/liposome/lipid–DNA complex
   1014–1019
   entry in cells   1016
   entry in nucleus   1019
   structure   1014–1016
cationic liposomes (lipoplex)   957
cationic polymer gene transfer system   961
cationic polymer   960
CBER, *see* center for biologics evaluation and
   research
CCK, *see* cholecystokinin
CD154   909

CD24   423
CD28   909
CD40   909
CD44   423
CD80   909
CD86   909
CDK, *see* cyclin-dependent kinase
cell   735, 738
   growth factors of   738–739
   shape   735–736
cell cycle   496, 756, 760
cell cycle checkpoints   704, 735
cell death   426
cell entry   839ff, 899
cell physiology   628
cell surface receptor   832ff
cellular adhesion   704, 734
cellular adhesion molecules (CAMS)   733
cellular level   149–151
cellular mediated immune response   589, 590
   immunoregulation   589
   NK cell   590
center for biologics evaluation and research
   (CBER)   946
central nervous system   363–370
cerebrospinal fluid   99
cerius   74
cetrorelix   129
CGAP, *see* cancer genome anatomy project
CGH, *see* comparative genomic hybridization
chaperone   507
charge density   838ff
charge interaction   844ff
charge state   248
chemical-exchange   278
chemical gene-transfection system   956
chemical genomics   338
chemical library   12ff.
chemical shift   226, 231, 232, 238, 241ff, 248,
   252, 259, 261, 275, 280
   ^{13}C   252
   amino acids   242
   definition   231
   perturbation   291, 292
   random-coil   241
chemical shift index   243, 244
chemical shift mapping   226, 269
chemical space   73, 185
chemical vector technology   957
chemokine receptor antagonist   570
chemokine receptor   988–989, 1053
chemokine   971, 977, 988–989
chemoprevention   704, 736–737
chemotherapy   141, 431, 432, 737

chimeric Ad vector   1060
chimeric antibody   476–477
chimeric transcription factor   901
chitosan   963
chloroquine   404–408
CHO (Chinese hamster ovary)   443
chol   835ff
cholecystokinin (CCK)   210
cholinergic receptor   328, 334
chromosomal translocation   628–629
chromosome 19q   892
chronic myelogenous leukemia (CML)   184,
   758
chronic pain   916
chylomicron   971f, 981, 986
circular DNA   964
circular pDNA   124
circulating protein   904
Clavulanic acid   385
clearance   94, 116
clinical gene therapy   941–945
clinical trial, hemophilia B patients   905
clinical trials   659
clofibrate   50
CLogP   70, 74
clotting factor   904f
CML, *see* chronic myelogenous leukemia
coalescence temperature   252
cold sore   895
collateral   644
colloidal property   833ff
colon cancer   729
combinatorial chemistry   12ff, 17, 18, 181
combinatorial libraries   18
CoMFA   73
committee for proprietary medicinal products
   (CPMP)   946
comparative genomic hybridization (CGH)
   721
complement   470, 483
complementation   494
complementing cells   887, 896
complex PK/PD models   128
compound databases   346
compound libraries   13ff
compound properties   340
compound sources   317, 348
   new chemical entities (NCEs)   317, 348
compounds   347, 349
   ABT-594   349
   epibatidine   349
computational chemistry   69
computer-aided structure prediction   185
concerted model   326

condensation 836
condense 835ff
conditionally replicating 913
conformational analysis 247
  NOE 247
conjugation reactions 41
conotoxin 240, 254, 365
constant region 470, 483
constitutive activity 328
contignasterol 402
controlled release 138, 141f
corticotropin-releasing factor (CRF) 206, 212
cost of goods sold (COGS) 445
cosuppression 609
COSY 233, 234, 298
coumarin anticoagulant 398
coupling constant 232, 239, 243, 247, 257, 261
  conformational analysis 247
covalent attachment 840ff
coxsackie/adenovirus receptor 900
CpG repeat sequences 901
CpG-immunostimulatory oligonucleotides
  697
cre−lox 500
CRF, *see* corticotropin-releasing factor
cryoelectron micrographs 834ff
cryoprobe 230, 235, 236, 246
CTLA-4 909
Curare 370−373
cyclin-dependent kinase (CDK) 714
cyclin 714
cyclosporin 233, 264, 410−411, 507
cyclosporin A 280
  cyclophilin complex 280
CYP1A1 42
CYP2D6 42
CYP3A 183
CYP3A4 95
CYPs 95
cystic fibrosis 889, 906, 953
cytochrome P-450 41ff, 511, 556, 562
cytochrome P-450 isozymes 191
  epoxidation 44
  genetic variability 42
  heteroatom oxidation 44
  hydroxylation 44
  nomenclature 42
  reductive reactions 45
cytokine 903, 972, 977, 988, 1011
  IFN-α 1028, 1029
  IFN-β 1024, 1028, 1029
  IFN-γ 1011, 1028, 1029
  IL-1 1011, 1028
  IL-2 1025

IL-4 1011
IL-6 1012, 1028, 1029
IL-8 1028
IL-10 1011, 1027
IL-12 1007, 1011, 1013, 1028, 1029
IL-18 1007
TGF-β1 1011−1013
TNF-α 1028, 1029
cytomegalovirus (CMV)-retinitis 954
cytotoxic chemotherapy 161
cytotoxic T-cell (CTL) 1007
cytotoxicity 808

d
D-ring 783
Danio rerio 495
date hub 715
daylight software 70
de novo design 188ff
de-nucleated virus 964
decamethonium 370−373
decoy approach 761
dedifferentiation 429f
defective interfering particle 898
delivery 837ff
dendrimer 138, 173, 962
  star- or tree-shaped, structure 962
dendronized polymer 173
density functional model 70
17α derivatives 787−788
7α and 11β derivatives 787
descriptor 69
deshielding 840ff
detection of gene expression 849ff
deuteration 271
DHFR 271, 273, 284, 286, 287
  trimetrexate complex 286
diabody 481
dicer 529, 602ff, 604
  PAZ domain 604
dicoumarol 398−399
dictyostelium 513
differentiation marker 422
diffusion editing 299
diffusion-filtered NMR screening 300
diflusinal 296
dihedral angle restraint 257
dihydrofolate reductase, *see* DHFR
1,4-dihydropyridine 13, 29, 30
dimethylbenzanthracene (DMBA) 708
diphtheria toxin (DT) 800

diploid   499
direct link PK/PD models   125
direct-link models   124
discriminant analysis   86
disease   495
dissociation constant, K_d 265, 343
distamycin   274
distribution   97, 114
disulfiram   47
DMP-323   288, 289
DMPK   65
DNA   258, 265, 269, 276ff
  ligand binding   265ff, 269
  minor groove binding   276
  structure determination   258
DNA alkylation   48
DNA vaccination   857
DNA-ligand binding   273
docetaxel   376–379
dopamine   53
dorsal root ganglia   916
dose-escalation schedule   914
dose-limiting toxicity   816
DOTAP liposome   959
DOTAP   835ff
DQF-COSY   233, 239, 240
Drosha   615
Drosophila   495
drug   183, 317ff, 495
  analog-based   255
  computer-assisted   341
  delivery   137–173, 664, 956
  design   19, 227, 228, 230, 232, 255, 756–758
  development   229, 236, 240
  discovery   214, 227, 228, 230, 232, 234, 318, 342, 393, 395
  ''druglike'' molecule   13, 16, 86
  mechanism-based   757–758
  metabolism   40, 58, 183
  receptor   30, 336
  resistance   704, 737–738
  structure-based   227, 228
  targeting   138, 141, 142
DT, *see* diphtheria toxin
dual targeting
  transcriptional   1064–1066
  transductional   1064–1066
duchenne muscular dystrophy   908, 953
dynamics   258, 281
dynamic combinatorial chemistry   17ff
dynamic libraries   18
dynamic process   278
dystonia   908
dystrophin   908

e
E2F   756
EAE, *see* experimental allergic encephalomyelitis
EAT, *see* experimental autoimmune thyroiditis   1008
EBV, *see* Eppstein–Barr virus
Echinocandins   392–393
efficacy, ε 324f, 329, 340
efficient delivery   831ff
EGFR, *see* Epidermal Growth Factor Receptor
Ehrlich, Paul   8
electrophilic 11β derivative   792–793
electroporation   956
electrostatic interaction   836
electrotopological state index   72
elimination   115
embryonic stem cell (ES)   501
EMEA, *see* European Agency for the Evaluation of Medicinal Products
emerging therapeutic agent   632
α-emitting compound   791
emphysema   906
enantiomers   31ff
encapsulation   835ff
encoded library   17
endocytic pathway   839ff
endocytosis   117, 119, 138, 149
endogenous fibroblast   905
endogenous ligand   152
endogenous RNAi   609, 611, 612
endorphin   364
endosomotropic   138
endothelial cell   643
endothelial progenitor cell   656
endothelin   244–246
endothelin antagonist   249
engineering antibody fragments   480
enigmatic vanilloid receptor   367
entropy   250
enveloped virus   898
enzyme induction   42
enzyme–substrate interaction   259
ephedrine   401–402
epidermal growth factor (EGF)   210, 758, 797
epidermal growth factor receptor   430, 720, 1013, 1021
epilepsy   508
epistasis   494
epithelial specific antigen   423
epothilones   379–380
epoxide hydrolase   41, 47
Eppstein–Barr virus (EBV)   1006, 1027
  EBV nuclear antigen-1 (EBNA1)   1006
eptifibatide   114

equine infectious anemia virus (EIAV)   940
ErbB   756, 758–759
ergodic   189
erythromycin macrolides   390–391
erythropoietin (EPO)   126, 443
ES, *see* embryonic stem cell
esterases   41, 47
estradiol binding   782f
estrogen binding capacity   784f
estrogen receptor level   785
estrogen receptor   783f
ethanol   46
etoposide   380–383
European Agency for the Evaluation of
    Medicinal products (EMEA)   448, 946, 953
exchange rate   275
exchange regime   260, 261, 264, 267
exocrine gland   906
exonuclease   123
exopeptidase   117, 118
expanded genetic code   34
experimental allergic encephalomyelitis (EAE)
    1011
experimental autoimmune thyroiditis (EAT)
    1011
exposure/response correlation   111, 124
expression   837ff
expression profiling   847
expression system   486
expression vector   859
extravasation   148, 836ff
extravascular space   148
extruded   838ff

f
^{19}F spectrum   283
Fab   470, 486
familial hypercholesterolemia   972, 983
familial hypoalphalipoproteinemia (FHA)   972,
    984
fas ligand   910
fast exchange   262, 264
fat   505
fatty streak   972, 977
Fc   470, 486
FDA, *see* food and drug administration
feline immunodeficiency virus (FIV)   940
FGF, *see* Fibroblast Growth Factor
FHA, *see* familial hypercholesterolemia
fiber   1046, 1060
Fibroblast Growth factor   649ff, 733
fibrous cap   972, 978
FID, *see* free induction decay
field carcinogenic event   710

fingerprint   71
first and second messenger   194, 210
first-pass metabolism   84
FISH, *see* fluorescence *in situ* hybridization
FIV, *see* feline immunodeficiency virus
FK506   264, 279, 280, 293
FK506 binding protein, *see* FKBP   279
FKBP   293, 300
flavoprotein monooxygenases   41ff
flexibility   257, 290, 837ff
FLIPR, *see* fluorescence imaging plate reader
flow NMR   236
fluorescence imaging plate reader (FLIPR)   344
fluorescence *in situ* hybridization (FISH)   721
fluorescence polarization (FP)   344
fluorescence resonance energy transfer (FRET)
    344
fluorescent oligonucleotide   690–691
fluoxetine   506
fluphenazine   47
foam cell   972, 977
food and drug administration (FDA)   111f, 124,
    448, 946
formalin test   917
fourier transform   231
fragile X mental retardation   908
fragment optimization   295
fragment-based screening   291
fragmentation method   295
free induction decay   231
FRET, *see* fluorescence resonance energy
    transfer
Friedreich's ataxia   907
frizzled   427
fruit fly   494
Fugu   513
functional genomic   337, 633
functional informatic   628, 634
fusiogenic peptides, *see also* peptides   960
fusion   839ff
fusion protein   164–166
Fv/scFv   470, 480f

g
G protein   210
G-CSF, *see* granulocyte colony stimulating factor
G-protein coupled protein   21
G-protein of vesicular stomatitis virus
    (VSV-G)   940
G-protein–coupled receptor (GPCR)   8ff, 182,
    317, 320, 328, 332, 333, 344, 496
GABA   321, 328, 333, 337
gain of function   908
GAL4   498

gallstone   972
gastrointestinal absorption   381
gastrointestinal cancer   1049–1050
gastrointestinal elimination   117
gastrointestinal stromal tumor (GIST)   758
GastroPlus   74
gel filtration (GF)   948
geldanamycin   764
gene amplification   629
gene delivery   34, 1004
   angiogenesis   1010
   autoimmune disease   1011
   cancer   1007, 1013, 1024–1026
   cationic lipid & cationic liposomes
      1013–1021
   chylomicron   1022
   Duchenne muscular dystrophy   1008, 1009
   electroporation   1011, 1012
   emulsion-mediated   1022, 1023
   ischemia   1010
   microelectroporation   1012
   myocardial diseases   1009
   nucleic acid vaccines (NAC)   1012
   skeletal muscle   1008, 1012
   stealth liposome   1023
   wound healing   1012, 1013
gene expression   846ff
gene function analysis   694–695
gene gun   956, 1012f.
gene switch   901
gene targeting   908
gene therapy   34, 142, 172, 661, 881, 944, 952,
   953, 969–996
   cardiovascular disease   979–987
   genetically modified organism   953
   growth factor   990–991
   infectious disease   944–945
   inflammatory target   987–991
   pain   916
   strategy   953
   transcription factors   993
   vascular target   987–991
   vector targeting   1045–1067
gene transfer   936, 941
gene validation   694–695
general solvation equation   91, 100
genetic algorithm   78, 189
genetic instability   628
genetic manipulation   952
genetic marker   721
genetic polymorphism   46
genetic programing   78
genetics   494
genomics   495, 723

German gene technology regulation   952
GFP, *see* green fluorescent protein
gleevec   629, 758
glial cell-line derived neurotrophic factor   911
global model   83
glomerular filtration   117
glucuronyl transferase   41, 48, 49
glutamic acid decarboxylase   911, 918
glutathione   41, 54, 56
glycogen synthase-3β 427
glycosylation   442, 486
GM-CSF, *see* granulocyte-macrophage
   colony-stimulating factor
good manufacturing practice (GMP)   442f, 946
GP120-CD4 interaction   568
GPCR, *see* G-protein coupled receptor
graft-versus-host disease (GvHD)   810
grafting   787
granulocyte colony-stimulating factor (G-CSF)
   115, 170
granulocyte-macrophage colony-stimulating
   factor (GM-CSF)   944
green fluorescent protein (GFP)   344, 454, 498
growth factor   704, 972, 977, 990–991
growth hormone–releasing factor (GRF)   198
guanine-nucleotide-binding protein-coupled
   receptor (GPCR)   570
guanylyl cyclase   8
guided missile   142
GvHD, *see* graft-versus-host disease
gynecological cancer   1054

h

HAART, *see* highly active antiretroviral therapy
HACA, *see* human antichimeric antibody
hairy cell leukemia (HCL)   811
half-life in the circulation   835ff
Hallervorden Spatz disease   908
HAMA, *see* human antimouse antibody
Hansch   88
hardware and automation   306
HDL, *see* high-density lipoprotein
head and neck squamous cell carcinoma
   (HNSCC)   709
heart   499
heat shock protein 90 (Hsp90)   764
helper function   893
hemarthrosis   904
hematological disease   903
hematopoietic stem cell (HSC)   424, 656, 914
hemophilias   904, 919
hemorrhage   972, 978
hemozoin   403
hepatic elimination   117

hepatocellular carcinoma   1050
hepatocyte   914
hepatocyte cell line   95
hepatocyte growth factor (HGF)   653ff
herpes simplex virus   894
hexachlorinated biphenyls   44
HGF, *see* hepatocyte growth factor
high-density lipoprotein (HDL)   972, 980
high-throughput genomics   632–633
high-throughput screening (HTS)   12, 16, 68, 338, 344, 347
highly active antiretroviral therapy (HAART)   556f
histamine H3   190
histone acetyltransferase (HAT)   725
histone deacetylase (HDAC)   725
HIV, *see* human immunodeficiency virus
HLA, *see* human leukocyte antigen
HMBC (heteronuclear multiple bond correlation)   239
HMQC-NOESY   280
Hoechst 33258   270, 273, 274, 277
homeostasis   319
homogenous   834
homologous recombination   848
hormone binding domain   777f
host range   887
Hox family   426
HSA   295, 296
HSC, *see* hematopoietic stem cell
Hsp90   756, 764ff
HSQC   226, 233, 234, 238, 263, 269, 291, 295, 297, 306
   chemical-shift mapping   269
HSV   895f, 912
HTS, *see* high-throughput screening
human antichimeric antibody (HACA)   477
human antimouse antibody (HAMA)   120, 475
human factor IX (hFIX)   1006
human genome   318, 495
human genome project   957
human immunodeficiency virus (HIV)   940
   HIV entry inhibitor   568
   HIV protease   20, 23, 257, 273, 285ff, 290
   HIV reverse transcriptase   182ff
   HIV therapeutics   555–571
   HIV-1 genome   887
   HIV-1 nucleocapsid protein   571
human leukocyte antigen (HLA)   814
human monoclonal antibody   477f
human serum albumin, *see* HSA
human therapeutics   837ff
humanized antibody   477
Huntington's disease (HD)   496, 538, 908

hybridoma   471, 474
hydrogen bond   186, 232, 279, 281, 289
hyperammonemia   913
hypertension   183, 502
hypertriglyceridemia   983
hypoxia   657
hypoxia-inducible factor-1α, HIF1α 910
hysteresis   125

i

IC$_{50}$ value   343
^{123}I and ^{125}I labeled compound   790f
ICH E4   111
iDEA   74
IDL, *see* intermediate density lipoprotein
IGF-1   115
IL-10   117, 909
immediate early functions   896
immune response   816, 831ff, 869
immune therapy   433
immunoadhesin   485
immunoassay   112, 121
immunoconjugate   138, 144
immunodominant   478
immunogenicity   120, 861
immunoglobulin (Ig)   471
immunoligand   484
immunoliposome   960
immunophilin   507
immunosuppressant drugs   279, 410–412
immunotherapy   141, 912
immunotoxin activity   812
immunotoxin therapy   795–818
in silico drug design   180ff
indirect link PK/PD model   124f
indirect-response PK/PD model   126
indium   213
indolethylamine *N*-methyltransferase   53
IND (investigative new drug application)   355
induced fit model   325
inducible promoter   847
inflammation   508, 655
inflammatory pain   916
Ink4a/Arf   430
insertional mutagenesis   886, 918
insertional oncogenesis   943
instrumentation   234
insulator element   900
insulin   112, 502
integrase inhibitor   567f
integration   847, 887
integrin, αVβ5   900
interactome   714
interferon-α 117

interferon-β 128, 911
interferon-γ 117, 989
interleukin   115, 117, 119, 125, 918, 989f
intermediate density lipoprotein (IDL)   973, 982
intermediate exchange   262, 266, 267
internal globus pallidus   911
internalization   832ff
intestinal absorption   89, 980f
intestinal epithelium   84
intima   973, 977
intracellular delivery   141
intracellular organelle compartmentation   149
intracellular receptor   335
intracellular targeting   155–159
intracoronary administration   910
intraepithelial neoplasia   704, 739
intravenous   833ff
intrinsic clearance   94
invertebrate   496
ion channel   8, 13ff, 21, 22, 25, 27, 209, 317, 496
ionic interaction   840ff
Iressa   759
ischemia   640ff, 973, 978, 987
ischemic heart disease   183, 910
isoniazid   52
isoprenaline   401–402
isotope editing   271, 272, 282
isotope filtering   271, 282
isotope labeling   227, 235

j
jaundice, neonatal   50

k
kallikrein-kinin system (KKS)   1008
key-based approach   71
khellin   399–401
kidney glomerulus   148
kinase   497
kinetics   259, 260, 264, 274
kininogen   1008
knob   1059
knockout   499
Koshland Nemethy Filmer sequential model   327
Kupffer cell   914

l
β-lactam   384–390
Langley, John Newton   8
latency   885, 895f
LC-NMR   235, 236, 246

LC/mass spectrometry   112
LCAT   985
LDL, *see* low-density lipoprotein
lead compound   347, 363
lead generation   6
lead optimization   6
lead structure   11
lentivirus   887ff
leukemia   504, 915
leukocyte counter receptor   987f
LH-RH (luteinizing hormone-releasing hormone)   114, 129, 131
library design   304
life span   504
ligand   317, 320, 325, 326ff, 338, 510
ligand dynamics   250
ligand library   294
ligand-based drug design   180ff, 237
ligand-binding domain   268, 778
ligand-coated complex   840ff
ligand-gated ion channels (LGICs)   8, 321, 327, 328, 333, 334, 337
   5HT$_3$ 328
   GABA$_A$ 321, 328, 337
   nicotinic cholinergic   328, 334
   NMDA receptor   334
line shape   232, 250
line width   238, 264
linear pDNA   124
linker lipid   841ff
Lipinski's "Rule of 5"   85, 346
lipodystrophy   556, 567
Lipofectin   958
lipoplex   1002, 1006, 1014–1019, 1023, 1024
   antisense plasmid   1025
   cancer   1023ff
lipopolyplex   1002, 1014, 1019–1021, 1024, 1029
   cancer vaccine   1024
   oligonucleotides (ODN)   1021
lipoprotein   502, 973, 977
lipoprotein lipase   973, 981ff
liposomes   138, 148, 161–164, 832ff, 959
liver   505
LMO2 gene   915
local minima   76
local model   83
lock and key   320
locus control region   900
LogD   70
LogP   70
LogPcyc   70
long terminal repeat (LTR)   935
long-term gene expression   847

lovastatin 393–396
low DNA transfer rates 964
low transfection rate 959
low-density lipoprotein (LDL) 980
low-density lipoprotein receptor 973
β-lyase 55
lysosomotropic 139

m
mAb, *see* monoclonal antibody
M-CSF 117, 119
macromolecular NMR 230
macromolecule–ligand interaction 259, 260
magnetization transfer experiment 297
MALDI-TOF (matrix assisted laser desorption
  ionization time of flight) 458
malignant melanoma 1055–1056
marine sources 383–384
marker expression 423, 429
master working cell bank (MWCB) 948
matrix attachment function 900
matrix metalloproteinase 273, 282, 658
MCP-1 655
MDCK 92
mechanistic model 75
media 973
medullary thyroid cancer (MTC) 1007
mefloquine 404–408
meis1 430
melanocyte stimulating hormone (MSH) 155
melanoma 502
melanoma inhibitory activity (MIA) 1055
melting temperature 680
membrane protein 259
membrane translocation 156
memory 502
meninges 911
messenger RNA (mRNA) 936
metabolic NMR 230
metabolic oxidation 407
metabolism 94, 116, 499
metastasis 502
metastatic ovarian carcinoma 164
meteor 74
methacrylate polymer 963
methotrexate 285, 287
methyl transferase 53
methylase 41
methylphosphonate linkage 686
metkephamid 115
2′-methoxy oligonucleotides 687
MGDF (megakaryocyte growth and
  differentiation factor) 738
MIA, *see* melanoma inhibitory activity

micelle 139, 152, 959
microarray 504
microinjection 1008
microRNA 612–617
microsome 95
milbemycin 408–410
minor groove 276
minoxidil 52
miRNA 612–617
miRNP 615–617
mitogen-activated protein kinase (MAP-kinase)
  1008
mixture design 305
MLV, *see* murine leukemia virus
model organism 495
modified vaccinia ancara (MVA) 936
Molconn-Z 74
molecular diffusion 299
molecular diversity 16
molecular mechanics 69
molecular oncology 703–750
monoamine oxidase 41ff, 45
monocarboxylic acid transporter 94
monoclonal antibody (mAb) 121, 800, 810
monocyte 511
Monod, Wyman, Changeux concerted model
  327
monogeneic congenital disease 34, 941
monomeric antibody 483
Monte Carlo simulation 75
morphine alkaloids 363–365
morphology 834ff
moss 457–460
mouse Moloney leukemia virus 885
MP2 70
MPF (maturation promotion factor) 714
MSH, *see* melanocyte stimulating hormone
MTC, *see* medullary thyroid cancer
MultiCASE 71, 74
multidrug resistance (MDR) 93, 166, 556f
multilamellar vesicle (MLV) 162, 834ff
multiple organ failure 913
multiple sclerosis 911
multitargeting 745–750
murine leukemia virus (MLV) 939
murine monoclonal antibodies 474–476
Mus musculus 495
muscarinic receptors 9ff
muscle 499
muscular dystrophy 504
mutations 494, 705, 740–741
MVIIA 240, 243, 245
Mycophenolate Mofetil 411–412
Mycophenolic acid 411–412

myocardial infarction   640ff, 973, 978
myocardium   910
myosin   1009f, 1024, 1028

n

N-acyl transferase   52
naked rodent antibody   631
naloxone   917
naltrexone   917
nanomedicine   139, 141, 159–160, 172f
nanoparticle   139, 166–167
nasal epithelium   906
natural killer (NK) cell   943, 1007, 1028
natural medicine   6
natural product   6, 11, 16, 238, 308, 379, 382, 404
necrotic zone   973, 978, 994
nematode   495
neopterin   128
neovascularization   910, 974
nerve growth factor (NGF)   210
NES, *see* nuclear export signal
netropsin   274
neural net   78
neurobiology   499
neurodegeneration   502
neurological disease   907, 911
neuromuscular blocking drugs   370–373
neuron   498
neuropathic pain   916, 917
neuropilin   646
neurotransmitter   365, 368
neutral endopeptidase (NEP)   214
neutral lipids   837
new chemical entities (NCEs)   349
nicotinic cholinergic receptor (nAChR)   328, 334
NIH rearrangement   44
nitric oxide (NO)   8, 1007
NK cell, *see* natural killer cell
NLS, *see* nuclear localization signal
NMDAR1 receptor   183
NMR   227f, 230, 235ff, 290, 306
   imaging   230ff, 281
   instrumentation   234, 246
   parameters   232, 261
   relaxation data   258
   screening   227, 228, 230, 235, 237, 290, 306
NNRTI, *see* nonnucleoside reverse transcriptase inhibitor
NO synthase II (NOS II)   1007
NOE (nuclear Overhauser effect)   227, 243, 247, 251, 257, 259, 272, 275, 282, 285, 292, 301
   conformational analysis   247

flexibility   251
   intermolecular   276, 282, 285
   structure determination   257
NOESY   234, 239, 240, 275, 282, 298, 301
   chemical-exchange cross peaks   275
non-hodgkin's lymphoma (NHL)   164
noninflammatory gene target   994–996
nonlinear modelling   77
nonnucleoside reverse transcriptase inhibitor (NNRTI)   562–563
nonnucleotidic modification   690
nonspecific ionic charge   839ff
nonviral gene-transfection   952ff, 964
nonviral vector   172, 831ff, 882, 901
Notch   426, 427
nuclear export signal (NES)   784
nuclear hormone receptor   496
nuclear localization signal (NLS)   784
nuclear Overhauser effect, *see* NOE   232
nuclear receptor   776, 777
nuclease   149
nucleic acid structure   258
nucleic acid-liposome complex   832ff
nucleoside   556, 560
nucleoside reverse transcriptase inhibitor (NRTI)   557–561
nucleotide reverse transcriptase inhibitor (NtRTI)   557–561
nucleotide   556, 560

o

obesity   502
occlusive thrombi   978
octreotid   114–116
oligodeoxynucleotide   680, 682, 683
oligonucleotide   35ff, 122, 265, 633, 679–698
   applications   691–695
   chemically modified   685–691
oligoribonucleotide   680, 683–685
omentum   905
oncogene   502, 628, 705, 739–740
oncolysis   1056
oncotoxin   800
opiate drug   916
opioid receptor   916
opsonization   148
optimization   189, 840ff
oral bioavailability   67, 84
1st, 2nd, 3rd order targeting   142
organometallic estradiol derivative   786–788
origin of replication   898
ornithine transcarbamylase   913, 940
orphan receptor   11, 317, 331, 335, 336
ortholog   496

orthosteric site   327
osmotic gradient   963
osteoarthritis   505
osteogenic protein   996
OTC, *see* ornithine transcarbamylase
overfitting   76, 80
oxidation   41

p
P element   498
p21^{cip1} 426, 428
pK_a 89
P-glycoprotein   93
P-gp   99
P450   95
p53   426, 756, 760f, 912
''packaging'' cell line   885
Paclitaxel   376–379
pain   508, 918
pancreas   906
paracellular   90
parathyroid hormone (PTH)   210
Parkinson's disease   496, 907, 911
party hub   715
passive targeting   148, 151f
pathological gene expression   695
PCA (principal components analysis)   77
PDGF   650ff
peak intensity   232
PEGylation   169, 835ff, 959
PEI-based gene transfer system   962
penetrate   833ff
penicillin   384
peptide   196, 204, 206, 208, 212
   biological function   208–212
   chemical synthesis   204–206
   pathophysiology   212–214
   therapeutic target   212–214
peptide library   206
peptide localization signal   159
peptide nucleic acid   688
peptide–receptor complex   210
peptidomimetics   23ff, 24, 194, 206, 556, 564
pericyte   644
peripheral ischemic vascular disease   641
peripheral vascular disease (PVD)   640ff
peritonitis   511
personalized medicine   191
petrozole   730
phage display   19
phage library   478–480
pharma algorithm   74
pharmaceutical   383, 412
pharmaceutical industry   180ff

pharmacodynamic (PD)   110, 728
pharmacogenetic   180ff
pharmacokinetic (PK)   110, 113, 123, 520, 534
   DNA   123
   peptides and proteins   113
pharmacological receptor   22
pharmacophore   13, 187, 212, 350
phase I/II trial   917
phenacetin   43
phenotype   500
philadelphia chromosome   629
phosphate linkage   685
3-phosphoadenosine-5′-phosphosulfate   51
phosphoamidate linkage   687
phosphoamidite   680f
phosphodiester linkage   680, 681
phospholipase C   9
phosphorothioate linkage   685–686
phosphothioate oligonucleotide (PON)   122
physical gene-transfection system   956
PK/PD modeling   110, 124
plant expression   445f, 460
plant toxin   801f
plant-based expression   441f, 446ff, 452, 454, 461
   biopharmaceuticals   441–462
   humanlike glycosylation   452–454
   risk assessment   448–452
   tobacco transfection   454–460
plasma lipoprotein
plasma membrane   155
plasma protein binding   97
plasmid   1005
   complementary DNA (cDNA)   1005
   CpG cytotoxicity   1028, 1029
   polyadenylation (poly A)   1005
   promoter   1005
   size   1005
plasmid DNA   123, 846ff, 935
plasmid DNA preparations   848ff
plasmid   846ff
platinum-based chemotherapy   433
PlGF   645
PLH/DNA complex   961
PLS (partial least squares)   77
PNA (peptide nucleic acid)   520, 531, 540f
podophyllotoxin   380–383
poly(2-dimethylamino) ethylmethacrylate   963
poly-L-lysine (PLL)   961
polyclonal antibody   474
polycyclic aromatic hydrocarbon   56
polycystic kidney disease   508
polyethylene glycol (PEG)   835ff
polyethyleneimine (PEI)   962

polyhalogenated hydrocarbon 44
polymer conjugate 167–171
polymer particle (polyplex) 960
polymer therapeutics 139, 167
polymer–drug conjugates 170–171
polymer–protein conjugates 169–170
polymerase chain reaction (PCR) 693, 812
polymeric gene transfer system 961
polymeric micelle 171–172
polymers 835ff
polymorphism 504
polyneuropathy 918
polypeptide 196
polyplex 140, 148, 1003, 1014, 1026, 1027
   dendrimers 1026, 1027
   polyethyleneimines (PEI) 1026–1028
pravastatin 393–396
precursor pool PK/PD Models 128
preventive vaccination 944
prialt 240, 248, 254
primary structure 194, 197
primer 692–694
privileged pharmacophore 351
probe 694
prodrug 47, 557
proenkephalin 916
progenitor cell 429
proliferation 425, 426, 428, 429
promoter 500, 522, 1046, 1053
promoter-enhancer 846ff
proopiomelanocortin 207
propranolol 397
proresid 382
protease 149, 497, 994f
protease inhibitor 563–567
   Kaletra 565
   nuclear sterol regulatory element binding
      protein (nSERBP) 567
proteasome 705, 741f, 768
protection group 680, 682
protein 181–185, 196
   binding 97, 115
   crystal structure 184
   data bank 181
   homology model 181
   misfolding 28
   three-dimensional structure 181f
   turnover 768
protein–ligand interaction 259
protein–protein interaction 27ff, 505
proteolysis 116, 777
proteomics 496, 723
proton sponge 157, 962
protooncogene 915

PSA 71, 90
pseudomonas exotoxin (PE) 800
PTH, *see* parathyroid hormone
pufferfish 513
pulse sequence 227
pulsed-field gradient 235–237
purine 690
pyrimidine 689–690

q
QikProp 74
QT prolongation 511
quality control 864, 865
quantitative structure–activity relationship
   (QSAR) 28ff
quantitative structure–property relationship
   (QSPR) mapping 76
quantum mechanics 70
quasi-species 523
quinine 404–408
quinone oxidoreductase 183

r
racemate 31
radiolabeled estradiol derivative 789–791
radiosensitization 912
radiotherapy 737
rapamycin 279, 280, 507
rate theory 326
Rattus norvegicus 495
reactive species 54
RDEB, *see* recessive dystrophic epidermolysis
   bullosa
real-time PCR (RT-PCR) 721
receptor 8ff, 317–320, 328–331, 341, 343, 496
receptor classes
   non-GPCR-linked cytokine receptors 335
receptor concepts 322, 323
   law of mass action 322
   occupancy theory 322
   Schild regression relationship 323
receptor dynamics 330
receptor nomenclature 331
receptor theory 325
receptor-based design 237, 256
receptor-binding assays 342
receptor-mediated 115
receptor-mediated elimination 119
receptor-mediated endocytosis 118
receptor-mediated internalization 155
recessive dystrophic epidermolysis bullosa
   (RDEB) 1007
recombinant antibody 796

recombinant immunotoxin   797, 801, 805,
   808–810, 815
   against leukemia and lymphoma   810–812
   against solid tumor   809–810
   design   801–808
recombinant peptide   194
recombinant virus   882
recombination   499
recursive partitioning   78
relaxation data   232, 250, 252, 258–261, 300
renal elimination   117
renin   208
reperfusion   640ff
replicase   892
replication   847
replication-competent adenovirus (RCA)   936
replication-competent lentivirus (RCL)   940
replication-competent plasmid   847
replication-competent retrovirus (RCR)   939
replication-defective lentivirus vector   889
reporter gene   501, 882
reproduction   499
respiratory disease   906
restenosis   910, 974, 987
retargeting   900, 1059
retinoblastoma tumor suppressor protein (pRb)
   761
retrovirus   885, 915
revascularization   640ff, 910
reverse NOE pumping   302
reverse transcriptase (RT)   184, 521, 557, 885
reversed phase (RP)   948
reversible masking   845ff
ribozyme   520, 533ff, 535f, 696
ring-current effect   277
RISC, *see* RNA-induced silencing complex
ritonavir   184ff
RNA   519, 521, 524, 530–533, 541, 543, 545
   clinical application   519–545
   metabolism   521–533
   pharmacokinetic   543–544
RNA aptamer   539f
RNA-dependent RNA polymerases   608, 609
   transitive RNAi   609
RNA drug   520, 523, 542f
RNA genome   523f
RNA-induced silencing complex (RISC)   529,
   607, 617
RNA interference (RNAi)   35, 36, 355, 498,
   520, 529, 536f, 617–619, 908
   miRNA   529–530, 619
   siRNA   529–530
   shRNA   619
   vs. cancer   537–538

   vs. genetic disorders   537–538
   vs. viruses   536–537
RNA polymerase (RNAP)   521
RNA splicing   524
   regulation by antisense RNA   524–526
RNAi, *see* RNA interference
robotics   633
ROESY   239
RT, *see* reverse transcriptase
RT-PCR, *see* reverse transcriptase
rule of five   12, 85, 304

s

saccharomyces   495
SAGE (serial analyses of gene expression)   847
SAHA (suberoylanilide hydroxamic acid)   763
salbutamol   401–402
SAR-by-NMR   228, 236, 291–294, 296, 303, 305
sarcoglycanopathy   908
sarcolemma   908
saturation transfer difference, *see* STD
scaffold   13
scavenger receptor   974, 977, 986, 992–993
scFv   480f
schizophrenia   183, 505
schizosaccharomyces   495
SCID, *see* severe combined immunodeficiency
   disease
screening   365, 412
screening bacteria   389
second messenger   210
secondary metabolite   361
secondary structure (conformation)   194, 197
selection   903, 904
selective estrogen receptor modulators (SERMs)
   780
selective growth advantage   904
semiempirical methods   70
   quantum mechanical   70
sensory ganglia   895
sensory nerve terminals   895
sequence   495
sequential or induced fit   326
serotonin   505
serum stability   842ff
severe combined immunodeficiency disease
   (SCID)   172, 886, 914, 940
SHAPES   296, 304, 305
shielding/deshielding compound   845ff
sickle cell anemia   953
sigmoid E_{max}-model   125
signal transduction   513, 955
simian immunodeficiency virus (SIV)   940
simulated annealing   189, 243, 257

simvastatin 393–396
single nucleotide polymorphism (SNP) 180ff
siRNA 35, 604, 605, 608, 697
sirolimus 410–411
site points 188ff
SIV, *see* simian immunodeficiency virus
SLATE 189
slime mold 513
slow exchange 261–263
small interfering RNA, *see* siRNA
small unilamellar vesicle (SUV) 834ff
SN-6999 270
SNP, *see* single nucleotide polymorphism
Sodium Cromoglycate 399–401
solubility 87
somatic gene therapy 933–949, 952
  clinical use 941–945
  regulatory aspects 945–948
somatostatin 114
somatotropin 112, 115, 120, 126–128, 209
sonic hedgehog 426
spaghetti effect 948
spatial 197
species differences 57
spectral assignment 240
spiegelmers 520, 531, 540
spin labeling 292, 302
spinobulbar muscular atrophy
  (SBMA) 538
spinocerebellar ataxia 908
spliceosome-mediated RNA trans-splicing
  (SMaRT) 527
splicing 524
SR-B1 receptor 986f
starburst – dendrimer 962
statin 974
statistical models 76
STD (saturation transfer difference) 292, 297,
  298, 303, 306
stealth delivery system 142
stem cell 421–431
stereochemistry 30ff
stereoselectivity 11
steric hindrance 835ff
steroid hormone 776
steroid receptor 8, 335, 777–781
STI-571 184
sticky protein 715
stoichiometry 238, 259, 263, 274
strand transfer 567
strengths, weaknesses, opportunities, and
  threats (SWOT) 446
streptogramin 391–392
stress protein 863

stromal cells and cancer 705, 742
stromelysin 283, 294
structural genomics 230
structure-activity relationship (SAR) 317–319,
  340, 345
structure-based drug design 11, 20, 180f, 227,
  236–238, 259, 284
substantia nigra 911
substrate 509
subthalamic nucleus 911
sugar 687f
suicide gene therapy 912
sulfamethazine 52
sulfotransferase 41, 51, 183
supercoiled pDNA 124
superconducting magnet 235
support vector machine (SVM) 78
sybyl 74
synteny 499
synthetic chemistry 140
synthetic cholesterol 837
synthetic peptide 193–221
synuclein 504
systemic injection 832ff
systems biology markup language
  (SBML) 716

t

T-cell 507, 869
t-PA 114f, 119f
tacrolimus 410–411
tal-1/SCL 426
tamoxifen 500
tangier disease 974, 984
target 504
target tissue 833ff
target validation 6, 11, 337, 339
target-accelerated synthesis 18
targeted delivery 832ff
targeted therapy 628, 629, 726, 732–750, 796
targeting moiety 817
tau 503
tautomerization 249
taxol 239, 247
TCF-4 428
TEMPO 303
tendamistat 251
tenecteplase 114
teniposide 380–383
teprotide 396–397
terephthalamide 270
ternary complex model 328
tertiary structure 197
test set 80

tetracycline 500
TGF-β 652ff, 910
Th1 response 909
Th2 response 909
therapeutic agent 359–417, 630–632
therapeutic antibody 631
therapeutic index 52, 318
therapy 756, 758
thermodynamic constant 265
thiopurine *S*-methyltransferase 183
three-dimensional structure 256
thrombosis 974
thyroid tumor 1055
thyroid-stimulating hormone (TSH) 209
thyrotropin (TSH) 213
thyrotropin-releasing hormone (TRH) 219
thyroxine 251
tissue plasminogen activator (TPA) 214
tissue tropism 172
tissue-specific promoter (TSP) 900, 954, 1049
titration analysis 238
TNF-α 989–990
tobacco mosaic virus (TMV) 450
TOCSY 239, 240, 298
toxicity 500
toxicology 499
TPA, *see* tissue plasminogen activator
transcellular 90
trans-cleaving ribozyme 526
transcription 1046, 1047
transcription factor recognition sequence 900
transcriptional control 900
transcriptional targeting 1046, 1048–1059
transduction protein 210
transductional targeting 1046, 1059–1064
transferred NOE, *see* TrNOE
transferrin receptor (TfR) 484
transgene 881
transgenic 442, 443, 496
transition state 556, 564
translational repression 614
translocating binding proteins 783
7-transmembrane (7-TM) GPCR 331
Transmissible Spongiform Encephalopathies 447
transplantation 581, 909, 919
transporter 94, 505
trans-splicing ribozyme 526
trastuzumab (Herceptin) 477
TRH, *see* thyrotropin-releasing hormone
trial by ordeal 6
trimetrexate 284, 285
triple resonance spectra 234
trisomy 21 (Down syndrome) 953

TrNOE 238, 255, 256, 284, 292, 301
  in screening 301
tropism 1046, 1059
TROSY 235, 236, 238, 256, 258
TSH, *see* thyroid-stimulating hormone
tumor 502, 943ff
tumor antigens 705, 743
tumor necrosis factor (TNF) 485, 918, 945, 988
tumor promoter 740
tumor suppressor 502, 705, 743–745
tumor therapy 935
tumor vaccination 936
tumor-associated antigen (TAA) 797
tumor-specific receptor expression 629–630
tumorigenesis 502
tumorigenic 421–424, 432, 433
turbidity 839ff
tyrosine kinase 8, 28, 184

u
ubiquitin-proteasome pathway 741
uncoating 882
unilamellar 162
unmasking 840ff
upper aerodigestive tract (UADT) 710
uptake 115
urea cycle 913
uridine-5′-diphospho-α-D-glucuronic acid 49
urological cancer 1053–1054
5′UTR-site 954

v
V_d 97
vaccination 855ff
variable region 471, 474
vascular endothelial growth factor (VEGF) 165, 645ff, 733
vascular leak syndrome (VLS) 816
vascular smooth muscle 644
vascular tone 995
vasculogenesis 641ff
vasopressin 117
vasospasm 974, 995
vector targeting 898, 919
vector 160–172, 882, 939–954
VEGF, *see* vascular endothelial growth factor
velcade 768
very low-density lipoprotein (VLDL) 974, 980, 986
vesicular stomatitis virus 886
vinblastine 373
viral fusion inhibitor 570
viral gene transfer system 964
viral transfection 455

viral vector   172, 882, 939–941
virosome   960
virtual library   82
virus-mediated gene transfer   882
VLDL, *see* very low-density lipoprotein (VLDL)
volsurf   74
voltage-gated ion channel   8
volume of distribution   97, 114

w
wall shear stress   657
warfarin   398–399
whole organism level   144
Wnt/β-catenin   426
Wnt/β-catenin pathway   428
Wnt/β-catenin signaling   427

worm   494
wrapping   837ff

x
X-ray crystallography   239, 256, 275, 291
X-ray diffraction   181
xenobiotics   40, 56
xenograft   1053
xenotransplantation   592f

y
yeast   496

z
zeta potential   959